Pierre R. Delaere

Laryngotracheal Reconstruction

From Lab to Clinic

With 264 Figures in 770 Separate Illustrations,
Mostly in Color

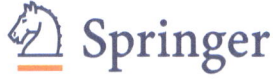

Pierre R. Delaere

Professor of Otolangyngology

Head and Neck Surgery

Katholieke Universiteit Leuven

Faculty of Medicine

Dept. ENT, HNS/Lab, Exp. ORL

Kapucijnenvoer 33

3000 Leuven

Belgium

Additional material to this book can be downloaded from http:// extras .springer .com .

ISBN 978-3-642-62245-8   ISBN 978-3-642-18684-4 (eBook)
DOI 10.1007/978-3-642-18684-4

Library of Congress Control Number: 2004105919

springeronline.com

© Springer-Verlag Berlin Heidelberg 2004
Originally published by Springer-Verlag
Berlin Heidelberg New York in 2004
Softcover reprint of the hardcover 1st edition

The use of general descriptive names, registered names, trademarks, etc. in this publication does not imply, even in the absence of a specific statement, that such names are exempt from the relevant protective laws and regulations and therefore free for general use.

Product liability: The publishers cannot guarantee the accuracy of any information about dosage and application contained in this book. In every individual case the user must check such information by consulting the relevant literature.

Editor: Marion Philipp, Heidelberg
Desk editor: Martina Himberger, Heidelberg
Production editor: Ute Pfaff, Heidelberg
Cover design: e STUDIO CALAMAR, Pau/Girona, Spain
Typesetting and layout: Dream Team, Loonbeek, Belgium
Printing and bookbinding: Mercedes-Druck, Berlin

Printed on acid-free paper
24/3150PF   5 4 3 2 1 0

In memory of my father

To my wife, Greet

And our children,
Anouck, Charlotte and Loïc

PIERRE DELAERE

'A surgical investigator is a bridge
tender, channeling knowledge from
biological science to the patient's
bedside and back again.
He traces his origin from both ends
of the bridge. He is thus a bastard
and is called this by everybody.
Those at one end of the bridge say
he is not a very good scientist,
and those at the other say that he
does not spend enough time in the
operating room. If only he is willing
to live with the abuse, he can
continue to do his job effectively.'
                    Francis D. Moore, 1958

Laryngotracheal Reconstruction: From Lab to Clinic presents the experimental and clinical aspects of tissue reconstruction of the larynx and trachea. The book reflects the development and implementation of a research-based clinical program. The experimental work was started in 1989 with the aim of improving the reconstructive possibilities in the following two clinical situations: (1) extended hemilaryngectomy defects after tumour removal and (2) tracheal stenoses that are impossible to repair by segmental tracheal resection. The two problems differ in localization (larynx, trachea), etiology (oncology, traumatic), and treatment possibilities. Extended laryngectomy defects cannot be reconstructed if parts of the cricoid cartilage are removed during the tumour resection, while the problem in tracheal stenosis treatment is formed by a long segment stenosis or by cases with recurrent stenosis at the anastomosis after previous segmental resection. The hypothesis set forward at the start of the experimental work was that improvement could come from reconstructive tissue having the three specific tissue requirements that are also available in the native laryngeal and tracheal tissue: (1) cartilage support, (2) mucosal lining and (3) vascularization. Special emphasis was placed on the blood supply of the reconstructive tissue because a reliable blood supply is lacking for most of the currently used reconstructive tissues (such as cartilage grafts).

Research on tracheal revascularization and transplantation provided a solution for the extended hemilaryngectomy defect that includes one half of the cricoid cartilage. Reconstructive tissue with the combined characteristics of a respiratory mucosal lining, a cartilage support and a reliable blood supply was made available after revascularization of segments of autologous trachea. The aim of the first part of this book (Chaps. I–V) is to provide experimental evidence and clinical guidelines for using the technique of tracheal autotransplantation in conservation laryngectomy. The shortcomings and complications of tracheal autotransplantation encountered in the initial patient series led to a modification of the technique. The modified autotransplantation technique proved to be reliable from a reconstructive, functional and oncological viewpoint.

In a second part (Chap. VI), healing aspects after repair of laryngotracheal defects are highlighted. The healing mechanisms of the cartilage support, the mucosal lining and the blood supply were studied for each tissue component individually. The step-by-step evaluation of tissue healing resulted in the development of artificially created tissue compositions. The composite tissue concept ('mucosal graft vascularization' and 'mucosal graft-cartilage graft vascularization') proved to be reliable in the management of difficult to treat airway stenosis.

This volume addresses tissue reconstruction of the larynx and trachea. It is written for ENT surgeons, head and neck surgeons and plastic and reconstructive surgeons with interest in reconstruction and wound healing of the larynx and trachea. I sincerely hope that this book will help in expanding organ-saving procedures in treating laryngeal cancer and will help in expanding our ability to treat tracheal stenosis.

I am indebted to the patients who have trusted me to operate on their larynx or trachea. This privilege has enabled me to learn much about laryngotracheal reconstruction. I will continue to devote my efforts to furthering my understanding while developing improved reconstructive techniques. I hope that the readers will find this comprehensive treatise as informative and stimulating as I have found its preparation. I would like to express my sincere appreciation to my colleagues who helped me with the experimental or clinical part of this project. I would also like to thank the Department of Otorhinolaryngology-Head and Neck Surgery and the Center for Experimental Surgery and Anaesthesiology.

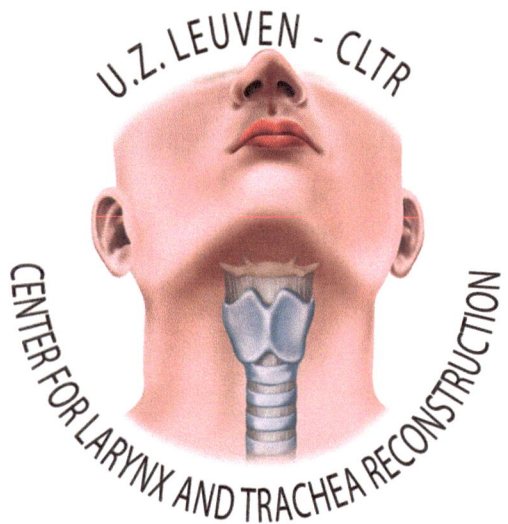

I would like to thank the research council of the Katholieke Universiteit Leuven (K.U. Leuven), the University Hospitals Leuven, and the Foundation for Scientific Research Flanders (FWO). This research would have been impossible without the funding obtained from these agencies.

Pierre Delaere
Center for Larynx and Trachea
Reconstruction (CLTR)
University Hospital Leuven - Belgium
www.uzleuven.be/cltr
Pierre.Delaere@uz.kuleuven.ac.be

This book is based on the following publications:

Delaere PR, et al. Epiglottoplasty for reconstruction of posttraumatic laryngeal stenosis. Ann Otol Rhinol Laryngol 1991;100:447-50.

Delaere P, et al. Results of full-thickness laryngotracheal wall reconstruction: a survey of the literature. Clin Otolaryng 1992;17:415-20.

Delaere PR, et al. Experimental transferable bed for laryngotracheal reconstruction. Ann Otol Rhinol Laryngol 1993;102:144-51.

Delaere PR, et al. Experimental tracheal tube created with vascularized fascia. Ann Otol Rhinol Laryngol 1993;102:935-40.

Delaere PR, et al. Experimental revascularization of airway segments. Laryngoscope 1994;104:736-40.

Delaere PR, et al. Vascularized fascia as transferable bed for experimental laryngeal reconstruction. Ann Otol Rhinol Laryngol 1994;103:215-21.

Delaere PR, et al. Tracheal autograft revascularization and transplantation. Arch Otolaryngol Head Neck Surg 1994;120:1130-6.

Delaere PR, et al. Revascularization of a salvage supraglottic laryngectomy. Ann Otol Rhinol Laryngol 1995;104:127-32.

Delaere PR, et al. Vascularized fascia as transferable bed for experimental laryngeal reconstruction-Letter to the Editor. Ann Otol Rhinol Laryngol 1994;103:916-7.

Delaere PR, et al. Experimental tracheal allograft revascularization and transplantation. J. Thorac Cardiovasc Surg 1995;110:728-37.

Delaere PR, et al. Vascularized fascia as transferable bed for experimental laryngeal reconstruction. Year Book of Otolaryngology Head and Neck Surgery 1995;160-1.

Delaere P, et al. Experimental tracheal revascularization and transplantation. Acta Otolaryngol Belg 1995;49:410-3.

Hermans R, et al. Magnetic imaging of experimental tracheal transplantation. Acad Radiol 1996;3:154-8.

Delaere PR, et al. Mucociliary clearance following segmental tracheal reversal. Laryngoscope 1996;106:450-6.

Delaere PR, et al. The role of immunosuppression in the long-term survival of tracheal allografts. Arch Otolaryngol Head Neck Surg 1996;122:1201-6.

Delaere PR, et al. Use of a composite fascial carrier for laryngotracheal reconstruction. Ann Otol Rhinol Laryngol 1997;106:175-81.

Delaere P, et al. Laryngotracheal reconstruction with tracheal patch allografts. Laryngoscope 1998;108:237-9.

Delaere P, et al. Tracheal autotransplantation: A reliable reconstructive technique for extended hemilaryngectomy defects. Laryngoscope 1998;108:929-34.

Delaere P, et al. Autotransplantation of the trachea: Experimental evaluation of a reconstructive technique for extended hemilaryngectomy defects. Ann Otol Rhinol Laryngol 1999;108:143-6.

Delaere P, et al. Progress in Larynx-sparing surgery for glottic cancer through tracheal transplantation. Plast Reconstr Surg 1999;104:1635-41.

Delaere P et al. Tracheal autotransplantation after extended hemilaryngectomy for advanced glottic cancer. Operative Techniques Otolaryngol-Head Neck Surg 1999;10:316-20.

Schutyser F et al. An image-based 3D planning environment for hemicricolaryngectomy and reconstruction by tracheal autotransplantation. Computer Aided Surgery 2000;5:166-74.

Delaere P, et al. Results of larynx preservation surgery for advanced laryngeal cancer through tracheal autotransplantation. Arch Otolaryngol Head Neck Surg 2000;126:1207-15.

Hardillo J, et al. An investigation of airway wound healing using a novel in vivo model. Laryngoscope 2001;111:1174-82.

Delaere P, et al. Prefabrication of composite tissue for improved tracheal reconstruction. Ann Otol Rhinol Laryngol 2001;110:849-60.

Delaere P, et al. Tubes of vascularized cartilage used for replacement of rabbit cervical trachea. Ann Otol Rhinol Laryngol 2003;112:807-12.

Delaere P, et al. Functional treatment of a large laryngeal chondrosarcoma by tracheal autotransplantation. Ann Otol Rhinol Laryngol 2003;112:678-82.

Delaere P, et al. Tracheal autotransplantation as a new and reliable technique for the functional treatment of advanced laryngeal cancer. Laryngoscope 2003;113:1244-51.

CHAPTER 1

Introduction

*Applied laryngeal anatomy and
physiology*

*Applied tracheal anatomy and
physiology*

1. Applied laryngeal anatomy and physiology

Understanding of the laryngeal functions (Fig. 1.1) and the subglottic tumor extension (Fig. 1.2) is important in the light of larynx reconstruction after extended hemilaryngectomy for glottic cancer.

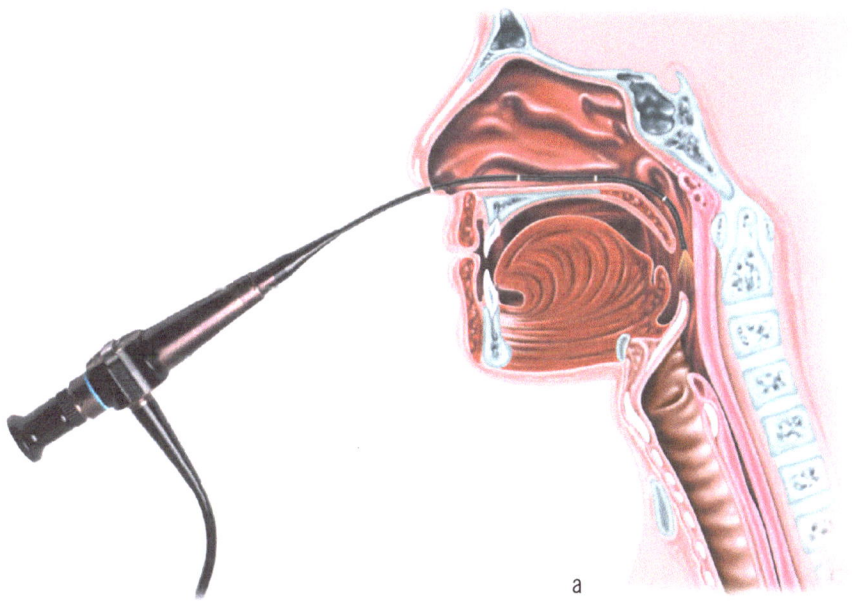
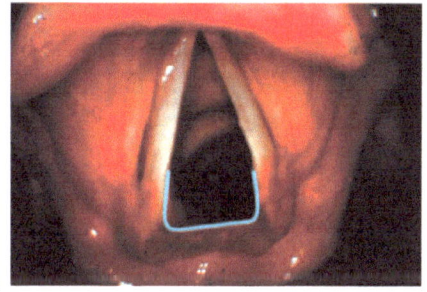
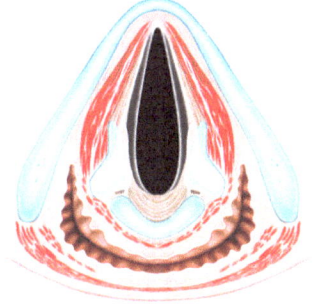

Figure 1.1. Functions of the larynx.
a. Laryngeal function can be evaluated during endoscopy. Indirect laryngoscopy (using a telescope or using a flexible laryngoscope) provides a clear image of the larynx, laryngopharynx and base of tongue.
b. b.1, b.2. Normal supraglottic and glottic structures during quiet respiration. The membranous vocal fold is *covered with stratified squamous epithelium, whereas the intercartilaginous portion of the glottis (blue line) is lined by pseudostratified ciliated epithelium (HIRANO et al. 1986). The supra- and subglottic larynx is also lined with pseudostratified ciliated epithelium.*

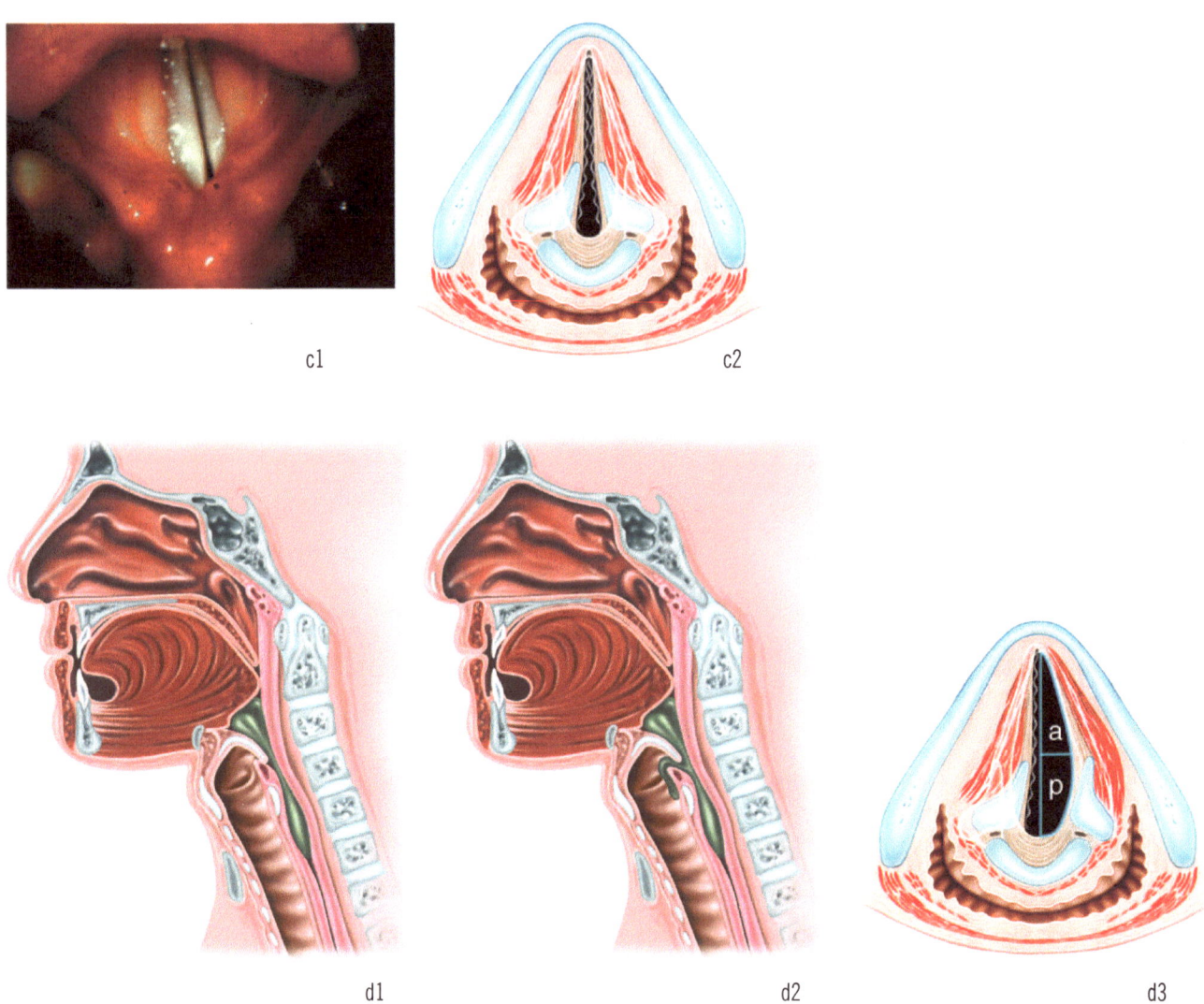

c1

c2

d1

d2

d3

Figure 1.1. Functions of the larynx (continued).
c. c.1, c.2. Normal larynx with vocal cords in adduction. The aryepiglottic folds define the anteromedial border of the pyriform fossae.
d. d.1.Pharyngeal phase of swallowing. Closure of the larynx involves three sphincters: the epiglottis and the aryepiglottic folds, the false vocal folds, and the true vocal folds. The epiglottis and aryepiglottic folds play a relatively minor role in protecting the airway and the true vocal folds play a major role.
d.2. Pharyngeal phase of swallowing. A food bolus is

penetrating the airway. Aspiration usually results from glottic insufficiency.
d.3. Unilateral vocal fold paralysis in abduction with glottic gap visible during phonation. An anterior glottic gap (a) will give a hoarse voice without aspiration. The epiglottis protects the larynx anteriorly during swallowing. A posterior glottic gap (p) will give a hoarse voice with aspiration. The epiglottis is not able to compensate for a posterior gap.

Tumor extent below the glottic level must be determined in assessing glottic cancer for its suitability for partial laryngectomy. The relationship of the glottic tumor with the superior border of the cricoid cartilage is demonstrated in Fig. 1.2.

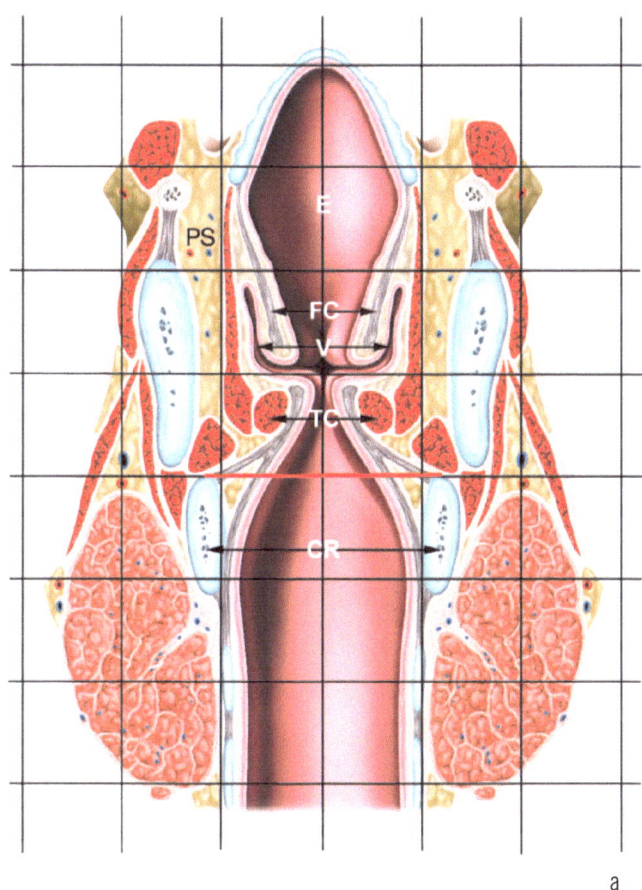

a

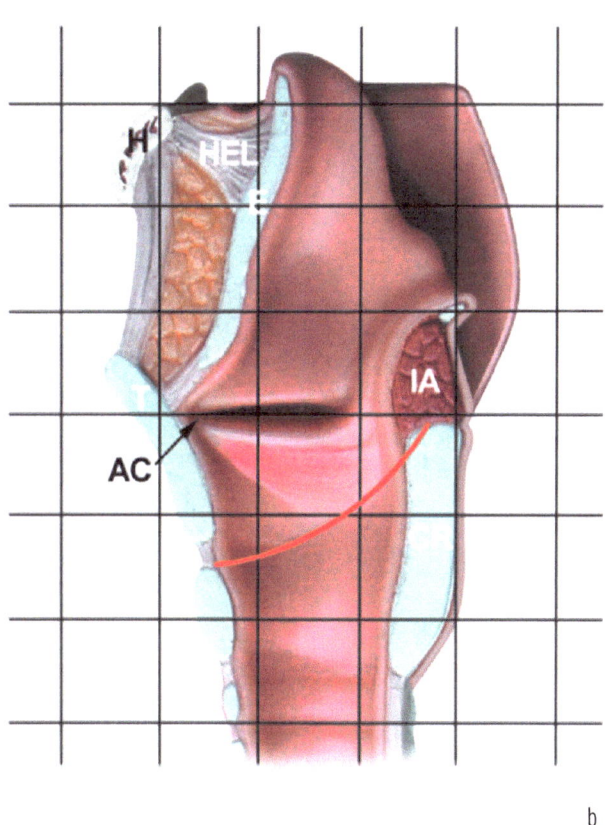

b

Figure 1.2. Subglottic tumor extension for glottic cancer.
a. Coronal section, mid-larynx. The 1-cm grid shows that the upper edge of the cricoid cartilage (CR) is about 1 cm below the free edge of the true vocal cord (TC). The paraglottic space (PS) is present as a strip along the inner surface of the thyroid ala above and below the ventricle. The lower margin of the currently available partial laryngectomy techniques is located at the superior margin of the cricoid cartilage (red line).
V=ventricle; FC=false cord; E=epiglottis.

b. Midsagittal section with 1-cm grid. The lower edge of the thyroid cartilage (T) lies about 1 cm below the anterior commissure (AC). The anterior portion of the cricoid cartilage is seen at about 17 mm below the commissure, whereas in the posterior larynx the top of the cricoid plate (CR) lies only a few millimetres below the glottic level. The top of the cricoid cartilage serves as the lower line of resection in conventional vertical hemilaryngectomy (SOM 1975) and in the various forms of supracricoid laryngectomy (LACCOUR-REYE et al. 1994) (red line). H=hyoid bone; HEL=hyoepiglottic ligament; E=epiglottis; IA=inter-arytenoid muscle.

Knowledge of the recurrent nerve anatomy is important in the light of both larynx reconstruction after extended hemilaryngectomy and tracheal reconstruction in cases of stenosis (Fig. 1.3). The recurrent laryngeal nerves are branches of the vagus. On the left, the nerve crosses the arch of the aorta while on the right it crosses the subclavian artery. Both pass posteriorly then superiorly to run in the tracheoesophageal groove to the cricothyroid joint where they enter the larynx. On both sides the nerve lies in close relation to the branches of the inferior thyroid artery.

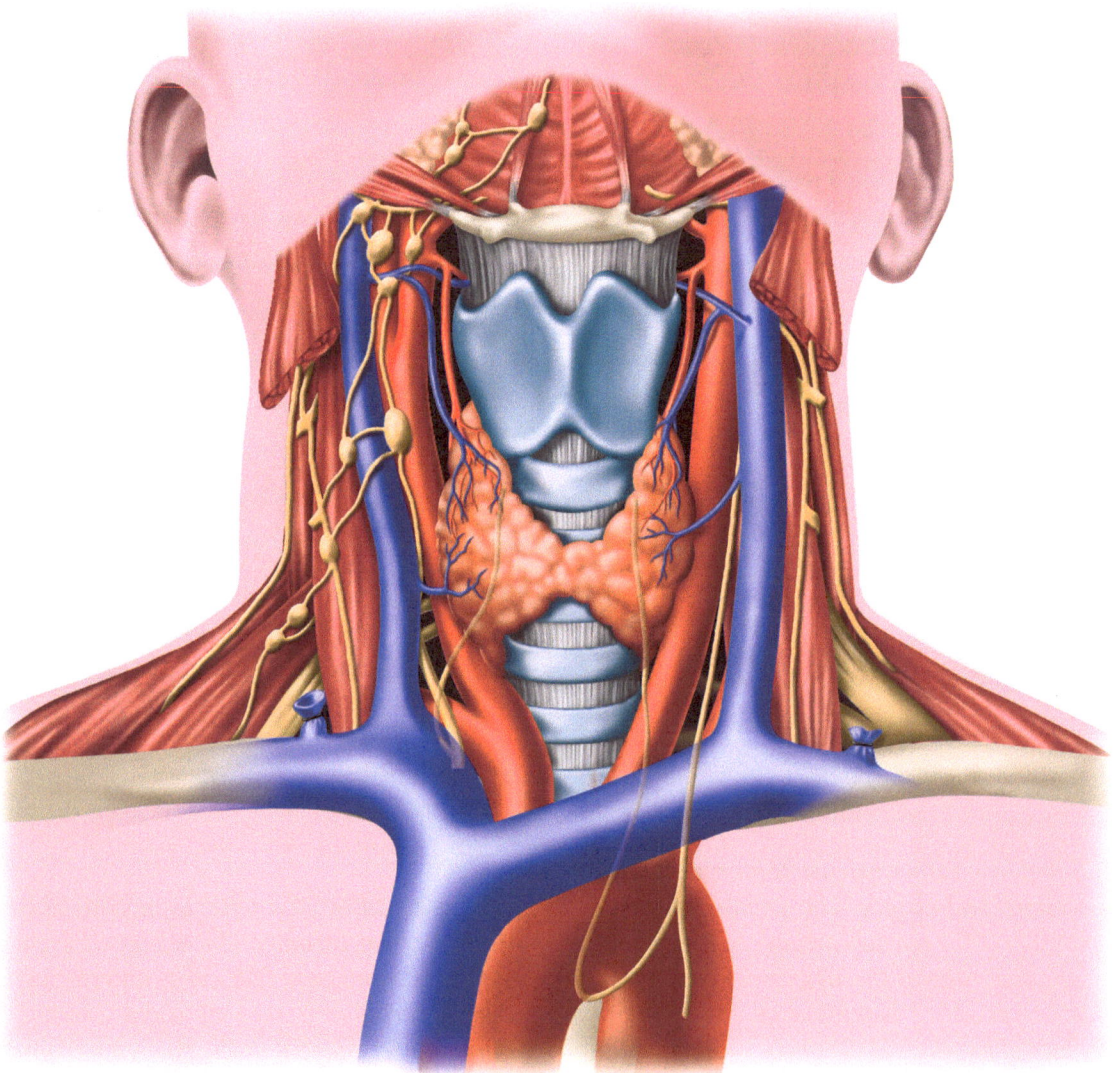

Figure 1.3. Anatomy of recurrent nerve.
This anterior view demonstrates the course of the recurrent nerves as they leave the vagus and descend the tracheo-oesophageal groove posterior to the thyroid gland to eventually enter the larynx at the cricothyroid area. On the left, the nerve crosses the arch of the aorta and lies close to the tracheo-oesophageal groove along its entire course. The right recurrent nerve loops around the subclavian artery and therefore approaches the tracheoesophageal groove from a more lateral position.

2. Applied tracheal anatomy and physiology

The adult male trachea averages 11.8 cm in length (range 10 to 13 cm) from the lower border of the cricoid cartilage to the top of the carinal spur, varying with the patient's height. There are usually from 18 to 22 cartilages within this length, approximating almost two rings per cm (GRILLO et al. 1964). The rings are normally C-shaped, with the posterior membranous wall connecting the arms of the 'C' in an essentially straight line. The mucosa is a ciliated pseudostratified columnar epithelium. Mucociliary transport provides a constant efflux of particulate matter, cellular debris, and secretions by the movement of cilia on the epithelium lining the airway. Disruptions to this process can cause pooling of secretions.

Understanding of the tracheal blood supply is important in the light of tracheal resection and transplantation (Fig. 1.4).

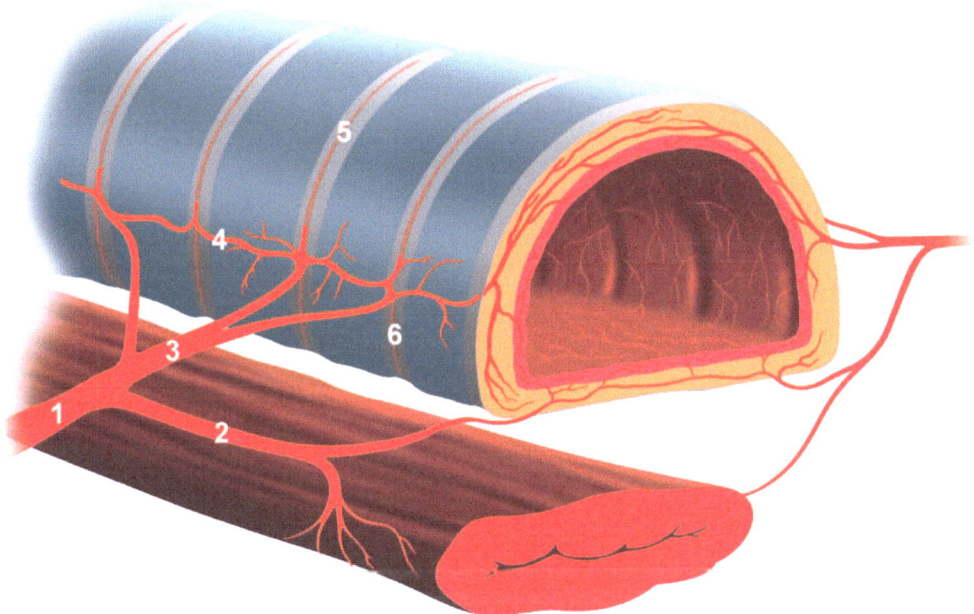

Figure 1.4. Tracheal blood supply (SALASSA at al. 1977). 1. Tracheoesphageal artery; 2. Primary esophageal artery; 3. Primary tracheal artery; 4. Lateral longitudinal anastomosis; 5. Anterior transverse intercartilaginous artery; 6. Posterior transverse intercartilaginous artery. The inferior thyroid artery supplies the lower portion of the thyroid gland and contributes importantly to the blood supply of the upper trachea (gives off 3 tracheoesophageal arteries). The middle and lower tracheal blood supply is derived in variable fashion from a brachiocephalic-subclavian system. Just lateral to the tracheoesophageal groove, the primary vessels divide into tracheal and esophageal branches. The tracheal branches pass directly to the tracheal wall, branching up and down over the width of several rings. These fine branches in turn connect with the branches of the next segmental vessels above and below. These vessels form a somewhat irregular but generally complete series of fine longitudinal anastomoses on the wall of the trachea.

From the vessels that reach the trachea, transverse intercartilaginous arteries extend deeply into the tracheal wall and anastomose with those from the opposite side at the midline. These vessels branch into the submucosa. Smaller intercartilaginous branches point posteriorly and terminate in the membranous tracheal wall. The posterior membranous wall of the trachea is also supplied by secondary small branches from the primary esophageal vessels branching from the tracheoesophageal arteries.

BIBLIOGRAPHY

Grillo HC, Dignan EF, Miura T. Extensive resection and reconstruction of mediastinal trachea without prosthesis or graft: an anatomical study in man. J Torac Cardiovasc Surg 1964;48:741-9.

Hirano M, Kurita S, Kiyokawa K, Sato K. Posterior glottis. Morphological study in excised human larynges. Ann Otol Rhinol Laryngol 95;1986:576-81.

Laccourreye O, Ross J, Brasnu D, Charbardes E, Kelly JH, Laccourreye H. Extended supracricoid partial laryngectomy with tracheocricohyoidoepiglottopexy. Acta Oto-Laryngol 1994;114:669-74.

Salassa JR, Pearson BW, Payne WS. Gross and microscopic blood supply of the trachea. Ann Thorac Surg 1977;24:100-7.

Som ML. Cordal cancer with extension to vocal process. Laryngocope 1975;85:1298-307.

CHAPTER 2

Limits in Laryngotracheal Reconstruction

Limits in larynx reconstruction after tumor resection

Limits in reconstruction of laryngotracheal stenosis

Hypothesis-reconstructive concept

> *Possibilities to resolve the limits in laryngotracheal reconstruction*
>
> *Autologous tissues used in laryngo-tracheal reconstruction*
>
>> *Vascularity: axial perfused fascia flap*
>> *Experimental: lateral thoracic fascia*
>> *Clinical: radial forearm fascia*
>>
>> *Mucosal lining*
>>
>> *Cartilage support*

1. limits in larynx reconstruction after tumor resection

At present, the indications for tissue reconstruction of the larynx in the functional treatment of laryngeal cancer are very limited. Tissue reconstruction is not necessary with the new endocopic approaches for early laryngeal carcinoma and the currently used conservation procedures are based on resection of parts of the larynx with primary closure of the created defect. An example is the supraglottic laryngectomy where closure between the glottic plane and the base of tongue is necessary after resection of the supraglottic structures.

The most extreme resections in partial laryngectomy without the need for tissue reconstruction are seen with supracricoid laryngectomees (SCPL). The supracricoid partial laryngectomy resects both true cords, both false cords, and the whole thyroid cartilage allowing for a functional treatment of selected glottic tumors. A more extensive procedure for selected supraglottic and transglottic carcinomas results in the resection of the true and false cords, the entire thyroid cartilage, and the whole epiglottis. After a supracricoid laryngectomy, the reconstruction is performed by suturing the cricoid to the epiglottis and the hyoid or cricohyoidoepiglottopexy (CHEP) (LACOUR-REYE et al. 1997). When the epiglottis is resected, the reconstruction is performed by suturing the cricoid to the hyoid, or cricohyoidopexy (CHP) (CHEVALIER et al. 1994). The addition of the technique of supracricoid laryngectomy has increased the options available to the surgeon for the successful management of larger laryngeal carcinomas while preserving the functions of speech and swallowing without a permanent stoma. As shown in figure 2.1, 2.2, 2.3, and 2.4, the caudal limit of a supracricoid laryngectomy is formed by the upper border of the cricoid cartilage which makes that T3 glottic cancer usually is not an indication for function sparing surgery.

The limiting factor in larynx reconstruction after

Figure 2.1.
Resection during CHEP. A SCPL-CHEP results in resection of both true vocal cords, both false cords, both paraglottic spaces, and, when required, one or part of one arytenoid cartilage. Grey area shows tumor extension visible in figure 2.2.

Figure 2.2.
CHEP-oncologic limits. CT scan of T3 glottic tumor with extension into subglottis. a = supraglottic plane, b = glottic plane, c = subglottic plane. Maximal amount of resection by a CHEP is indicated. The postero-inferior margin (arrows) of the resection is not sufficient to remove the T3 glottic tumor with safe margins.

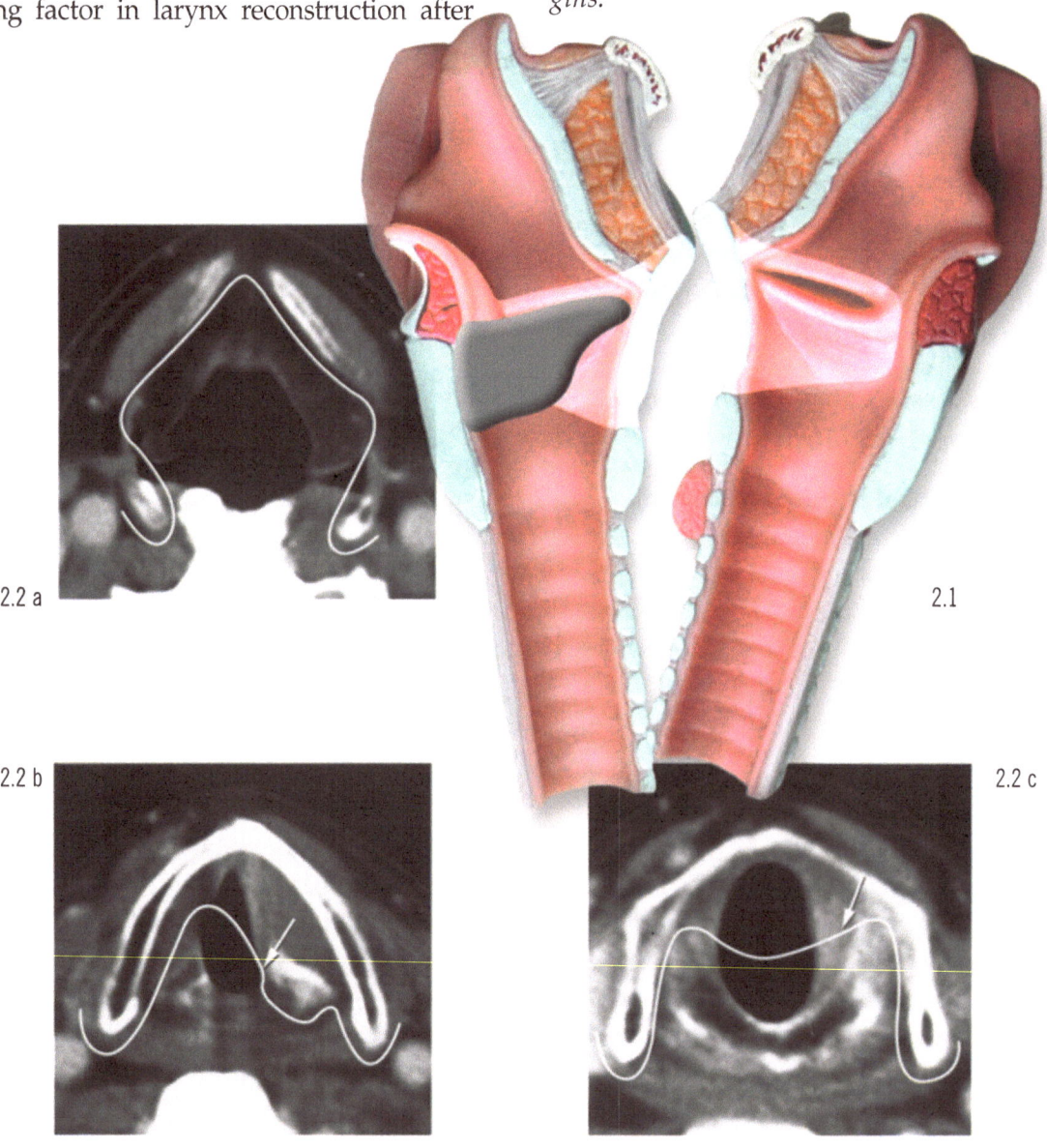

2.2 a

2.1

2.2 b

2.2 c

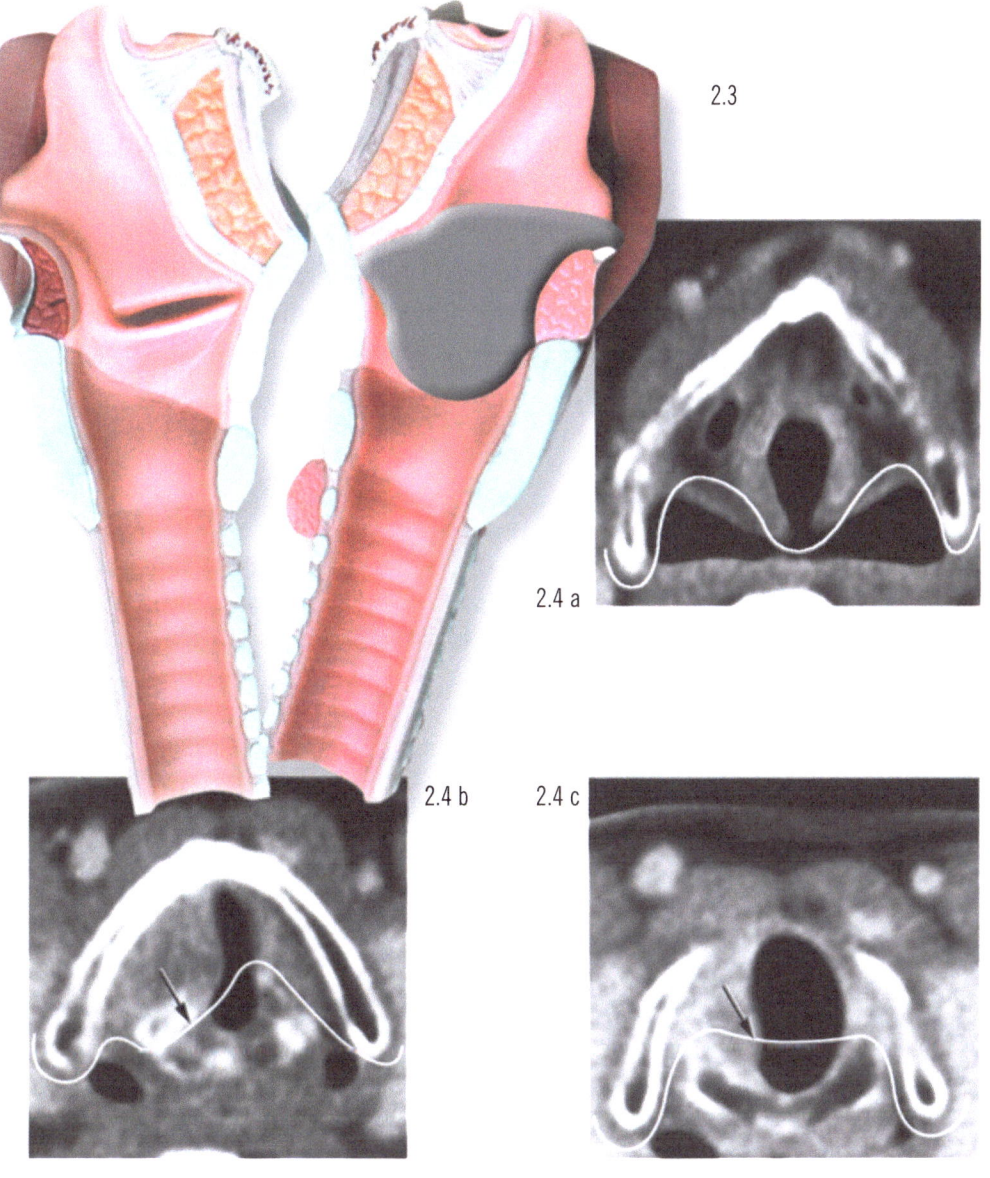

2.3

2.4 a

2.4 b

2.4 c

Figure 2.3.
Resection during CHP. A SCPL-CHP results in resection of both true vocal cords, both false cords, both paraglottic spaces, the epiglottis, and, when required, one or part of one arytenoid cartilage. Grey area shows tumor extension visible in figure 2.4.

Figure 2.4.
CHP-oncologic limits.
CT scan of T3 transglottic tumor. a = supraglottic plane, b = glottic plane, c = subglottic plane.
Maximal amount of resection by a CHP is indicated. The postero-inferior margin of the resection is not sufficient to remove a T3 transglottic tumor with safe margins (arrows).

tumor resection is formed by the cricoid cartilage. Major problems are encountered when parts of the posterior cricoid needs resection (BILLER et al. 1986, BILLER et al. 1977). All the currently used conservation laryngectomees have their caudal resection at the upper margin of the cricoid cartilage. This means that the tumor may have 8 to 9 mm of subglottic extension from the anterior to the midportion of the true cord but no more than 3 to 4 mm of subglottic extension posteriorly because the cricoid

lamina is located immediately below the arytenoid. A reliable reconstruction technique after resection of parts of the posterior cricoid cartilage is not yet available. The limited reconstructive possibilities make a total laryngectomy frequently necessary because of reconstructive shortcomings rather than for oncological reasons.

The laryngeal structures are shown from a posterolateral view in Fig. 2.5. The glottic tumor shown in Fig. 2.2 and 2.4 may be resected safely if 1 side of the cricoid cartilage is included in the resection. The resulting defect can however not be reconstructed reliably because reconstructive tissues to repair cricoid defects are not yet available.

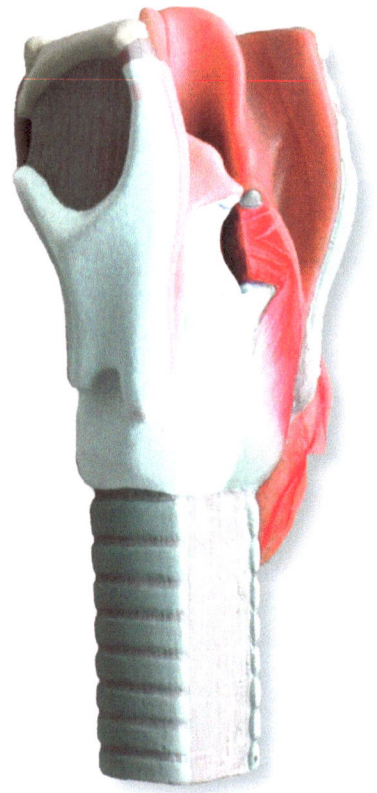

Figure 2.5.
Model showing the extent of thyroid and cricoid resection necessary to remove the tumor shown in Fig. 2.2 and 2.4.

2. Limits in reconstruction of laryngotracheal stenosis

Most cases of laryngotracheal stenosis may be treated by segmental resection of the stenotic segment and end-to-end reanastomosis. In general this may be done safely after resection of up to one half of the trachea in adults and one third in infants and small children.

A tracheal resection (GRILLO 1990, DeLORIMIER

1990) (Fig. 2.6) can be performed for tracheal stenosis; a cricotracheal resection (PEARSON et al. 1975, MONNIER et al. 1998) can be performed when the cricoid cartilage is also involved in the stenosis; and a slide tracheoplasty (GRILLO 1994) may be used as a primary reconstruction technique for correction of long-segment congenital tracheal stenosis (circumferential cartilage rings). The advantage of tracheal resection, cricotracheal

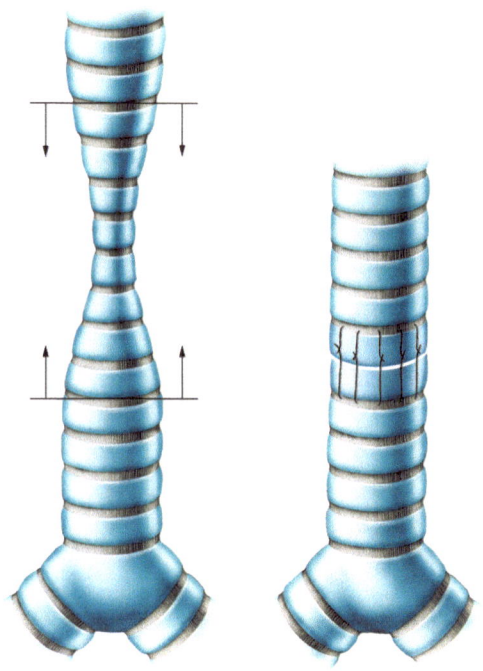

Figure 2.6.
Tracheal stenosis treated by segmental resection and end-to-end reanastomosis.

resection , and slide tracheoplasty is that no graft is necessary and that there is no need for prolonged endotracheal intubation.

Augmentation of the tracheal lumen by inserting local, regional, or distant tissue is necessary when a tracheal resection is not possible as for example in long segment stenoses (more than half of the tracheal length) (Fig. 2.8) or in cases of restenosis after tracheal resection (Fig. 2.7). A stenosis of more than half the tracheal length is rather exceptional. However, because the indications for tracheal resections are growing, it can be anticipated that restenosis at the anastomotic site will become a more frequently encountered problem.

Restenosis poses a therapeutic problem because further resection is usually not possible and mostly, reconstructive tissue has to be used to augment the problematic airway segment.

Tracheal reconstruction by using repair tissue is a second choice solution because the optimal repair tissue is not available clinically. The most frequently used reconstructive tissues consist of cartilage grafts, pericardium (IDRISS et al. 1984), and

muscle flaps (used as a carrier for skin (ELIACHAR et al. 1987), periosteum, or bone). Results obtained with these reconstructive tissues are not constant because they all lack 1 or more requirements for optimal tracheal repair. Optimal tracheal repair tissue should resemble the native tracheal tissue as close as possible and be composed of a cartilaginous support, an internal lining consisting of respiratory mucosa, and a reliable blood supply. This optimal repair tissue can not be found outside the airway. As a consequence, all the currently used reconstructive options are missing one or more basic requirements.

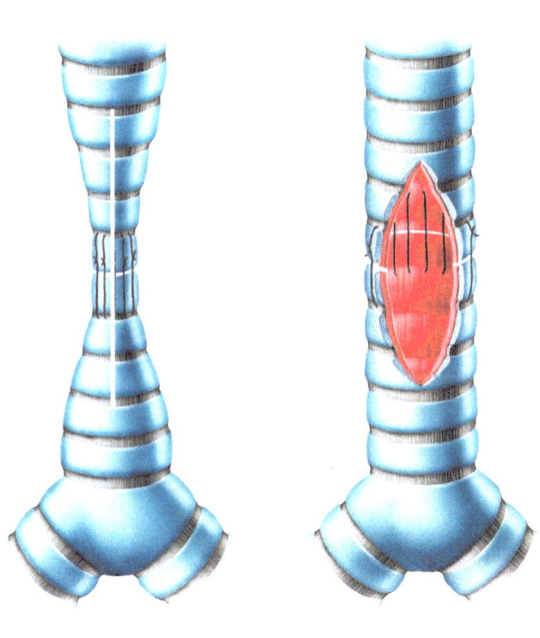

Figure 2.7.
Restenosis after segmental resection.
A complication of a segmental tracheal resection is that an anastomotic stricture may develop. These strictures are usually related to excessive tension at the anastomosed site. The restenosis may be treated by longitudinal incision, expansion of the stenotic area and insertion of repair tissue.

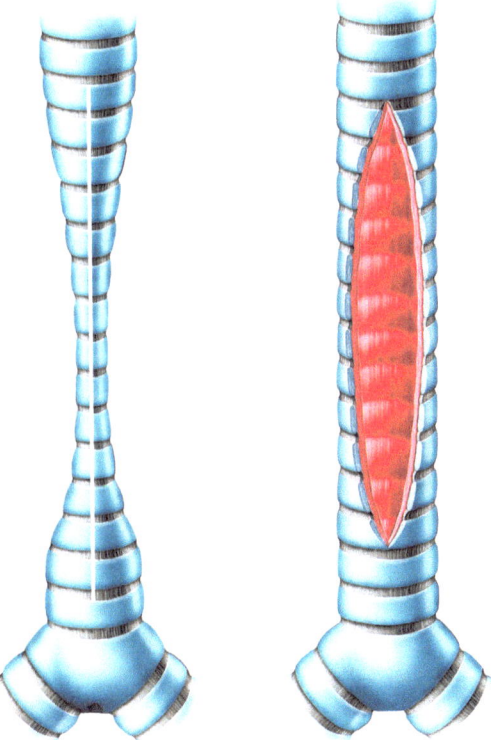

Figure 2.8.
Long segment tracheal stenosis. For an augmentation tracheoplasty, new material has to be inserted in an anterior airway defect after longitudinal incision and expansion of the stenotic segment.

3. Hypothesis-reconstructive concept
3.A. Possibilities to resolve the limits in laryngotracheal reconstruction

A rational ablation for a unilateral T3 glottic cancer removes the paraglottic space and its contiguous structures, including the cricoid and thyroid cartilages. The remaining larynx then consists of one thyroid ala with the corresponding true vocal cord and one half of the cricoid with one mobile arytenoid. One functional hemilarynx may be sufficient to assure all laryngeal functions. Speech, respiration, and swallowing may remain almost intact in cases of unilateral abductor laryngeal paralysis with the paralysed vocal fold immobilized in a position close to the midline (Fig. 2.9). Unilateral glottic cancers with vocal fold fixation may fall within the scope of partial laryngectomy if the laryngeal remnant consisting of a part of one thyroid ala with the corresponding vocal cord remnant and one half of the cricoid, with one mobile arytenoid, can be reconstructed. After resection of 1 side of the cricoid cartilage, the patient will be able to preserve his laryngeal functions if the laryngeal defect is restored in a way that is comparable to the unilateral paralysis in the midline (Fig. 2.10).

In analogy with the native laryngeal tissues, possible repair tissues for these extended laryngeal defects should be well vascularized and should

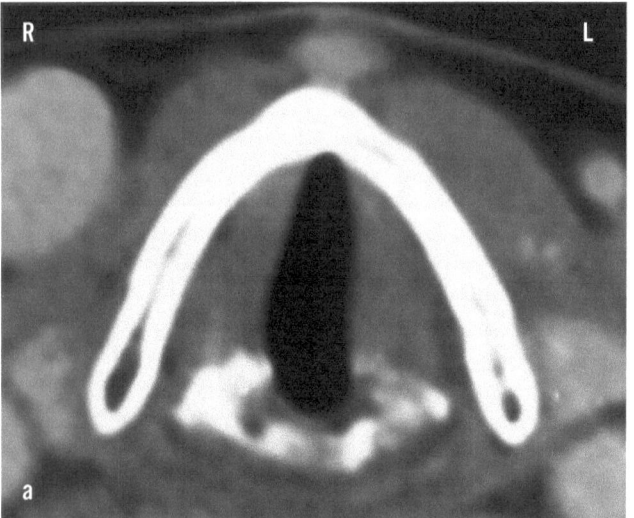 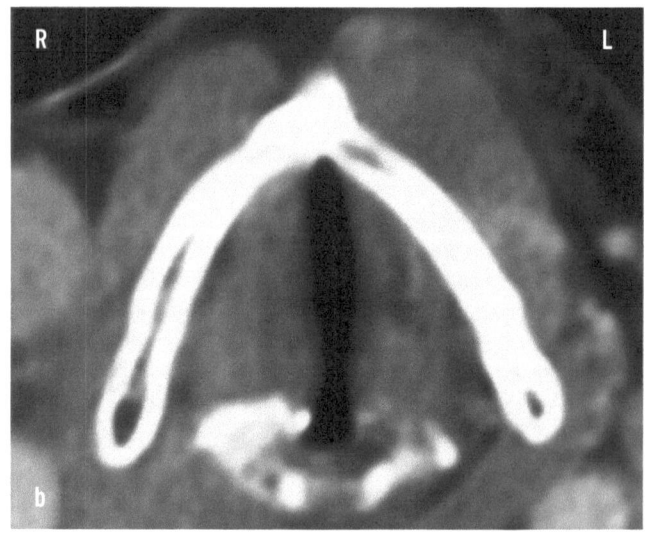

Figure 2.9. Axial CT scan of left vocal fold paralysis. The left vocal fold is immobilized in a paramedian position. a. Axial CT scan during quiet breathing. b. Axial CT scan during phonation.

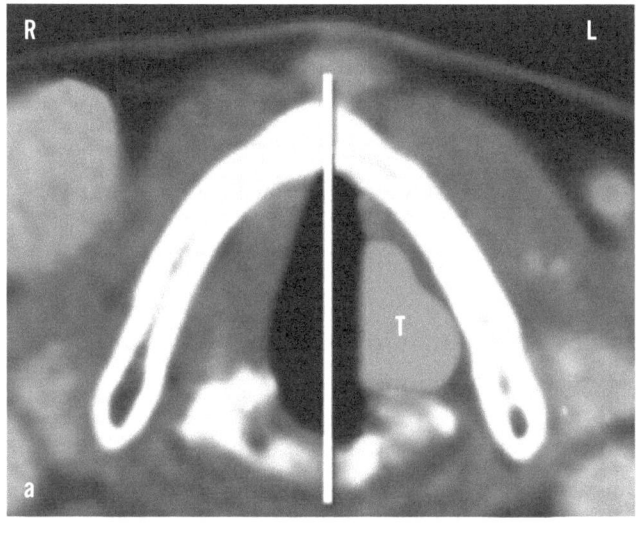

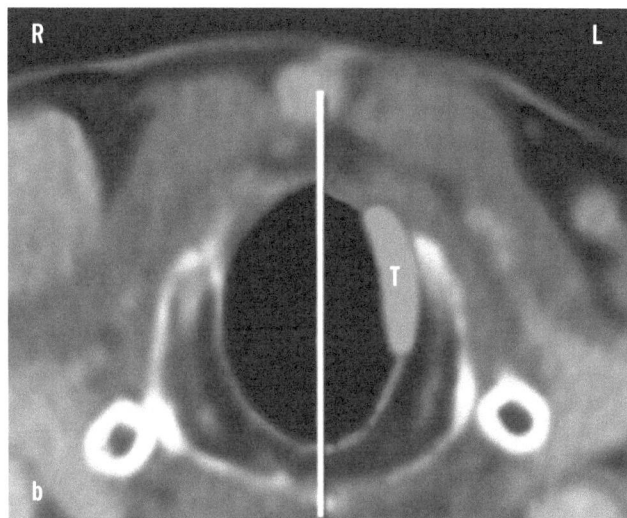

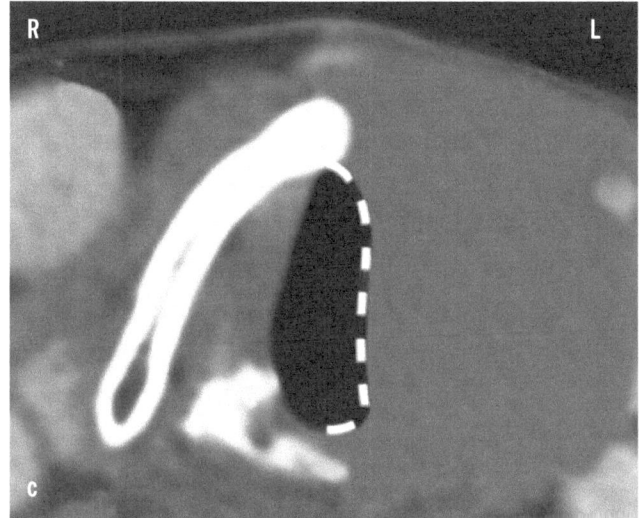

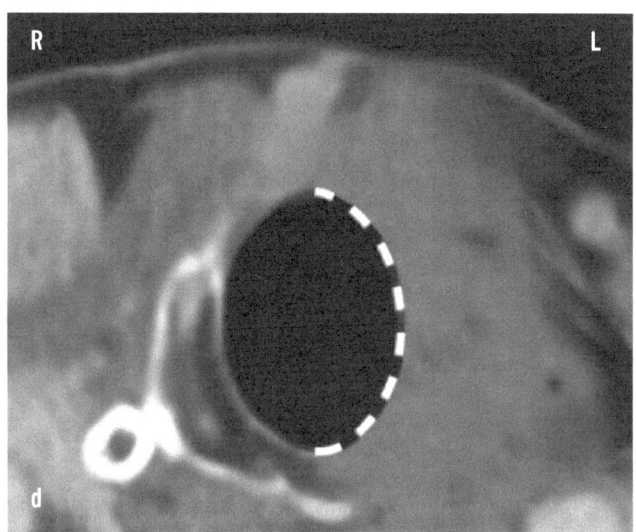

Figure 2.10.
CT scan with suggestion of left T3 glottic cancer (T)
with subglottic extension-Same CT scan as under 2.9.
Glottic (a) and subglotic (b) level with proposal for
resection. The extent of laryngeal resection necessary
for tumor removal is outlined. Glottic (c) and subglotic

(d) level with proposal for reconstruction.
Theoretically, the laryngeal remnant may fullfil all
laryngeal functions if the defect is transformed into a
situation comparable to a unilateral paralysis in the
paramedian position. The desired position of the
reconstructive tissue is indicated with a dotted line.

provide for an internal mucosal lining in combination with an external cartilaginous support.

The limits in larynx reconstruction may be resolved if transplantation of the larynx would become an option or if better reconstructive tissue would become available. Larynx allotransplantation poses problems of immunologic rejection, revascularization, and reinnervation and is beyond the scope of this book. However, the laryngeal defect seen in Fig. 2.10 may probably be reconstructed with parts of laryngeal allografts as visible in fig. 2.11. The main theoretical obstacle of this approach is the necessity for immunologic suppressive treatment in a cancer patient.

Another possibility to resolve the limits in larynx reconstruction is to look for autologous tissue composed of vascularized mucosa and cartilage (Table 2.1).

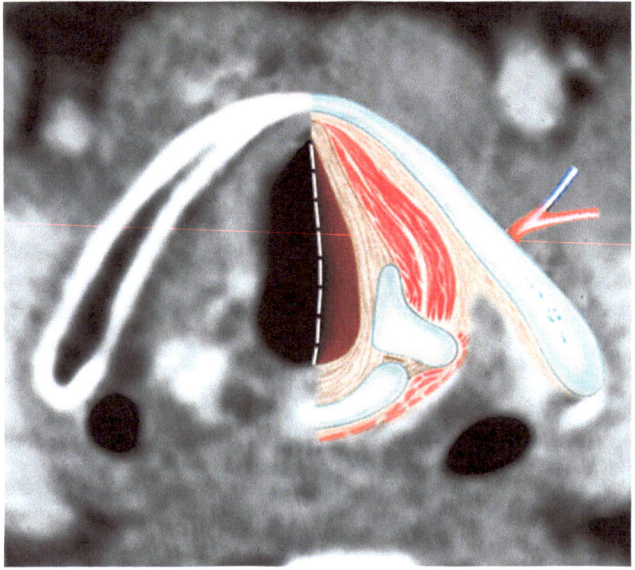

Figure 2.11.
Reconstruction of hemicrico-hemilaryngectomy defect with a partial laryngeal allotransplant. The theoretical reconstruction visible in Fig. 2.10 can probably be performed with a part of a laryngeal allograft that is revascularized by suturing the vascular pedicle of the hemilarynx to the neck vessels. Optimal function may be obtained with the vocal fold immobilized in a midline position (white line).

The limits in reconstruction of tracheal stenosis may be resolved if transplantation of the trachea would become an option or if better autologous, composite tissue would become available.
Research was directed in the following way:

• An experimental model of tracheal transplantation was developed to study the potential role of allotransplantation in improving laryngeal or tracheal reconstruction.

• Search for autologous, composite tissue.
The individual tissue used in the experimental composite tissue model are:
- Vascularized fascia as vascular source
- Buccal mucosa as epithelial lining and
- Ear cartilage as cartilaginous support
The 3 tissue components (vascularized tissue, tissue with mucosal lining, and supportive tissue) were studied individually and after combining the different tissues in a composite tissue concept.
The hypothesis was that the reconstructive possibilities inside the larynx and trachea might be improved if tissue with the combined characteristics of a mucosal lining, a cartilage support, and a reliable vascularity would become available (Table 2.2, Fig. 2.12).

Table 2.1. Possibilities to resolve the limits in L.T. reconstruction

LARYNX (cancer):	- Parts of laryngeal allografts?
	- Autologous composite tissue?
TRACHEA (stenosis):	- Tracheal allograft?
	- Autologous composite tissue?

Table 2.2. Tissue requirements for optimal laryngotracheal reconstruction

- Mucosal lining
- Cartilage graft as supportive tissue
- Blood supply to preserve the viability of the mucosal and cartilage component

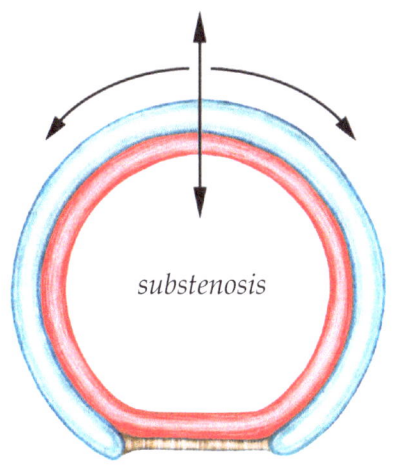

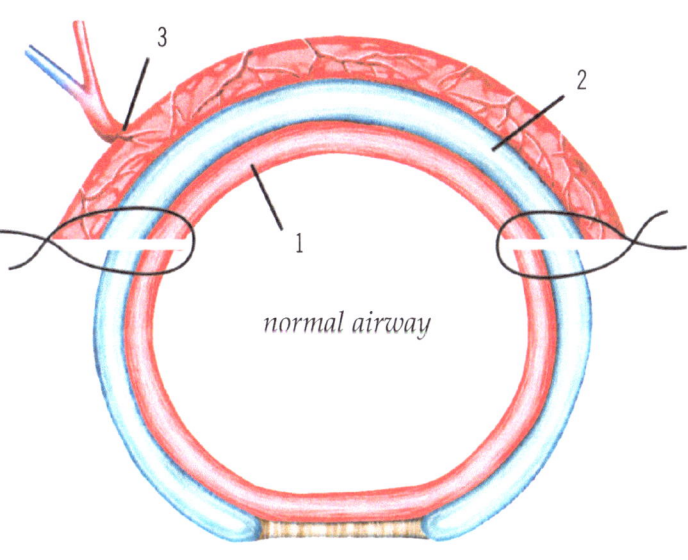

Figure 2.12.
Optimal repair of a patch defect after longitudinal incision (double arrow) and expansion (arrows) of a long segment stenosis or after longitudinal incision of a restenosis. Theoretically, repair of a normal airway lumen is possible when using tissue with a respiratory mucosal lining (1), an elastic type of cartilage support (2), and a reliable vascular pedicle (3) perfusing the reconstructive tissue. Vascularized fascia was chosen as vascular component of the reconstruction (3).

3.B. Autologous tissues used in laryngo-tracheal reconstruction

The most appropriate individual tissues that provide for vascularization, lining, and support were defined in the experimental (rabbit) and in the clinical situation. Some of these tissues or tissue combinations may have the potential to improve laryngotracheal reconstruction.

3.B.1. Vascularity: Axial perfused fascia flap

As in other areas of reconstructive surgery, the key factor in laryngotracheal reconstruction is a reliable blood supply to the reconstructive tissues. The option was to use the thinnest vascularized tissue sheet that is currently available in order to minimally interfere with the bulk of the reconstruction. A vascularized fascia flap was used as vascular supply to the reconstructive tissues.

In rabbits, the lateral thoracic fascia flap (Fig. 2.13, 2.14) provides for a reliable fascial connective tissue. The option was to use the radial forearm fascia (Fig. 2.15, 2.16) as a clinical counterpart for the lateral thoracic fascia flap.

3.B.1.a. Experimental: Lateral thoracic fascia

A thin, axially perfused fascia flap is available in the lateral thoracic area of the rabbit.

The fascial flap can be used as a 'vascular bed' for the cartilaginous and the mucosal component of the reconstructive tissues. A buccal mucosa graft, a cartilage graft, and a full-thickness graft of trachea have no intrinsic vascularity that allows for viable transplantation to the airway. A possible way for survival of these tissues is to provide for a vascular bed in the form of a fascia flap. The amount of vessel outgrowth and revascularization from the fascia flap may be followed by injection of the lateral thoracic artery with blue silicone dye (Microfil®, Canton Bio-Medical Products Inc., Boulder, Colo.).

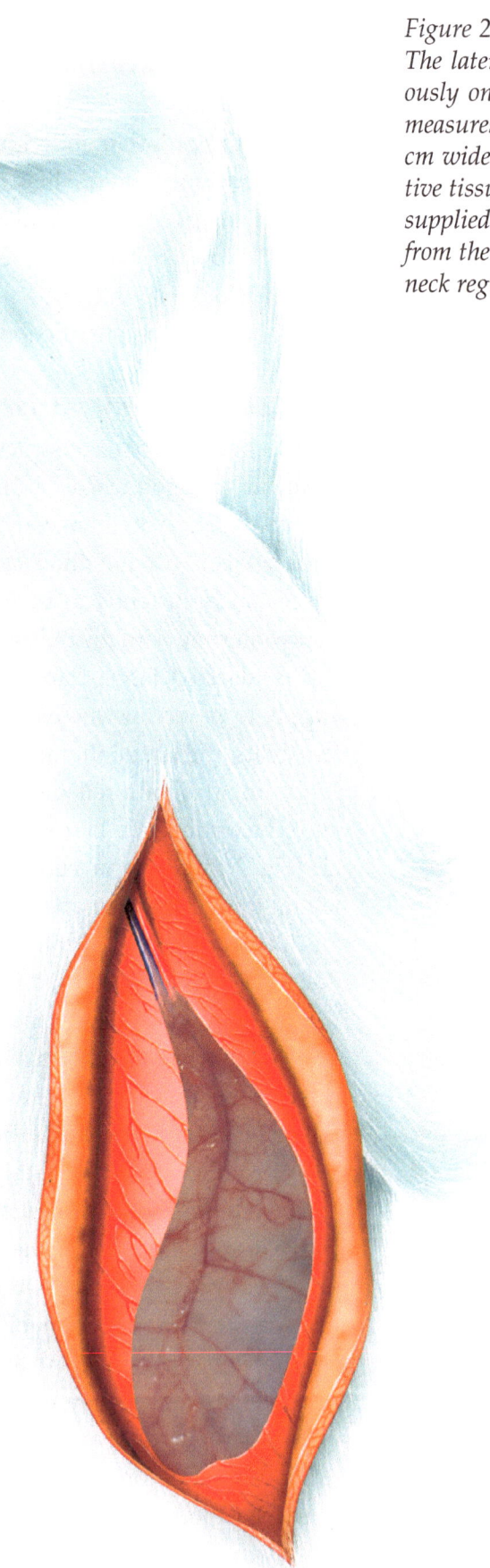

Figure 2.13.
The lateral thoracic fascial flap is situated subcutaneously on the lateral chest wall. The craniocaudal axis
measures 15 cm; in ventrodorsal direction the flap is 5
cm wide. The flap consists mainly of a fascial connective tissue containing the vascular network. The flap is
supplied by the lateral thoracic vessels which emerge
from the axillary vessels. The flap can be rotated to the
neck region with preservation of the vascular pedicle.

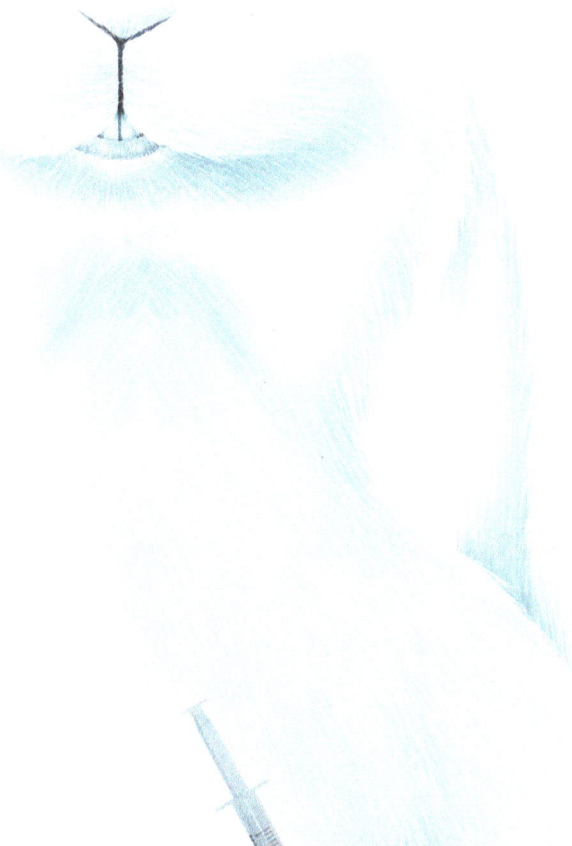

Figure 2.14.
The lateral thoracic fascial flap after injection with blue silicone (Microfil®). The lateral thoracic artery can be injected with blue silicone dye to better visualize the vascularity of the fascial flap. The dorsal branch of the lateral thoracic artery and vein (arrow) runs in the middle of the fascia flap, axially towards the iliac crest. The tissue is less than 1 mm thick and is extremely pliable.

Inset: Histology of fascial flap after injection of blue silicone. The fascia is densely perfused by blood vessels and forms an optimal environment for reperfusion of ischemic and avascular tissues. A small muscle layer is connected with the deep surface of the fascial flap. This small muscle, known as the cutaneous trunci muscle, is part of the panniculus carnosus and covers the whole trunc of the rabbit.

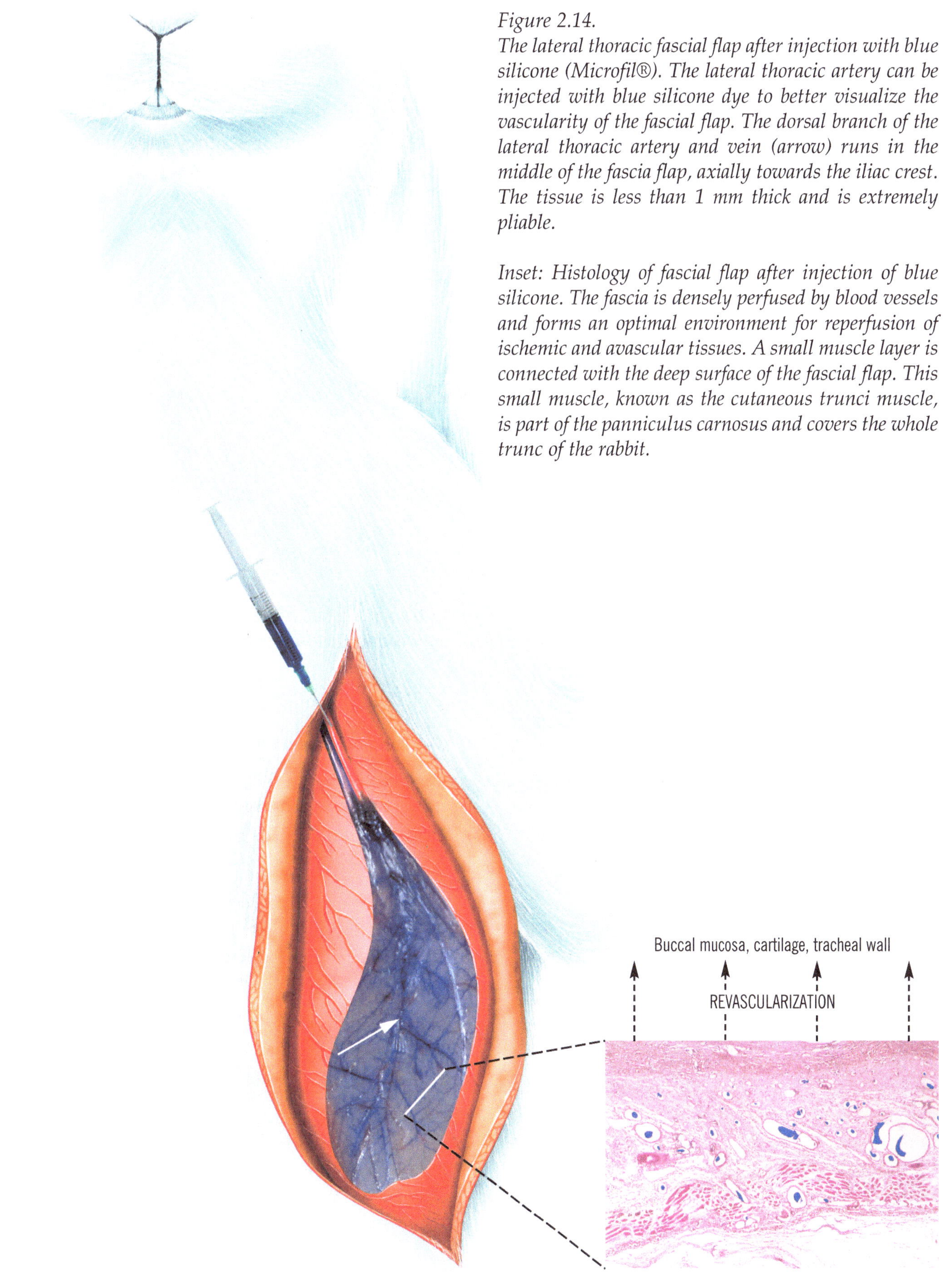

Buccal mucosa, cartilage, tracheal wall

REVASCULARIZATION

3.B.1.b. Clinical: Radial forearm fascia

A clinical counterpart was sought for each tissue that was used experimentally in order to make a translation of the experimental results into a clinical application (from 'bench to bedside') easier. The subcutaneous fat (with or without overlying skin) and fascia of virtually the entire forearm, extending from the antecubital fossa to the flexor crease of the wrist, may be harvested. The radial artery, with its venae commitantes, runs in the lateral intermuscular septum and gives of different fascial branches in the forearm.

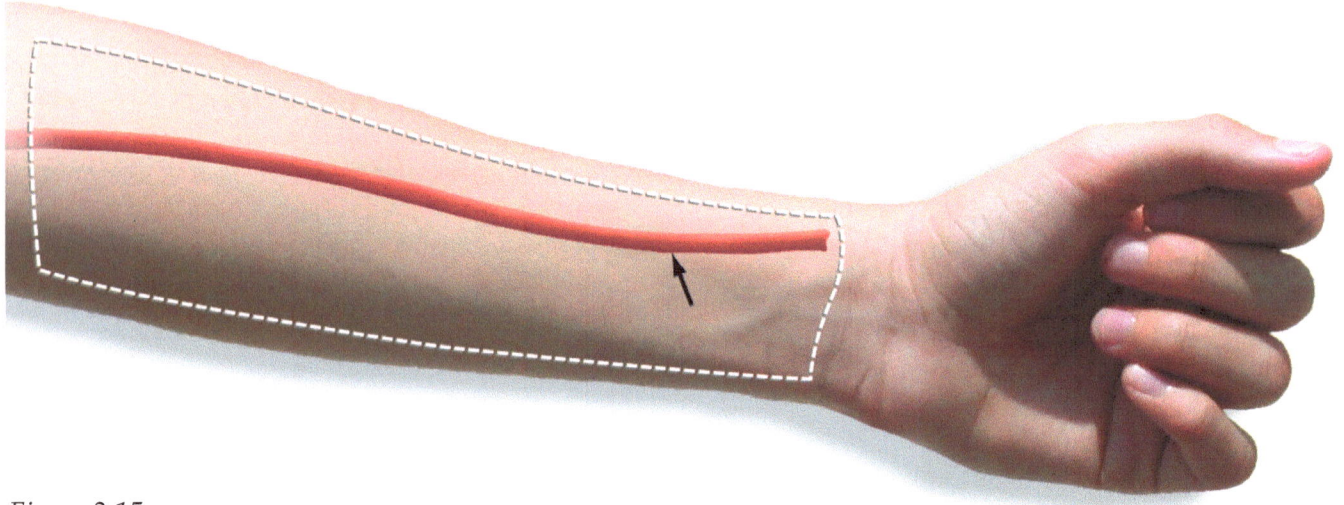

Figure 2.15.
A fascia flap may be taken in large amounts at the volar site of the forearm after incision and dissection of the overlying skin. This tissue is axially supplied by the radial artery and vein (arrow) and can be transferred to the neck by microvascular anastomosis of the vascular pedicle.

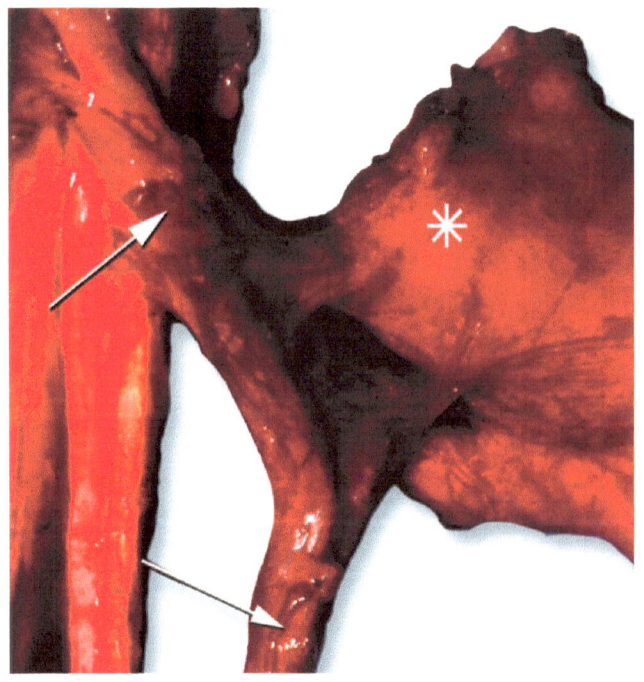

We preferred the radial forearm fascia over other fascia donor sites (temporal, lateral arm) because of the large surface area of the flap and because of the long and reliable vascular pedicle (Fig. 2.15, 2.16).

The experimental and clinical fascial flap have similar characteristics: they are thin and pliable, have a large flap surface area, and are axially perfused by a long and reliable vascular pedicle. The experimental and clinical flap differ in their way

Figure 2.16.
View on radial vascular pedicle (arrows) and undersurface of dissected fascia. The radial artery and veins supply the fascia of virtually the entire forearm so that the deep fascia (asterisk) and subcutaneous tissue can be harvested without the overlying skin.

of transfer to the neck: the radial forearm flap needs microvascular transplantation whereas the lateral thoracic fascia flap can be brought into the neck by rotation of the (lateral thoracic) vascular pedicle.

3.B.2. Mucosal lining

The mucosal lining of the reconstructive tissue may consist of respiratory epithelium or of squamous epithelium. A respiratory epithelial lining is available when using tracheal transplants.

Respiratory epithelium is not available outside the airway so that buccal mucosa may be considered as the internal lining of 'second choice' when other tissues than tracheal transplants are used (Fig. 2.17, 2.18). Buccal mucosa is better than skin because skin may give crusting, desquamation and hair growth within the airway. Oral mucosa can be taken at the left and right buccal area and can be used as a full-thickness graft in laryngotracheal reconstruction. The fascial flap may serve as a 'transferable bed' in order to bring the mucosal graft viably inside a laryngotracheal defect.

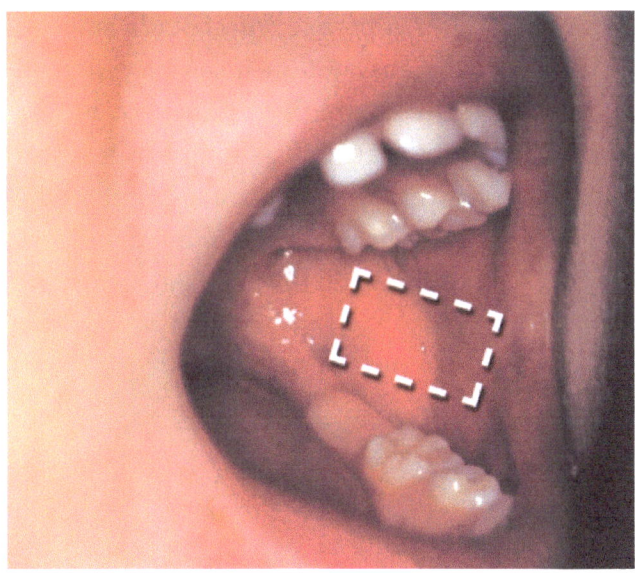

Figure 2.18.
Donor site of full-thickness buccal mucosal graft in humans. The outlined area of mucosa can be taken at 2 sides. Care must be taken to avoid injury to the parotid duct.

3.B.3. Cartilage support

An airway defect can be repaired with or without cartilage support. The best result that can be obtained without using cartilage is a flat reconstruction of the airway defect (Fig. 2.19).

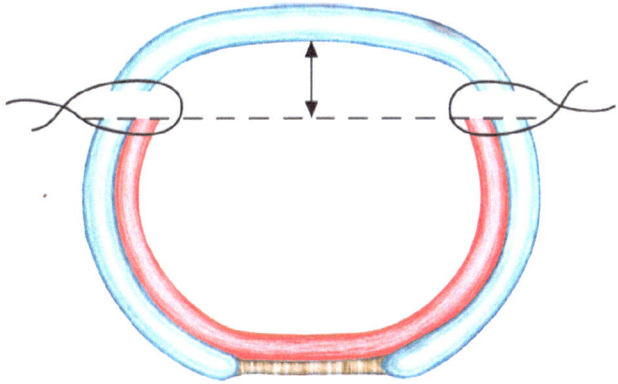

Figure 2.19.
Definition of cartilage support in airway reconstruction. A flat reconstruction of an airway defect is shown (dotted line). Additional expansion of the airway lumen (double arrow) is only possible when using cartilage.

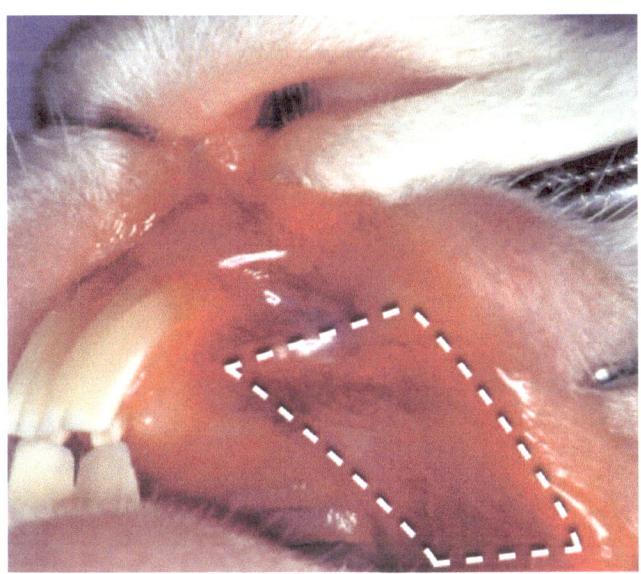

Figure 1.17. Donor site of full-thickness buccal mucosal graft in rabbits. The outlined area of mucosa can be taken at 2 sides.

A cartilaginous supportive effect with anterior expansion of the airway lumen can be provided by tracheal cartilage, by rib cartilage, or by ear cartilage. Tracheal cartilage is found in tracheal transplants and gives an optimal support to the airway lumen. Cartilage grafts for airway reconstruction can be found in the outer ear and in the rib. Fibrocartilage is available in large quantities in the human rib (Fig. 2.20). Large amounts of elastic cartilage can be found in the outer rabbit ear (Fig. 2.21); only small amounts are available in the human outer ear (Fig. 2.22).

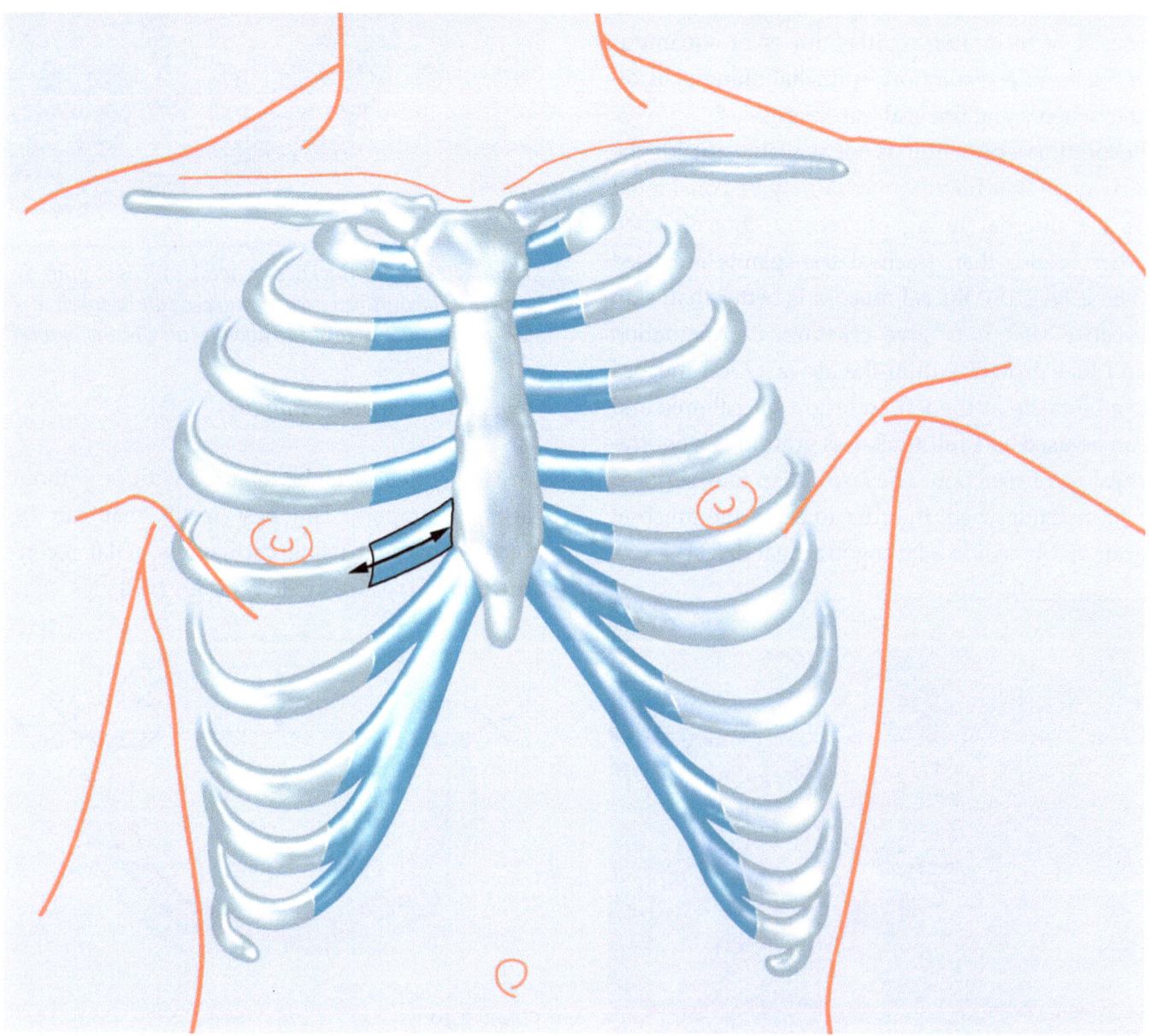

Figure 2.20. Donor site of rib cartilage in humans.
Through an incision overlying the right fifth rib (double arrow), the subcutaneous tissue and underlying muscle is divided to expose the lateral surface of the rib. The cartilage is incised laterally at its bony junction and medially as it inserts into the sternum.

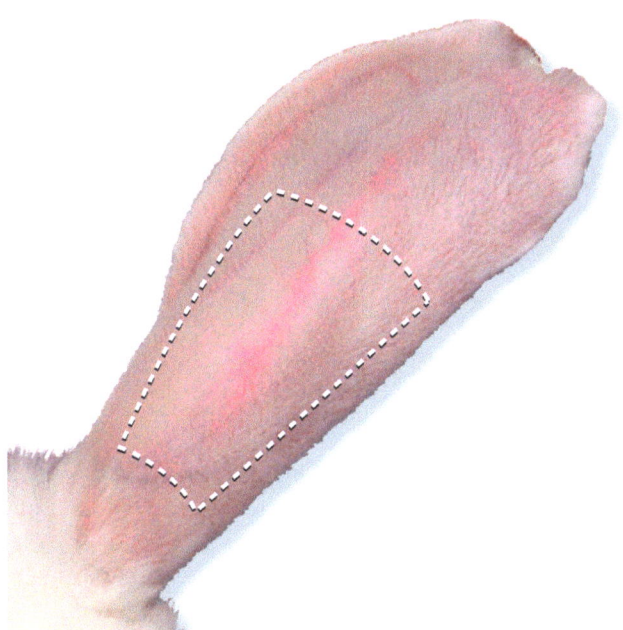

Figure 2.21.
Donor site of elastic cartilage in rabbits.
The outlined area of cartilage can be taken.

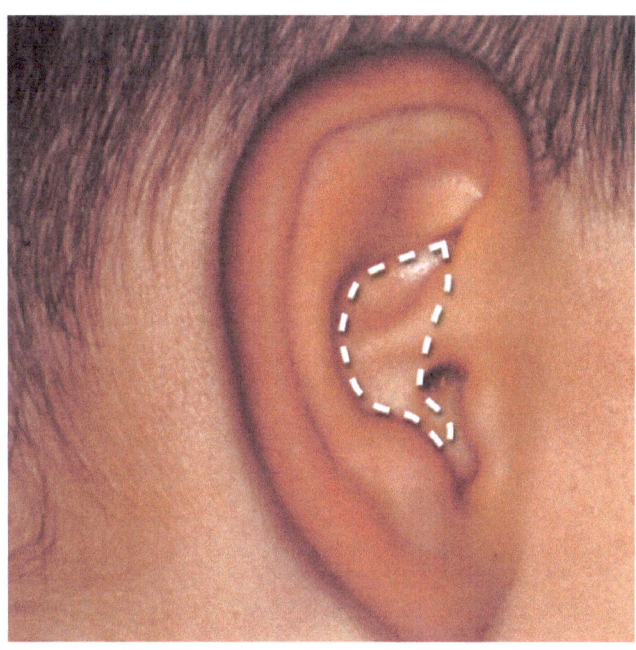

Figure 2.22.
Donor site of elastic cartilage in humans. In humans, an auricular graft with dimensions approaching 2 x 5 cm may be harvested without creating a deformity of the external ear. The outlined area of cartilage can be taken at 2 sides.

BIBLIOGRAPHY

Biller HF, Lawson W. Partial laryngectomy for vocal cord cancer with marked limitation or fixation of the vocal cord. Laryngoscope 1986;96:61-4.

Biller HF, Som ML. Vertical partial laryngectomy for glottic carcinoma with posterior subglottic extension. Ann Otol 1977;86:715-21.

Chevalier D, Piquet JJ. Subtotal laryngectomy with cricohyoidopexy for supraglottic carcinoma: review of 61 cases. Am J Surg 1994;168:472-3.

DeLorimier AA, Harrison MR, Hardy K, et al. Tracheobronchial obstructions in infants and children. Experience with 45 cases. Ann Surg 1990;212:277-85.

Eliachar I, Roberts J, Hayes J, et al. Laryngotracheal reconstruction: Sternohyoid myocutaneous rotary door flap. Arch Otolaryngol Head Neck Surg 1987;113:1094-7.

Laccourreye O, Muscatello L, Laccourreye L, et al. Supracricoid partial laryngectomy with cricohyoidoepiglottopexy for 'early' glottic carcinoma classified as T1-T2N0 invading the anterior commissure. Am J Otolaryngol 1997;18:385-90.

Grillo HC. Tracheal replacement. Ann Thorac Surg 1990;49:846-5.

Grillo HC. Slide tracheoplasty for long-segment congenital tracheal stenosis. Ann Thorac Surg 1994;56:613-21.

Idriss FS, DeLeon SY, Ilbawi MN. Tracheoplasty with pericardial patch for extensive tracheal stenosis in infants and children. J Thorac Cardiovasc Surg 1984;88:527-36.

Monnier P, Lang F, Savary M. Partial cricotracheal resection for severe pediatric subglottic stenosis: Update of the Lausanne experience. Ann Otol Rhinol Laryngol 1998;107:961-8.

Pearson FG, Cooper JD, Nelems JM, et al. Primary tracheal anastomosis after resection of the cricoid cartilage with preservation of recurrent laryngeal nerves. J Thorac Cardiovasc Surg 1975;70,806-16.

Tracheal Transplantation Research

The possibility of tracheal allotransplantation was explored as a possible solution to resolve the limits in laryngotracheal stenosis treatment.

1. *Experimental tracheal transplantation - current knowledge*

Restoration of the tracheal blood supply is necessary when attempting tracheal transplantation. Revascularization can be performed by *direct* or *indirect* techniques and in an *orthotopical* or a *heterotopical* position.

Direct revascularization of tracheal transplants is difficult because, at first sight, the trachea has no vascular pedicle that can be used for microvascular anastomosis. Anatomic studies in both mammals (GETTY 1975) and humans (SALASSA

et al. 1977), demonstrated a rich tracheal vascular network that derived from the superior thyroid artery and traversed the thyroid gland. Khalil-Marzouk (KHALIL-MARZOUK 1993) demonstrated that the superior thyroid artery could serve as a vascular supply for a canine trachea and reported a vascularized tracheal transplant model. However, his model was established without a venous pedicle. It was not until 1999 that Gannon (GANNON et al. 1999) demonstrated that the internal jugular vein could be consistently located within the investing fascia of the trachea and that the internal jugular system reliably drained the trachea. Long segments of circumferential trachea, based on the superior thyroid artery and internal jugular vein could be autotransplanted in the canine model (Fig. 3.1).

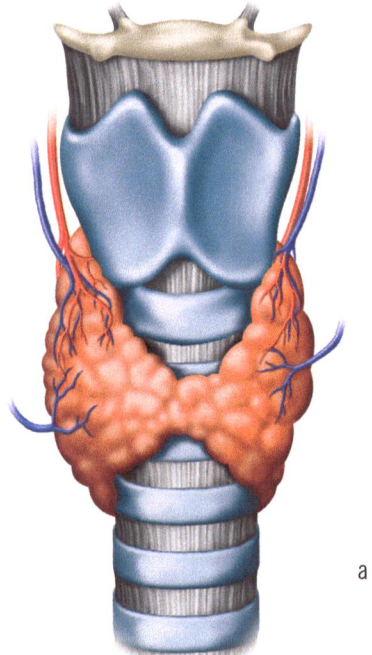

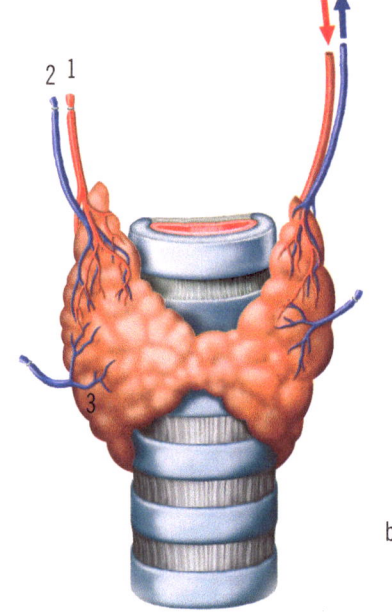

Figure 3.1. Direct revascularization of the trachea.
a. Vascular anatomy of thyroid gland.

b. The cervical trachea is presented as a vascularized transplant on the left superior thyroid vessels.
(1) Superior thyroid artery
(2) Superior thyroid vein
(3) Middle thyroid vein

A possibility is to transplant the thyroid gland on a thyroid artery and vein together with the cervical trachea which is attached to the thyroid gland. There are only few experimental reports on direct tracheal transplantation because of the practical problems encountered when attempting direct revascularization (MACCHIARINI et al. 1994, GANNON et al. 1999, GENDEN et al. 2003). A recent publication from Mount Sinai-New York (ZUR et al. 2003, URKEN 2003) reported on 3 cases where a segment of the patient's own trachea was transferred on the superior and inferior thyroid vessels to resolve a subglottis stenosis.

Transplantation of the trachea using the superior and inferior thyroid vessels may be used in selected cases. It is however not an attractive option to repair extended hemilaryngectomy defects after tumor resection. The main reason is that the ipsilateral thyroid gland is resected together with the

tracheoesophageal lymph nodes in cases of advanced glottic carcinoma. The majority of the studies concerning tracheal transplantation were done with indirect revascularization (BALDERMAN et al. 1987, OLECH et al. 1991, BORRO et al. 1992). The omentum has been used intensively in *indirect* tracheal revascularization with different results. In indirect revascularization, the isolated tracheal graft is wrapped in vascularized omentum outside the airway (heterotopic) or inside the airway (orthotopic). For indirect , orthotopic revascularization it is necessary to transpose the omentum towards the neck. The majority of the studies on indirect tracheal revascularization were done *orthotopically* with tracheal autografts that were isolated and immediately reimplanted wrapped by the transposed omentum (Fig. 3.2.).

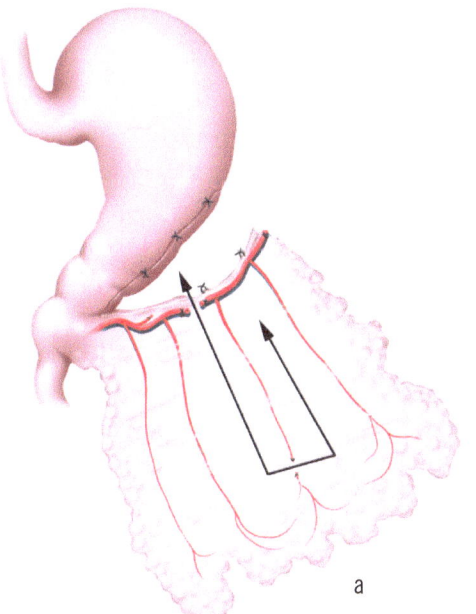

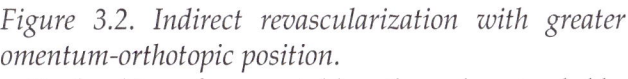

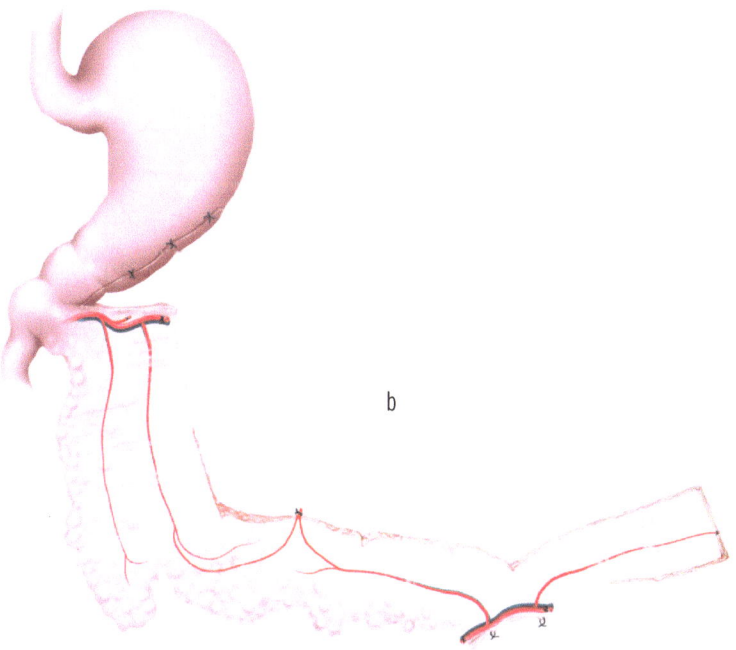

Figure 3.2. Indirect revascularization with greater omentum-orthotopic position.
a. For local transfer, omental length can be extended by ligation and division of the gastroepiploic arterial arch (double arrow).

b. Omental length can be increased without damage to the blood supply.

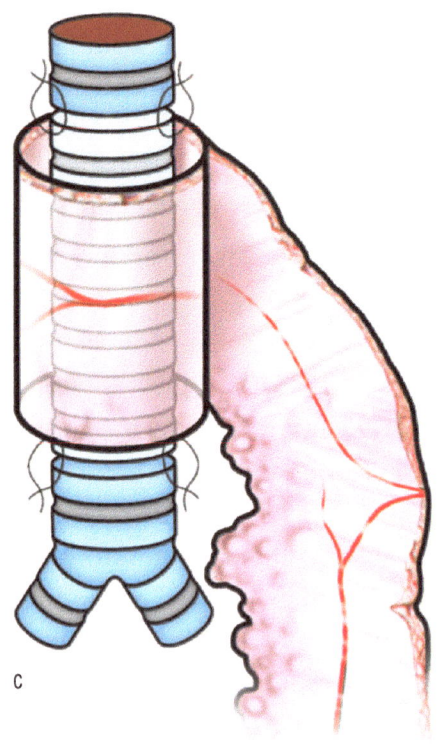

c

Figure 3.2. Indirect revascularization with greater omentum-orthotopic position (continued).
c. A tracheal transplant can be wrapped in the orthotopic position after transfer of the greater omentum into the neck area.

In the orthotopic position, the blood supply of the grafts may come from two sources:
• the neovascularity from the recipient trachea at both ends of the graft and
• the supply from the omentum.
From these studies, it became clear that the blood supply that comes from the omentum and from the recipient trachea is not sufficient to keep the tracheal transplant viable (NAKANISHI et al. 1992). The main reason is that the graft moves with each respiration and swallowing act (movement between omentum and tracheal transplant prevents outgrowth of blood vessels) and that the mucosal lining is exposed to the airway during revascularization.
A better place for indirect revascularization of tracheal transplants is the *heterotopic* position. Although only the supply from the omentum may reperfuse the trachea heterotopically, this revascularization position is more successful because the immobility between transplant and surrounding tissue guarantees a better outgrowth of blood vessels to the transplant.
Successful revascularization of tracheal allotransplants after indirect, heterotopical and direct orthotopical revascularization (MACCHIARINI, et al. 1995) have been reported when the receptor animal was immunosuppressed.
We developed a tracheal revascularization and transplantation model in the rabbit by using an *indirect technique* and by using an axial perfused *fascia flap* as the vascular source for the avascular allotransplant.
This model allowed us to study:
• Heterotopic revascularization of tracheal allografts.
• Acute and chronic rejection of revascularized allografts.
• Orthotopic transplantation of tracheal allografts after full revascularization.

2. Heterotopical revascularization of tracheal allografts

Tracheal revascularization was studied through a day-by-day evaluation of isolated tracheal allografts wrapped by vascularized fascia in immuno-suppressed animals. A 2 cm segment of cervical trachea was brought from 1 animal to the lateral thoracic area of another, immunosuppressed (cyclosporin 10 mg/kg, intramuscular injection), animal as shown in Fig. 3.3. The avascular tracheal segment was circumferentially wrapped by the fascial flap. The amount of revascularization of the tracheal allografts was studied after injection of the artery of the fascial flap with blue silicone dye (Microfil®) after revascularization periods varying from 2 to 28 days. The silicone cures following injection to form a cast of the vascular architecture of the fascial flap and the established vascular connections with the tracheal segment.

The submucosal blood vessels of the tracheal transplant undergo thrombosis after isolation from the donor animal. Because of ischemia of the mucosal layer, the respiratory epithelium will undergo desintegration except for some individual 'reserve' cells that remain on top of the

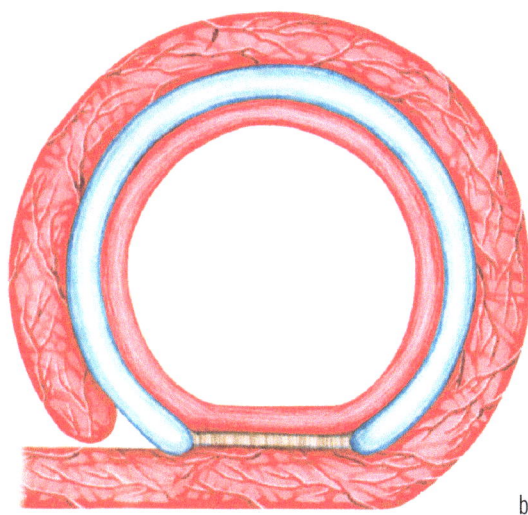

a

b

Figure 3.3.
Tracheal revascularization.
a. A 2 cm segment of cervical trachea is brought to the lateral thoracic area and wrapped with fascia (dotted arrows) in an immunosuppressed receptor animal. The skin of the lateral thoracic area is closed (arrows) and the transplant is studied after different follow-up periods.
b. Axial section through tracheal segment wrapped by fascia.

thrombosed mucosa. The vascularized fascia around the transplant will prevent avascular necrosis and will induce the revascularization pro-cess. The first revascularization signs are visible after 4-6 days as shown in Fig. 3.4 and 3.5.

Figure 3.4.
a. Routes of tracheal revascularization. Two routes of revascularization are possible: (1) the membranous trachea and (2) the intercartilaginous ligaments. Histology of outlined area is visible in Fig. 3.4b. After follow-up, the lateral thoracic artery is injected with blue silicone. b. Axial section through tracheal transplant after 6 days of revascularization. Blue silicone injected tracheal transplant. The area distant from the membranous trachea (1) shows desintegration with some isolated epithelial cells visible on top of an edematous submucosa with congestion and thrombosis of blood vessels. The area which is orientated towards the membranous trachea (2) shows early signs of revascularization. Revascularization takes place by recanalization (visible as blue silicone spots) of thrombosed subepithelial vessels. The reepithelialization follows the revascularization process: at the area of early revascularization (2), the epithelial lining consists of squamous epithelium while a denuded epithelium is seen in the area without revascularization (1). The first signs of revascularization are seen posteriorly near the membranous trachea (HE, x20). A longitudinal section (white line) through the transplant at the area of early revascularization is visible in Fig. 3.5.

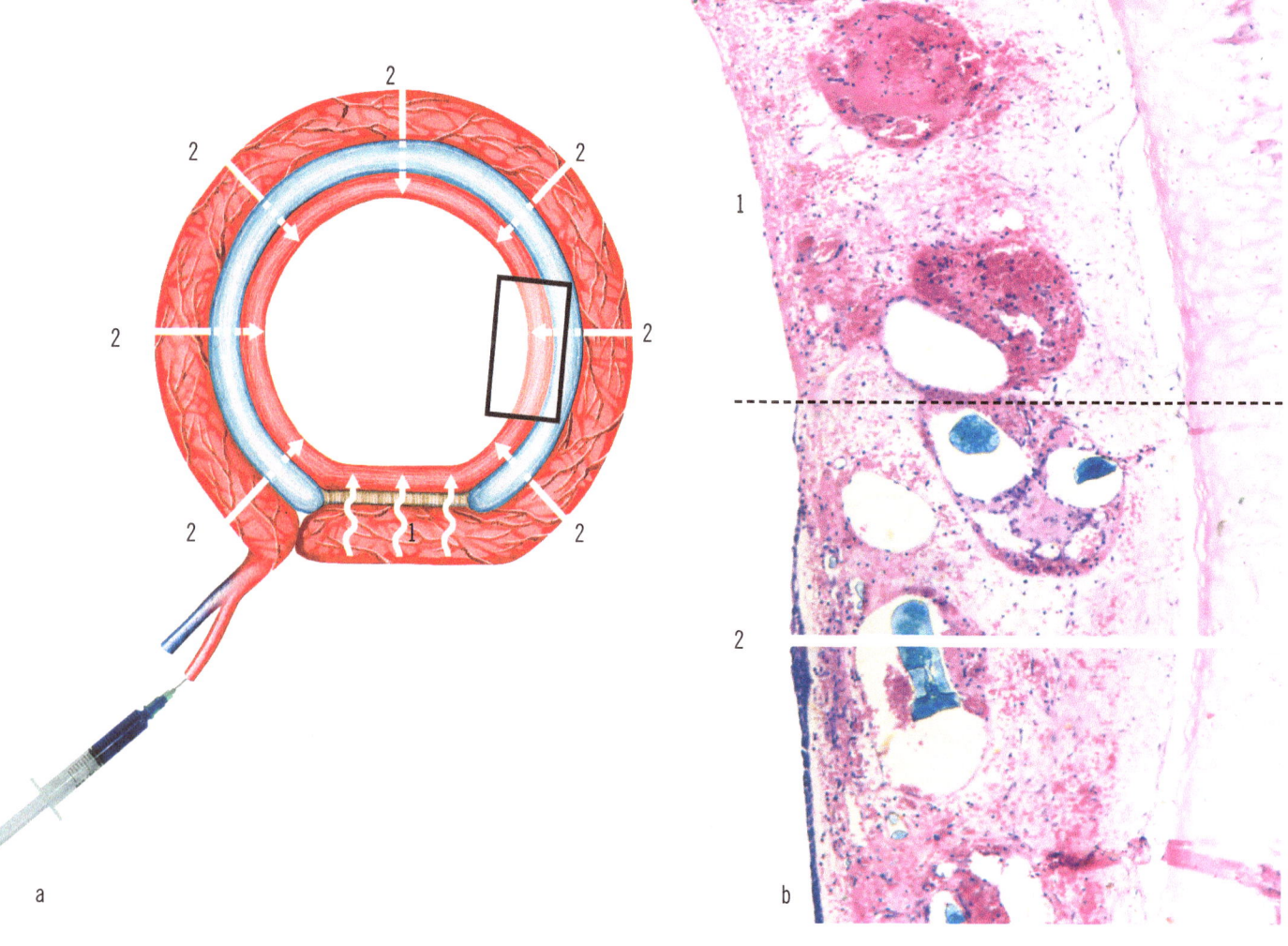

a

b

As shown in Fig. 3.6 and 3.7, avascular segments of the rabbit's trachea are revascularized over the total fascia-enwrapped area in a heterotopical position. The mechanism is based on revascularization of thrombosed mucosal vessels and regeneration of respiratory epithelium over the revascularized lamina propria. Two routes of revascularization may be distinguished: the membranous region and the intercartilaginous ligaments.

A significant link exist between tracheal revascularization and epithelial regeneration. Recovery (from the isolated epithelial cells on top of the thrombosed mucosa) of nonciliated (squamous) epithelium is seen at the sites of early revascularization while ciliated cells are visible after full revascularization.

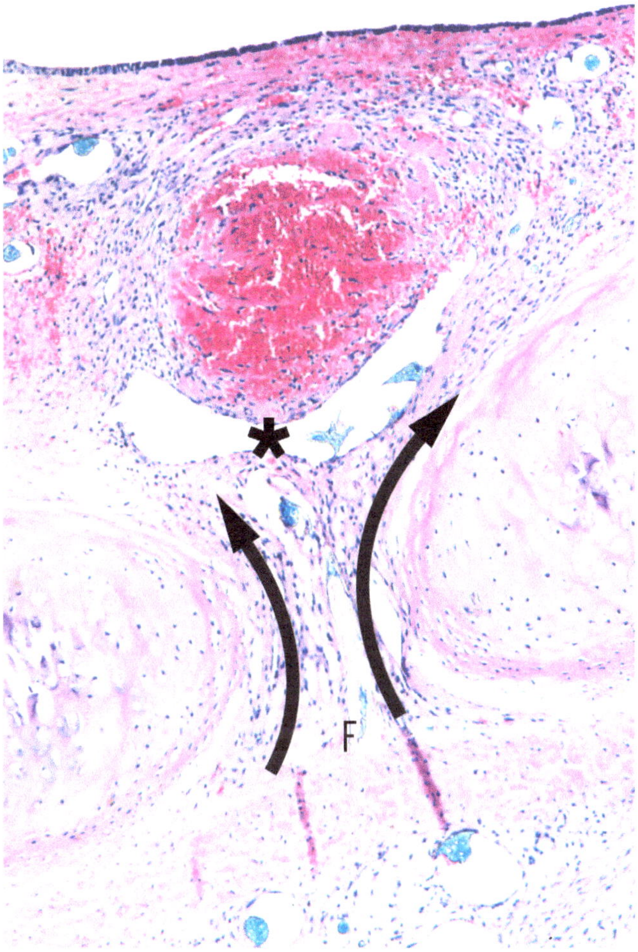

Figure 3.5.
Longitudinal section through tracheal transplant after 6 days of revascularization. Blue silicone injected tracheal transplant. Silicone spots are visible inside a thrombosed mucosal vessel (asterisk). The airway lumen is lined with a confluent layer of squamous epithelium. Outgrowth of blood vessels from the fascia to the submucosal layer of the transplant occurs through the intercartilaginous ligaments (arrow) because cartilage do not allow vessel ingrowth. F=fascia flap. (HE, x20).

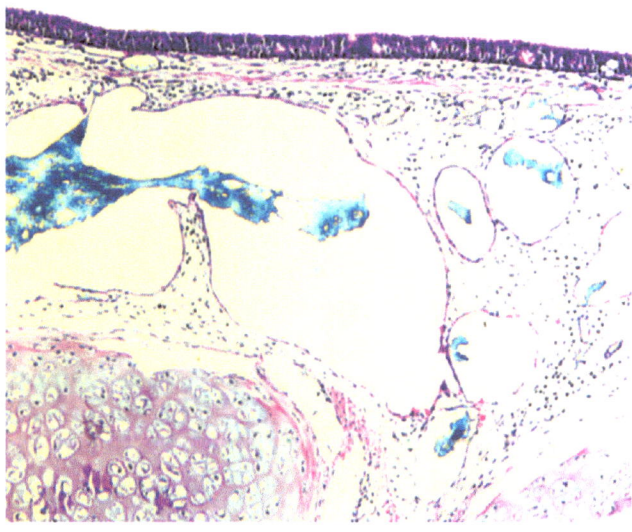

Figure 3.6.
Longitudinal section through tracheal transplant after 14 days of revascularization. Blue silicone injected tracheal transplant. Recovery of ciliated epithelium over fully revascularized submucosal layer. (HE, x20).

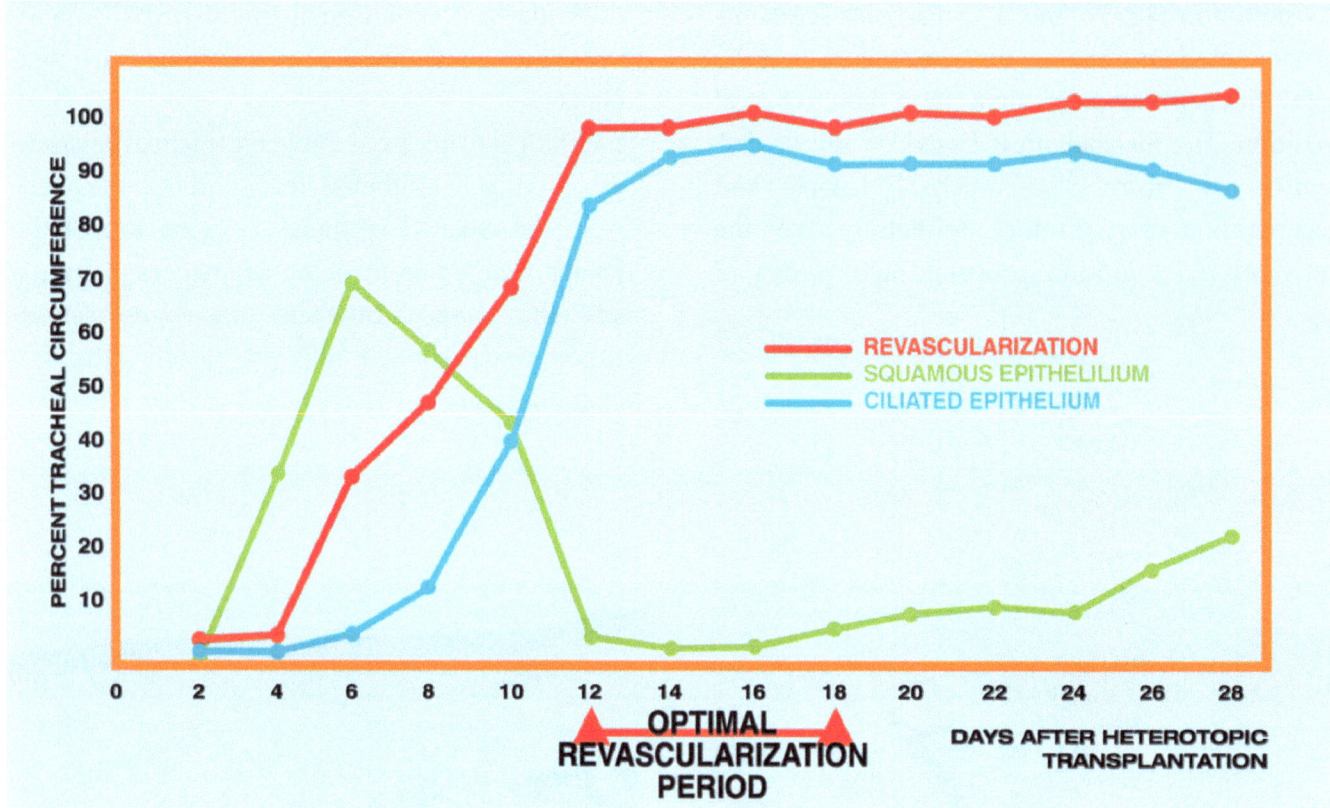

Figure 3.7. Time table of tracheal heterotopical revascularization and epithelial regeneration.
Blue line = respiratory epithelium; green line = squamous epithelium; red line = mucosal revascularization. The period of maximal revascularization and optimal ciliated epithelial recovery is situated between 14 and 20 days after graft isolation. Ninethy percent of the tracheal circumference is revascularized after 14 days. A recovery of respiratory epithelium of about 90% is obtained after 14 days with a small area of squamous epithelium remaining in the most anterior part of the tracheal segment. Mucosal desintegration is seen if the grafts are isolated for a longer period because of stagnation of respiratory secretions and intraluminal infection.

As shown in Fig. 3.7, optimal revascularization of the tracheal transplant is reached after 14 days.

The revascularization process of tracheal allografts is an example of a mucosal healing process by *regeneration*. Healing by regeneration results in a return to the normal histologic and functional architecture of the damaged tissue. The ability of a tissue to regenerate depends on the regenerative capacity of the cells involved (respiratory epithelium) and the stromal integrity of the tissue involved (lamina propria).

Table 3.1. Key features of heterotopical revascularization

1. Vascular and epithelial REGENERATION.

2. Routes of revascularization:
- Membranous trachea (from posterior to anterior)
- Intercartilaginous ligament

3. Optimal revascularization after 14 days.

3. Orthotopical transplantation of tracheal allografts

Tracheal allografts under continuous immunosuppression with cyclosporin, 10 mg/kg per day, show no rejection during heterotopic revascularization. After a 14 day revascularization period, the allograft is fully revascularized and may be transplanted orthotopically on the newly created vascular pedicle of the fascia flap as shown in Fig. 3.8.

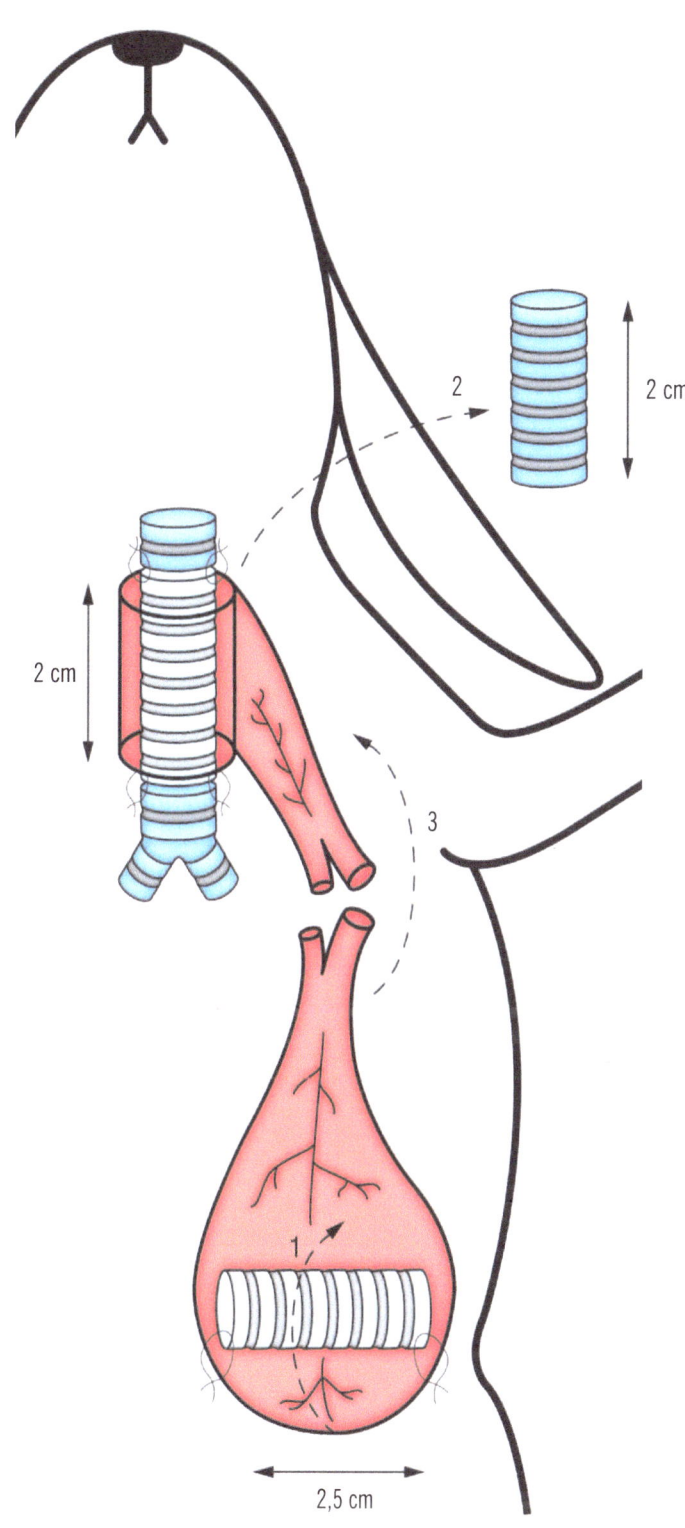

Figure 3.8.
Schematic presentation of orthotopic tracheal allotransplantation. 1, Tracheal allograft, stretched to its original length (2.5 cm), is wrapped by fascial flap for heterotopic revascularization.; 2, resection of 2 cm segment of native trachea; 3, transplantation of 2 cm revascularized allograft segment by transposition of pedicled fascial flap after 14-day revascularization period.
The tracheal segment and its surrounding fascia are dissected and the composite island flap pedicled on the lateral thoracic vessels is subcutaneously rotated to the neck region. The mucosal overgrowth at both ends of the allograft is removed and the remaining tracheal allograft of 2 cm length is orthotopically transplanted after resection of a 2 cm long segment of native trachea. Polypropylene (Prolene, Ethicon Inc) sutures are used for both anastomoses. The transplant is oriented in its original proximal-distal direction to allow for mucociliary clearance over the transplanted region.

Table 3.2. Key features of experimental orthotopical transplantation

1. Possible after 14 days of heterotopical revascularization
2. Cyclosporin at 10 mg/kg preserves the morphologic and functional integrity of the tracheal allotransplant

As shown in Fig. 3.9 and 3.10, the viability of the tracheal allograft after orthotopic transplantation is preserved with a minimal daily immunosup- pressive dose of 10 mg/kg cyclosporin. The tracheal allograft is fully vascularized by the vascular pedicle of the fascia flap as shown in Fig. 3.11.

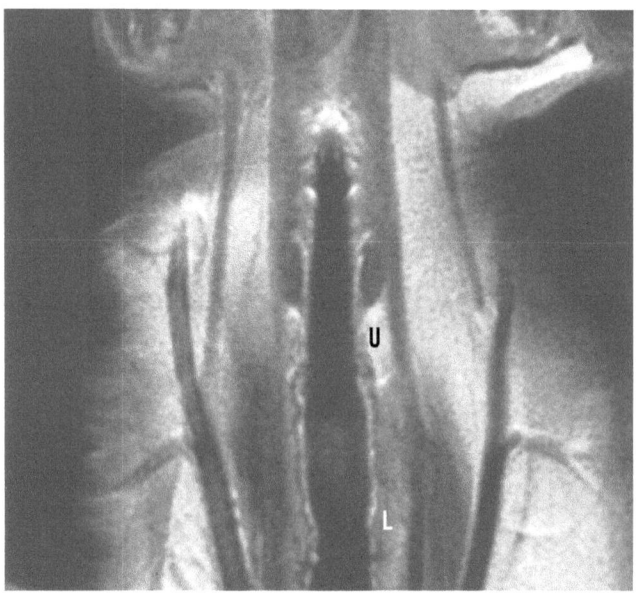

Figure 3.9. Coronal T1-weighted spin echo MRI sec- tion through tracheal transplant (gadolinium-enhan- ced) shows upper (U) and lower (L) transplant anasto- mosis. Transplanted region (2 cm) represents majority of cervical trachea.

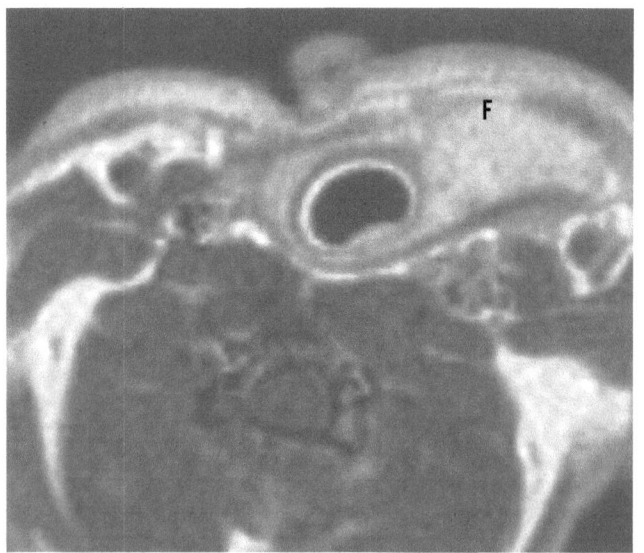

Figure 3.10. Axial enhanced T1-weighted spin echo MRI demonstrates tracheal segment with fascial wrap. Tracheal segment is lined by hyperintense ring repre- senting revascularized mucosa. F = fascia flap.

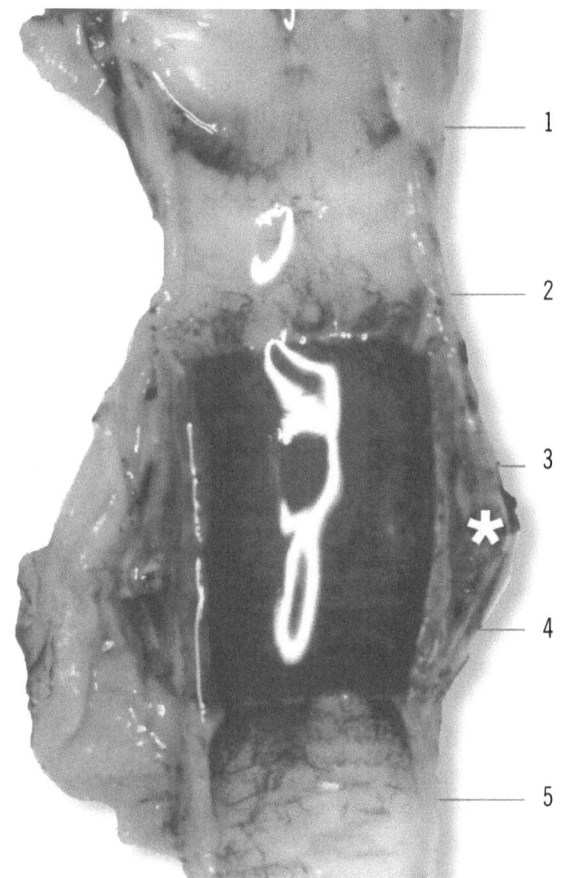

Figure 3.11.
Postmortem macroscopy of tracheal allograft. The vas- cular pedicle of the fascial flap was injected with blue silicone dye and the laryngotracheal complex was inci- sed posteriorly. Intact revascularized tracheal allograft. Fascia (asterisk) and mucosal lining of tracheal trans- plant are uniformly colored by blue silicone dye. The upper and lower transplant anastomoses are free of granulation tissue. Scale in cm.

Cyclosporin at 10 mg/kg is not only capable of preserving the morphologic integrity of the trans- planted trachea, also the mucociliary function remains preserved as shown in Fig. 3.12.

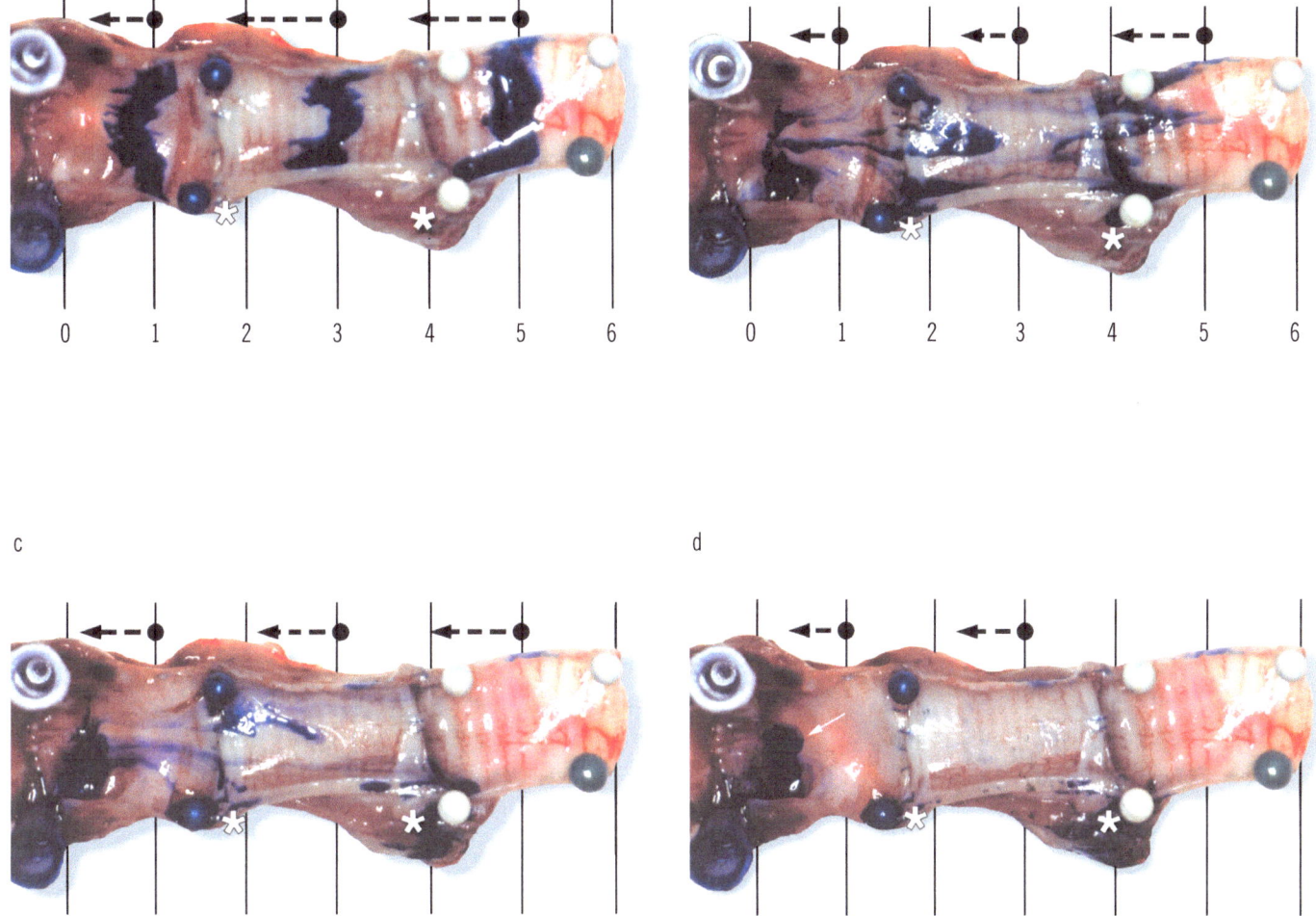

Figure 3.12. Mucociliary clearance of transplanted allografts.
Three spots of silicone particles are deposited on the air-
way mucosa of a vertically placed segment immediately
after removal of the laryngotracheal complex (incised
posteriorly over the entire length). The spots are flowing
down in a vertical direction because of gravity (a).
Asterisks indicate transplant anastomoses. Dotted
arrows indicate direction of mucociliary flow.

All silicone particles are displaced towards the larynx
without interfering with the transplant anastomoses
(b, c). The tracheal transplant is completely cleared after
10 minutes with the silicone located in the subglottic
area (arrow) (d). Scale in cm.

4. Acute and chronic transplant rejection

4.A. Unprotected revascularization -acute rejection

Immunologic rejection will occur during *revascularization in non-immunosuppressed animals*. The rejection can be followed in a day-by-day fashion during the heterotopical revascularization process (Fig. 3.13). During unprotected revascularization, the allograft shows similar initial revascularization signs as during immunosuppressed revascularization during the first 6 days. The initial revascularization and epithelial regeneration will be damaged in non-immunosuppressed revascularization because activated lymphocytes attack the regenerated microcirculation with rethrombosis of the microcirculation and necrosis of the mucosal layer (Fig. 3.14).

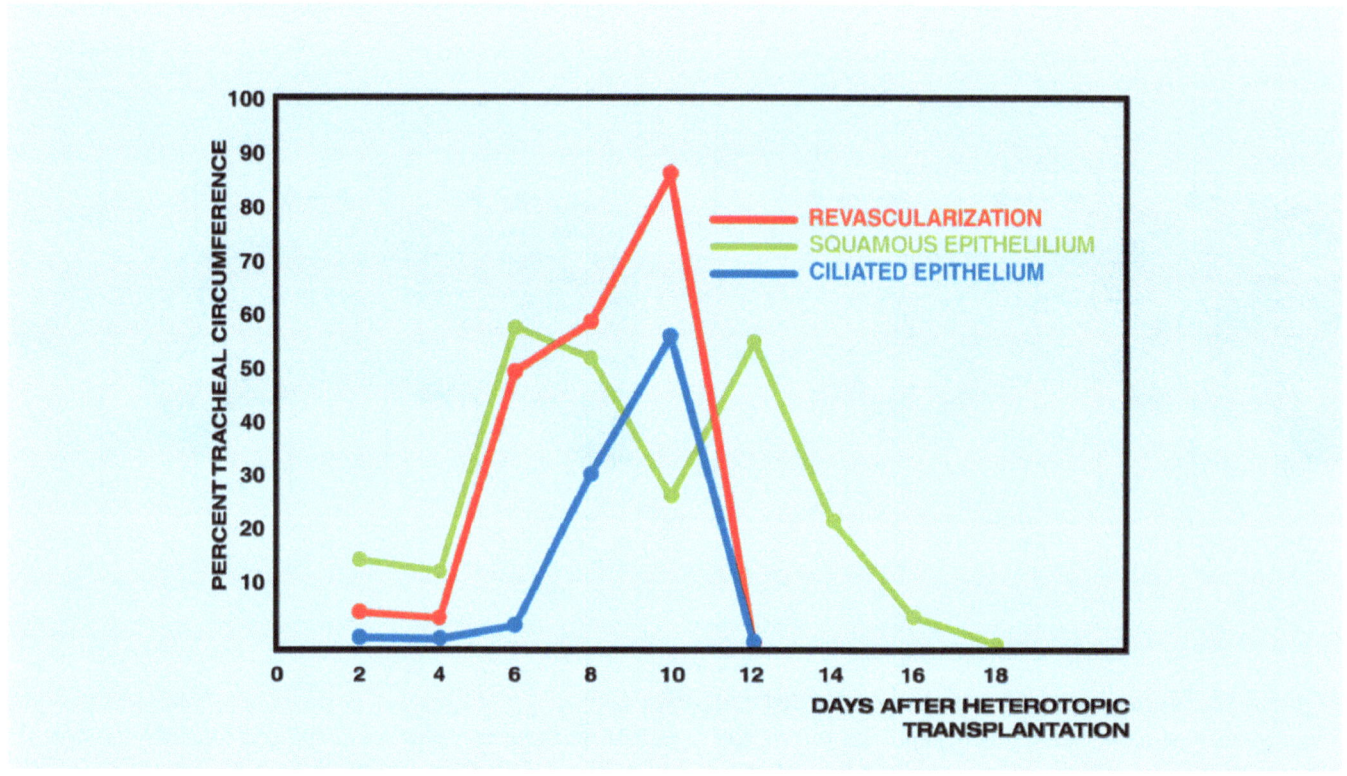

Figure 3.13. Acute tracheal allograft rejection during heterotopic revascularization.

Allograft revascularization, squamous and ciliated epithelium regeneration expressed as percent of tracheal allograft circumference. Allograft revascularization score acutely decreases after 10 days and after initial progressive reperfusion. Epithelial regeneration from squamous to ciliated cells is seen with progressive vascularization.

Ischemic mucosal degeneration evolves from ciliated cells over squamous cells and basal cells to completely denuded avascular submucosa. Revascularization with mucosal regeneration and rejection-mediated cessation of microcirculation with mucosal dedifferentiation are significantly linked. Rejection process terminates when submucosal capillaries of graft involute and can no longer deliver fresh immune cells.

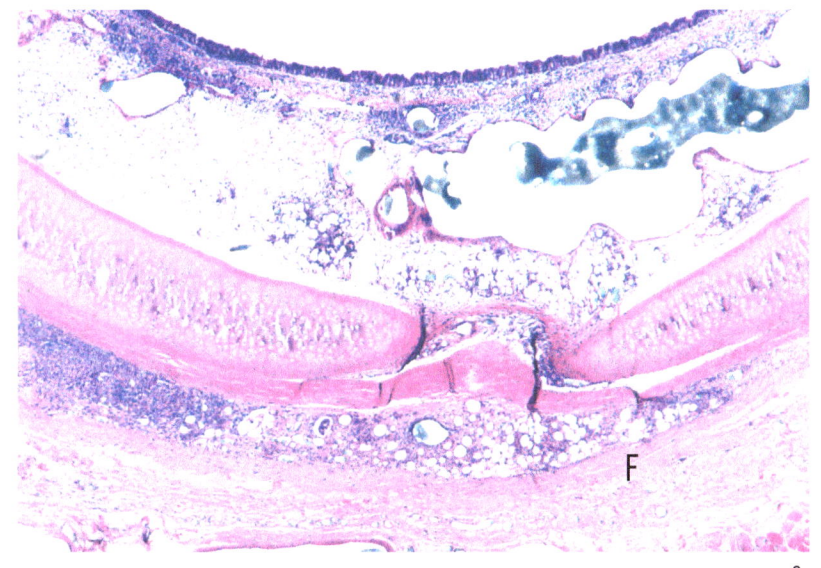

Figure 3.14.
Photomicrographs of acute allograft rejection during revascularization on day 10 and on day 16.
a. Photomicrograph (axial section) of allograft revascularization and rejection after 10 days (H&E, x20) shows well-defined perivascular mononuclear cell infiltration on both sides of cartilage graft. F = fascia flap.

a

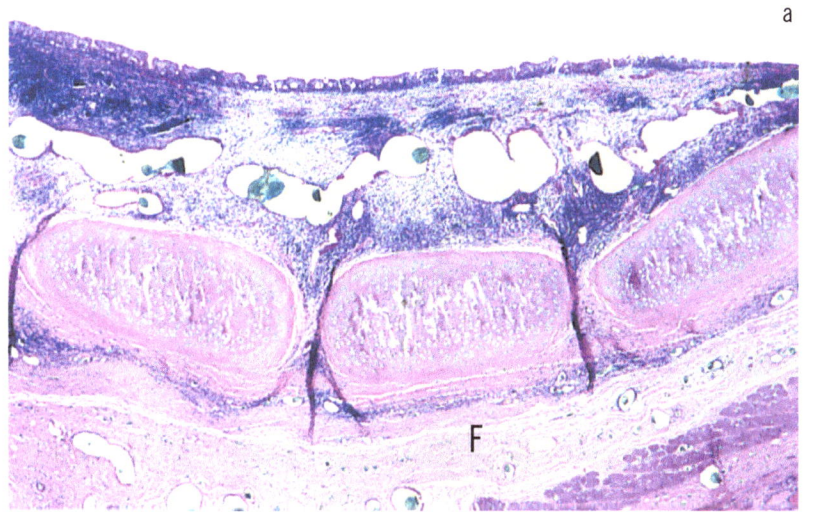

b. Photomicrograph (longitudinal section) of allograft revascularization and rejection after 10 days (H&E, x 20). The regenerated capillaries on both sides of the cartilage ring are attacked by lymphocyts. F = fascia flap.

b

c

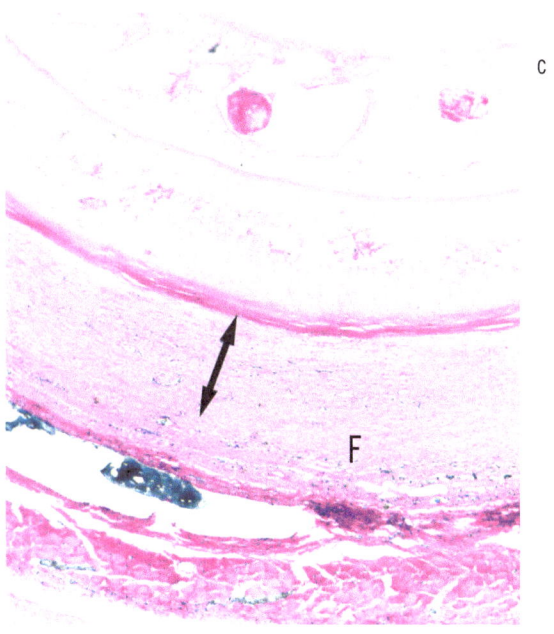

c. Photomicrograph of allograft after 16 days of revascularization (H&E, x 20). End stage of tracheal rejection with cartilage allograft surrounded by two nearly avascular bands. Lamina propria contains vasculonecrotic lesions with significant fibrinoid materal. Epithelial lining has completely disappeared. Cartilage allograft and fascia are separated by fibrous connective tissue (double arrow). Cartilage component shows early signs of ischemic necrosis with eosinophilic ground substance and resorption. F = fascia flap.

As shown in Fig. 3.14, tracheal rejection occurs in a morphologically well defined sequence of events evidenced by damage to the endothelial cells and cessation of microcirculation. The respiratory cells and the cartilaginous component desintegrate secondary to the immunologically induced submucosal and pericartilaginous ischemic necrosis and are not rejected directly by the immunologic attack.

The trachea is an organ subject to the same immunologic laws as all other allogenic tissues. The most important component in tracheal rejection appears to be cell-mediated rejection and the presumed prime target cell population is allograft endothelium. Microvascular thrombosis is the end point in acute tracheal rejection after initial progressive revascularization and mucosal regeneration.

The mucosal rejection process is related to the submucosal microcirculation. Mononuclear cells, provided by the revascularized submucosal blood vessels, attack the lamina propria and destroy the vessel wall with thrombosis and blockage of the microcirculation and subsequent mucosal degeneration.

The cartilaginous component of the allograft is rejected, like the epithelial cells, as a result of vascular changes. The cell-mediated vascular rejection occurs at both sides of the cartilage component. The revascularized connective tissue between cartilage and fascial flap displays microvascular rejection signs similar to those of the tracheal submucosa with mononuclear vasculitis and thrombosis. The immunologically induced avascularity around the cartilage rings isolates the cartilaginous component in a fibrous cocoon with problematic metabolic diffusion. Cartilaginous ischemic necrosis results from pericartilaginous avascularity.

The endothelial cells of the capillary network, at both sides of the tracheal cartilage, are derived from donor vascular endothelial cells. The donor endothelial cells reline the revascularized thrombi during initial revascularization and this regenerated endothelium is the site of the prime manifestation of the rejection process.

4.B. Acute rejection of an orthotopically transplanted allograft

Acute transplant rejection will also occur after cessation of immunosuppression in a rabbit with orthotopic transplantation of a revascularized tracheal segment.

Acute rejection will be seen shortly after orthotopic transplantation when all immunosuppression is stopped in a rabbit that received immunosuppression during the heterotopic revascularisation period and during a short period (7 days) after orthotopical transplantation (Table 3.3).

Immunosuppression is delivered during the 14 days revascularization process and during the first week after orthotopic tracheal transplantation. The first clinical sign of rejection (dyspnea) is visible 10 days after cessation of immunosuppression.

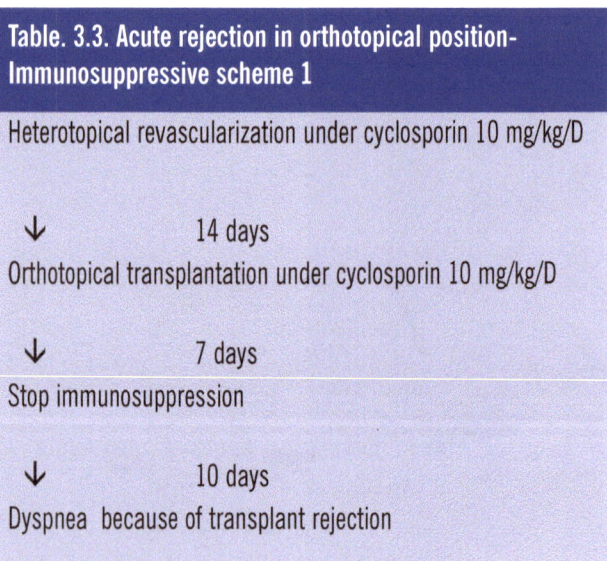

Table. 3.3. Acute rejection in orthotopical position-
Immunosuppressive scheme 1

Heterotopical revascularization under cyclosporin 10 mg/kg/D

↓   14 days
Orthotopical transplantation under cyclosporin 10 mg/kg/D

↓   7 days
Stop immunosuppression

↓   10 days
Dyspnea because of transplant rejection

The first histological signs of immunologic rejection become visible shortly after cessation of immunosuppression (Fig. 3.15).

The immunologic induced lymphocytes attack the microcirculation of the transplant. The immunologic rejection leads to necrosis of the mucosal layer (Fig. 3.16) over the full surface area of the transplant. Necrosis of the mucosal layer leads to respiratory distress after an average period of 10 days after cessation of immunosuppression.

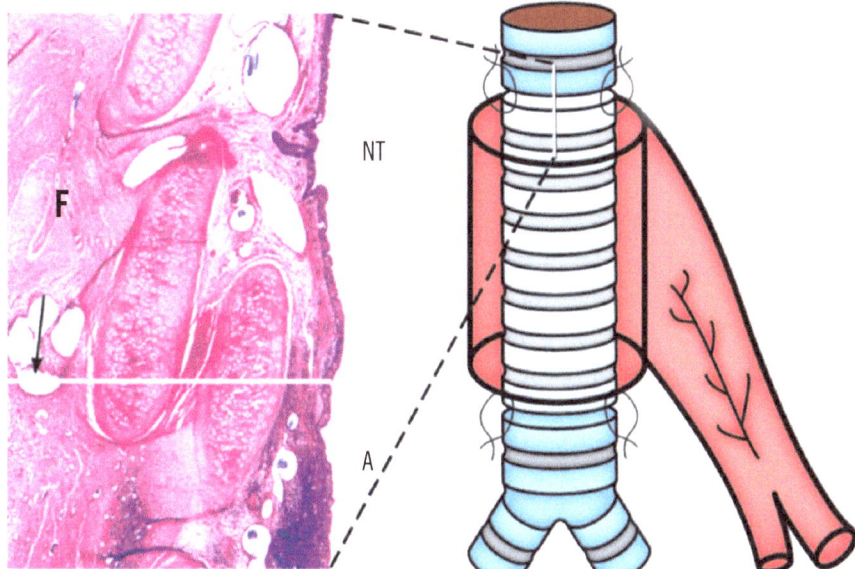

Figure 3.15.
Acute rejection of tracheal allograft in orthotopical position. Photomicrograph of transplant anastomosis 5 days after cessation of immunosuppression (H&E, x 10). Dense, silicone injected submucosa and lymphocytic infiltration of lamina propria allow for identification of transplanted allograft.

Mononuclear cells are present at both sides of the cartilage component in the transplanted segment. No signs of rejection are visible at the site of the native trachea. A, allograft; NT, native trachea; F, fascia. Arrow indicates polypropylene suture.

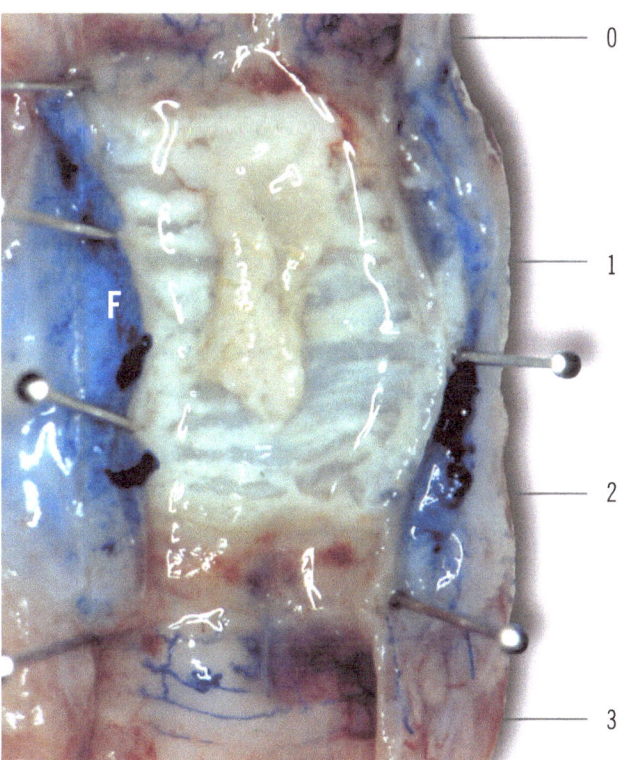

Figure 3.16.
Acute rejection of tracheal allograft in orthotopical position.
Posteriorly incised tracheal transplant 10 days after cessation of immunosuppression. Situation after desquamation of necrotic mucosal layer. Fascia flap (F) is injected with blue silicone. In contrast with the blue silicone-colored fascia around the transplant, no silicone dye-injected mucosal vessels can be distinguished on the transplanted site, indicating a complete avascularity of the transplant. Collateral submucosal vessels injected with blue silicone dye are observed on the native trachea near the anastomosis.

4.C. Chronic rejection

Chronic rejection can be studied when immunosuppression is stopped after a relatively long period of continuous immunosuppression (Cyclosporin 10 mg/kg daily). The chronic rejection studies were performed between New Zealand white rabbits and Dutch-belted rabbits (Fig. 3.17).

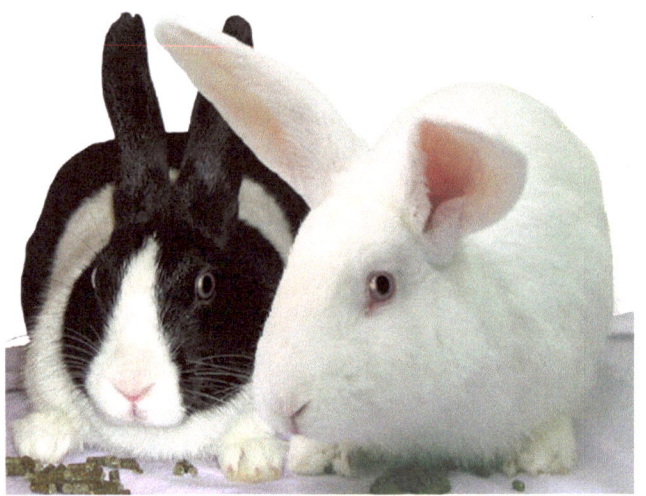

Figure 3.17. Rabbits for chronic rejection studies. New Zealand white rabbits served as recipients and Dutch-belted rabbits were the donors.

These 2 different rabbit strains enabled us to use a well visible skin transplant that served as an external monitor for the immunologic rejection process (Fig. 3.18).

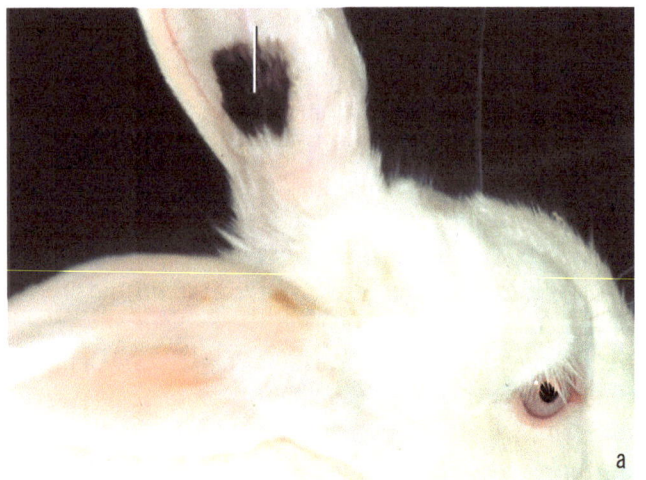

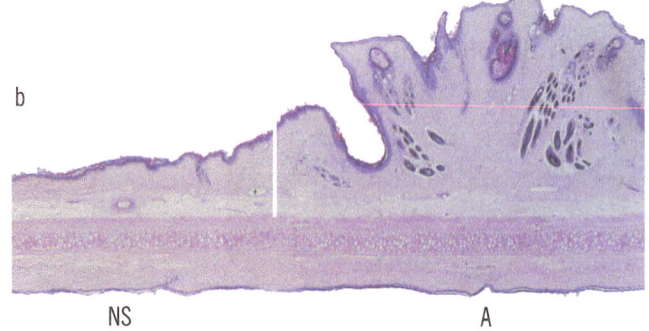

NS   A

Figure 3.18.
External ear of transplanted New Zealand rabbit.
a. piece of abdominal skin (Dutch-beleted) is sutured into an external ear defect of a receptor (New Zealand) rabbit at the time the tracheal allograft is transplanted to the lateral thoracic area for heterotopic revascularization. This skin graft serves as an external monitor during the chronic rejection studies.
b. Histology of skin allograft. The allograft can be identified by the black colored hair follicles. NS = native skin; A = allograft.

For the chronic rejection studies, all immunosuppression was stopped after an initial period of continuous immunosuppression (varying from 4 to 8 weeks). The animals were followed until the first signs of respiratory distress became apparent. Animals received immunosuppressive treatment during 28 days (scheme 2).

Table 3.4. Chronic rejection in orthotopical position-Immunosuppressive scheme 2

Heterotopical revascularization under cyclosporin 10 mg/kg/D
↓   14 days
Orthotopical transplantation under cyclosporin 10 mg/kg/D
↓   14 days
Stop immunosuppression
↓   7 days
Start rejection skin graft
↓   14 days
Dyspnea because of transplant rejection

This *immunosuppressive scheme 2* (Table 3.4) led to rejection of the skin graft, a process that started 7 days after cessation of immunosuppression (Fig. 3.19).

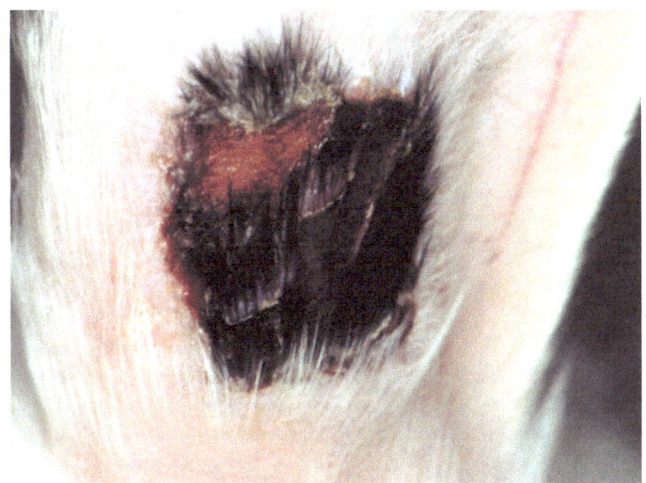

Figure 3.19.
Chronic rejection-Rejection of skin graft.
Skin graft rejection is visible as progressive skin graft necrosis.

The macroscopical and histological evaluation of the tracheal transplant 2 weeks after the first signs of skin rejection and at the moment the rabbit showed the first signs of respiratory distress is shown in Fig. 3.20.

Figure 3.20.
Chronic rejection-Morphology of tracheal transplant after immunosuppressive scheme 2 and after injection of vascular pedicle with blue silicone dye. Photomicrograph of section at anastomotic region. (H&E, x 20).
Illustration of the different histologic patterns at anastomotic (2 mm) and middle transplant sites, sharply separated from each other.
Part A. Native trachea with normal submucosal blood vessels and respiratory epithelium. Arrow indicates Prolene suture between native trachea and allotransplant.
Part B. Indicates anastomotic site of transplant. The anastomotic site of the transplant shows a lamina propria mucosae populated by several blue silicone dye-injected, small capillaries. The submucosa is populated by lymphocyts and lined with ciliated respiratory epithelium.
Part C. The submucosal blood vessels show an immunologic induced thrombosis and a complete avascularity (absence of blue silicone inside vessels) of the mucosal lining. The mucosal lining is not injected with blue silicone because of immunologic rejection and thrombosis of the submucosal blood vessels.
The mucosal lining of the tracheal transplant is characterized by a different vascular pattern at both anastomotic sites, sharply demarcated from the middle, avascular transplant site.

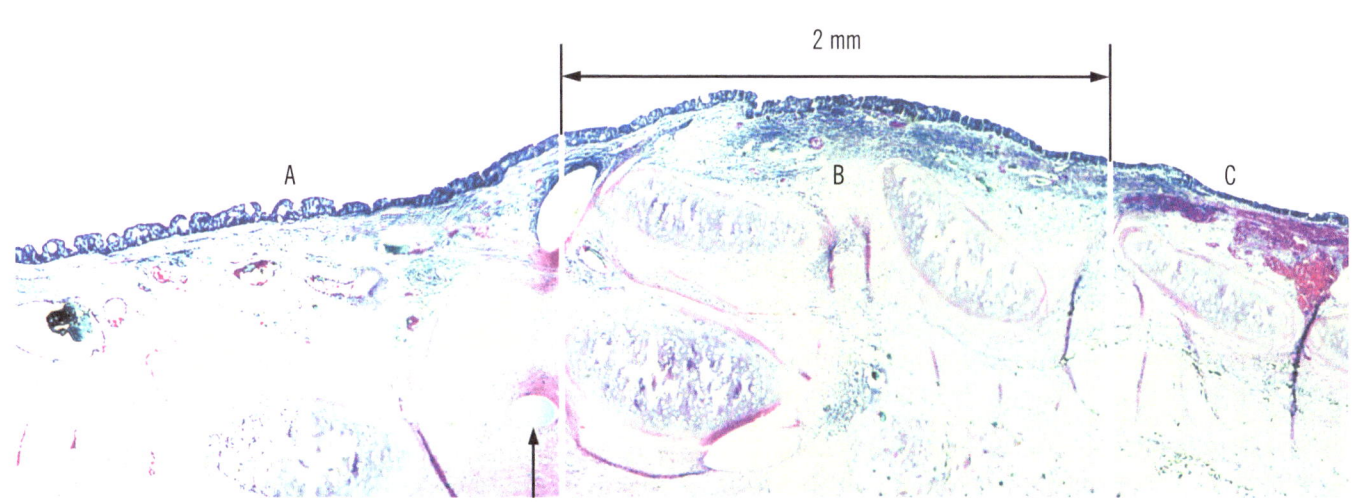

The difference between B and C sites of the tracheal transplant in Fig. 3.20 can be explained by an endothelial repopulation of the transplant. Capillaries from the native trachea are growing into the anastomotic sites of the transplant and these capillaries resist the immunologic attack because the endothelial lining is from receptor origine.

With another immunosuppressive scheme (3), animals received immunosuppression during a longer period of 56 days.

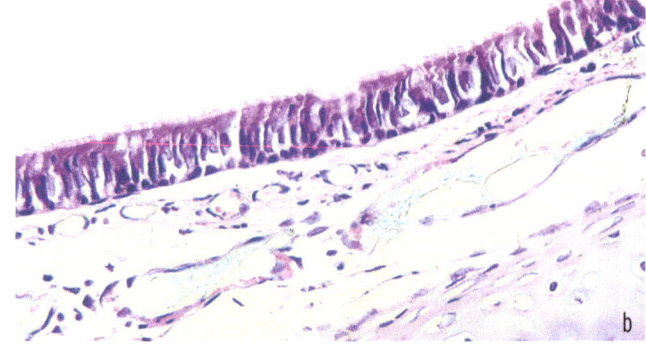

Table 3.5. Chronic rejection in orthotopical position-Immunosuppressive scheme 3
Heterotopical revascularization under cyclosporin 10 mg/kg/D
↓   14 days
Orthotopical transplantation under cyclosporin 10 mg/kg/D
↓   42 days
Stop immunosuppression
↓   14 days
Start rejection skin graft
↓   35 days
Dyspnea because of transplant rejection

With the *immunosuppressive scheme 3* (Table 3.5), the period between cessation of immunosuppression and the start of the rejection process of the skin and the trachea became longer. A period of 6 to 7 weeks elapsed between tracheal symptoms of rejection (dyspnea) and cessation of the immunosuppressive protocol which consisted of 8 weeks of continuous administration of cyclosporin.

Macroscopical evaluation of the transplant at the time the animal showed dyspnea (Fig. 3.21) showed a chronically rejected segment with signs of endothelial repopulation at the anastomotic sites. The middle part ot the transplant showed necrosis with loss of cartilage support.

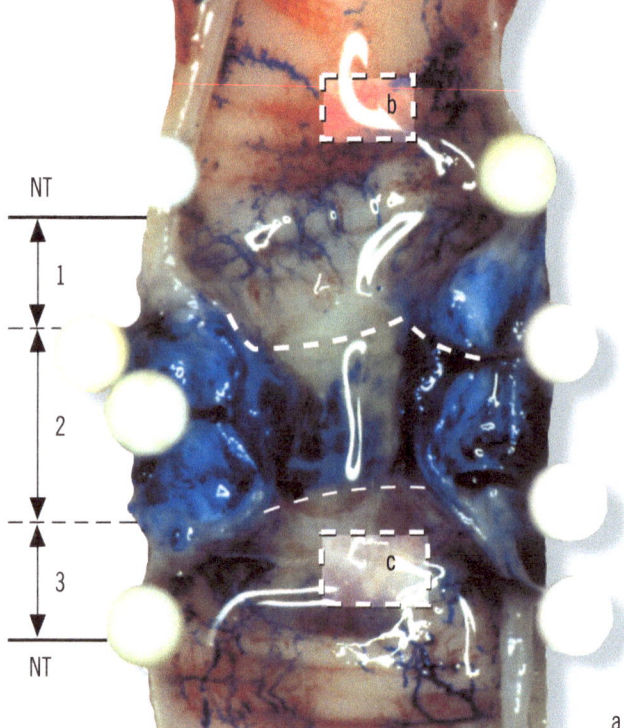

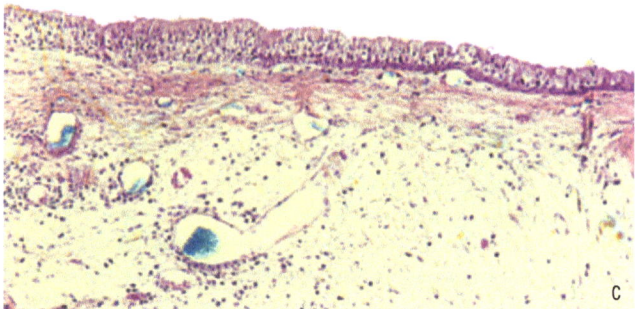

Figure 3.21.
Chronic rejection-Macroscopy of tracheal transplant after immunosuppressive scheme 3.
a.The anastomotic site (1 and 3) shows endothelial repopulation from the native trachea (N.T.) ; the central area (2) shows necrosis with loss of the airway

lumen. Silicone-injected blood vessels are present on both sides of the anastomoses. The middle part shows necrosis with loss of support and luminal stenosis and is sharply separated from the anastomotic sites (dotted lines). The middle part of the transplant is blue colored because the fascia flap forms the internal lining after necrosis of the mucosal and cartilage component.
b.Histology of native trachea. Lamina propria is lined with ciliated epithelium and is vascularized by capillaries with large diameter (H&E x 20).
c.Histology of anastomotic site showing endothelial repopulation. Lamina propria is lined with ciliated epithelium and is vascularized by (regenerated) capillaries with small diameter (H&E x 20).

Studies on chronic rejection provided evidence for the possibility of tracheal allograft endothelial repopulation. However, this repopulation process was seen over a distance of maximal 3 mm and was not sufficient to preserve the complete morphological and functional integrity of the tracheal allograft.

When considering graft repopulation, orthotopic tracheal transplantation on a vascular carrier has some specific characteristics not available in most other tissue transplantations. The tracheal transplant is in contact with the native trachea at both anastomoses and is wrapped circumferentially in well-vascularized tissue of the host. This location of the transplant makes it amenable to host cell repopulation with possible induction of graft tolerance.

Repopulation signs in chronic rejected tracheas are first observed at the anastomotic tracheal transplant areas. After chronic rejection, the capillaries at the anastomotic sites originate from receptor capillary outgrowths. This assumption is supported by the capillaries' resistance to rejection and their first appearance at the interface with the native trachea.

It can be assumed that chronic, rejection-induced ischemia promotes angiogenesis leading to graft endothelial repopulation. This phenomenon, however, is not sufficient to preserve the complete morphological integrity of the tracheal transplants. Only the anastomotic areas over a distance of 2-3 mm were revascularized to a level that allowed preservation of ciliated epithelium. The morphological findings of the mucosal vasculature suggest that the capillary networks at the anastomoses originate from the native trachea. It seems that the angiogenic capacity from the native trachea is length dependent and confined to the anastomotic regions.

Two different processes of revascularization can be distinguished in the tracheal transplants showing endothelial repopulation. They are first revascularized in a heterotopical position under protection with immunosuppression after isolation from the donor animal. Unlike whole organ grafts that provide the preformed autochtonous microvascular system, the avascular tracheal allografts require the process of revascularization to reestablish nutritional blood vessels by recanalization of previously existing but thrombosed capillaries. The endothelial cells of the submucosal network of the transplant are derived from donor vascular endothelial cells. The donor endothelial cells reline the revascularized thrombi, a phenomenon induced by the fascial wrap. The vessel diameter of these revascularized submucosal vessels is comparable with the preexisting vessels and with the submucosal vessels of the native trachea. A second revascularization stage is observed during chronic rejection of the initially revascularized capillary network of the allograft. This revascularization stage is characterized by true angiogenesis with receptor capillary sprouts advancing across the graft-host junction with vascular reperfusion of the chronically rejected submucosal layer. The endothelial cells of the induced vascular network are resistant to rejection and thus originate from the receptor.

Revascularization of a preexisting but thrombosed capillary network and true angiogenesis defined as the formation of capillary outgrowths represent 2 distinct reperfusion processes responsible for survival of the unrejected and the chronically rejected tracheal allografts, respectively.

> Blood vessel repopulation
> of the transplant anastomoses
> occurs over a distance
> of maximal 2-3 mm.

Currently, transplantation of tracheal segments has no clinical relevance. Only tracheal allotransplantation in the rare case of long tracheal stenosis (> 6 cm) could be useful but the need for chronic immunosuppression makes this option not attractive at this moment.

The clinical feasibility of allotransplantation of a vascularized tracheal allograft depends on reducing immunosuppression and its associated toxicity for the graft recipient. The significant morbidity associated with chronic immunosuppression is difficult to justify in non-life-threatening situations.

Another problem may be the degree of revascularization of the human trachea when wrapped with fascia in a heterotopical position. The human tracheal wall is much thicker than the rabbit's trachea and it remains questionable whether the avascular, human trachea would revascularize with the same ease as the rabbit's trachea.

5. Formation of tracheal patch

We redirected our research from allotransplantation of tracheal tubes to allotransplantation of tracheal patches. We wanted to know whether it is possible to transform a revascularized tube of trachea into a revascularized patch and use the patch for anterior reconstruction of the larynx and trachea.

5.A. Optimal vascular patch design

The optimal vascular patch design was studied on heterotopically revascularized tracheal allografts in immunosuppressed (Cyclosporin A 10 mg/ml) animals. Depending on the site of incision of the trachea and the fascia flap, four possible patch designs may be created on the fascial enwrapped allograft after 14 days of heterotopic revascularization.

The amount of patch revascularization was evaluated after longitudinal incision of the fascia flap and the tracheal transplant (Fig. 3.22).

The amount of surface area that was colored by blue silicone after patch formation and after blue Microfil® injection of the vascular pedicle was a measure for the vascular supply to the patch.

Figure 3.22.
Schematic presentation of different tracheal patch designs.
Patch 1. Patch created by division of cartilage ring and incision of fascial flap at its proximal end (a). P= proximal end of fascia near vascular pedicle D=distal end of fascial flap. After longitudinal incision, the arterial vascular pedicle of the different patch designs was injected by blue Microfil®
Dotted double arrow indicates mean amount of mucosal surface area that was injected with blue silicone for each patch design. Blue spots are mucosal vessels perfused by fascial flap (b). A morphologic picture after injection of blue silicone shows that about 25% of the patch surface area is perfused by the fascia. The membranous ligament (arrowheads) is included in the patch (c)
Patch 2. Patch created by division of membranous trachea and incision of fascial flap at its proximal end (a). P = proximal end of fascia near vascular pedicle. D = distal end of fascial flap. This patch is completely supported by cartilage with only a small area near the proximal site of the fascia flap that is perfused by silicone (b).

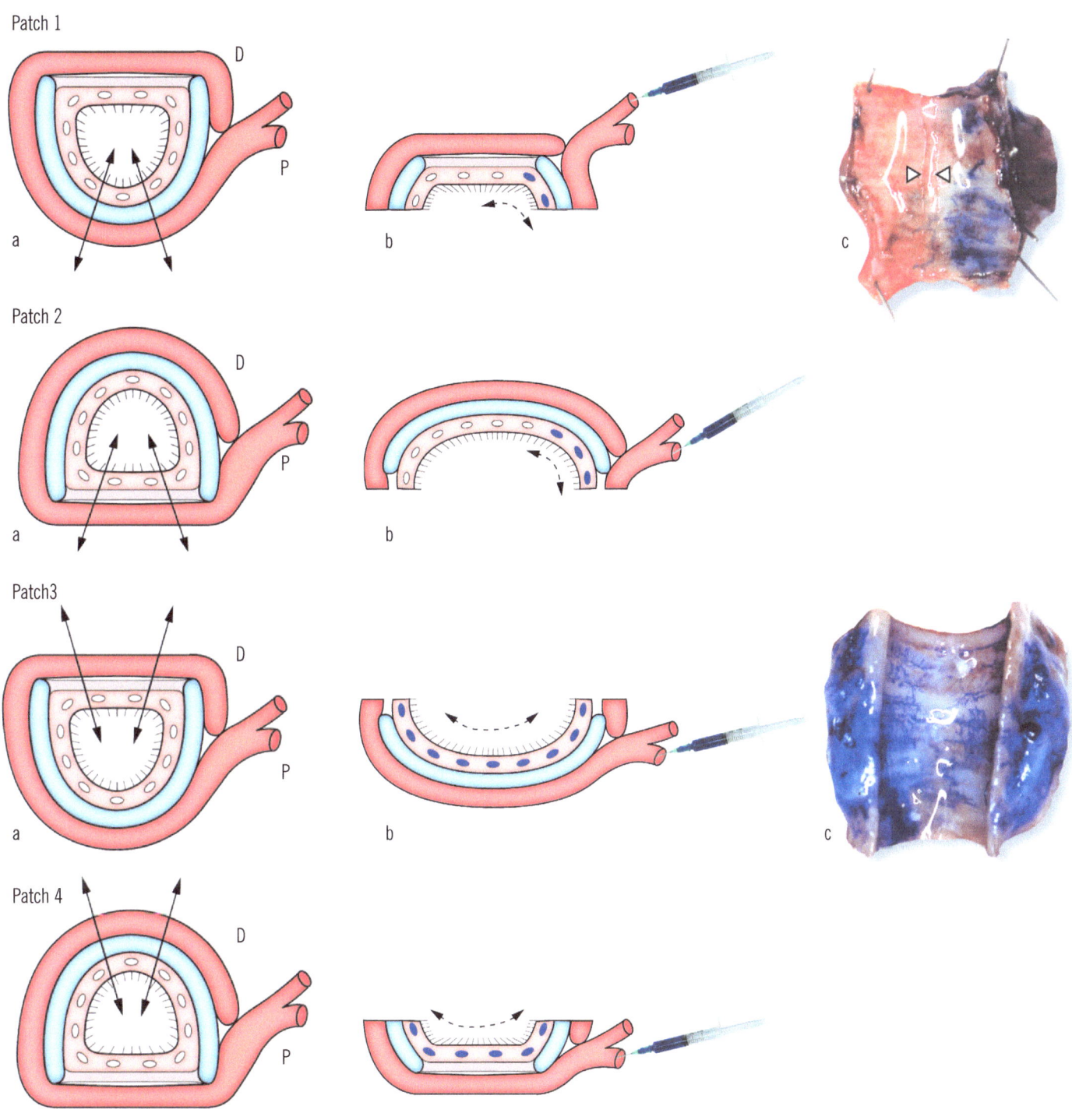

Patch 1

Patch 2

Patch3

Patch 4

Patch 3. Patch created by division of membranous trachea and incision of fascial flap at its distal end (a). P = proximal end of fascia near vascular pedicle. D= distal end of fascial flap. This patch is completely supported by cartilage and completely perfused by the fascia (b, c)

Patch 4. Patch created by division of cartilage ring and incision of fascial flap at its distal end (a). P = proximal end of fascia near vascular pedicle. D = distal end of fascial flap. This patch is completely perfused by the fascia flap with inclusion of the membranous ligament (b). Patch 3 and patch 4 show full vascularization and provide for the optimal vascular patch design.

As expected, group 3 and group 4 patches showed a blue colored mucosal surface area of more than 75% (between 75-100%) after a distal incision of the fascia flap while less than 25% (between 0-25%) of the patch surface area was colored after a proximal incision (group 1 and 2) of the fascia flap. It was concluded that a reliable vascular patch supply can be obtained after a distal transsection of the circumferentially applied fascial flap.

5.B. Optimal morphologic patch design

Patches with a reliable blood supply (Group 3 and 4 patches) were used for repair of anterior laryngotracheal defects in order to examine which patch design could provide for the optimal post-reconstructive morphologic situation (Fig. 3.23). The two patch designs were evaluated morphologically (MRI and postmortem macroscopy) 4 weeks after transplantation into the anterior laryngotracheal defect (Fig. 3.24, 3.25).

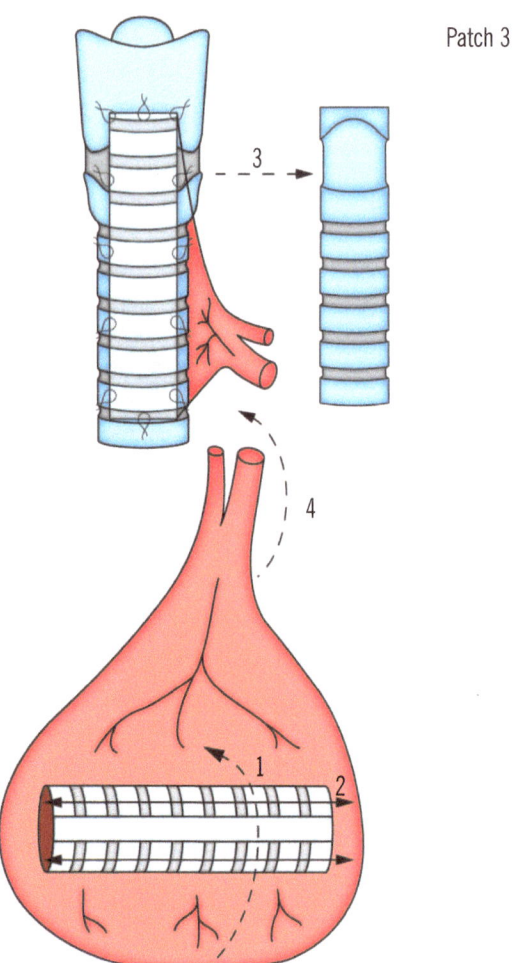

Patch 3

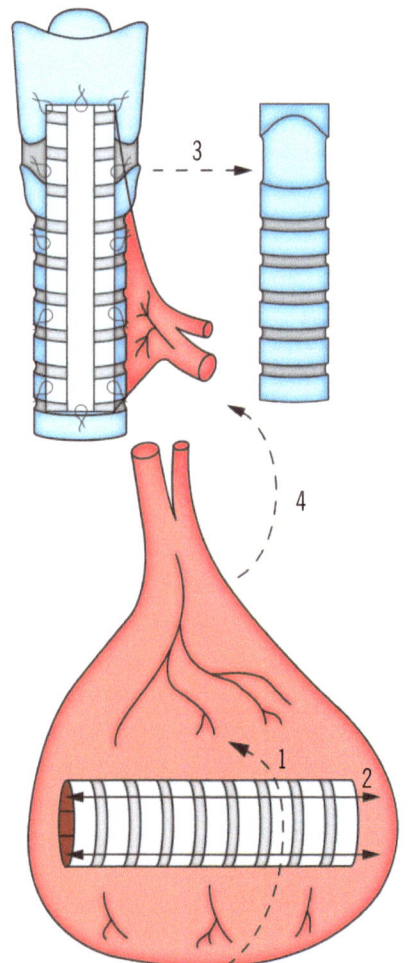

Patch 4

Figure 3.23.
Schematic presentation of laryngotracheal reconstruction with patch 3 and patch 4.
1, Tracheal allograft stretched to its original length (3 cm), is wrapped by fascial flap for heterotopic revascularization. 2, longitudinal incision of tracheal allograft and fascial flap incision at its distal end to create patch

3 (full cartilage support) and patch 4 (membranous trachea included) after a 14 days revascularization period; 3, resection of 2.5 cm laryngotracheal anterior wall; 4, transplantation of tracheal patch (length 2.5 cm) by transposition of pedicled fascial flap.

Full cartilaginous supported patches (patch 3) are needed to optimally restore the airway lumen. The tracheal patches containing the membranous trachea (patch 4) show a localized prolaps inside the lumen at the membranous region.

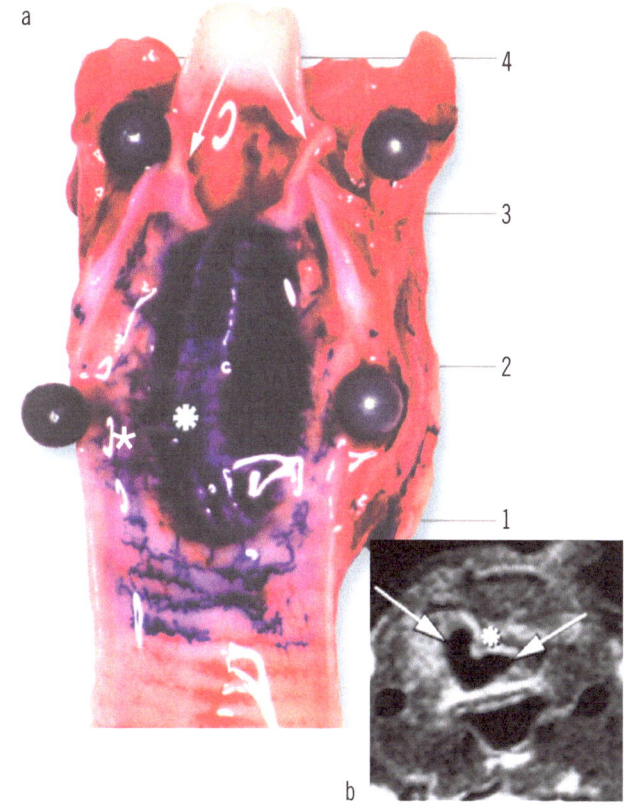

Figure 3.24. Morphology of patch 3.
a. Patch 3 postmortem macroscopy after longitudinal incision posteriorly. The vascular pedicle of the fascia flap is injected with blue Microfil®. Abrupt transition area is seen between patch and native larynx and trachea. The tracheal patch is injected with silicone dye through the lateral thoracic artery and is intensely stained. Some collateral supply is visible on the native airway. No granulation tissue has formed at suture lines with all the knots of the Prolene sutures lying on the outside. The patch provides for an optimal anterior wall reconstruction. Arrows indicate arytenoids.
b. Patch 3 morphology of reconstruction on axial images. Axial gadolinium-enhanced T1-weighted MR image demonstrates revascularized tracheal patch between 2 arrows. The lumen is lined anteriorly by an enhancing area representing revascularized mucosa of tracheal patch (area between 2 arrows). The support provided by the cartilaginous component secures restoration of a nearly normal airway lumen.

Figure 3.25. Morphology patch 4.
a. Patch 4 postmortem macroscopy. Internal lining of tracheal patch is colored by silicone dye, indicating normal mucosal viability. Prolapsing membranous trachea is indicated by asterisk. Arrows show arytenoids.
b. Patch 4 morphology of reconstruction on axial images. Axial gadolinium-enhanced T1 weighted MR image shows anterior patch between 2 arrows. The membranous ligament (asterisk) shows prolaps inside the lumen.

An optimal patch design may be obtained by excision of the membranous trachea and by a distal transection of the circumferentially applied fascial flap (Table 3.6).

The results after reconstruction of anterior airway defects using vascularized allotransplants show that complications may be avoided when using tissues that fullfil the requirements for optimal

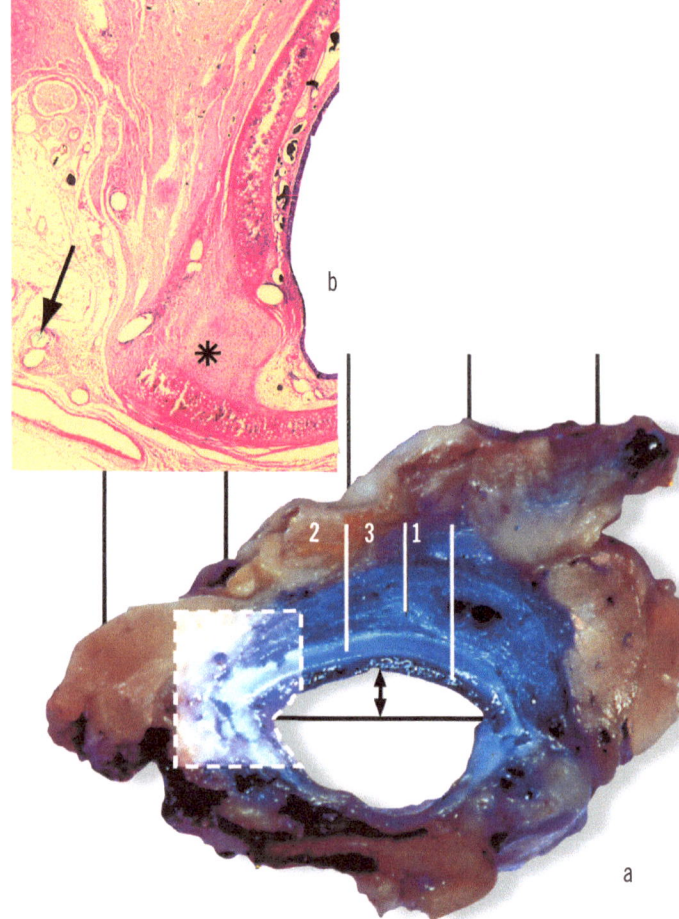

Table 3.6. Key features of the optimal tracheal patch design
1. Optimal morphology of patch: Longitudinal incision of membranous trachea 2. Optimal vascularization of patch: Distal transection of fascia flap

laryngeal reconstruction. The frequently reported complications after laryngeal reconstruction such as graft extrusion, granulation tissue formation, and stenosis are not inherently linked with airway repair. These complications are not seen when using optimal repair tissues.

The clinical importance of the improved reconstructive possibilities with allogenic tracheal patches remain low because of the need for continuous immunosuppression. The revascularized allograft stands for the definition of the optimal reconstruction of anterior laryngotracheal defects (Fig. 3.26). The optimal reconstruction may serve as 'the ideal example' against which other autologous composite tissues for airway reconstruction have to be weighted.

Because of the impressive results obtained with tracheal allotransplants, autologous donor sites for tracheal transplantation were explored in an attempt to bring the experimental results closer to clinical application. It was hypothetized that tracheal autotransplantation may have the potential to improve larynx reconstruction after extended hemilaryngectomy.

Figure 3.26.
Morpholopgy of patch 3 on axial section.
a. The 3 tissue components: respiratory epithelium (1), cartilage support (2), and vascularization (3) provide for a primary healing with additional anterior airway lumen expansion (double arrow). Scale in cm.
b. Photomicrograph of transition area between native airway and patch reconstruction (H&E x 20). The connection between the patch and the margins of the airway defect appears solid and is fibrous or cartilaginous (asterisk) in nature. The polypropylene (Prolene 6.0, ethicon) sutures (arrow) provides immediate patch support at the suture lines. Healing at the anastomoses is not necesary for obtaining a stable reconstruction.

6. Revascularization and transplantation of tracheal autografts

Revascularization and transplantation of tracheal autografts were explored as a possible way to improve the reconstruction of hemicricoid defects after tumor removal.

6.A. Orthotopic revascularization

The orthotopic position is not a good place for revascularization of avascular tracheal transplants because the movement of the transplant during respiration and swallowing interferes with the critical revascularization process of a completely avascular tracheal graft. The situation is however different when considering revascularization of tracheal autografts. Tracheal autografts may become revascularized in a progressive way without going through a critical period of total avascularity. The orthotopic position provides the optimal place for a staged revascularization of an ischemic but still perfused tracheal segment. For wrapping the trachea in vascularized fascia, it is necessary to isolate the trachea from its surrounding tissue connections with disruption of the extrinsic blood supply that is provided by small tracheoesophageal vascular branches. The autologous trachea may be wrapped without incision of the trachea so that the intrinsic mucosal blood supply of the trachea remains preserved. A moderate ischemic trachea is beneficial for promoting angiogenesis with outgrowth of blood vessels between fascia flap and trachea. The preserved intrinsic tracheal's blood supply makes that revascularization can occur without the risk for avascular necrosis (Fig. 3.27).

Experimentally, the orthotopic position was found to be the optimal place for staged revasculariza-

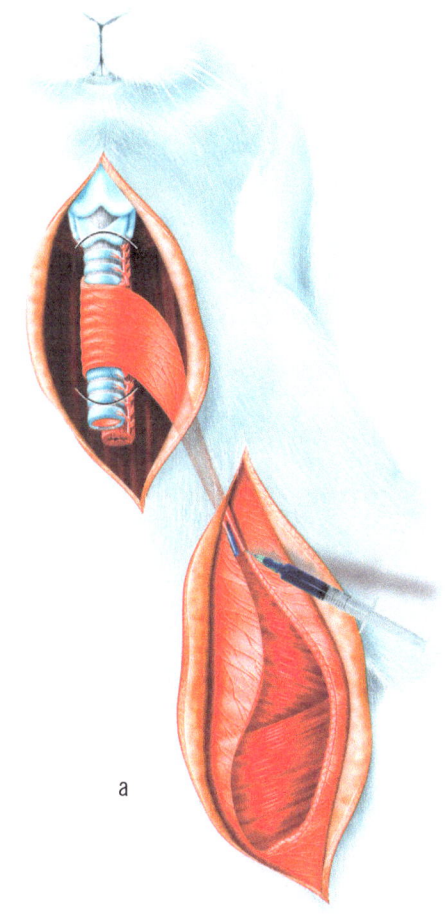

Figure 3.27.
Orthotopic tracheal revascularization.
a. Schematic presentation of orthotopic revascularization of segments of autologous trachea. The cervical trachea is reached through a midline neck incision and dissected over 2 cm from the underlying esophagus. The left thoracic fascial flap is isolated on the lateral thoracic vessels and subcutaneously rotated to the neck region. The cervical trachea is then wrapped by the transposed lateral thoracic fascial flap. To allow for circumferential wrapping by the vascular carrier, the trachea has to be isolated from its surrounding tissue connections that results in ischemia due to disruption of the tracheal's extrinsic segmental blood supply. Tissue ischemia leads to angiogenic stimulation driving new vessels from the vascularized fascial flap to the isolated tracheal segment. Tracheal revascularization occurs without risk for necrosis because the intrinsic mucosal perfusion remains intact.
The amount of tracheal revascularization is visualized after two weeks and after injection of blue silicone into the artery of the fascial flap.

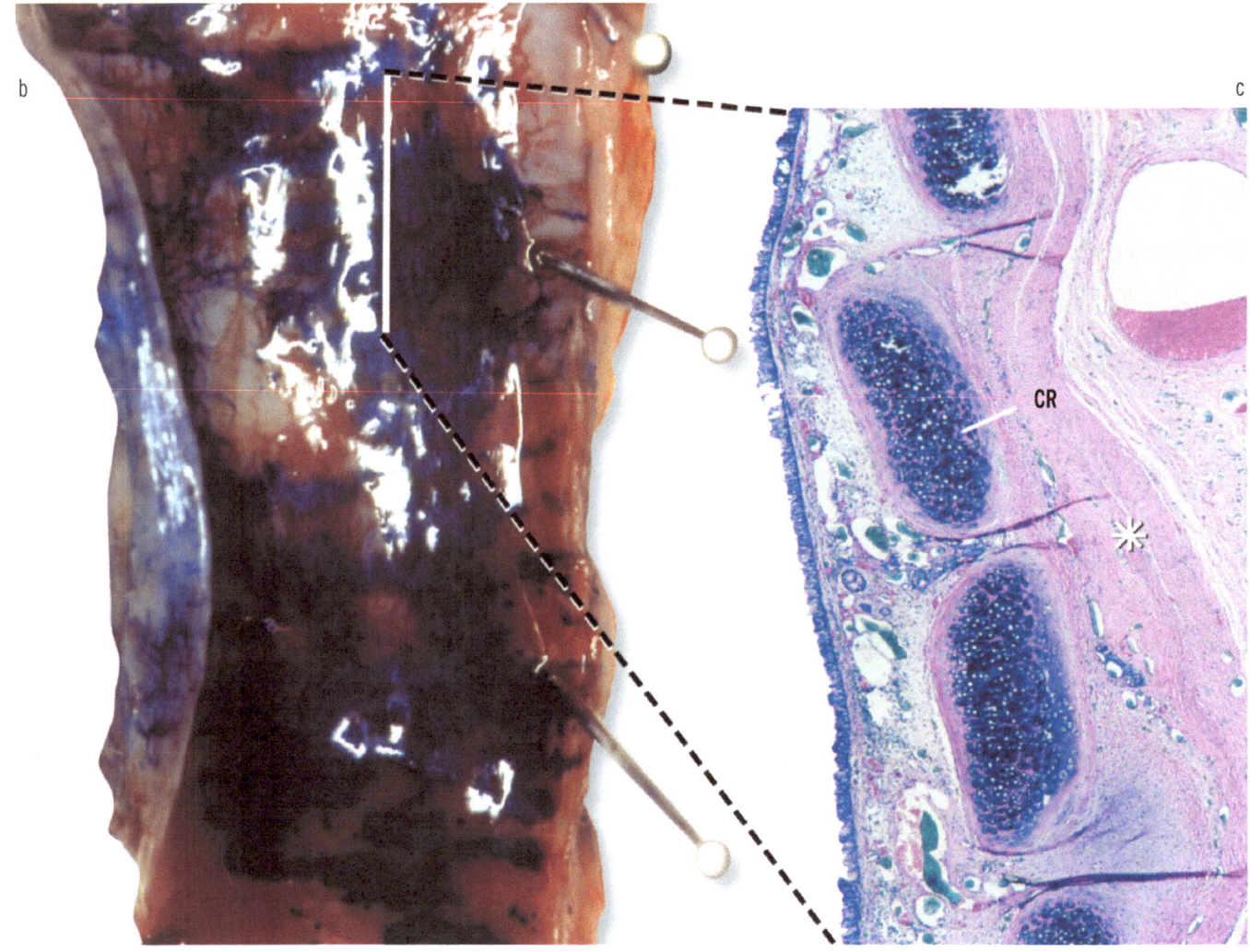

Figure 3.27. Orthotopic tracheal revascularization (continued).

b. Macroscopic evaluation of orthotopic revasculariza-tion process. After a 14 days period, the neck is reopen-ed and the trachea is isolated from the airway, only con-nected with the vascular pedicle of the fascial flap. After injection of blue silicone into the artery of the fas-cial flap, and after posterior longitudinal incision of the trachea, the mucosal lining reveals a 2 cm segment of trachea intensely stained by the blue silicone. The stai-ning is more pronounced at the intercartilaginous liga-ments. The segment is not completely stained by the blue color because the intrinsic blood supply remained intact.

c. Photomicrograph of a longitudinal incision of Fig. 3.27 b. - The vessels supplied by the fascia flap (aste-riks) have a blue staining. They reach the mucosal lining of the tracheal segment through the intercarti-laginous ligaments. The largest mucosal blood vessel concentration is present at the intercartilaginous liga-ments (H.E. x20). CR, cartilage ring.

tion of ischemic but still perfused tracheal autografts. Optimal tracheal autograft revascularization was obtained by a 2-stage approach and by using a thin, pliable, and axially perfused fascial envelope. The large tracheal surface area, the relatively thin tracheal wall, the adherence between tracheal cartilage and fascia after 14 days, and the presence of intercartilaginous ligaments allowing vessel ingrowth and mucosal perfusion contributed to the success of the staged revascularization technique. The initially preserved intrinsic, mucosal blood supply could be interrupted and the trachea could rely completely on the fascial blood supply after the revascularization period.

6.B. Recovery of mucociliary clearance function after reversed tracheal transplantation

The technique of tracheal autotransplantation after staged orthotopic revascularization could be used to examine the mucociliary clearance following segmental tracheal autotransplantation in a reversed position. It remains a question whether transplant orientation is important for preserving the right direction of the mucociliary clearance process. With the model of tracheal autotransplantation, we were able to answer the following question: are the cilia within tracheal transplants programmed to beat in a given direction indefinitely, or are they influenced by cilia in adjacent tracheal segments to beat in line with the entire laryngotracheal complex?

Segments of rabbit cervical trachea were reversed 2 weeks after orthotopic revascularization (Fig. 3.28). Mucociliary clearance was examined 1 month after tracheal reversal. After posterior longitudinal incision of the laryngotracheal complex, the

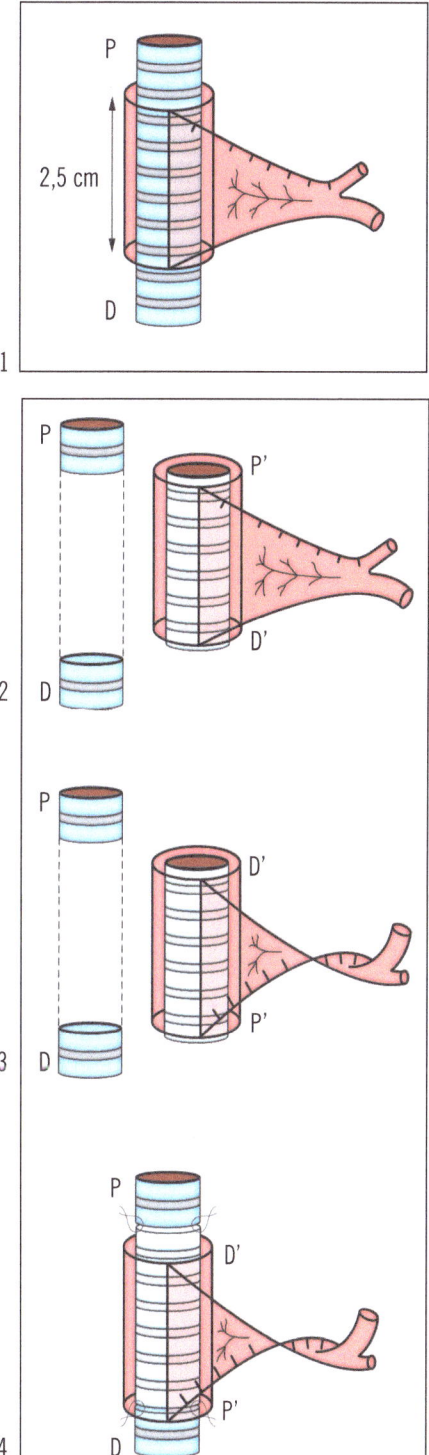

Figure 3.28.
Staged tracheal inversion by vascular fascial induction. 1. In the first stage, the cervical trachea is wrapped by the fascial flap. Section (2) and reversal (3) of the segment occurs after 14 days. Continuity after reversal is reestablished (4) (P and P'= proximal; D and D'= distal).

movement of silicone particles was evaluated immediately postmortem. It was shown on these reversely transplanted tracheas that both mucociliary orientation and coördination fully recovers after transplantation of respiratory epithelium. Surgical reversal of a tracheal segment however did not reprogram the polarity of cilia, indicating that this polarity is not influenced by external factors such as airflow and mucus flow in the tracheal lumen (Fig. 3.29).

Because the originally programmed direction and coördination of the ciliary beat is maintained and

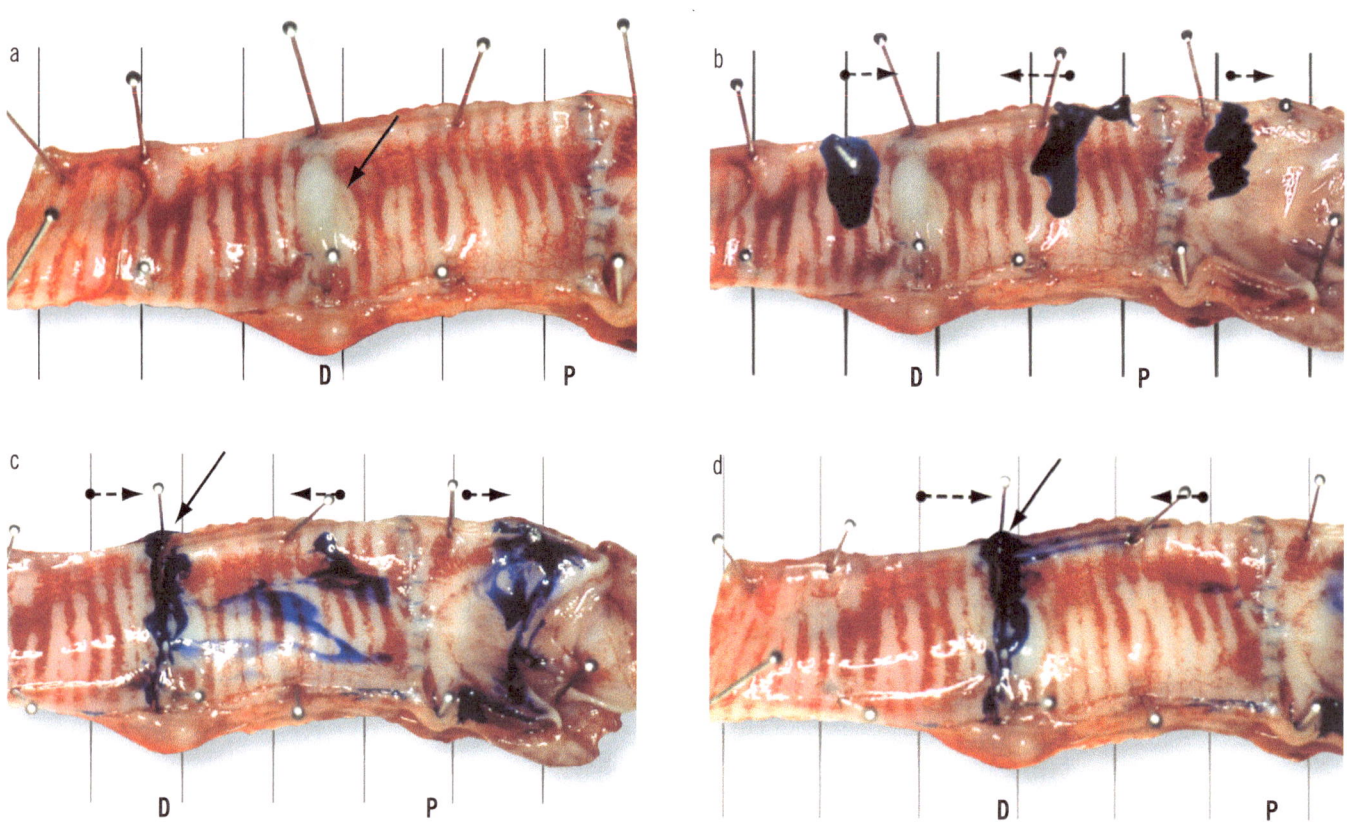

Figure 3.29. Measurement of mucociliary clearance in reversed tracheal segments by deposition of silicone particles.
a. Postmortem macroscopy before silicone deposition. A mucus plug is visible at the distal anastomosis, providing evidence for the presence of opposite mucociliary flow in the region of the distal anastomosis. (P = proximal anastomosis; D = distal anastomosis)
b. Macroscopy of mucociliary clearance in a laryngotracheal complex immediately after silicone deposition. Silicone spots are deposited at 3 locations. The spots are flowing down due to gravity. Dotted arrows indicate directions of mucociliary flow. (P = proximal anastomosis; D = distal anastomosis).
c. Macroscopy of mucociliary clearance in a laryngotracheal complex 2 minutes after silicone deposition. The upper silicone spot is displaced upward until the glottic level is reached. The middle spot is moved downward until the distal anastomosis is reached. The lower spot is displaced upwards, with silicone stagnation (arrow) at the distal anastomosis (p = proximal anastomosis; D = distal anastomosis).
d. Macroscopy of mucociliary clearance in a laryngotracheal complex 10 minutes after silicone deposition. The inverted tracheal segment is cleared, with the middle and lower silicone spots completely displaced toward the distal anastomosis (arrow) (P = proximal anastomosis; D = distal anastomosis).

is not altered or reprogrammed by adjacent ciliated cells in normal segments of trachea, tracheal transplants must be orientated in the appropriate direction to obtain a normal mucosal clearance.

7. Transplantation of autologous tracheal patches to laryngeal defects
7.A. Two-stage procedure

No clinical indications exist for autotransplantation of tracheal tubes. Patches of tracheal tissue however might be useful in the reconstruction of extended laryngeal defects.

The question raised if revascularized tracheal segments could be transformed into patches suitable for hemilaryngeal reconstruction after hemicricohemilaryngectomy.

As shown in Fig. 3.30 and Fig. 3.31, full cartilaginous supported patches may be formed on revascularized tracheal segments wrapped with fascia after distal longitudinal incision of the fascia flap and after removal of the membranous trachea.

For optimal repair of extended laryngeal defects, it is important to have tracheal patches with cartilage support over their whole surface area.

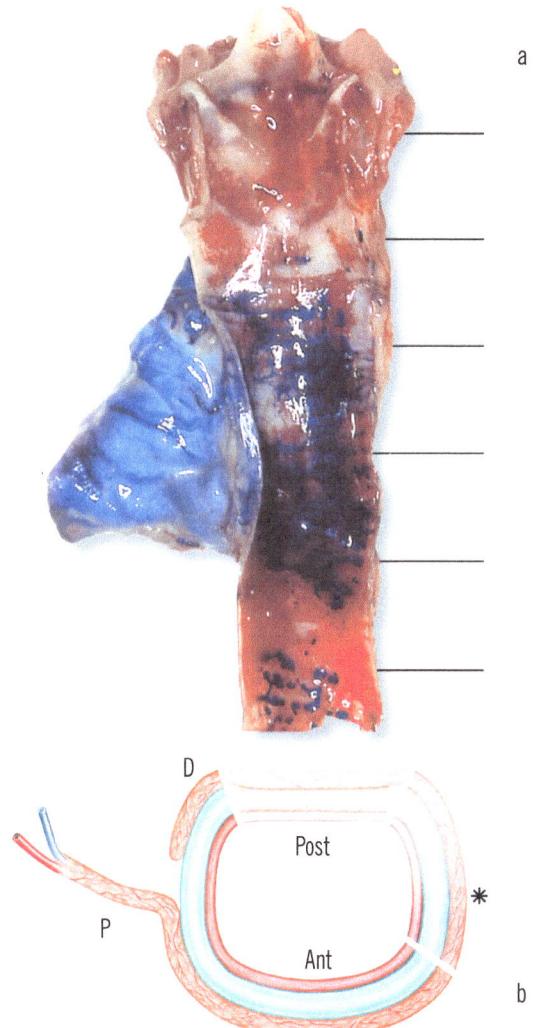

Figure 3.31.
Formation of autologous tracheal patch.
a. Revascularized tracheal patch. View on laryngotracheal complex after posterior longitudinal incision and after blue Microfil® injection of fascial flap. After 14 days of revascularization, the fascial enwrapped segment shows a reliable revascularization
b. Axial section of tracheal tube wrapped by fascia. A sufficient blood supply to the patch is guaranteed when the fascia flap wrapping the trachea is incised distally. It is important that the anterior tracheal wall is wrapped by the proximal end of the fascial flap in order to prevent interferention with the fascial blood supply of the tracheal patch after longitudinal incision. The cartilaginous portion can be shortened (asterisk) until the desired anterior-posterior patch length (matching the laryngeal defect) is obtained. Ant = anterior tracheal wall; Post = posterior trachea; P = proximal end of fascia flap; D = distal end of fascia flap.

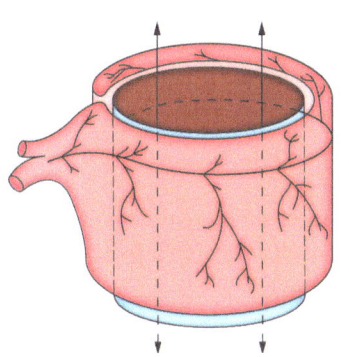

Figure 3.30.
Schematic presentation of formation of tracheal patch.
Frontal view on tracheal tube wrapped by fascia. A well vascularized tracheal patch is obtained after posterior longitudinal incision of a revascularized tracheal segment and after distal incision of the fascia flap. A full cartilaginous supported patch is obtained after removal of the membranous trachea (double arrows).

After revascularization, the fascial enwrapped segment was completely isolated from the airway, transformed into a patch, and then used to repair a laryngeal defect after hemicrico-hemilaryngectomy (Fig. 3.32, 3.33).

After suturing the patch into the laryngeal defect, the laryngotracheal continuity was repaired by an upwards tracheal mobilization and a reanastomosis between the trachea and the reconstructed caudal cricoid cartilage (Prolene 5.0, Ethicon).

As shown in Fig. 3.34, autotransplantation of revascularized patches allowed for reconstruction of extended hemilaryngectomy defects in rabbits. The patch vascularity, the respiratory mucosa, and the full cartilaginous patch support are responsible for the reliability of the technique.

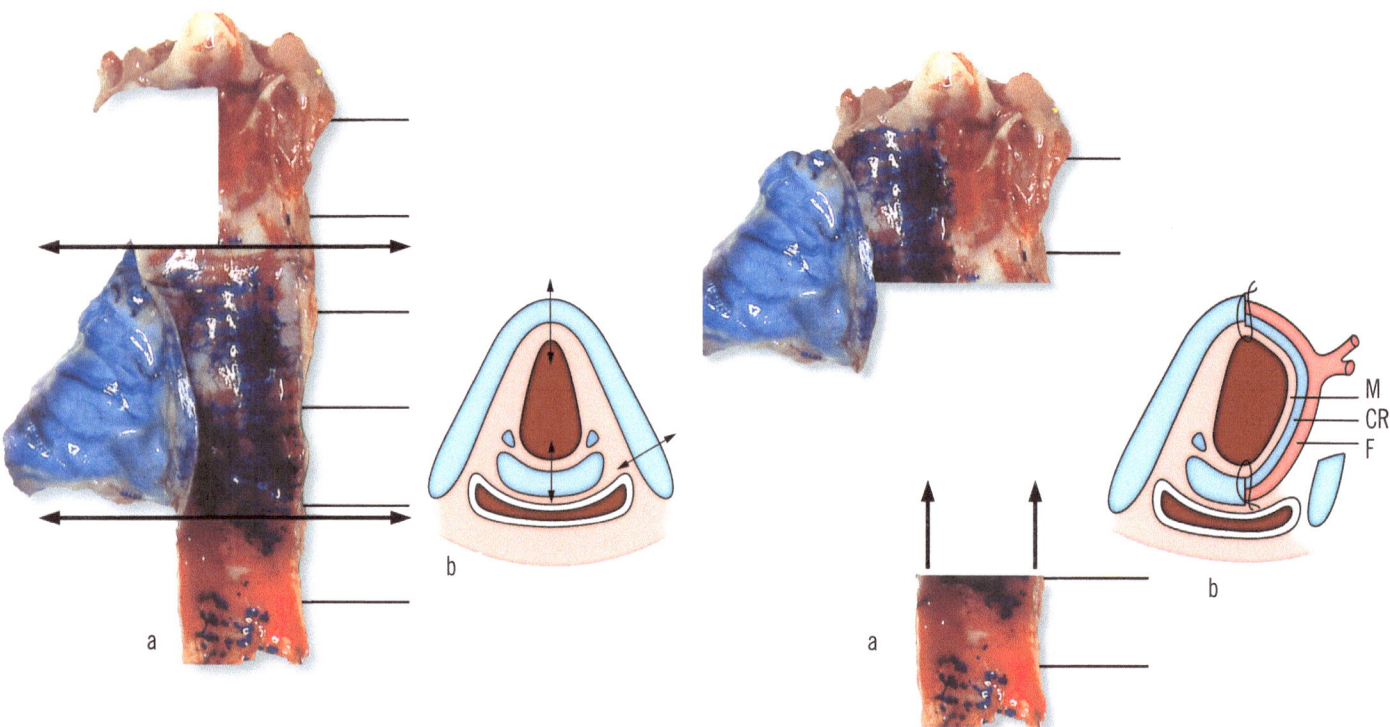

Figure 3.32.
Tracheal autotransplantation of laryngeal defect.
a. Revascularized tracheal patch. A hemilaryngectomy with inclusion of the cricoid cartilage is made after a 2 weeks revascularization period. The revascularized trachea is isolated on the fascial pedicle (double arrows).
b. Schematic presentation of tracheal autotransplantation. Resection includes left thyroid cartilage, left half of cricoid, and left arytenoid.

Figure 3.33.
Tracheal autotransplantation to laryngeal defect.
a. Revascularized tracheal patch. The patch is displaced to the laryngeal defect. The trachea is closed by end-to-end anastomosis (arrows).
b. Reconstruction with tracheal patch pedicled on the left thoracic fascial flap. The patch consists of 3 layers: mucosa (M), cartilage ring (CR), and fascia (F).

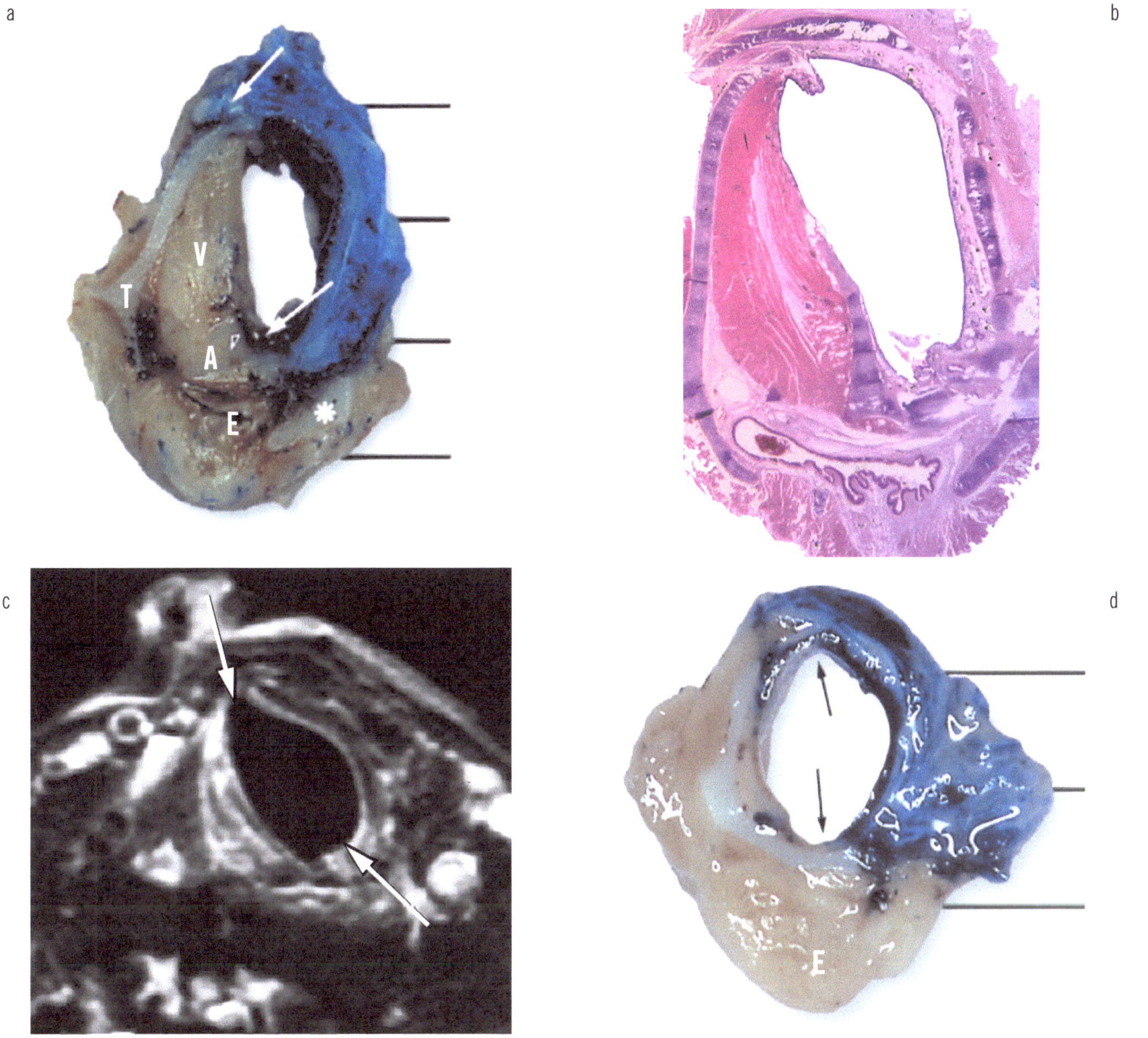

a

b

c

d

Figure 3.34. Morphology of tracheal autotransplantation to the larynx.

a. Postmortem cross-section of hemilaryngeal reconstruction at glottic level after silicone dye infusion of the vascular fascial pedicle. Tracheal patch, between two arrows, repairs the left laryngectomy defect, including left arytenoid and cricoid cartilage.

Posterior glottis is restored to ensure a competent glottic sphincter. A = right arytenoid ; V = right vocal cord; T = right thyroid lamina ; E = esophagus. Asterisk indicates remnant of left thyroid cartilage. Scale in cm.

b. Postmortem histology of hemilaryngeal reconstruction at glottic level (H.E. x 5).

c. Postreconstruction MRI of tracheal autotransplantation to the larynx. Gadolinium-enhanced axial T1 weighted image shows tracheal patch between 2 arrows.

d. Postmortem cross section of hemilaryngeal reconstruction at subglottic level after silicone dye infusion of the vascular fascial pedicle. The tracheal patch, between two arrows, is completely perfused by the fascial flap. Note the preservation of the near normal subglottic laryngeal lumen with no buckling or collapse at the reconstruction. E = esophagus. Scale in cm.

The concept of tracheal autotransplantation challenges the current statement that the cricoid cartilage needs preservation to allow for decannulation after laryngeal reconstruction. Although autotransplantation of tracheal patches may help in resolving the limits of larynx reconstruction, the question whether a one-stage procedure could be feasible still remains. Before introducing the concept of tracheal autotransplantation into the clinic as a means for extending the limits of conservation laryngeal surgery, we attempted to answer the question if a the two-stage approach is realy necessary in tracheal autotransplantation.

Two theoretical possibilities are possible when thinking about a 1-stage reconstruction with autologous trachea:

• Transplantation and revascularization with fascial wrapping of the transplanted patch in a 1-stage procedure.

• Advancing the upper segment of cervical trachea inside the larynx without complete isolation from the airway so that revascularization is not necessary.

7.B. Is 1-stage transplantation and revascularization a possibility?

To answer this question, patches with 4 different degrees of vascular supply were studied experimentally and it was shown that fascia enwrapped tracheal autografts showed reliable revascularization through the intercartilaginous ligaments only when a 2-stage revascularization technique was used.

Four different patch designs were used to reconstruct anterior tracheal defects (Fig. 3.35).

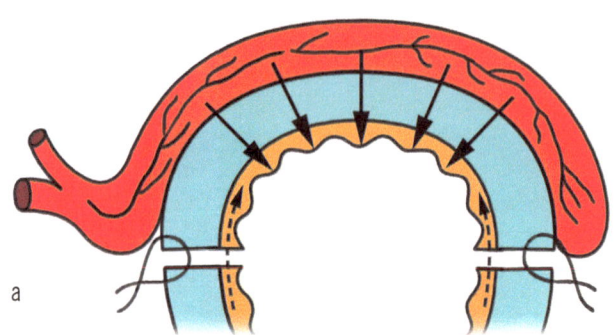

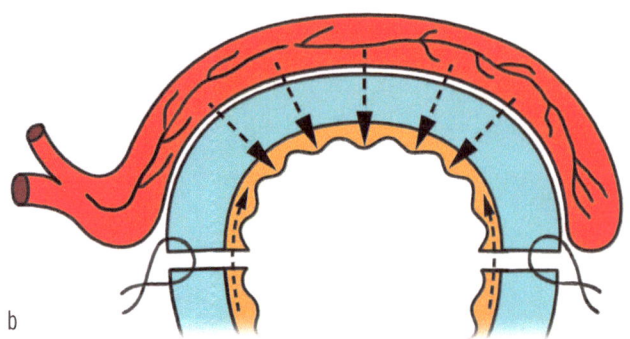

Figure 3.35.
Schematic presentation of different patch groups.
a. 2-stage revascularization (group A - Design 1). Patch vascularity originates from established vascular connections with the fascia flap (full arrows) and from the margins of the defect (dotted arrows).Two weeks elapsed between revascularization and transplantation.
b. 1-stage revascularization. (group B - Design 2) Patch vascularity originates from non-established vascular connections with the fascia flap (interrupted arrows) and from the margins of the defect (dotted arrows).

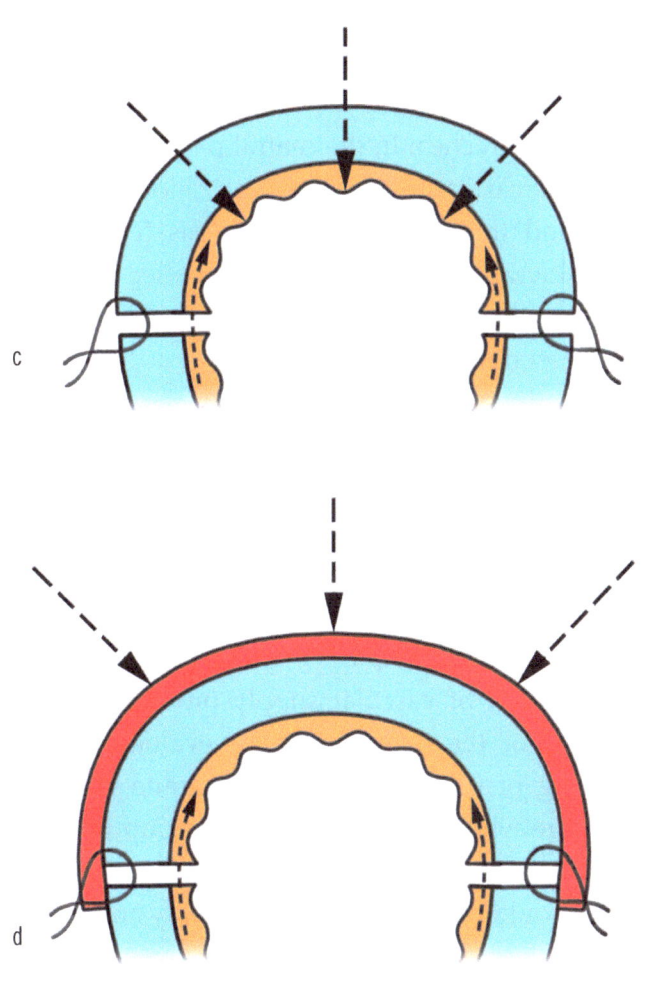

A segment of trachea (previously wrapped in vascularized fascia in group A) was excised and transformed into a patch. The trachea was closed by end-to-end reanastomosis and an anterior airway defect was created. The tracheal patch (previously wrapped in vascularized fascia in group A) was sutured into the airway defect. The lateral thoracic fascia was sutured over the tracheal patch in group B (1 operation stage) and a Gore-Tex® membrane was sutured over the tracheal patch in group D after suturing the tracheal patch into the defect. The tracheal patch remained uncovered in group C.

Patches were evaluated 2 weeks after repair of the anterior airway defect.

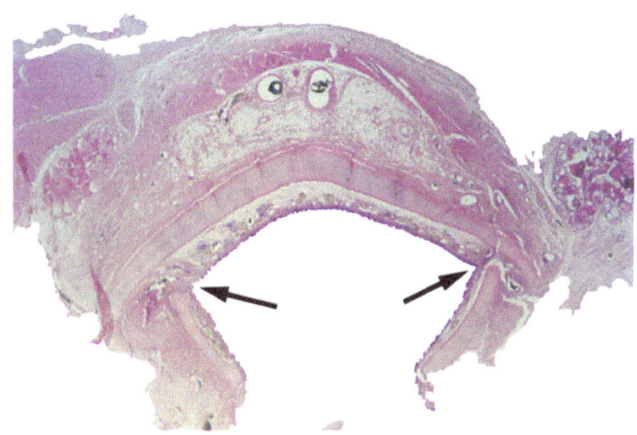

Figure 3.35 (continued).
Schematic presentation of different patch groups.
c. Free patch. (Group C - Design 3) Patch vascularity originates from non-established vascular connections with the surrounding neck tissues (interrupted arrows) and from the margins of the defect (dotted arrows).
d. Free patch covered with Gore-Tex®. (Group D - Design 4) Patch vascularity originates from the margins of the defect (dotted arrows).

Figure 3.36.
Histology of patch after 2-stage revascularization (group A) (H&E original x 10). Tracheal patch is located between arrows. The suture lines between patch and trachea are sharp without granulation tissue. Full viability of cartilaginous and mucosal component of the patch. The fascial and submucosal blood vessels are injected with blue silicone dye.

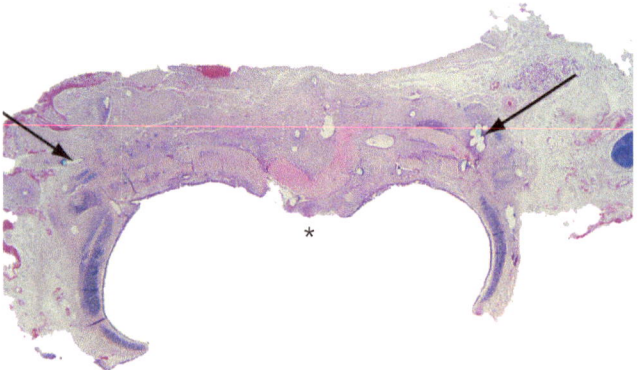

Figure 3.37.
Histology of 1-stage revascularization (Group B) and of free patch (Group C) (H&E original x 10). Tracheal patch is located between arrows, pointing to prolene sutures. The patch near both anastomoses is vital and lined with respiratory epithelium. The central part of the patch (asterisk) is ulcerated with disruption of the mucosal lining.

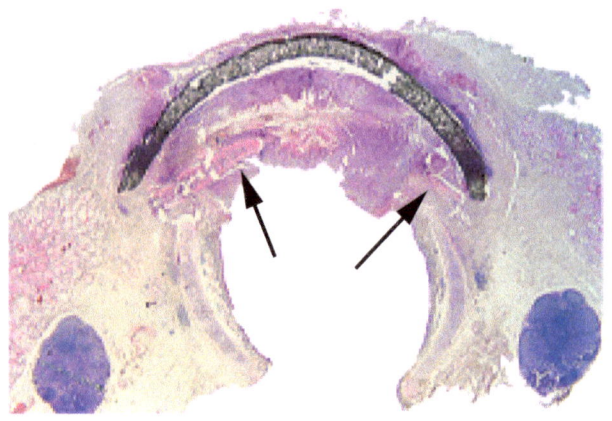

Figure 3.38.
Histology of free patch covered with Gore-tex® (Group D) (H&E original x 10). Full thickness necrosis of the tracheal patch with some cartilaginous remnants near the anastomoses (arrows). The Gore-tex sheet is visible on top of the tracheal patch.

From these experiments it became clear that optimal tracheal autograft revascularization is obtained by a 2-stage approach and by using a thin, pliable, and axially perfused fascial envelop (group A - Design 1) . The 2-stage technique guarantees a successful outcome of orthotopic transplanted tracheal patches (Fig. 3.36).

Survival of avascular tracheal patches is unpredictable in cases of 1-stage transplantation (group C) with partial or complete patch necrosis. Graft viability was preserved at the suture lines because of the synergistic effect of both the intercartilaginous revascularization and the revascularization from the intact trachea. In the central part of the graft, only intercartilaginous revascularization was possible and this area showed necrosis (Fig. 3.37). Fascial wrapping did not result in better revascularization of avascular tracheal grafts (group B). The reason can be found in the orthotopic revascularization position with the trachea moving with each respiration and swallowing act. The mobility between the completely avascular trachea and the fascia flap is responsible for the fact that no positive revascularization effect results after fascial wrapping in the orthotopic position (result group B = result group C).

The amount of vascular supply provided at the margins of the defect could be evaluated after blocking of the intercartilaginous route through coverage with a Gore-Tex® sheet (group D). The vascular supply provided at the margins of the defect could not maintain graft viability and resulted in full necrosis of the patch (Fig. 3.38).

Clinically, tracheal autografts are intended to be used for repair of extended hemilaryngectomy defects resulting after removal of advanced laryngeal cancer. The posterior larynx has an average height of about 4 cm so that a segment of trachea of 4 cm will be sufficient for laryngeal repair after extended hemilaryngectomy. It is extremely important to obtain revascularization results that approach a 100% success rate because a tracheal segment of 4 cm can be taken only once. With the staged revascularization technique, the intrinsic, mucosal blood supply prevents ischemic necrosis even in the case of failure of the fascial flap. In cases of failure of the fascial flap, a second vascular carrier can be applied without compromising the vitality of the dissected tracheal segment. During the second operation stage, the vascular risk for the isolated trachea will be low because the trachea can be transplanted to a regional airway defect without further manipulation of the vascular pedicle of the fascia flap.

The trachea has unique vascular characteristics making it the optimal tissue for staged revascularization and transplantation. The extrinsic and intrinsic blood supply can be disrupted separately which allows for progressive revascularization without periods of complete avascularity.

7.C. Is it possible to bring the trachea inside an extended laryngeal defect in a 1-stage advancement procedure?

Due to the proximity of the cervical trachea to the larynx, a possible 1-stage reconstruction after extended hemilaryngectomy may lay in a simple advancement of 4 cm of trachea with preservation of the tracheal continuity. To accomplish this upwards mobilization of the trachea, the trachea has to be mobilized from the surrounding tissues over about 8 cm which means that this segment will have its extrinsic blood supply interrupted. The vascularity will further diminish after removal of the upper 4 cm of membranous trachea (for patch formation) and interruption of the anterior wall for placement of a tracheostomy (extended hemilaryngectomy will be impossible in humans without placing of a tracheostomy) (Fig. 3.39). After these manoeuvres, it is difficult to imagine how the upper 4 cm of cervical trachea will survive inside the laryngeal defect. Even in non-irradiated cases, advancement of a tracheal patch would inevitably lead to patch necrosis.

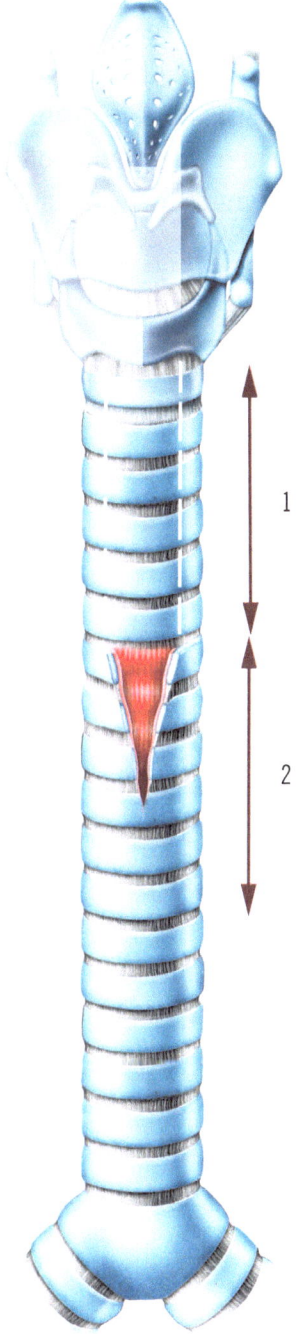

Figure 3.39.
Laryngotracheal complex.
Extended hemilaryngectomy defect reconstructed with advancement of 4 cm of cervical trachea. The upper 4 cm (double arrow-1) is mobilized and transferred into a patch by removal of the membranous trachea (dotted lines). Another segment of 4 cm (double arrow-2) has to be mobilized to allow for upper movement. A tracheostomy has to be placed.

For clinical use, we were convinced that only the technique of tracheal autotransplantation after a 2-stage revascularization and transplantation procedure could lead to successful outcome in repairing extended laryngeal defects (table 3.7).

Table 3.7. Key features of tracheal autotransplantation

-2 stages:
- Revascularization stage (14 days)
- Transplantation stage

-During revascularization stage:
- Extrinsic tracheal blood supply interrupted
- Intrinsic tracheal blood supply intact
- Progressive fascial revascularization

-During transplantation stage:
- Extrinsic tracheal blood supply interrupted
- Intrinsic tracheal blood supply interrupted
- Fascial blood supply intact

-Length of transplant = length that still allows for primary closure
- 1.5 cm in rabbits
- 4-5 cm in humans

8. Conclusion

Research on tracheal transplantation was started with the aim of resolving the limits in treating laryngotracheal stenosis. The vascularity of tracheal allotransplants could be restored in the experimental setting but it remains a question whether human tracheal allografts would revascularize in a similar way. The human tracheal wall is much thicker and revascularization of avascular allografts could be more difficult than in rabbits. Moreover, immunosuppressive therapy is necessary to preserve the full viability of a revascularized tracheal allotransplant because repopulation of the allotransplant occurred over only a short distance at the anastomotic regions. Therefore, tracheal allografts will not be able to improve laryngotracheal reconstruction for difficult to treat stenoses.

The excellent reconstructive results obtained with patches of tracheal allografts led to the idea of using tracheal autografts in repairing laryngeal defects. A tracheal autograft may become revascularized in an orthotopical position without going to a period of complete avascularity. It can be stated that human tracheas will undergo revascularization in a similar way after being wrapped with vascularized fascia. There is no risk for necrosis because the tracheal continuity and the intrinsic blood supply are preserved during the revascularization period.

After experimental documentation of the feasibility of tracheal autotransplantation, the use of tracheal autografts in the repair of extended hemilaryngectomy defects was explored in depth (Fig. 3.40).

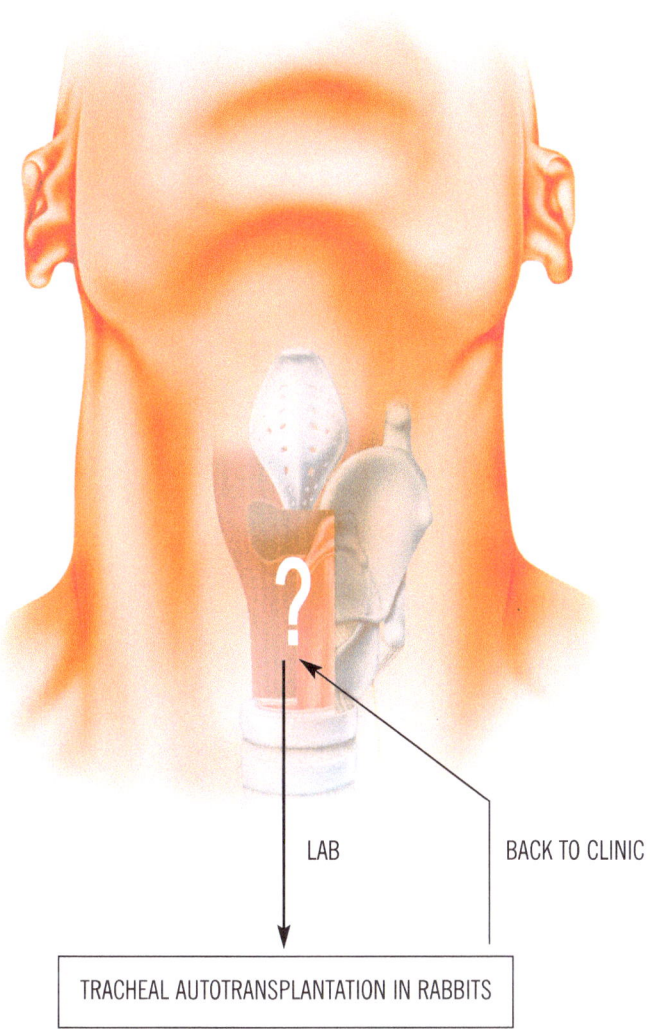

Figure 3.40.
From the bedside to the lab and back again.
The clinical problem (reconstruction of extended hemi-laryngectomy defects) was taken to the laboratory, where the feasibility of tracheal autotransplantation was demonstrated. The results were brought back to the patient in 1997.

LAB

BACK TO CLINIC

TRACHEAL AUTOTRANSPLANTATION IN RABBITS

BIBLIOGRAPHY

Balderman SC, Weinblatt G. Tracheal autograft revascularization. J Thorac Cardiovasc Surg 1987;94:434-41.

Borro JM, Chirivella M, Vila C, et al. Successful revascularization of large isolated tracheal segments. Eur J Cardiothorac Surg 1992;6:621-3.

Gannon P, Costantino P, Lueg EA, et al. Use of the peritracheal fold in the dog tracheal transplantation model. Arch Otolaryngol Head Neck Surg 1999;125:959-63

Genden E, Gannon P, Smith S, Deftereos M, Urken M. Microvascular transplantation of tracheal allografts in the canine model. Ann Otol Rhinol Laryngol 2003;112:307-13.

Getty R. Anatomy of the neck. In: Grossman SA, ed. Anatomy of domestic animals. Philadelphia, Pe:WB Saunders, 1975:416-620.

Khalil-Marzouk JF. Allograft replacement of the trachea. Experimental synchronous revascularization of composite thyrotracheal transplant. J Thorac Cardiovasc Surg 1993;105:242-6.

Macchiarini P, Lenot B, De Montpreville V, et al. Heterotopic pig model for direct revascularization and venous drainage of tracheal allografts. J Thorac Cardiovasc Surg 1994;108:1066-75.

Macchiarini P, Mazmanian GM, de Montpréville V, et al. Experimental tracheal and tracheoesophageal allotransplantation. J Thorac Cardiovasc Surg 1995;110:1037-46.

Nakanishi R, Shirakusa T, Mitsudomi T. Maximum length of tracheal autografts in dogs. J Thorac Cardiovasc Surg 1992;106:1081-7.

Olech VM, Keshavjee H, Chamberlain W, et al. Role of basic fibroblast growth factor in revascularization of rabbit autografts. Ann Thorac Surg 1991;52:258-64.

Salassa IR, Pearson BW, Payne WS. Gross and microscopical blood supply of the trachea. Ann Thorac Surg 1977;24:100-7.

Urken M. Advances in head and neck reconstruction. Laryngoscope 2003;113:1473-6.

Zur K, Urken M. Vascularized hemitracheal autograft for laryngotracheal reconstruction: a new surgical technique based on the thyroid gland as a vascular carrier. Laryngoscope 2003;113:1494-8.

CHAPTER 4

From Bench to Bedside:

Implementing tracheal autotransplantation as organ saving procedure after extended hemilaryngectomy

1. Introduction

It is generally accepted that tumors with vocal fold fixation are unsuitable for conservation surgery because the lower resection margin of a partial laryngectomy is confined to the upper part of the cricoid cartilage. Preservation of the cricoid is essential to allow for postoperative decannulation, whereas a rational ablation of a T2 (extending subglottically) and T3 glottic cancer necessitates the resection of the paraglottic space and its contiguous structures, including the thyroid and cricoid cartilages. Currently, the surgical treatment of advanced, unilateral glottic cancer consists of a total or a near-total laryngectomy, with a resulting permanent tracheostomy. Advanced, unilateral glottic cancers may fall within the scope of partial laryngectomy, if a laryngeal remnant consisting of one thyroid ala with the corresponding true vocal cord and one half of the cricoid, with one mobile arytenoid, can be reconstructed. The desired repair tissue for this difficult defect may be found inside the trachea. The amount of autologous tracheal tissue available for laryngeal reconstruction is similar to the amount of trachea that can be resected with tracheal reanastomosis of the created defect. Tracheal resection in cases of stenosis has shown that segments of up to 5 cm may be resected. A tracheal length of 4 cm should be sufficient for repair of hemicrico-hemilaryngectomy defects since the average height of the larynx (from caudal border of cricoid to apex of arytenoid) is about 4 cm. The mean height of the posterior cricoid cartilage has been reported as measuring 21.0 mm-SD=1.6 in females and 23.3 mm-SD=1.6 in males (RANDESTAD et al. 2000) (Fig. 4.1, 4.2)

The tracheal cartilage with its respiratory mucosal lining forms the optimal composition for use inside the larynx and experimental research on

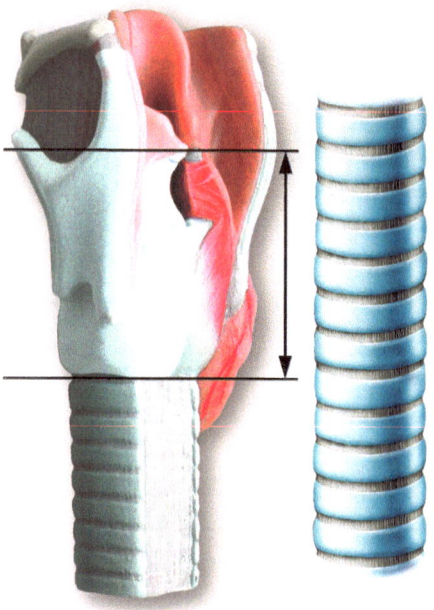

Figure 4.1.
Outlining of hemicrico-hemilaryngectomy defect. The average height of the larynx in male patients is about 4 cm (double arrow). A segment of trachea of 4 cm can be used to repair the hemicrico-hemilaryngectomy defect.

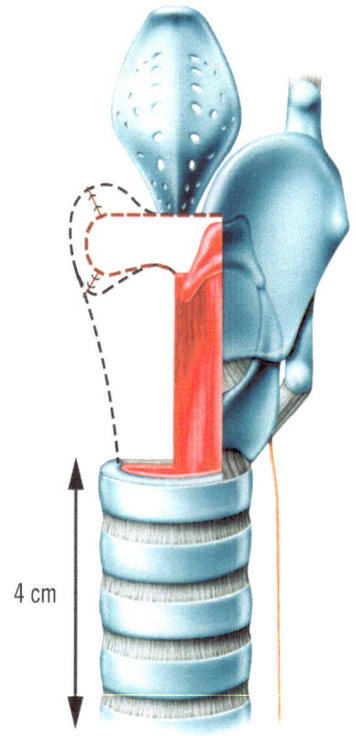

Figure 4.2.
Defect after hemicrico-hemilaryngectomy.
The upper 4 cm of trachea will be used to reconstruct the laryngeal defect.

tracheal transplantation showed that the tracheal tissue components can be revascularized after being wrapped in vascularized fascia. The trachea consists of a hollow tube and this is not the optimal configuration for use inside a laryngeal defect. The optimal reconstructive configuration is visible in figure 4.3.

The optimal position of the reconstructive tissue is different at the glottic and subglottic regions. A convex-shaped reconstruction at the subglotic level (for restoration of the airway lumen) in combination with a reconstruction approaching the midline at the glottic level (for speech and swallowing rehabilitation) may provide for an optimal situation. A straight midline position of the reconstructive tissue would be too close to stenosis while the convex-shaped reconstruction would lead to glottic insufficiency.

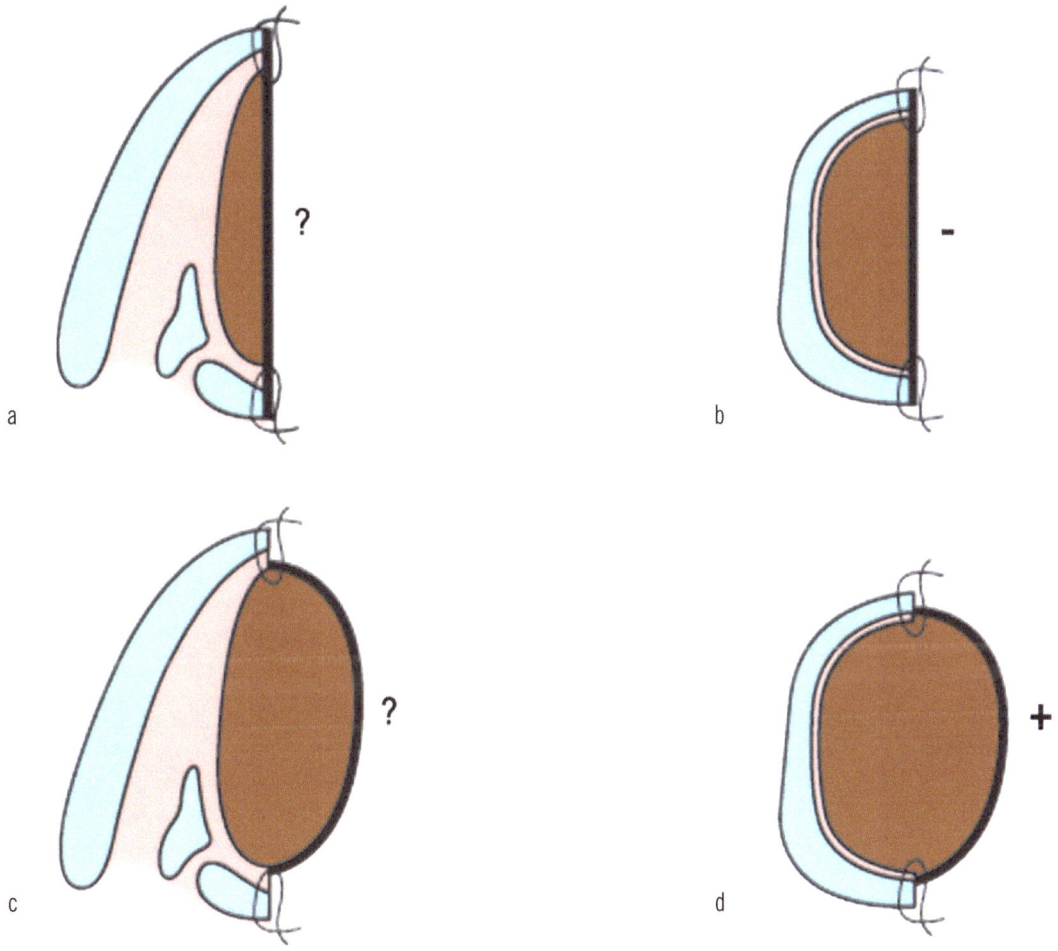

Figure 4.3. Position of reconstructive tissue in hemicrico-hemilaryngectomy defect.

Postreconstructive situation at glottic (a, c) and subglottic (b,d) level. At the glottic level, a midline position of the reconstruction (a) would provide for excellent sphincteric function during speech and swallowing. This position may however predispose to laryngeal stenosis. The midline position at the subglottic level (b) would lead to laryngeal substenosis.

At the subglottic level, restoration of the laryngeal lumen (d) would provide for an excellent airway. The convex-shaped reconstruction at the glottic level would lead to glottic insufficiency (c).

At the glottic level, the optimal position of the reconstructive tissue is situated between the position seen in 3.a and the position seen in 3.c.

For optimal repair at the glottic level, a situation comparable to the situation of a unilateral vocal fold paralysis in a paramedial position (between straight and convex-shaped) should be obtained after reconstruction (Fig. 4.4).

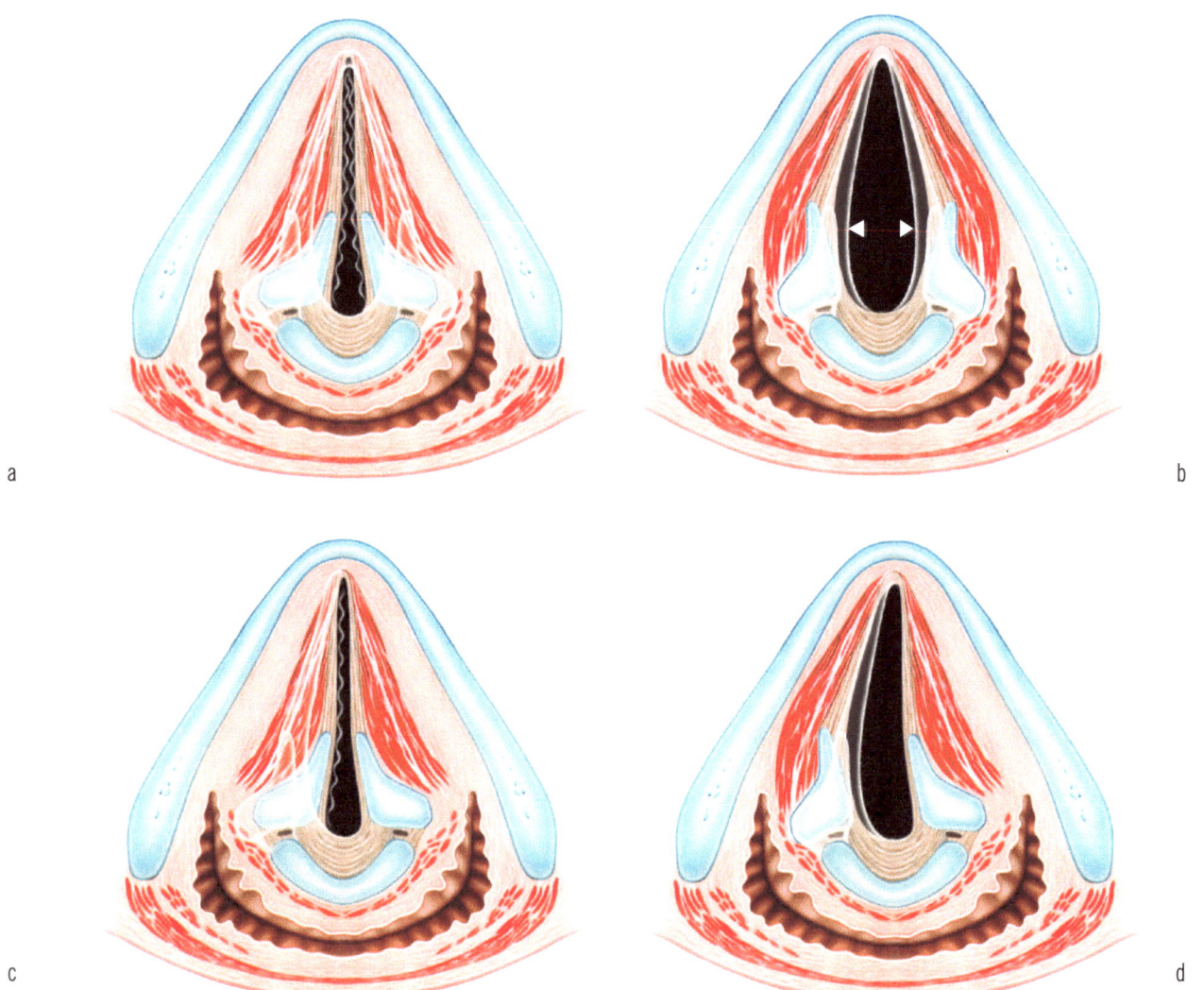

Figure 4.4. Search for an optimal reconstructive configuration.

a. Axial section during phonation. During phonation pulmonary air power supplied to adducted vocal folds is transduced into acoustic power as the vocal fold vibrates passively. This vibration is enabled through an ingenious layer structure of the two vocal folds.

b. Axial section during deep inspiration. Vocal folds are in lateral position. Intermediate position is the vocal fold position during quiet breathing (arrowheads).

c. Axial section during phonation with paralysis of left vocal fold in paramedial position. A near normal voice production remains possible.

d. Axial section during deep inspiration with paralysis of left vocal fold in paramedial position. A sufficient airway lumen is preserved.

A vocal fold paralysis in the paramedial position guarantees a preservation of the sphincteric function during speech and swallowing with a sufficient airway during respiration.

The tracheal tube has to be transformed into a patch in order to obtain the optimal configuration for larynx reconstruction. The concavity of the tracheal patch forms the optimal configuration for reconstruction at the subglottic level but the tracheal patch concavity is not the desired configuration for reconstruction at the glottic level. At the glottic level, it will be necessary to unfold the patch so that it can be placed in a position close to the midline (Fig. 4.5).

An optimal configuration of the reconstructive tissue within the laryngeal defect may lead to a successful reconstruction if the reconstructive tissue maintains its vitality within the defect.

Experimental studies showed the reliability of vascular induction of the trachea by wrapping the trachea in vascularized fascia. A patch of trachea can be brought into the larynx with intact blood supply by using a 2-stage reconstruction procedure. The reason for the 2-stage reconstruction is the necessity for a revascularization period of a least 14 days.

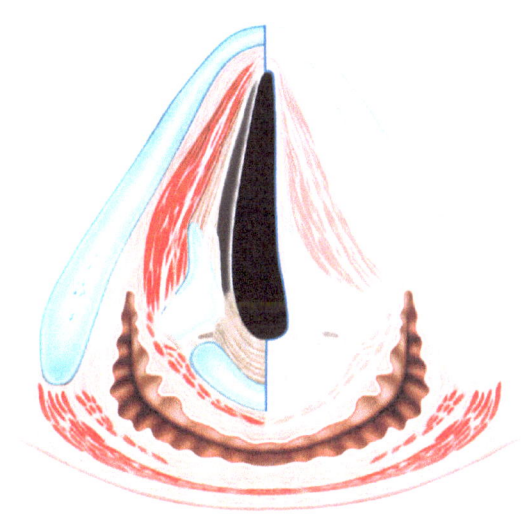

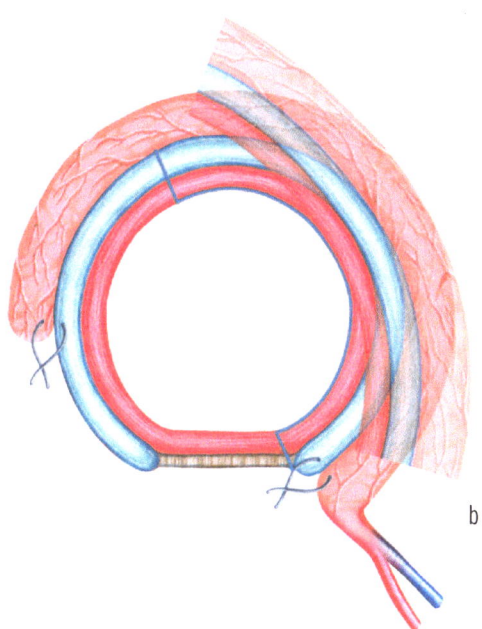

a

b

Figure 4.5. Optimal reconstructive configuration. Glottic level with indication of optimal reconstruction in paramedial position (a)+Axial section trachea (b). A segment of the cartilaginous trachea can be used to reconstruct the larynx in a paramedial position at the glottic level. The cartilaginous trachea has to be unfolded to obtain the desired reconstructive configuration.

2. Initial concept of tracheal autotransplantation

The initial design of the surgical procedure consists of 2 interventions with 2 weeks elapsing between the first and second procedure. Neck dissection and wrapping of the trachea with vascularized fascia is done in the first operation while resection of the primary tumor and tracheal autotransplantation occurs in the second operation (Table 4.1).

This initial design was based on the following 3 assumptions:

1/ The need for a 2 weeks revascularization period.

2/ The impossibility to place a tracheotomy during tracheal revascularization because the upper 4 cm of cervical trachea is used for reconstruction.

3/ The consideration that reconstruction of all laryngeal functions after extended hemilaryngectomy is only possible with revascularized tracheal autografts.

The initial patient series treated with tracheal autotransplantation is based on the clinical records of 40 patients undergoing primary or salvage hemilaryngectomy for laryngeal (36) and pyriform sinus (4) cancer (Table 4.2). Thirty six patients (33 men, 3 women), ranging in age from 28 to 79 years, were diagnosed as having cancer of the larynx. Four male patients displayed a tumor of the pyriform sinus with extension into the apex. All of the primary laryngeal tumors were staged T2 or T3 and the pyriform sinus tumors were staged T2. All tumors were carcinomas with exception of 1 chondrosarcoma of a cricoid and 1 synovial sarcoma of the hypopharynx. Twenty-three patients in this series had received preoperative radiotherapy. Six patients received postoperative radiotherapy. The patients were treated during a 4 year period (1997-2001). Forty patients underwent tracheal revascularization but only 38 underwent tracheal autotransplantation. Two patients underwent a total laryngectomy during the second operation stage because the tumor was larger than expected and hence not suitable for an extended hemilaryngectomy.

Table 4.2. Patient series tracheal autotransplantation-Initial concept

- 40 patients tracheal revascularization
- 38 patients tracheal autotransplantation
    - 32 T2-3N0 glottis-subglottis
        23 radiation failures
        6 not irradiated
        3 postoperative radiotherapy
    - 4 T2-N0-2b pyriform sinus
        1 not irradiated
        3 postoperative radiotherapy
    - 2 T3N0 transglottis
        2 not irradiated

Table 4.1. Initial concept for tracheal autotransplantation

Stage 1:	- Neck dissection
	- Tracheal revascularization
Stage 2:	
After 14 days	- Resection of primary tumor
	- Tracheal autotransplantation
	- Tracheostomy
Closure of tracheostomy 5-6 weeks after autotransplantation	

2.A. Overview of the procedure

Tracheal autotransplantation after extended hemi-laryngectomy will have a serious impact on the swallowing function. A gastrostomy tube is placed at the beginning of the first operation to avoid the potential negative influence of a nasogastric tube on the swallowing recovery of the reconstructed larynx (Fig. 4.6).

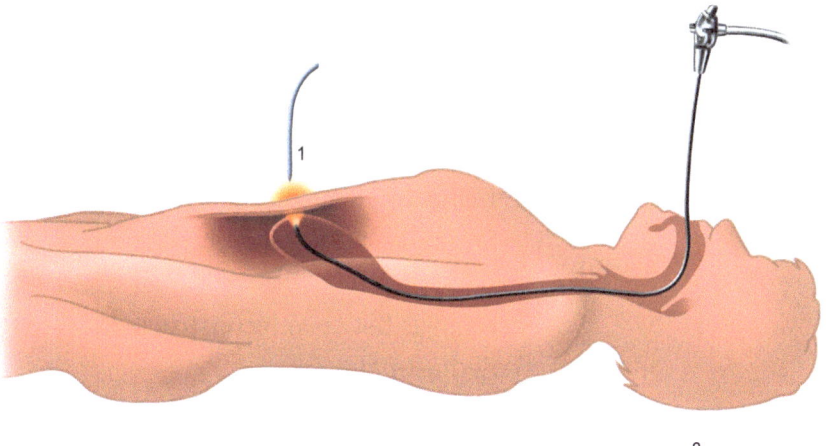

a

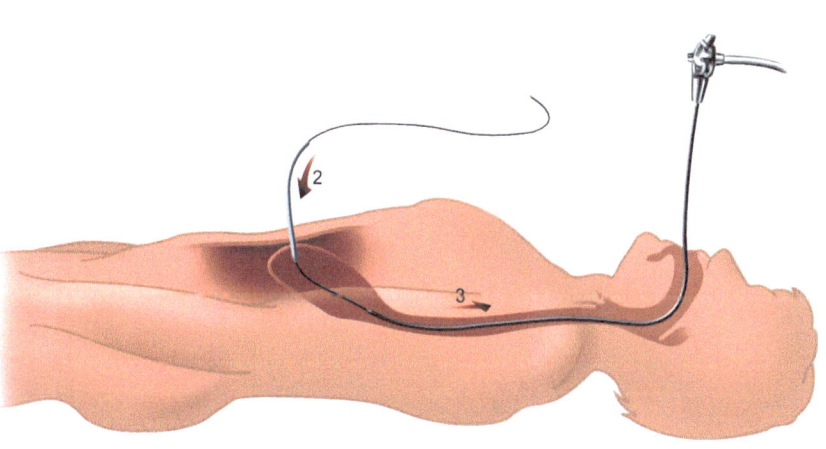

b

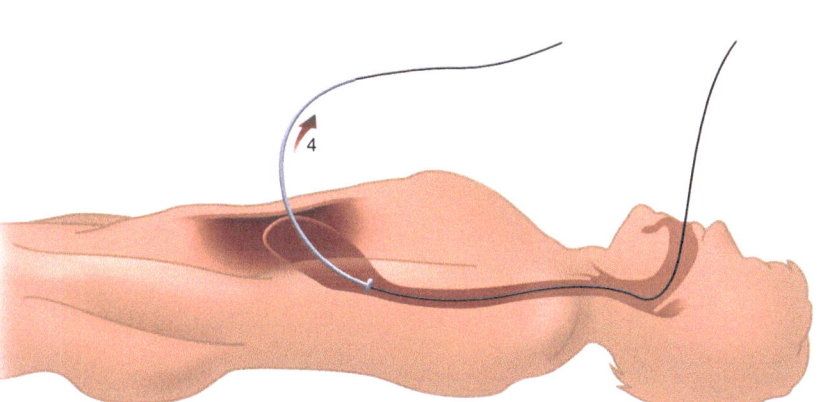

c

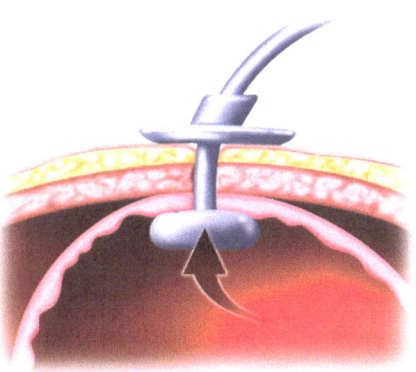

d

Figure 4.6.
Percutaneous endoscopic gastrostomy tube placement.
a. The scope is introduced and the abdominal wall is transilluminated by the scope for positioning of the percut-aneous needle (1).
b. The needle is inserted percutane-ously into the stomach (2). A guide-wire is passed through the needle and pulled out the mouth with the endo-scope (3).
c. The gastrostomy tube is pulled over the guidewire (inside to outside) (4).
d. Gastric tube in place.

The radial forearm fascia flap was chosen for tracheal revascularization. The radial donor site provides for a fascia flap with a large surface area (5 x 20 cm can easiliy be taken) and with a long and reliable vascular pedicle (radial artery and vein). The following operative steps are necessary in a first operation stage:

- Neck dissection.
- Thyroidectomy on tumor-bearing side.
- Identification of recurrent nerves.
- Circumferential mobilization of upper 4 cm of cervical trachea.
- Dissection of radial forearm fascia.
- Wrapping of forearm fascia around upper 4 cm of trachea.
- Closure of the neck and the forearm donor site.

Similar as in the experimental setting, circumferential wrapping with vascularized fascia was done because of the belief that circumferential wrapping guarantees the most complete revascularization. The cervical trachea was allowed to revascularize during a 14 days period.

After revascularization, the following steps were made in a second operation stage:

- Extended hemilaryngectomy.
- Isolation of revascularized cervical trachea. and tracheal patch formation.
- Insertion of tracheal patch into laryngeal defect.
- Anastomosis between reconstructed larynx and mediastinal trachea.
- Formation of tracheostome.
- Closure of the neck (Fig. 4.7., Fig. 4.8).

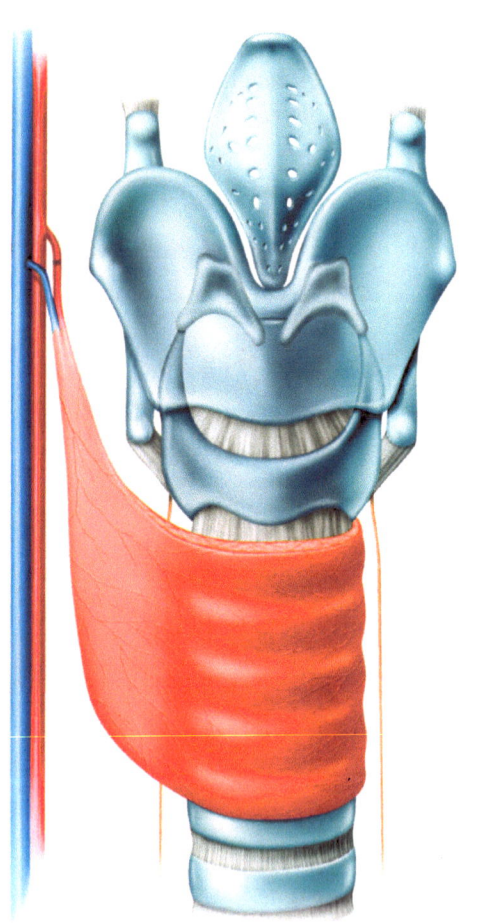

Figure 4.7.
Surgical steps tracheal autotransplantation initial concept - first operation.
The cervical trachea is wrapped by the radial fascial flap. The vascular pedicle of the flap is reanastomosed to the neck vessels at the same side as the laryngeal tumor. Usually, the superior thyroid artery (end-to-end) and the internal jugular vein (end-to-side) are used.

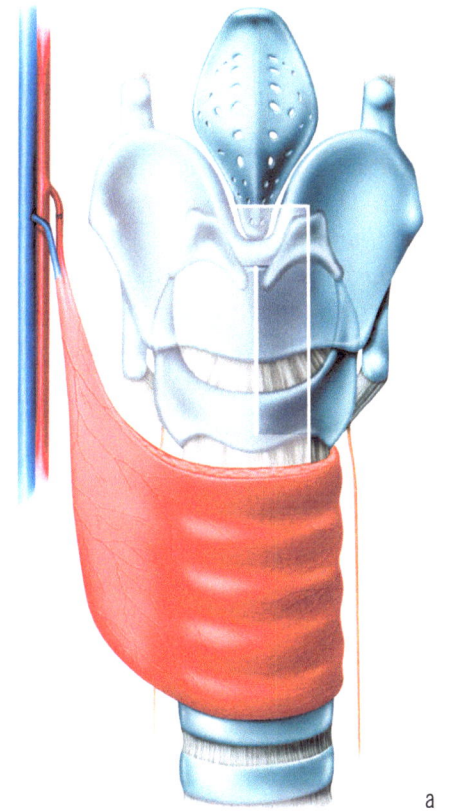

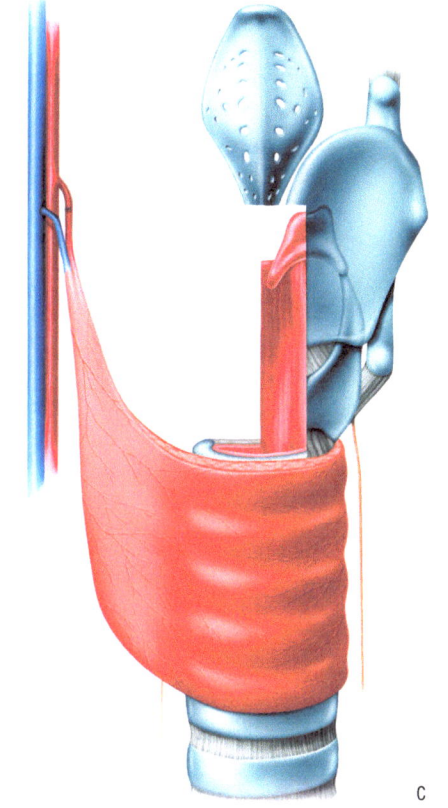

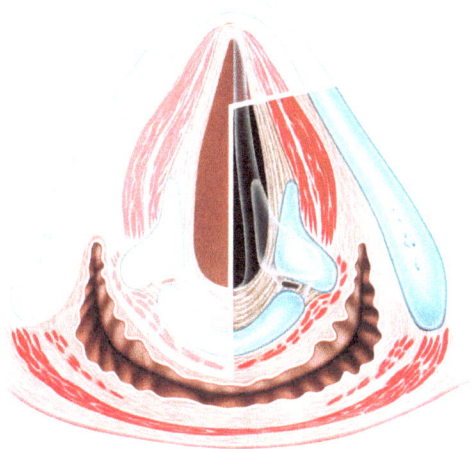

Figure. 4.8.
Surgical steps tracheal autotransplantation initial concept - second operation.
a. Outlining of resection-frontal view. Resection of unilateral glottic cancer reaching the anterior commissure. The cricoid is incised in the midline posteriorly. Anteriorly, the thyroid and cricoid cartilages are incised with inclusion of the anterior commissure (b).
c. Frontal view after resection. The remaining larynx consists of one functional arytenoid with a remnant of vocal fold.

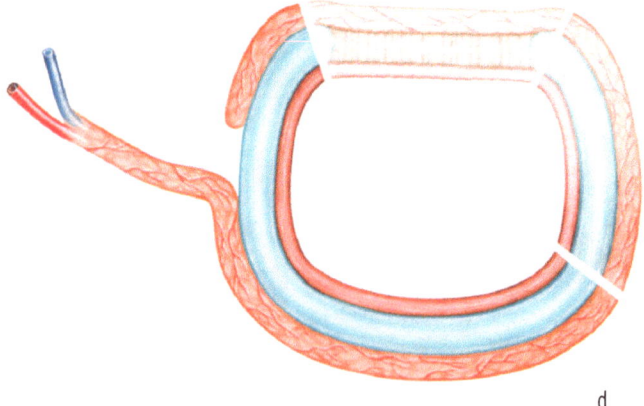

d

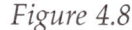

Figure 4.8.
Surgical steps tracheal autotransplantation initial concept - second operation (continued).
d. The revascularized trachea is completely mobilized on the fascial flap. The membranous trachea and a part of the cartilaginous trachea are removed.
e. The tracheal patch is displaced upwards and sutured into the defect. The vascular anastomosis of the fascia flap (superior thyroid artery end-to-end to radial artery and radial vein end-to-side to internal jugular vein) allows for upper movement of the tracheal patch without further manipulation of the vascular pedicle. The mediastinal trachea is sutured to the reconstructed larynx.
f. Schematic presentation of cross-section at the level of the vocal folds after transplantation. Optimal paramedial patch placement with the transplant serving as a buttress of apposition for the remaining mobile arytenoid and vocal fold remnant.

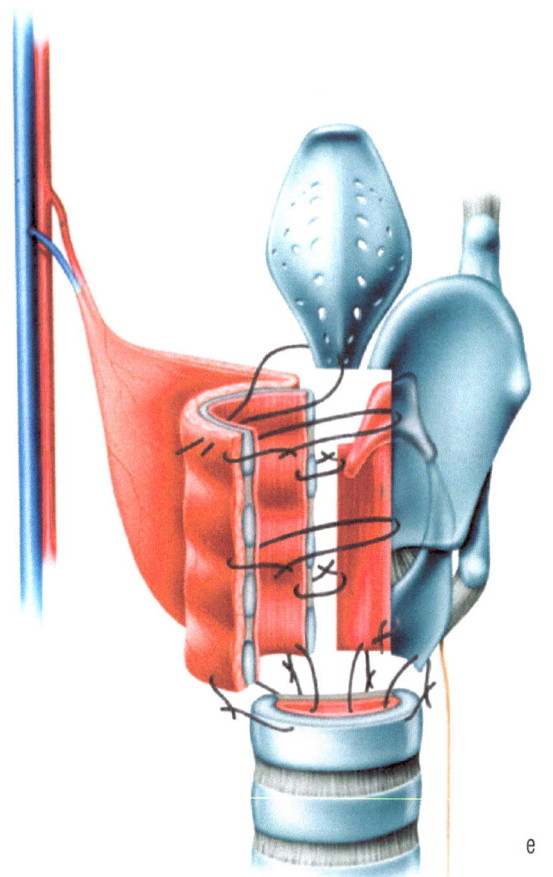

e

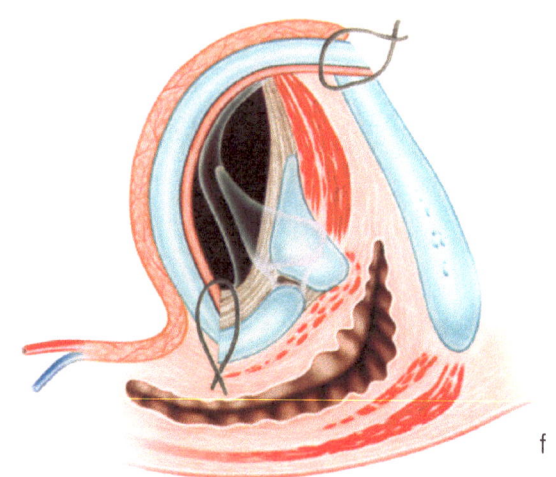

f

2.B. First operation

2.B.1. Neck dissection

A standard apron incision is placed at the level of the second tracheal ring (Fig. 4.9). The superiorly based subplatysmal flap is elevated to approximately 2 cm superior to the hyoid bone. The operation is started with a neck dissection. The extension of the neck dissection depends on the extent and location of the primary tumor. An ipsilateral neck dissection of levels 2 to 5 is performed for tumors of the pyriform sinus, transglottic tumors, and N+ necks. A contralateral neck dissection (levels 2 to 4 for N0) is performed for transglottic tumors with supraglottic extension over the midline. An ipsilateral neck dissection of levels 2 to 4 is performed for a T3N0 glottic cancer. It is important to preserve the internal jugular vein in all cases to allow for venous drainage of the fascia flap at the tumor-bearing side. After performing the appropriate neck dissection, the thyroid gland and the tracheoesophageal lymph nodes at the tumor bearing side are removed. The isthmus of the thyroid gland is divided in the midline. The cervical trachea is mobilized over a length of 4 cm with creation of a plane between trachea and esophagus after identification of the recurrent laryngeal nerves and after thyroid lobectomy and clearance of the tracheoesophageal lymph nodes at the tumor-bearing side.

The recurrent nerve at the non-tumor-bearing side will be responsible for the function of the neolarynx so that its preservation is of upmost importance. The recurrent nerve at the tumor-bearing side will be sacrificed during the resection phase. It is usually preserved during the first operation to avoid problems with aspiration or impaired respiration during the 2 weeks revascularization period.

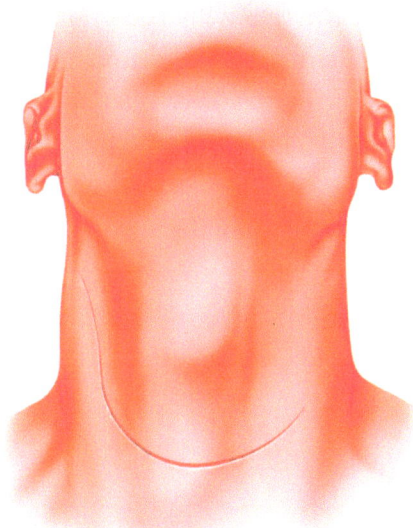

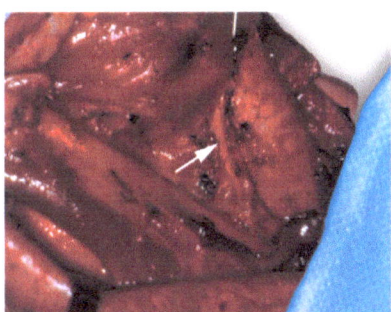

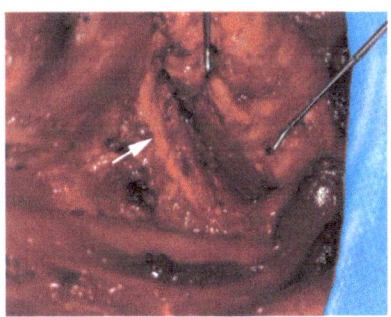

Figure 4.9.
Neck dissection and dissection of cervical trachea.
a. Outlining of skin incision. The apron incison is extended towards the mastoid at the side of neck dissection.
b. The recurrent nerve (arrow) at the tumor-bearing side is preserved.
c. The upper 4 cm of cervical trachea is dissected from the esophagus to allow for circumferential wrapping by the fascia flap. Arrow points to recurrent nerve.

2.B.2. Wrapping of cervical trachea

A radial forearm flap with a de-epithelialized paddle of 4 x 12 cm is dissected under tourniquet on the radial vascular pedicle. The flap dissection can be done simultaneously with the neck dissection if a 2-team approach is used. Since the flap will be buried, a proximal monitoring skin paddle is har-

vested for placement in the cutaneous suture line of the neck to assess the vascular supply during the postoperative period. The donor defect of the fascia flap is closed primarily. A small, full-thickness skin graft is applied on the defect created by the monitoring flap (Fig. 4.10).

a

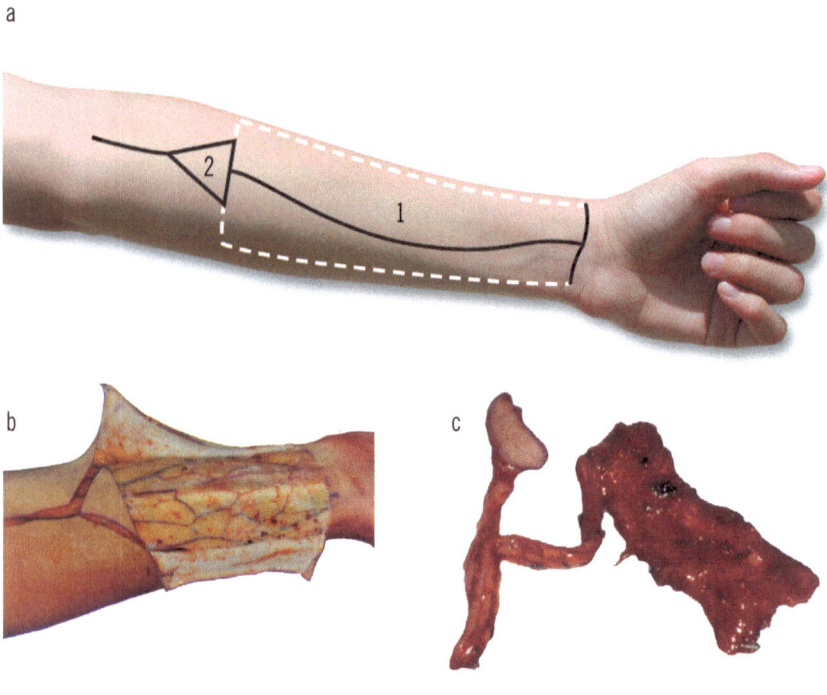

b

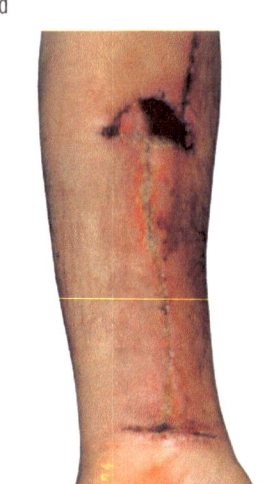

c

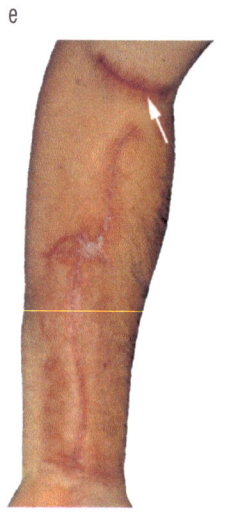

d

e

Figure 4.10.
Radial forearm fascia flap.
a. Outlining of fascia flap. The distal skin is incised in the midline. Both skin flaps are raised in a subdermal plane and are left attached laterally. A paddle consisting of fascia and subcutaneous tissue (4 by 12 cm) is taken with inclusion of a small cutaneous portion proximal from the facial flap. 1=paddle of fascia for tracheal wrapping (dotted line), 2=monitoring skin paddle. The skin incisions are marked with a full line.
b. Situation after skin incision and elevation of skin flaps from underlying fascia flap.
c. A radial forearm flap with a desepithelialized paddle of 4 by 12 cm is dissected on the radial vascular pedicle. A small skin paddle is included to serve as a monitor. The tracheal wall will be wrapped by the upper (skin) site of the fascia flap.
d. A tension free closure of the donor site is important. Therefore, a full-thickness skin graft (donor place indicated by arrow in Fig. 4.10.e) is included in the closure (sutured onto the defect created by the monitor flap) to diminish traction when closing the distal skin flaps. The full-thickness skin graft and the longitudinal skin incision may show some small wound healing problems.
e. Situation after healing of the donor site. Arrow points to the place where the skin graft was taken.

The forearm fascial flap is wrapped around the 4 cm segment of cervical trachea. The upper surface of the fascia (skin site) is lying against the tracheal wall. The anterior part of the trachea is wrapped by the proximal site of the de-epithelialized forearm flap, whereas the membranous trachea is wrapped by the distal site of the fascial flap.

A Gore-Tex sheet (Gore-Tex patch 0.1 mm, W.L. Gore and Associates, Inc. Flagstaff, AZ) is applied over the fascia flap that wraps the trachea. The Gore-Tex membrane will prevent adhesions between flap and surrounding tissue and will facilitate dissection after the revascularization period. A second sheet of Gore-Tex is placed between fascia and neck vessels. The fascial flap is revascularized by reanastomosis of the radial artery to the superior thyroid artery (end-to-end) and the radial vein to the internal jugular vein (end-to-side) at the same site as the laryngeal tumor. Ipsilateral revascularization is necessary to allow for transfer of the trachea to the larynx without further manipulation of the vascular pedicle during the second operation. The small proximal skin island is inserted in the neck incision, providing a monitor for the buried fascial flap (Fig. 4.11). A CT scan of the fascial enwrapped trachea is visible in Fig. 4.12.

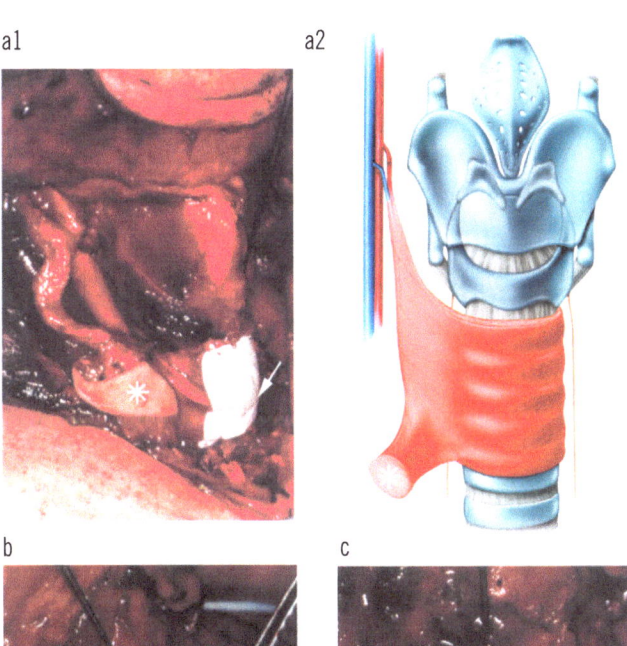

Figure 4.11.
Tracheal revascularization.
a. Fascial wrapping-Overview neck (a1) and schematic presentation (a2). The monitor skin paddle is indicated with an asterisk. The radial artery and vein are reanastomosed to the neck vessels at the level of the thyroid cartilage at the tumor-bearing side. The cervical trachea is circumferentially wrapped by the fascia flap. The upper side of the fascia is lying against the tracheal wall while the undersurface of the flap is covered with the Gore-Tex membrane (arrow).
b. The trachea is wrapped by fascia and the monitoring skin paddle (asterisk) is attached to the lower neck skin flap. A second Gore-Tex sheet (arrowhead) is placed between internal jugular vein and fascia flap.
c. Fascial wrapping-Detail. The fascia is wrapped around the trachea in a counterclock wise direction (dotted arrow) for a tumor situated on the right side. The fascia flap wraps a segment of 4 cm. The prolene suture (full arrow) caudal from the enwrapped trachea serves as an orientation point during the second operation. The second Gore-Tex sheet between fascia and neck vessels (arrowhead) will facilitate the upwards mobilization of the revascularized trachea during the second operation.

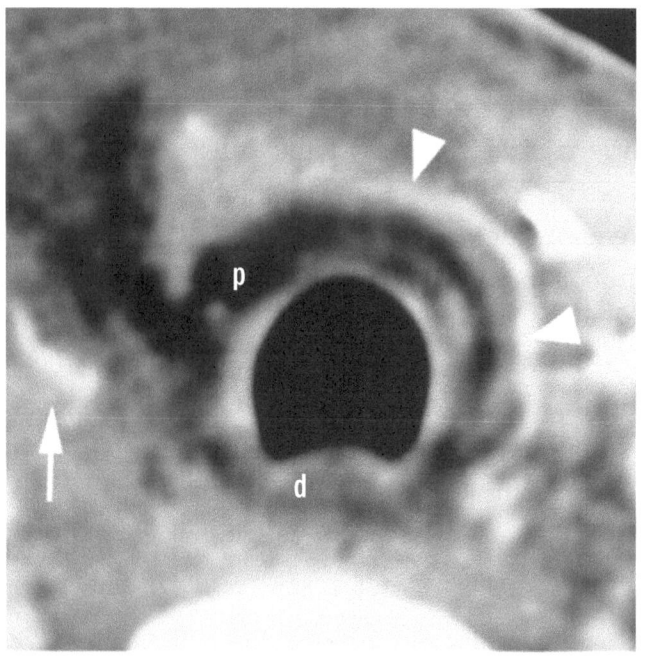

Figure 3.12.
CT scan of cervical trachea between the first and second operation.
The fascia flap is visible as a radiolucent band around the trachea. The radioopaque area on top of the fascia flap (arrowheads) represents a Gore-Tex sheet which is placed over the fascial flap to prevent adhesions between flap and surrounding tissue. Another Gore-Tex sheet is placed between fascia and neck vessels (arrow) to facilitate dissection during the second operation stage.
p = proximal site of fascia flap; d = distal site of fascia flap. The vascular pedicle is reanastomosed to the right neck vessels. This design is suitable for a laryngeal reconstruction at the right side.

2.B.3. Wound healing after first operation

The situation of the patient after the first intervention is visible in Figure 4.13.

Hematoma formation and the necessity for reintubation were 'minor complications' seen after the first operation stage. After the first intervention, the patient can mostly be extubated immediately and he can retake oral feeding 1 day postoperatively. Discharge from hospital follows 3 or 4 days postoperatively. Four patients needed reintubation and remained intubated on the intensive care unit for the 2 weeks revascularization period. Reintubation was necessary because of the bulk of the tumor in combination with the impact of intubation and surgery. A tracheotomy placed at the level of the cervical trachea is not compatible with tracheal revascularization and reintubation has to be considered after the first intervention especially in patients with a bulky tumor after irradiation. Also 3 patients needed a re-exploration after the first operation because of hematome formation.

In our series, 1 free flap failed due to venous thrombosis. A second flap was taken without compromising the vitality of the unique tracheal transplant. The trachea will not become necrotic even in cases of flap failure because the preserved, intrinsic mucosal vascularity of the trachea is sufficient during the 2 weeks after the first operation stage. The two stage approach of tracheal autotransplantation contribute to the safety of the reconstructive procedure because the unique tracheal transplant is not lost after failure of the microsurgical anastomosis. One patient developed a hematome between the flap and a part of the underlying trachea. In this patient, the vascular connections between fascia and trachea were still sufficient for survival of the whole autotransplant (Fig. 4.14).

Healing of the radial forearm donor site usually occurs uncomplicated. The forearm is immobilized and a splint is applied for 1 week. Small wound healing problems may be seen at the skin graft and at the longitudinal incision over the donor site of the fascial paddle (Fig. 4.10.d).

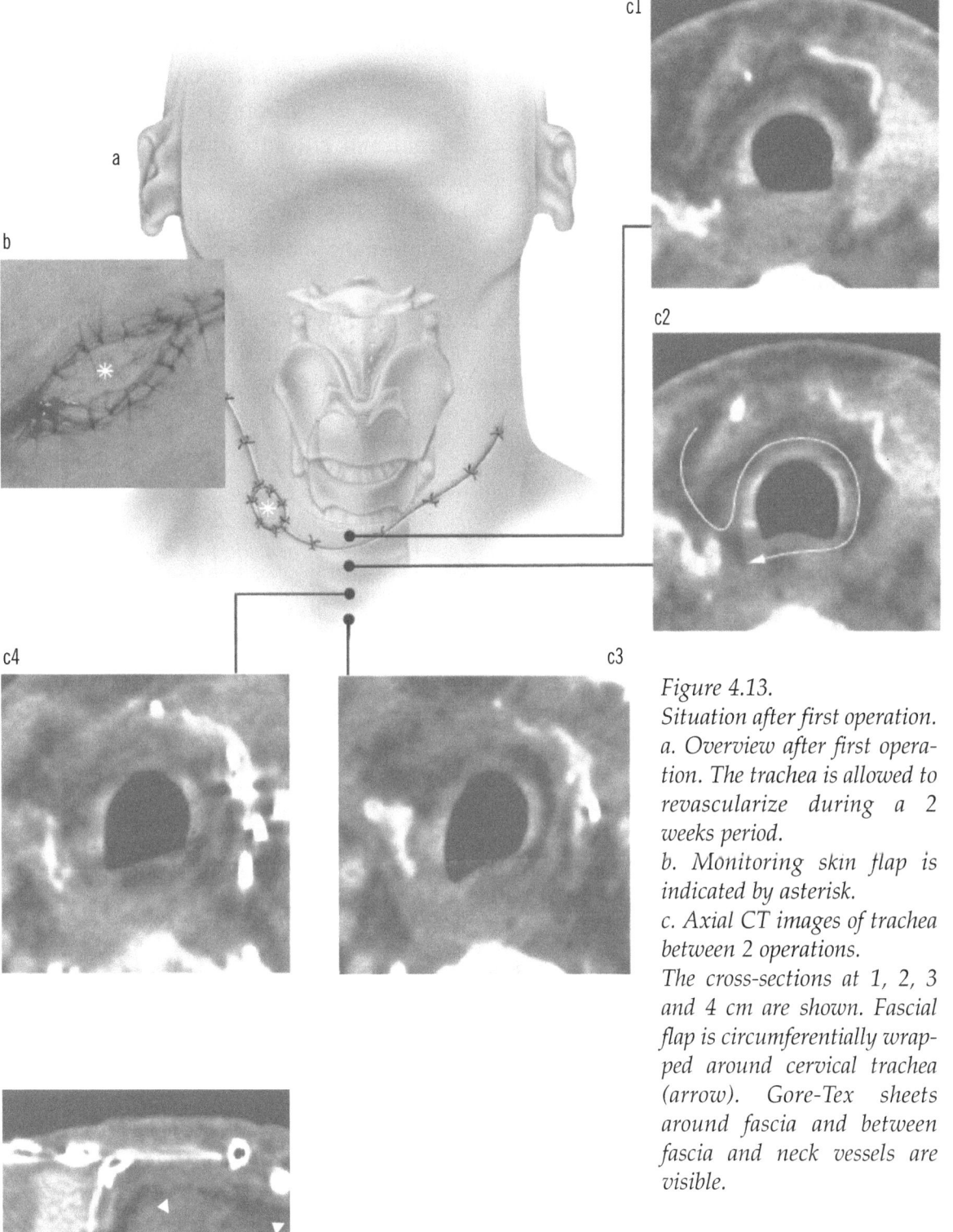

Figure 4.13.
Situation after first operation.
a. Overview after first operation. The trachea is allowed to revascularize during a 2 weeks period.
b. Monitoring skin flap is indicated by asterisk.
c. Axial CT images of trachea between 2 operations.
The cross-sections at 1, 2, 3 and 4 cm are shown. Fascial flap is circumferentially wrapped around cervical trachea (arrow). Gore-Tex sheets around fascia and between fascia and neck vessels are visible.

Figure 4.14.
Hematome formation between fascia and trachea.
Hematome is indicated by arrowheads. Only a small amount of the tracheal cartilage ring was wrapped by fascia (double arrow). This amount was sufficient for survival of the whole transplanted autograft.

2.C. Second operation

2.C.1. Tumor resection

The following operative steps are made during the second operation stage (Fig. 4.15):

- The cricotracheal membrane is incised in the midline along the inferior border of the cricoid cartilage. The oroendotracheal tube is removed and a tracheal tube is inserted via the cricotracheal incision.
- Anterior laryngeal section line placed in the midline at the level of the thyroid and cricoid cartilage (anterior commissure included if tumor reaches anterior site of vocal fold).
- Section of petiole of epiglottis and mobilisation of lateral edge of thyroid cartilage.
- Dissection of pyriform sinus mucosa from thyroid and cricoid cartilage at the tumor-bearing side.
- Incision of posterior cricoid lamina in the midline and removal of resection specimen.

2.C.2. Tracheal autotransplantation

Isolation of the revascularized trachea and patch formation are shown in figure 4.16.

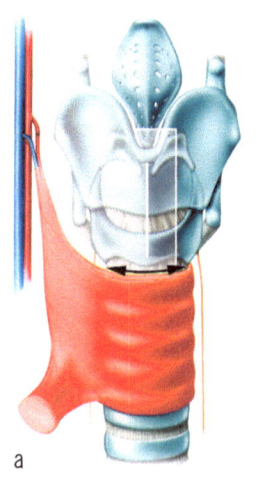
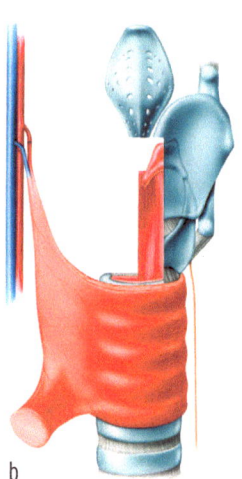
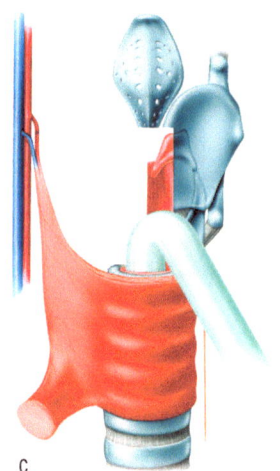

a

b

c

Figure 4.15.
Schematic presentation of tumor resection.
a. Outlining of defect. Anterior commissure is included in resection. The intubation tube is placed in a cricotracheal incision (double arrow) during tumor resection.
b. Situation after resection.
c. Situation after resection - the intubation tube is placed in the proximal cervical trachea.

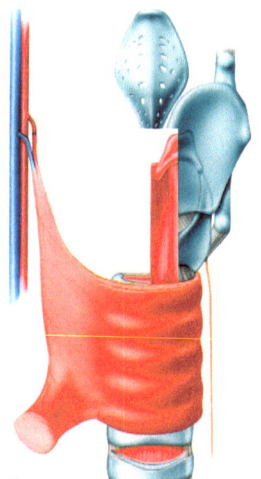
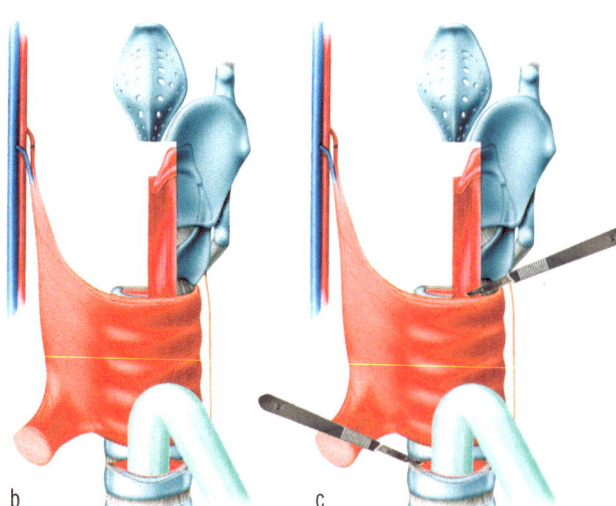

a

b

c

Figure 4.16.
Tracheal isolation and patch formation.
a. The trachea is incised below the revascularized segment.
b. Intubation tube placed below revascularized segment.
c. Tracheal isolation. The fascial enwrapped cervical trachea is completely isolated from the airway tract. Care is taken to preserve the recurrent nerve at the left (opposite tumor) side.

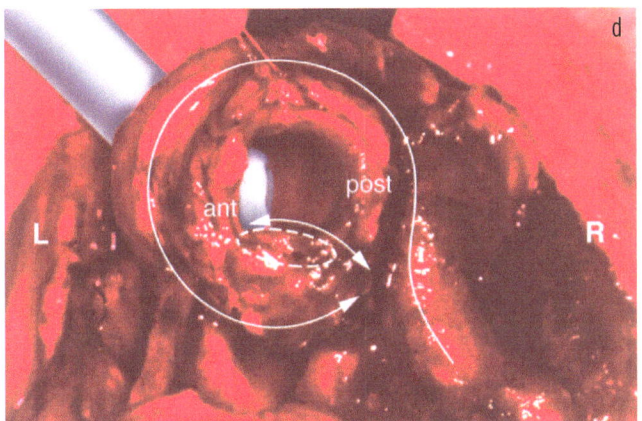

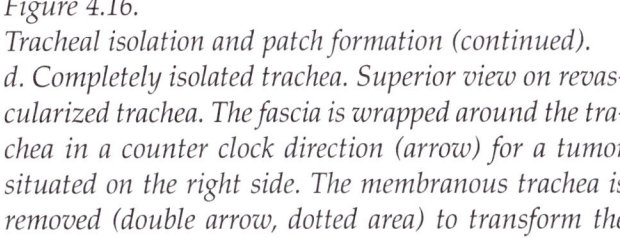

Figure 4.16.
Tracheal isolation and patch formation (continued).
d. Completely isolated trachea. Superior view on revascularized trachea. The fascia is wrapped around the trachea in a counter clock direction (arrow) for a tumor situated on the right side. The membranous trachea is removed (double arrow, dotted area) to transform the tube into a patch. R = right; L = left.

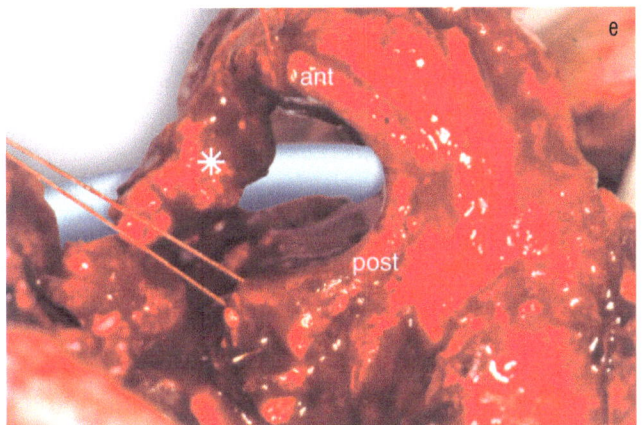

e. Tracheal patch-configuration for reconstruction at subglottic level. The revascularized trachea is visible after removal of the membranous trachea. The distal end of the fascia (asterisk) will cover the anterior suture line. The convex shaped configuration is useful for restoration of the subglottic larynx. The posterior (post) site of the patch will be sutured to the posterior cricoid resection margin; the anterior (ant) site of the patch will be sutured to the anterior section margin of the cricoid cartilage.

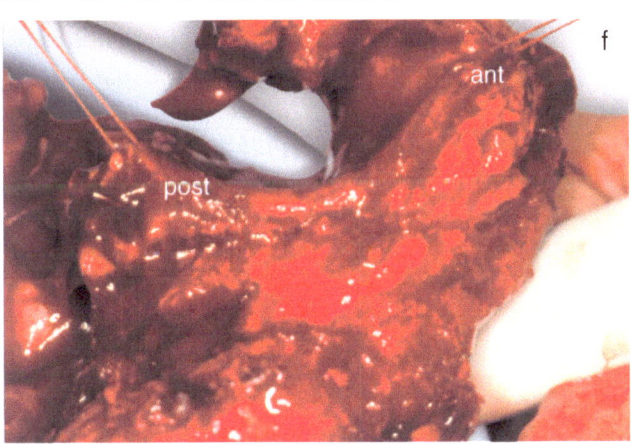

f. Tracheal patch-configuration for reconstruction at glottic level. The same tracheal patch as under e is visible after pulling on the anterior and posterior end of the tracheal patch. The curvature of the cartilaginous tracheal ring can be flattened. This is important to obtain the desired configuration at the glottic level. The anterior site of the cartilaginous portion of the tracheal patch (ant) can be shortened without interference with the blood supply of the patch. The anterior site (ant) of the tracheal patch will be sutured to the anterior laryngeal section line while the posterior site (post) of the tracheal patch will be sutured to the posterior laryngeal section line.

After tumor resection, the fascial enwrapped segment of cartilage is completely removed from the airway so that it is only connected with the vascular pedicle of the fascia flap. Isolation of the tracheal segment occurs by transsection between the cricoid and the first tracheal ring at its upper site and transsection caudad to the 4 cm of cervical trachea at its lower site. A 4-cm length is chosen to correspond with the average laryngeal height. After isolation of the cervical trachea, the intubation tube is placed in the sectionned mediastinal trachea. Then, the revascularized tracheal tube is transformed into a patch through a distal incision of the fascia flap and through a removal of the membranous trachea and a part of the cartilaginous trachea.

Autotransplantation of the tracheal patch is shown in figure 4.17.

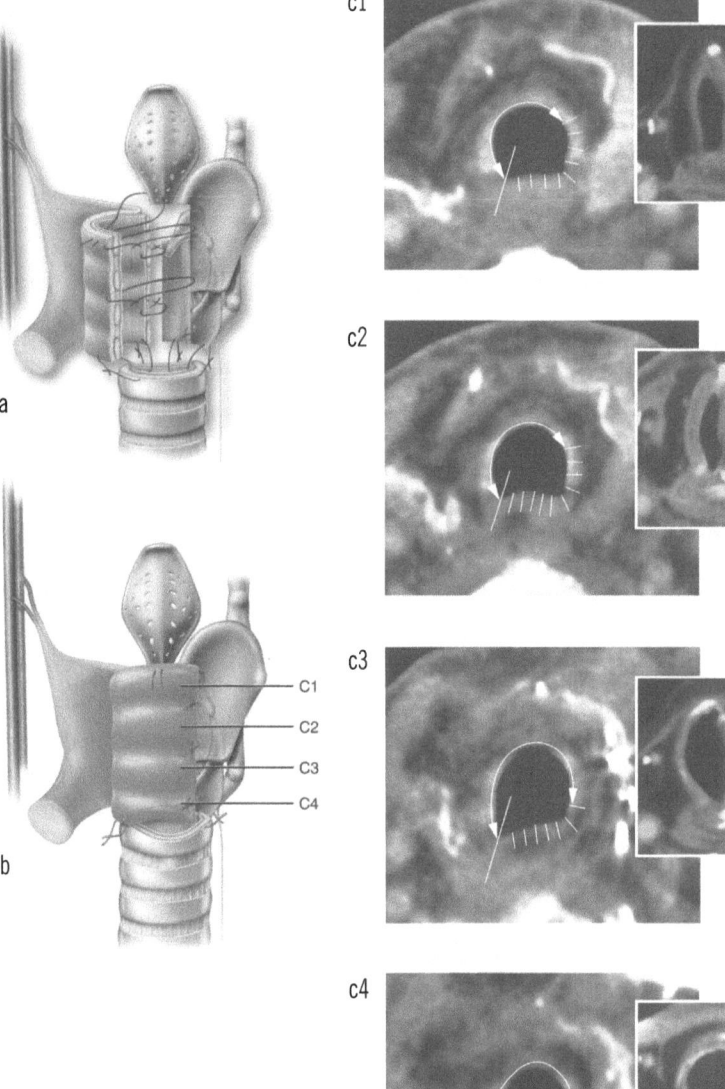

Figure 4.17.
Autotransplantation of tracheal patch.
a. Patch is sutured into defect.
b. Situation after suturing of patch into defect. The mediastinal trachea is brought up to restore the airway continuity.
c. Axial CT scans before and after reconstruction
1. Supraglottic level. The reconstruction allows for posterior closure at the level of the arytenoid. The amount of cartilaginous trachea included in the reconstruction (double arrow) is indicated.
2. Glottic level. The amount of cartilaginous trachea included in the reconstruction (double arrow) is indicated.
The cross-sections at 0 and 2 cm correspond with the level of reconstruction at the false and true vocal folds. The membranous trachea and a segment of cartilaginous trachea are removed at these levels to obtain a patch that will be placed in a paramedial position.
3. Subglottic level-high. The amount of cartilaginous trachea included in the reconstruction is indicated (double arrow).
4. Subglottic level-low. The amount of cartilaginous trachea included in the reconstruction is indicated (double arrow). The optimal reconstruction in the subglottic region is formed by the internal site of the original airway lumen-the caliber of the airway is the important factor in the subglottic region. The cross-section at 4 cm corresponds with the level of reconstruction at the caudal margin of the cricoid cartilage. The membranous trachea is removed and the full amount of cartilage ring is used at this level to restore the original airway lumen. More patch length is included at the subglottic level.

The tracheal patch can be brought upwards without further manipulation of the vascular pedicle. The tracheal patch is sutured into the laryngeal defect. The posterior site of the tracheal patch is sutured to the posterior cricoid (2-0 Vicryl) with the knots of the sutures placed away from the airway lumen. At this point, the posterior-anterior length of the patch can be adapted by excision of a part of the cartilaginous trachea. The upper border of the tracheal patch is then sutured to the pyriform sinus mucosa and to the epiglottic petiole. The anterior site of the patch is sutured to the anterior laryngeal section line from superior to inferior. After reconstruction of the larynx, it is necessary to re-establish the airway continuity by bringing the mediastinal trachea to the caudal end of the reconstructed larynx. A blunt finger dissection is performed to release the tracheal wall down into the mediastinum. This is the same finger dissection of the cervicomediastinal trachea done for tracheal resection anastomosis. The stump of the remaining trachea is reanastomosed posteriorly and laterally toward the cricoid cartilage and to the hemilaryngeal patch.

2.C.3. Wound healing after second operation
2.C.3.a. Wound healing problems around tracheostome
The anastomosis between mediastinal trachea and cricoid is left open anteriorly. A tracheostome is created by suturing the cervical skin to the anterior defect. A cuffed Shiley cannula is placed in the tracheostome.

Wound healing problems were seen when the Shiley cannula was placed in the anterior laryngotracheal anastomosis (Fig. 4.18). The design of the tracheostome was changed because the Shiley cannula produced pressure necrosis on the lateral sites of the tracheostome. The anterior site of the mediastinal trachea was incised over 3 cartilage rings in a way that the Shiley cannula could be placed in a more caudal position. The tracheal cannula was placed in a position immediately under the anastomosis so that less pressure was exercised on the suture line that connects the mediastinal trachea with the reconstructed larynx (Fig. 4.19).

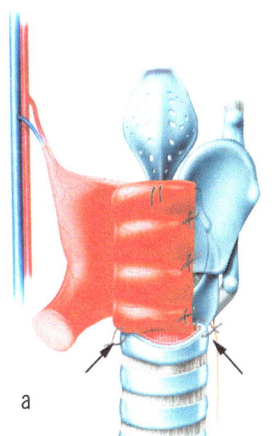 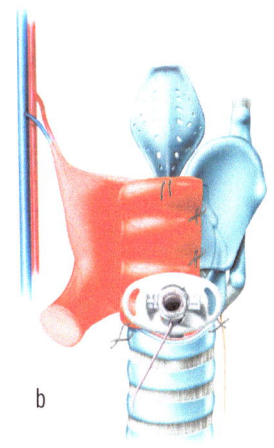 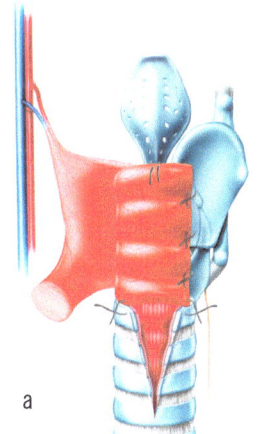 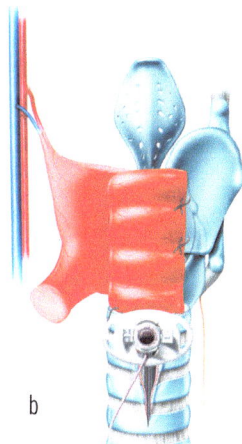

Figure 4.18.
Tracheostome in anterior anastomosis.
a. Situation without cannula.
b. Situation with cannula. Pressure effects exercised by the cannula will give wound healing problems at the lateral sites of the tracheostome (arrows in Fig. 4.18.a).

Figure 4.19.
Tracheostome located caudal of anterior anastomosis.
a. Situation without cannula. The mediastinal trachea is incised over 3 cartilage rings.
b. Situation with cannula. The cannula is located caudal from the laryngotracheal anastomosis.

The neck is closed with the flap monitor still present in the neck incision. Due to the bulk of the fascia flap, it is not always possible to bring the upper skin flap to the superior margin of the tracheostome. In cases of too much flap bulk, the lower site of the fascia is left uncovered and is allowed to heal by secondary intention (Fig. 4.20, 4.21). A paraffin gauze dressing covers the bare fascia for the first postoperative days.

Aspiration of saliva has to be expected during the first weeks. To prevent infection of the tracheostome, it is advisible to treat the patient with antibiotics (Metronidazole 3x500 mg/d and Cefadroxil 3x1 g/d) during the first week after tracheal autotransplantation.

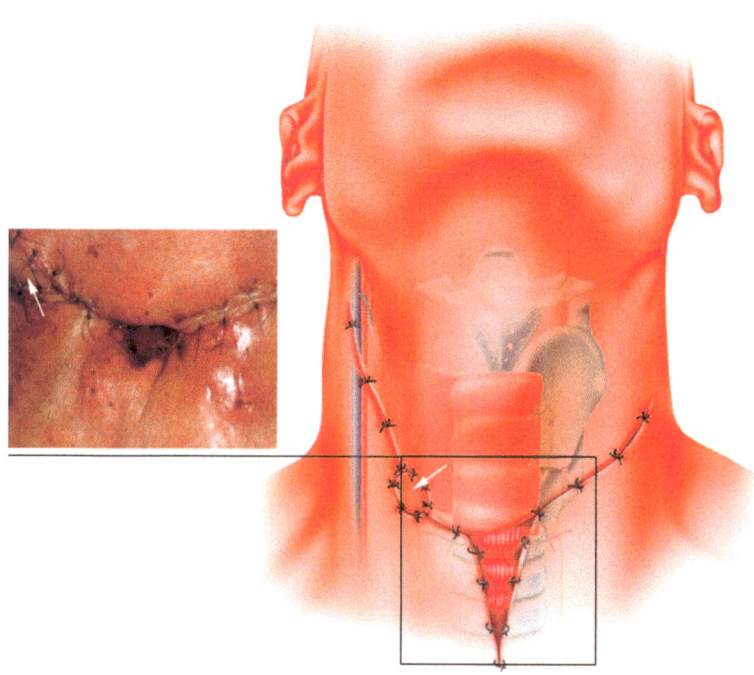

Figure 4.20.
Anterior view of tracheostoma-skin lined tracheostome.
The upper skin flap is sutured to the reconstructed cricoid anteriorly. The lower skin flap is sutured to the mediastinal trachea anteriorly. Arrow points to skin monitor.

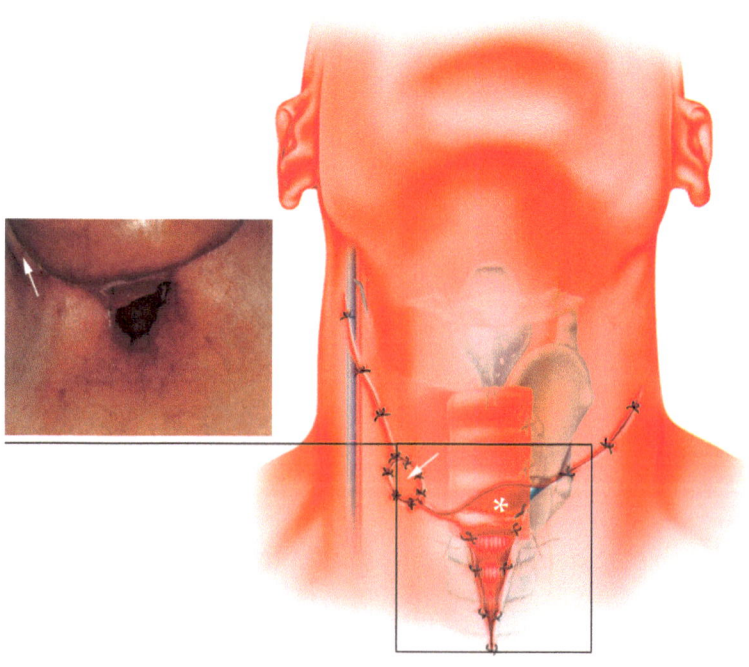

Figure 4.21.
Anterior view of tracheostoma-bare fascia.
The upper skin flap can not always be sutured towards the anterior, lower margin of the reconstructed larynx. The fascia can be left uncovered in cases with too much flap bulk. At the upper site of the tracheostome, a part of the uncovered fascia flap is visible (asterisk). Arrow points to skin monitor.

2.C.3.b. Flap failure after second operation

The risk to compromise the vascularity of the transplanted trachea during the second stage is very low because no manipulation of the vascular pedicle of the radial forearm flap is necessary during the transplantation stage. Within the initial series, 1 patient had an interruption of the venous anastomosis of the radial forearm flap during re-elevation of the skin flap. The tracheal transplantation was performed with a fascia flap and with a tracheal transplant showing venous congestion. Our initial hope was that new venous connections, formed during the 2 weeks period, would be suf-ficient for flap survival. Over the next 2 days how-ever, the fascia flap showed evolution to complete necrosis. The necrotic fascia flap was removed and the neck was packed with a pedicled pectoralis muscle in an attempt to obtain a secondary vas-cularization of the tracheal transplant by the sur-rounding well vascularized pectoralis muscle. The neolarynx however showed evolution to stenosis because of a complete necrosis of the tracheal transplant. This patient is now able to speak with a permanent cannula in place. The functional sta-tus of the patient is comparable to a near total laryngectomy (Fig. 4.22, Fig. 4.23).

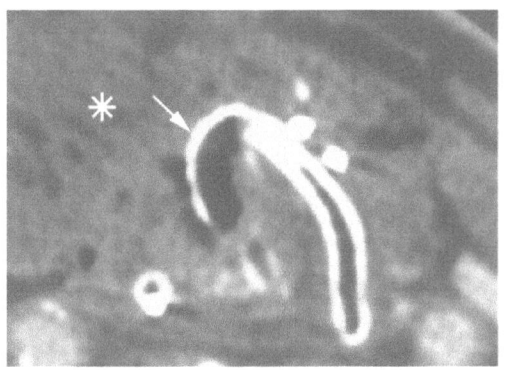

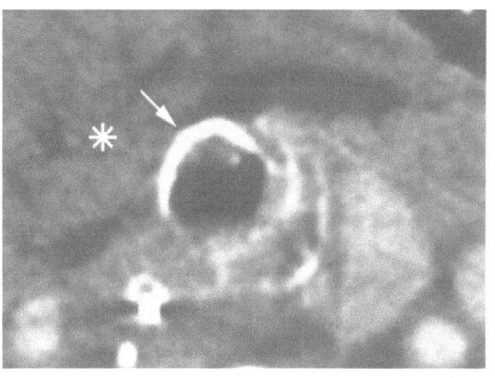

Fig. 4.22. Postreconstruction CT scan 1 week after transfer of the pectoralis major flap.
a. Glottic level. Arrow points to tracheal patch; pecto-ralis flap is indicated by an asterisk.

b. Subglottic level. Arrow points to tracheal patch; pectoralis flap is indicated by an asterisk.
A pectoralis major muscle was placed in an attempt to save the tracheal autotransplant.

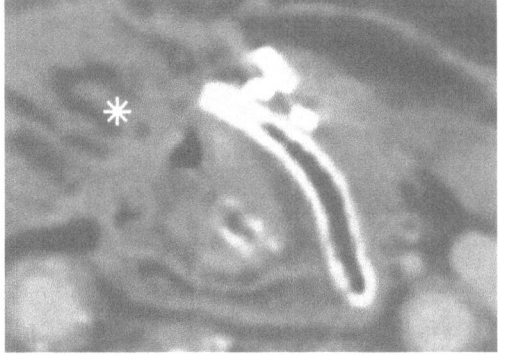

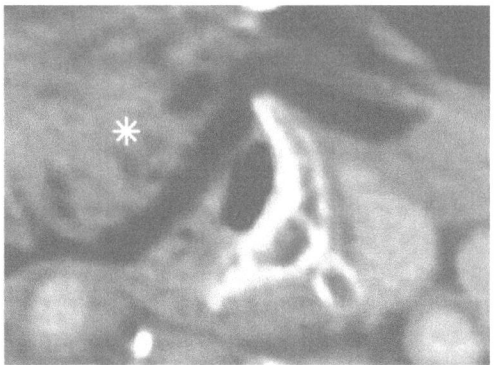

Fig. 4.23. Postreconstruction CT scan 2 months after transfer of the pectoralis major flap.
a. Glottic level. Pectoralis major flap is indicated by an asterisk. The tracheal patch has completely disappeared.

The remaining laryngeal lumen serves as a speaking valve. b. Subglottic level. Pectoralis major flap is indi-cated by an asterisk. The tracheal patch has completely disappeared.

This flap failure during the second operation emphasizes once again that tracheal transplantation without a reliable (2-stage) revascularization approach is not possible.

2.D. Postoperative course and closure of tracheostomy

During the first 2 weeks, the patients were fed by using the percutaneous endoscopic gastrostomy (PEG) tube. The tracheostomy tube is removed as soon as possible after the second operation so that the patient can speak during closure of the tracheostome. The patient is discharged at approx-

imately 1 week postoperatively. Retake of oral feeding is started after 10 days under supervision of the speech therapist. The patient works with the speech-language pathologist for speech and swallowing as an outpatient. A pureed diet is started and liquids are introduced after a few days. Normal oral feeding without aspiration is usually possible 1 to 2 weeks postoperatively. The anterior tracheostome progressively diminishes without cannula and the remaining tracheostome is closed under local anesthesia several weeks (usually 4 to 6) after the patient is discharged from hospital (Fig. 4.24).

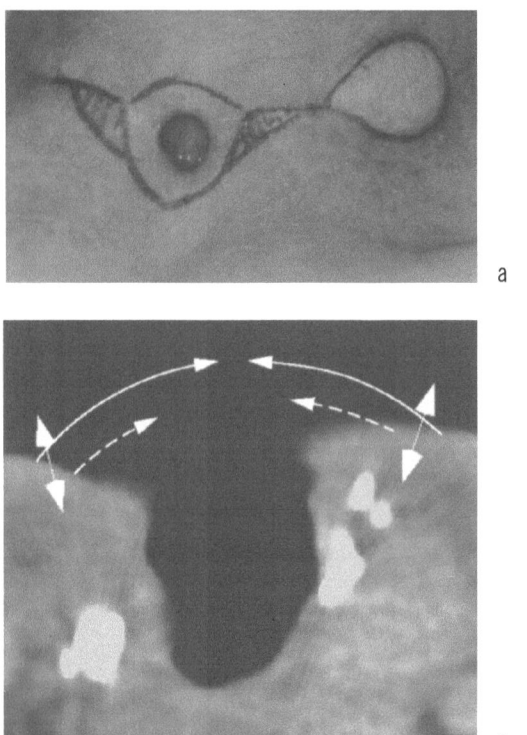

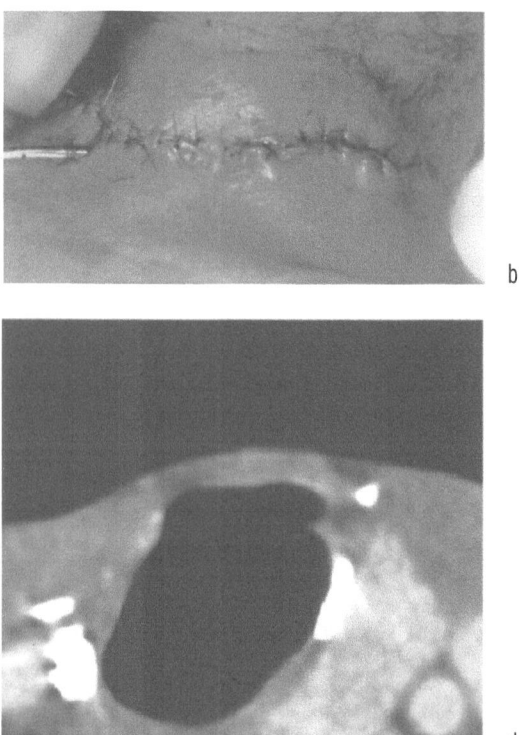

Figure 4.24. Closure of tracheostomy.
a. Outlining of skin flaps. The tracheostome is closed several weeks after the tracheal transplantation following the 'trough principle'. Skin flaps around the tracheostome are incised and inverted; the lower and upper skin flap are sutured over the skin lined tracheostome. The monitor flap is removed simultaneously.
b. Situation after tracheostomy closure.

c. CT scan before tracheostomy closure. Double arrows indicate skin incision. Dotted arrows show closure of anterior tracheostome by inverting the neck skin. Arrows show how the cervical skin is advanced over the closed tracheostome.
d. CT scan after tracheostomy closure. The anterior tracheal wall is lined by cervical skin.

2.E. Indications for tracheal autotransplantation

2.E.1. T2-T3 glottic cancer

An important indication for tracheal autotransplantation is the unilateral T2 and T3 glottic tumor with subglottic extension but without extension towards the ventricle. Selection criteria for extended hemilaryngectomy include glottic squamous cell carcinoma that did not involve the ventricle, false vocal fold, petiole of the epiglottis, interarytenoid space, or the cervical trachea. Hemilaryngectomy with tracheal autotransplantation is suitable for unilateral glottic tumors with arytenoid cartilage fixation and infraglottic tumor extension reaching the upper border of the cricoid cartilage, two major contraindications for all 'classical' conservation procedures.

The posterior incision is always placed in the midline. Depending on the place of the anterior section line, two different situations may be distinguished:

- The anterior section line is placed in the anterior commissure if the tumor has a posterior localization.
- The anterior commissure is included in the resection if the tumor reaches the anterior commissure (Fig. 4.25).

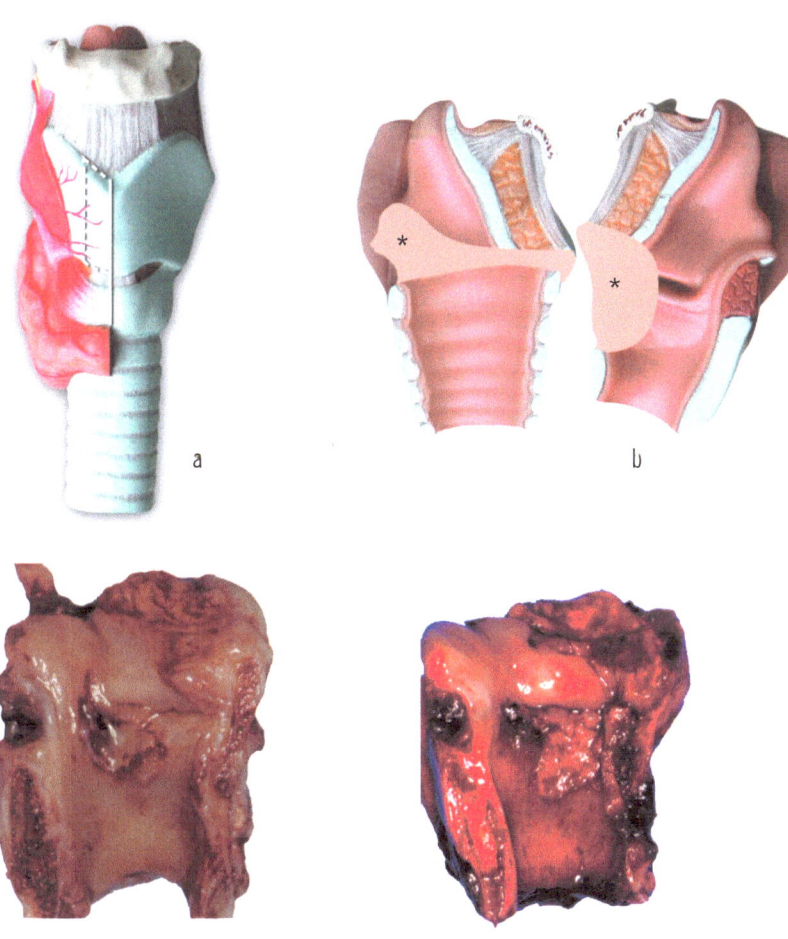

Figure 4.25.
Extent of resection.
a. Laryngeal model-anterior view. Midline sagittal section of thyroid and cricoid cartilage. The anterior commissure can be included (dotted lines) if the tumor reaches the anterior site of the vocal fold: 1 cm of the contralateral thyroid cartilage and 1 cm of the contralateral vocal fold is then resected.
b. Longitudinally incised laryngeal model showing the extent of resection and reconstruction. Internal view after midsagittal incision. The resection includes one half of the cricoid and thyroid cartilages and the true and false vocal folds. The anterior commissure is included if the tumor reaches the anterior site of the vocal fold. The amount of reconstruction by the tracheal transplant is shown. The areas indicated by an asterisk are closed primarily.
c. Resection specimen after extended hemilaryngectomy for glottic cancer.
c.1. The anterior section line is placed in the anterior midline for a glottic tumor with subglottic extension and with posterior localization.
c2. The anterior commissure is included in the resection if the tumor reaches the anterior commissure.

2.E.2. Pyriform sinus cancer

An extended hemilaryngectomy can be combined with a removal of the medial and lateral wall of 1 pyriform sinus. Selected pyriform sinus tumors that involve the pyriform sinus apex can be resected with inclusion of the hemicricoid cartilage as long as the hypopharyngeal mucosa can be closed primarily. The hypopharyngeal mucosa can be closed primarily when the section lines are not beyond the anterior and posterior midline (Fig. 4.26).

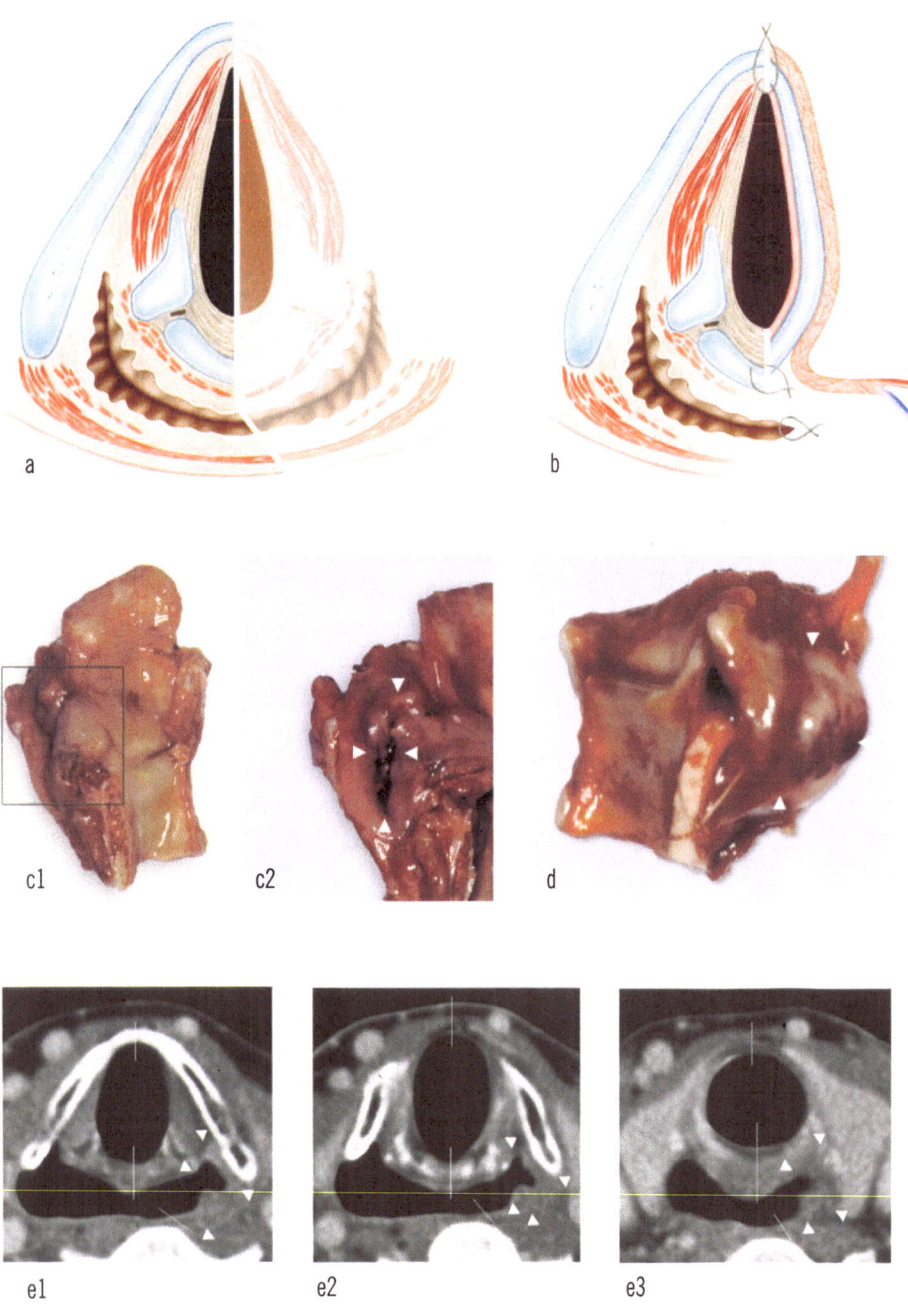

Figure 4.26.
Extended hemilaryngectomy for pyriform sinus tumor.
a. Schematic presentation of resection. Resection of 1 hemilarynx (between anterior and posterior commissure) with 1 pyriform sinus.
b. Schematic presentation of reconstruction. Tracheal patch is used for reconstruction of the hemilarynx. Pharyngeal defect is closed primarily.
c. Resection specimen of pyriform sinus tumor with involvement of apex. C1: overview, C2:detail. Tumor extension is indicated by arrowheads. The tumor was resected by removal of the ipsilateral thyroid, vocal folds, cricoid, pyriform sinus, aryepiglottic fold, and part of the epiglottis.
d. Resection specimen. Synovial sarcoma with involvement of arytenoid.
The submucosal located synovial sarcoma (arrowheads) was resected by removal of the ipsilateral thyroid, vocal folds, cricoid, and pyriform sinus.
e. CT preoperative, glottic (1), subglottic level (heigh-2; low-3) during valsalva. Tumor extension is indicated with arrowheads. This tumor extension allows for extended hemilaryngectomy with inclusion of 1 pyriform sinus.

2.E.3. Lateralized chondrosarcoma

Laryngeal chondrosarcomas occur infrequently. They account for only 0.5% to 1% of all laryngeal tumors. Laryngeal chondrosarcomas most often occur in patients between the ages of 50 to 70, with a male to female ration of 3 to 1 (NIKOLAI et al. 1990).

Laryngeal chondrosarcoma most commonly arises from the cricoid cartilage, with a predilection for the posterior or posterolateral lamina. The presenting symptoms are progressive hoarseness, dyspnea, and dysphagia, varying according to tumor location. Surgical excision with maximal function preservation is regarded as the treatment of choice (FERLITO et al. 1984, KOZELSKY et al. 1997).

A case of a large, unilateral chondrosarcoma of the cricoid cartilage with involvement of 1 cricoarytenoid joint was included in the initial series. The tumor was removed by performing an extended hemilaryngectomy. After 2 weeks of tracheal revascularization, the cervical trachea was used to repair the laryngeal defect. The tumor was completely resected and all laryngeal functions (swallowing, voice, respiration without tracheostomy) were restored.

Case Report. A 53-year-old women was referred with hoarseness lasting several months and progressive worsening dyspnea during the previous 3 weeks. Indirect laryngoscopy revealed a tumor in the right hemilarynx, narrowing the laryngeal lumen and covered by an apparently intact mucosa. The right hemilarynx was fixed. On direct laryngoscopy, a large right-sided laryngeal mass was visible which appeared submucosal in nature, extending from the aryepiglottic fold superiorly down to the subglottic region. A biopsy specimen was reported to be chondrosarcoma. A CT scan was obtained and revealed an expansile lesion in the cricoid cartilage. Irregular ringlike calcifications were noted in the mass suggestive for a tumor of cartilaginous origin. There was involvement of the right cricoarytenoid joint (Fig. 4.27).

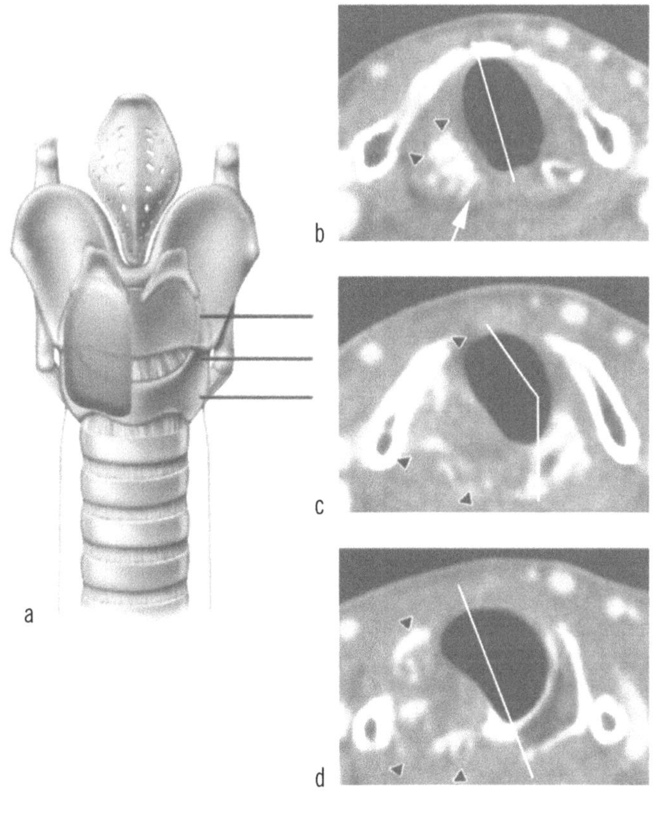

Figure 4.27. Extent of tumor resection.
a. Schematic drawing of larynx and cervical trachea. The tumor extension in the right hemilarynx is indicated. The levels of the CT scans b, c, anb d are indicated.
b. CT scan glottic area. Axial contrast-enhanced CT image. Tumor involvement of right cricoid and arytenoid. The intratumoral calcifications (arrowheads) reveal extension to the level of the true vocal cord and posterior displacement of the arytenoid cartilage (arrow). Section margins are indicated.
c. CT scan subglottic area (high). The chondrosarcoma involving the posterolateral lamina of the right cricoid is visible (arrowheads). An expansile, relatively low-density lesion in the right cricoid arch is visible. Section lines to remove the tumor are indicated.
d. CT scan subglottic area (low). The chondrosarcoma (arrowheads) involving the posterolateral lamina of the right cricoid is visible. Section lines to remove the tumor are indicated.

Resection of at least 1 half of the cricoid cartilage was necessary to remove the tumor completely and it was attempted to preserve all laryngeal functions by performing a tracheal autotransplantation in a 2-stage procedure (Fig. 4.28).

After 5 days, the Shiley cannula was removed and the patient started swallowing under supervision of the speech therapist. Voicing was stimulated by thumb closure of the tracheostome. The anterior tracheostome was closed 5 weeks after the larynx reconstruction under local anesthesia.

On a CT scan, taken 6 weeks after the reconstruction, it was shown that the tracheal autotransplant restores the glottic and subglottic laryngeal airway lumen in a way that closure during speech and swallowing remains possible (Fig. 4.29).

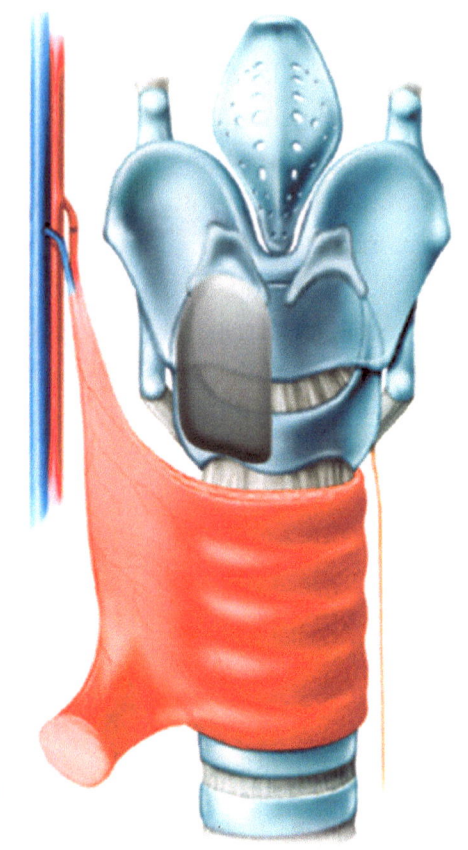
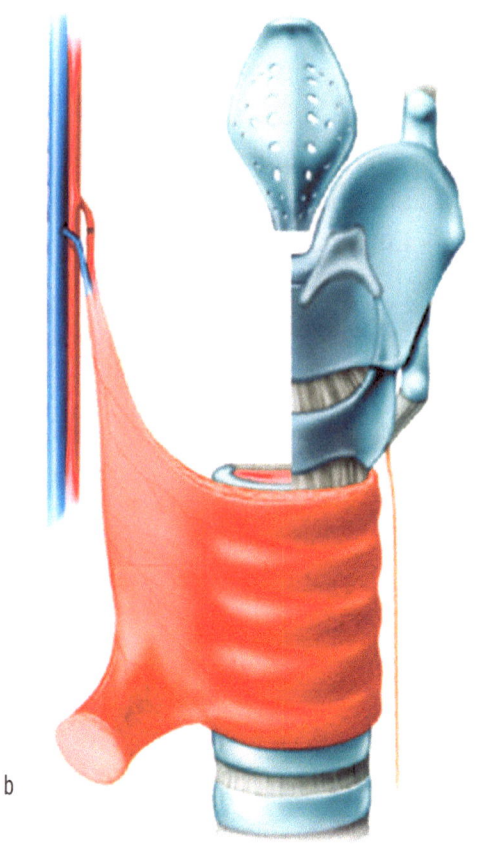

a

b

Figure 4.28. Operative procedure.
a. First operation. During the first operation, the cervical trachea (4 cm segment) is mobilized from surrounding tissues and wrapped by vascularized fascia flap. The neck is closed and the fascia flap is allowed to make vascular connections with the trachea during a 2 weeks period.

b. Second operation.
The neck is reopened after 2 weeks. The tumor is resected by performing a right-sided extended hemilaryngectomy.

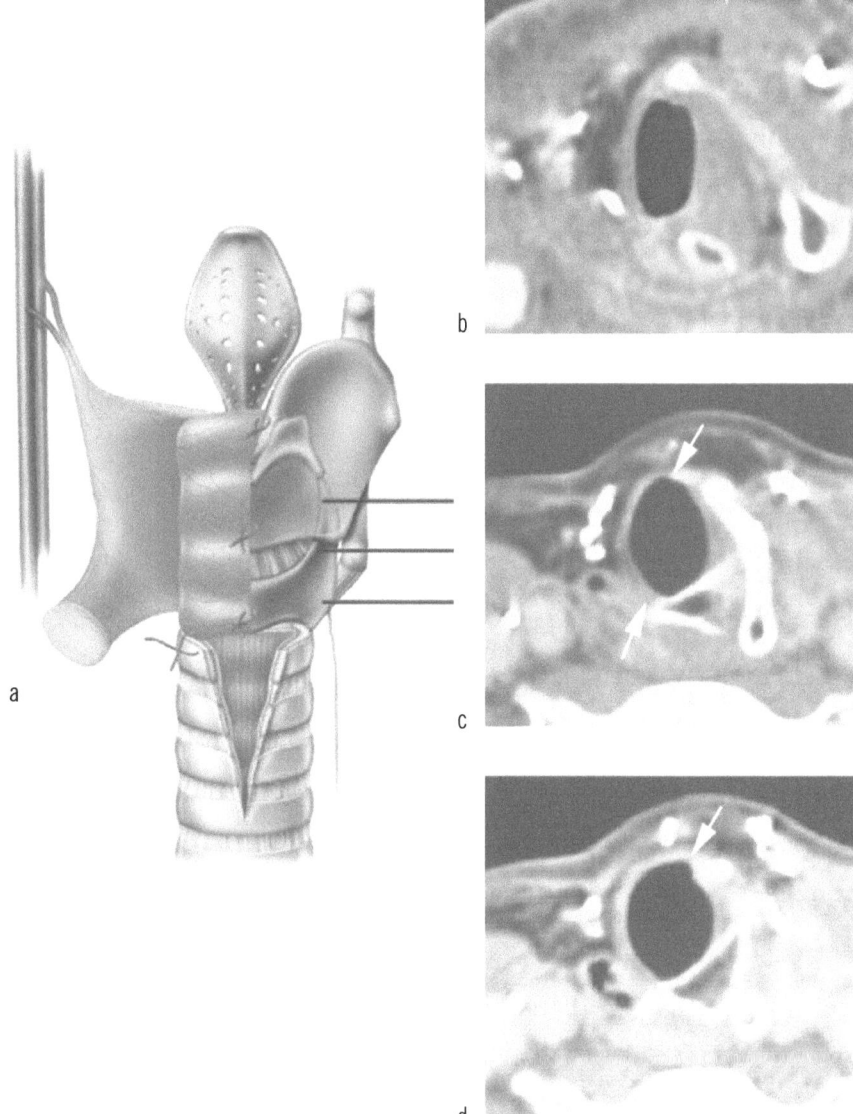

Figure 4.29.
Situation after tracheal autotransplantation.
a. Schematic drawing of larynx and cervical trachea.
The revascularized trachea is isolated on the fascia flap, transformed into a patch and transplanted into the laryngeal defect. The trachea is brought up to close the continuity defect of the airway tract. A tracheostomy is constructed for the first postoperative weeks. The levels of the CT scans b, c, and d are indicated.
b. CT scan Glottic area. At the glottic level, the tracheal transplant was placed in a position close to the midline. c. CT scan subglottic area (high). The tracheal transplant (between arrows) repairs the right hemicricoid defect. The airway lumen is optimally restored.
d. CT scan subglottic area (low). Tracheal transplant is located between 2 arrows.

All laryngeal functions were preserved and the patient remains tumor free since 3 years. Chondrosarcoma of the larynx has a different biologic behavior from those lesions found elsewhere in the body (BURKEY et al. 1990). They are usually more well differentiated and clinically less aggressive than lesions found at other sites and for these reasons should be treated differently. The most frequent site of laryngeal chondrosarcomas is the cricoid cartilage, where 72% to 75% of these lesions are identified. The majority of these lesions

arise from the posterior or postero-lateral aspect of the cricoid.

Laryngeal chondrosarcomas are generally low grade and do not metastasize. Surgical excision is the treatment of choice because radiation and chemotherapy have not proven to be beneficial in cases of primary disease. The tumor should be excised widely with special attention to excision of the external perichondrium, along with a margin of normal tissue, in order to ensure eradication of the tumor. Piecemeal excisions sparing the external perichondrium predispose to local recurrence (HICKS et al. 1982). The possibility for a conservative approach will depend on the extent of cricoid involvement. Less extensive involvement of the cricoid have been managed conservatively with excision of the involved cartilaginous segments. The cricoid is the cornerstone of the larynx and full height cricoid defects will interrupt the laryngeal support. No reliable reconstructive tissues are currently available for repair of full height cricoid defects and a total laryngectomy may be necessary because of the inability to repair the defect. Tracheal autotransplants have unique reconstructive charateristics for use inside the larynx. They can be used for repair of hemilaryngectomy defects including the full height of 50% of the circumference of the cricoid cartilage. Total laryngectomy should still be performed for lesions involving greather than 50% of the cricoid.

2.F. Morphometrical and functional evaluation of tracheal autotransplantation after extended hemilaryngectomy

2.F.1. Evaluation of reconstructive procedure
The amount of resection and reconstruction in patients treated for T2-T3 glottic cancer or pyriform sinus cancer is visible in Figure 4.30. The initial patient series treated with tracheal autotransplantation was studied morphometrically and functionally. This was done in an attempt to evaluate if tracheal autotransplants could approach a situation of 'theoretical optimal' reconstruction of extended hemilaryngectomy defects.

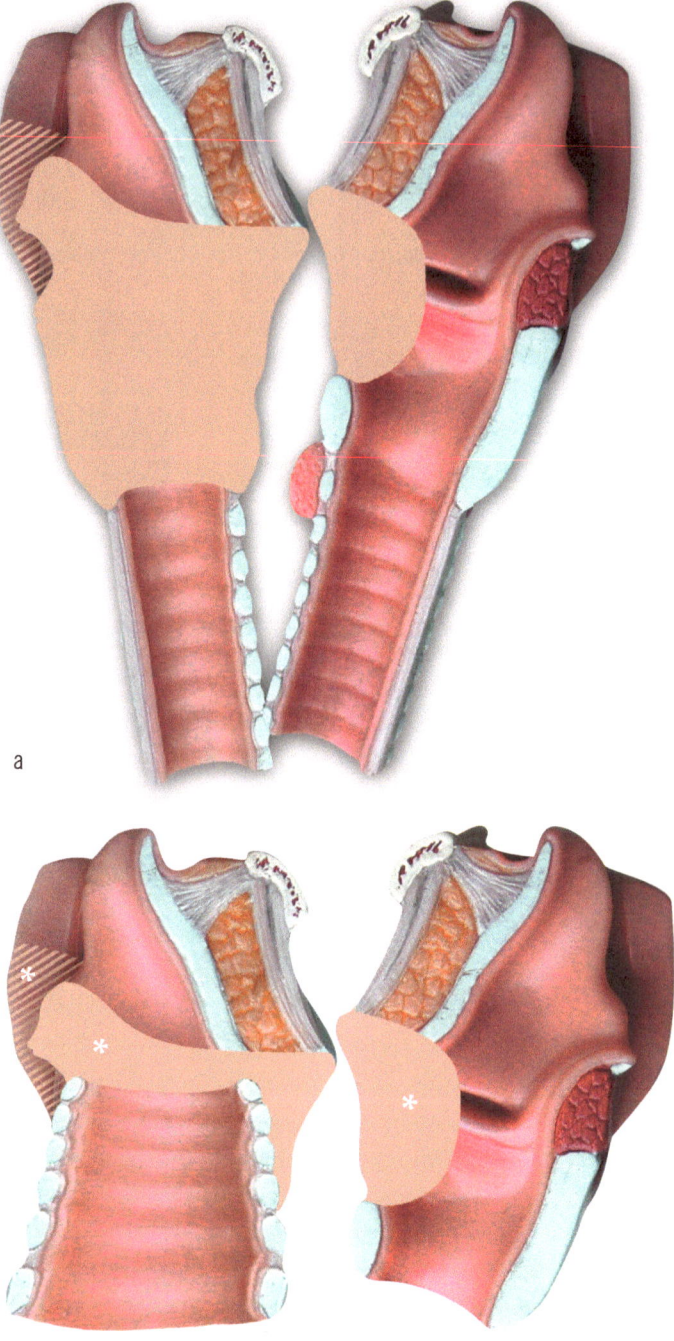

a

Figure 4.30.
Schematic presentation of extent of resection and reconstruction.
a. Amount of resection for T2-T3 glottic cancer or pyriform sinus cancer (additional resection of pyriform sinus indicated by lined area).
b. Amount of reconstruction with a 4 cm tracheal autotransplant. The areas indicated by asterisk are closed primarily.

2.F.2. Development of CT-based morphometrical model

The laryngeal function after reconstruction will be determined by the position of the tracheal transplant in relation to the laryngeal remnant. To define the optimal position (=position leading to good functional results) of the reconstructed tissue, we made use of CT scans taken during quiet respiration and during phonation (Fig. 4.31 and 4.32). A phonation CT scan was made during vocalizing of the sustained vowel /i/ at a comfortable pitch and loudness level during about 6 seconds (time necessary for scanning of the larynx using a multislice helical CT scanner). The theoretical optimal reconstruction of a laryngeal defect that extends from the anterior to the posterior commissure is by reconstructive tissue that is placed in a similar position as the free margin of a vocal fold paralysed in adduction. Minimal impairment of speech, swallowing, and respiration is seen when dealing with a unilateral vocal fold paralysis in adduction. Phonation CT scans were used to define the 'optimal position' of the reconstructive tissue at the glottic level. On CT scan, the position of a vocal fold paralysis in adduction is comparable to the position of the vocal fold during phonation. The laryngeal CT scans of normal larynges were used to define the optimal place of the reconstructive tissue within the larynx.

On the CT scans during phonation, a complete closure between the left and right laryngeal segments is seen at the supraglottic level between the medial surfaces of both arytenoids (Fig. 4.31 A2, B2). At the glottic level, a small gap remains between the free edges of the vocal folds. The smallest gap exists at the transition between membranous and cartilaginous site of the vocal fold (Fig. 4.31 D2).

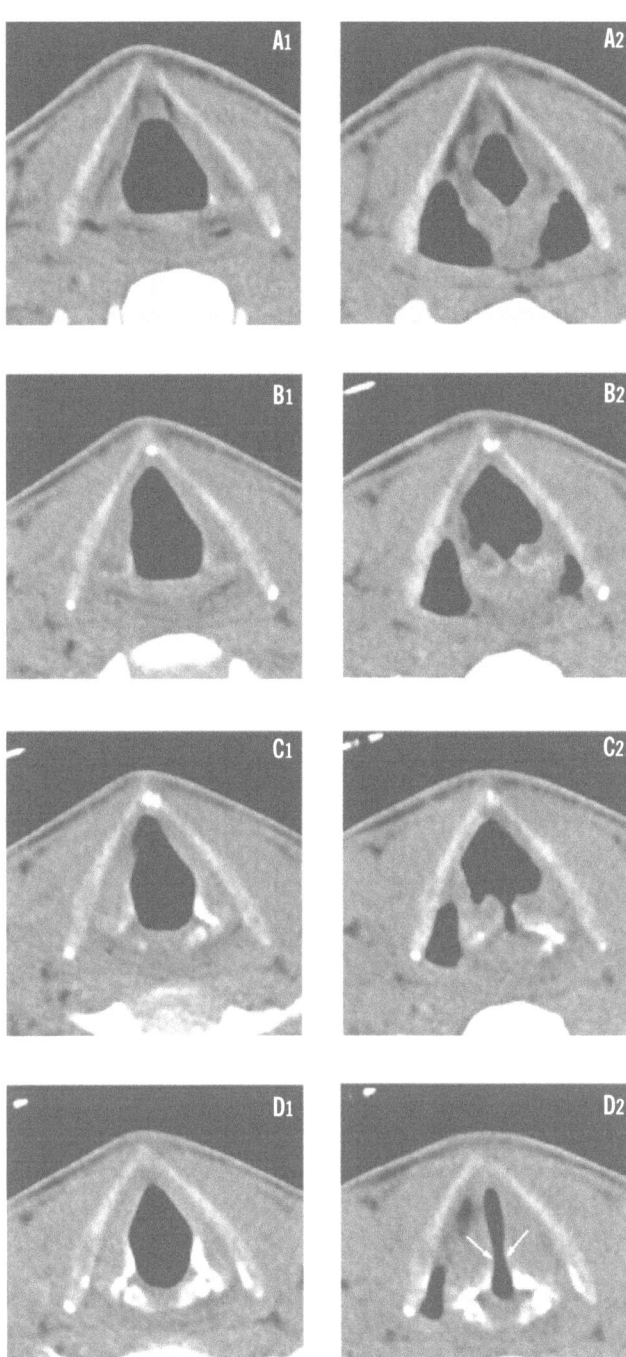

Figure 4.31.
Axial CT scan of the larynx during quiet respiration (1) and during phonation (2).
Sections A to D represent axial sections from superior to inferior (A, B, C: supraglottic level; D: glottic level). An elongation of the glottic chink is noted during phonation (D).
Arrows indicate the site of smallest glottic gap during phonation.

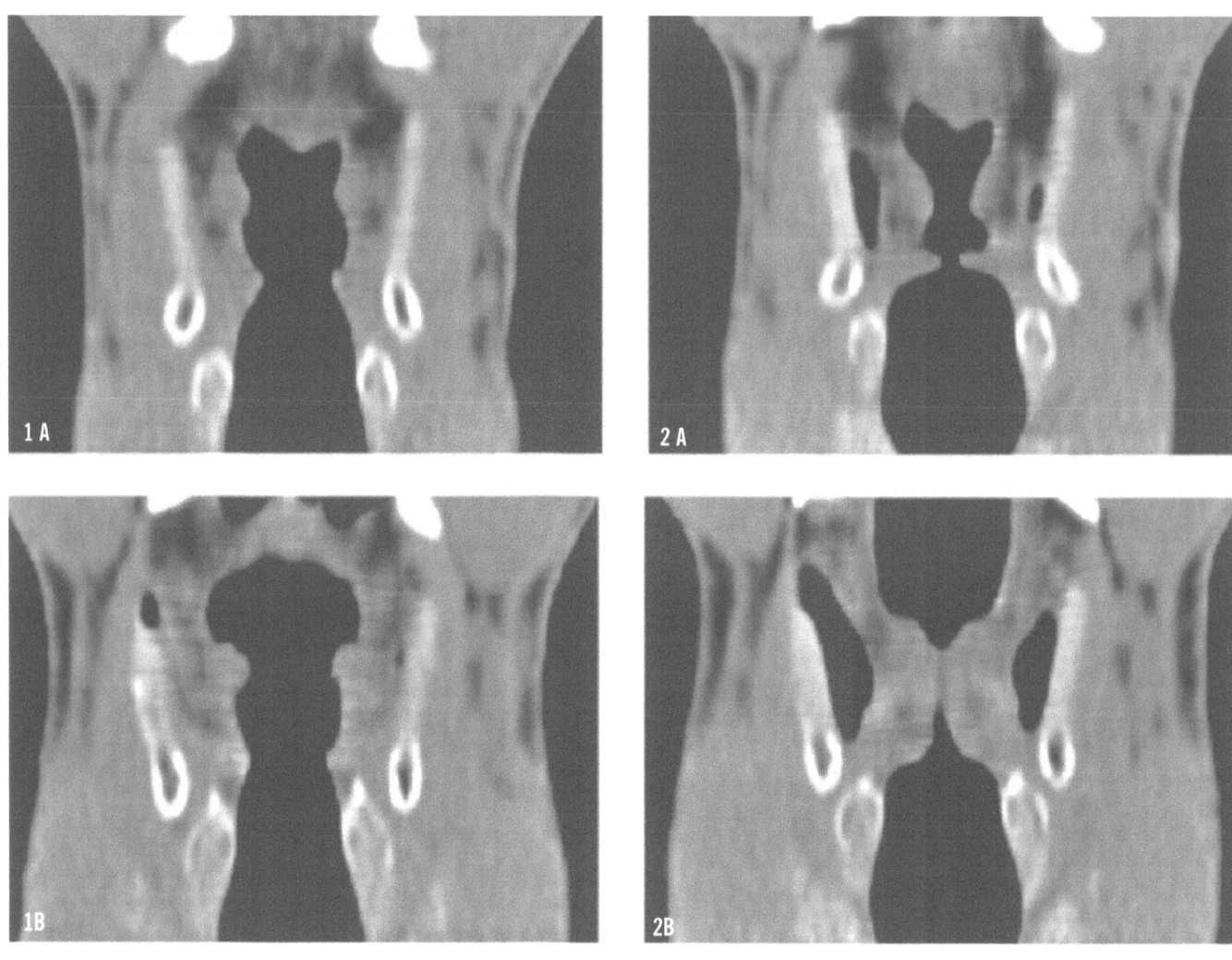

Figure 4.32. The coronal reformation of the larynx during quiet breathing (1) and during phonation (2).

Section A: level of membranous vocal fold. A small gap remains between the free edges of the vocal folds. During quiet respiration, the true and false vocal cords are opposed (1.A). During phonation, the laryngeal ventricle is filled with air and separates the two cords (2.A).

Section B: level of arytenoid. A complete closure between the left and right laryngeal segments is seen at the supraglottic level between the medial surfaces of both arytenoids.

The morphology of the reconstruction after repair of a hemilaryngeal defect should correspond to the radiological morphology of a vocal fold during phonation in order to obtain a competent larynx. The free margin of the vocal fold, which is visible on CT scan during phonation, was defined as the optimal position for the reconstructive tissue after extended hemilaryngectomy. This position is comparable to the vocal fold paralysis in a paramedial position and it was supposed that this position should lead to the best possible function (Fig. 4.33, 4.34).

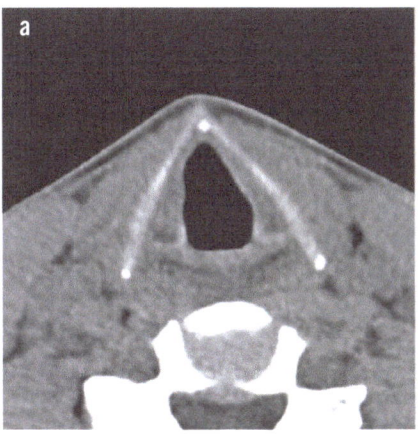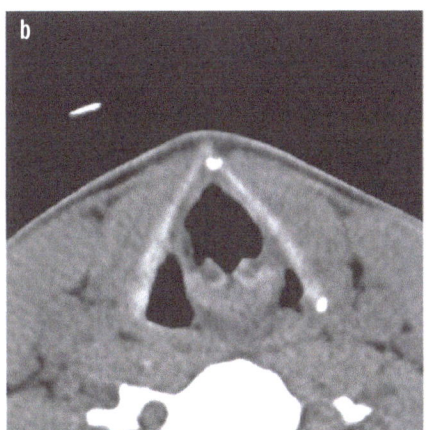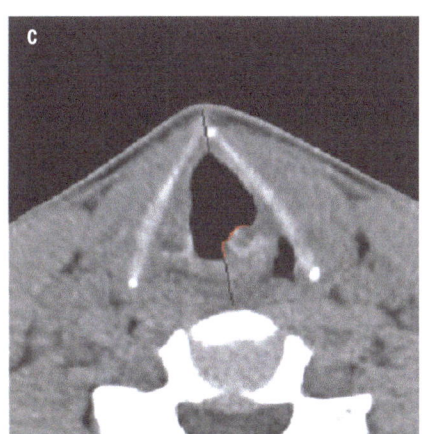

Figure 4.33. Combination of CT scan during quiet respiration and during phonation at supraglottic level a. CT during during quiet respiration. b. CT during phonation. c. Simulation of left extended hemilaryngectomy with replacement of the resected hemilarynx by the left hemilarynx during phonation. The free margin of the arytenoid during phonation (red line) forms the optimal position for the reconstructive tissue at the supraglottic level.

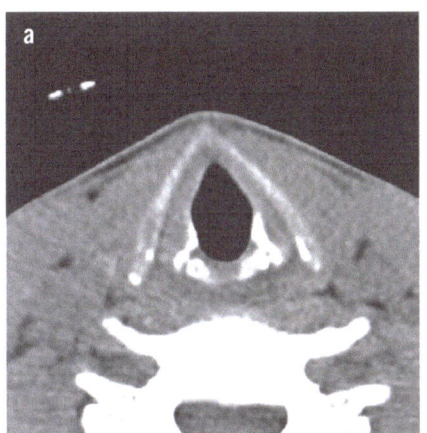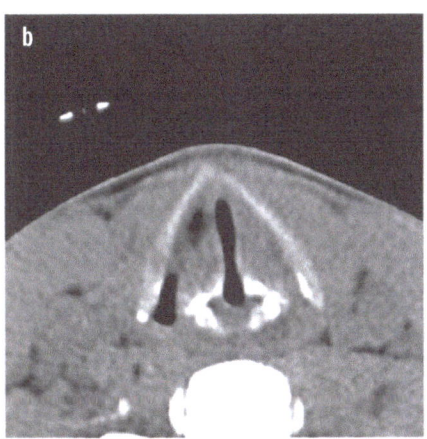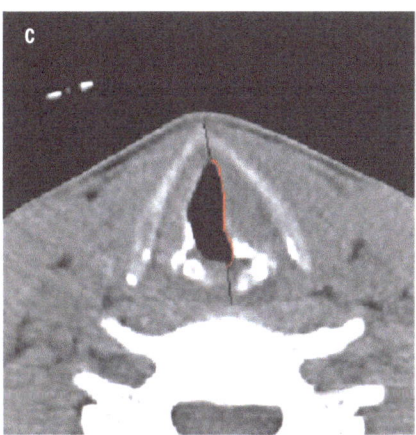

Figure 4.34. Combination of CT scan during quiet respiration and during phonation at glottic level a. CT during during quiet respiration. Axial section at glottic level of normal CT scan during quiet respiration. b. CT during phonation. c. Simulation of left extended hemilaryngectomy with replacement of the resected hemilarynx by the left hemilarynx during phonation. The free margin of the vocal fold during phonation (red line) forms the optimal position for the reconstructive tissue at the glottic level.

The optimal position for the reconstruction after extended hemilaryngectomy was defined for the subglottic, glottic, and supraglottic level:
° The optimal place for the reconstructive tissue in the **subglottic region** is formed by the internal site of the original airway lumen- the calibre of the airway is the important factor in the subglottic region.

°The free margin of the vocal fold visible on a phonation CTscan forms the optimal place for the reconstructive tissue at the **glottic level**.
°At the **supraglottic level**, the reconstruction has to allow for posterior closure at the level of the arytenoid. Providing posterior bulk in the region of the resected arytenoid will be important during reconstruction.

The radiological position of the free margin of the vocal fold on the CTscan during phonation was defined as the optimal position for the reconstructive tissue. A graphical model to find this 'optimal position' was constructed using the glottic gaps as visible on the CT scan taken during quiet respiration and during phonation (Fig. 4.35). The graphical model was constructed by using the mean values of 5 normal male larynges taken during quiet breathing and during phonation. The graphical model was used to evaluate the larynx after reconstruction and to link the morphological data to data of respiratory and sphincteric function.

The position of the points A, M, B, I, II, III, and IV and the angle of the lines (expressed in degrees in relation to the sagittal plane) A-I, A-II, A-III, and A-IV were defined on the CT scans (during quiet respiration and phonation) of 5 normal males. The images were stacked as layers in Adobe Photoshop in order to match the pre- and postoperative images. The glottic gap during phonation was projected within the glottic gap during respiration at the same axial level.

Figure 4.35. Morphologic definition of optimal position of tracheal transplant at glottic level.
a. CT scan during quiet respiration. Axial section at glottic level of normal CT scan during quiet respiration.
b. CT scan during phonation. Axial section at glottic level of normal CT scan during phonation. The patient vocalizes the vowel /i/ during the scanning procedure (6 seconds). On the CT scans during phonation, a small gap remains between the free edges of the vocal folds due to the specific vibration pattern of the vocal folds. The smallest gap exists at the transition between the membranous and the cartilaginous site of the vocal fold (arrows). The free margin of the vocal fold is defined as the optimal position for the tracheal transplant.
c. CT scan during quiet breathing. The glottic gap visible on the CTscan during phonation is projected on the CT image during quiet respiration. Matching was done on the anterior-posterior midline and the anterior commissure which were projected over each other. The thick white line represents the optimal position of the reconstructive tissue after a left sided hemilaryngectomy (='optimal position' for tracheal transplant). Compared to the situation during quiet breathing, the anterior-posterior diameter of the glottic gap showed a lengthening of 9.5 % during phonation (double arrow). R=right; L=left.
d. Image-based optimal reconstruction model.
Schematic presentation of the glottic gap during quiet respiration and the glottic gap during phonation projected over each other. The following reference lines and points are drawn:

- The anterior-posterior midline (AC = anterior commissure; PC = posterior commissure on CT during quiet respiration).
- Horizontal line dividing the glottic gap (of CT during quiet respiration) into a posterior gap and into an anterior gap (Length AC-M= 2/3 length M-PC).
R = contact point with free margin of right vocal fold during quiet respiration.
L = contact point with free margin of left vocal fold during quiet respiration.
M = contact point with anterior-posterior midline.
A = contact point with free margin of right vocal fold during phonation.
B = contact point with free margin of left vocal fold during phonation.
I=contact point of glottic gap during phonation with glottic gap of CT scan during quiet respiration on right anterior site.
II = contact point of glottic gap during phonation with glottic gap of CT scan during quiet respiration on left anterior site.
III = contact point of glottic gap during phonation with glottic gap of CT scan during quiet respiration on left posterior site.
IV = contact point of glottic gap during phonation with glottic gap of CT scan during quiet respiration on right posterior site.
Line A-I= line connecting point A with point I.
Line B-II= line connecting point B with point II.
Line B-III= line connecting point B with point III.
Line A-IV= line connecting point A with point IV.

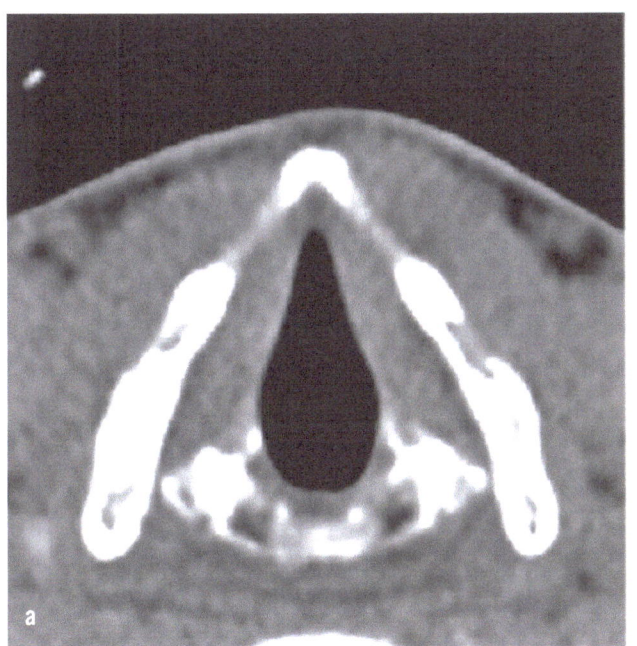

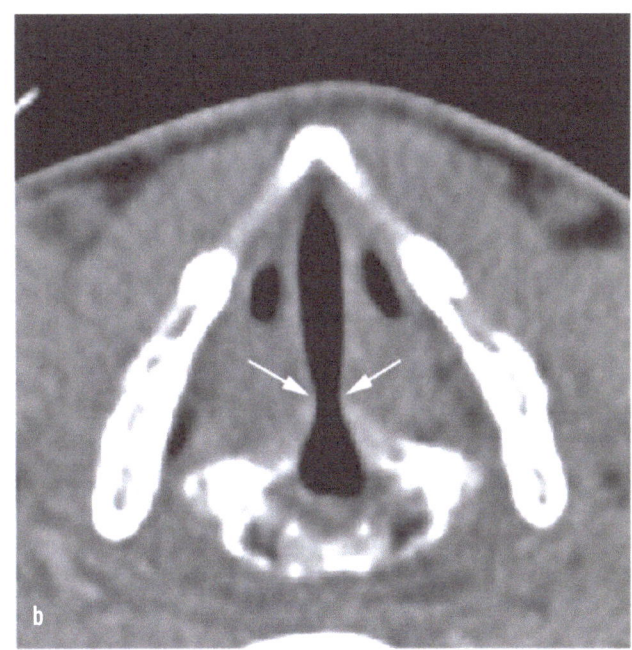

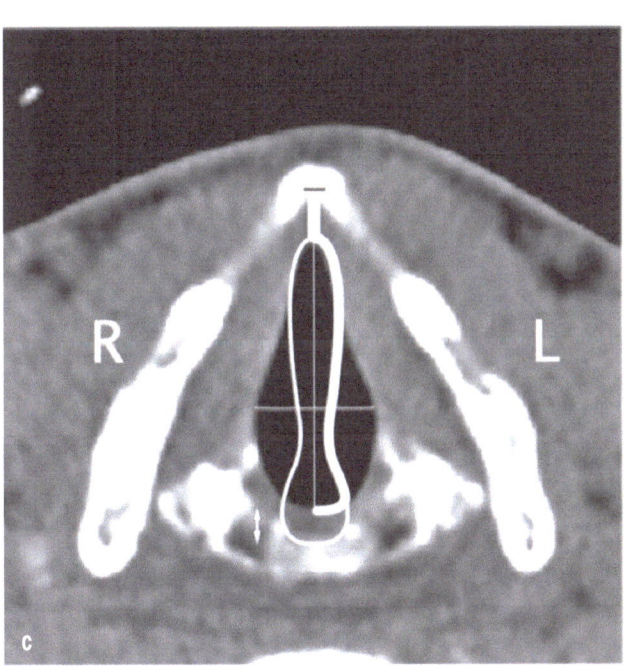

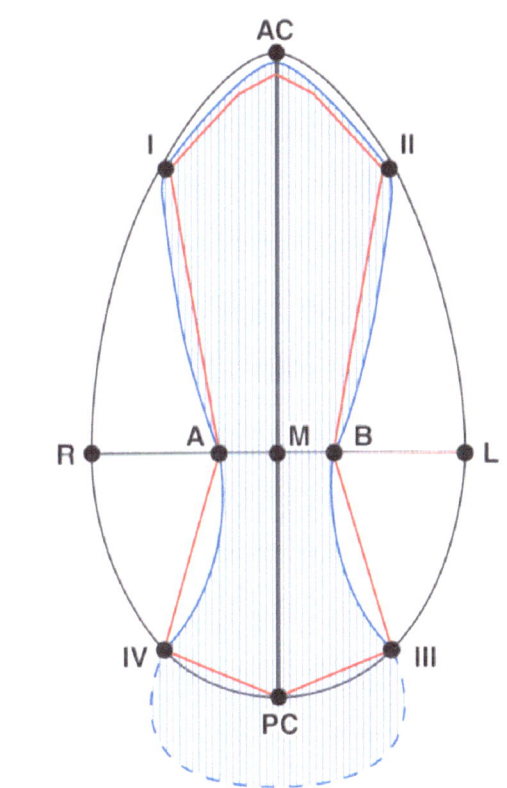

From these digitalized images, the quantitative measures were calculated. The purpose was to develop an image-based model and to determine the 'optimal position' for the reconstructive tissue in each individual patient using the healthy hemi-laynx before operation. The anterior-posterior diameter of the glottic gap showed a lengthening of 9.5 % (mean-SD=5.0) during phonation. The narrowest area of the glottic gap during phonation (points A and B) was located at the tip of the arytenoid cartilages at the transition between cartilaginous and membranous vocal fold (Fig. 4.35). The mean, relative values for points A and B were: length of AM= 25.2 % length RM (SD=4.3) and length of BM=27.2 % length LM (SD=5.6). One relative value (= 26% of length of RM or LM) for the points A and B was adopted to be used in the graphical model.

The angle of the lines A-I, B-II, B-III, and A-IV was expressed in degrees in relation to the sagittal plane. The mean values for the 5 larynges were: A-I= 8.6° (SD= 2.4); B-II= 6.8° (SD= 2.9); B-III= 9.6°

(SD= 3.3); A-IV= 8.8° (SD= 2.8) abduction. One value for the 4 lines was adopted to be used in the graphical model: 8° abduction in relation to the sagittal plane.

These 2 values (26% and 8°) enabled us to determine the 'optimal position' for the reconstructive tissue in an approximative and relatively easy way on the preoperative CT scan of each patient. The 'optimal position' was calculated on the hemilarynx opposite the tumor as visible on the axial CT scan at the glottic level before operation (Fig 4.36 a).

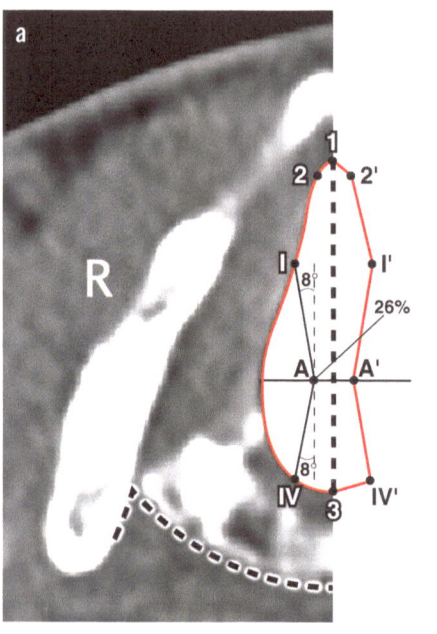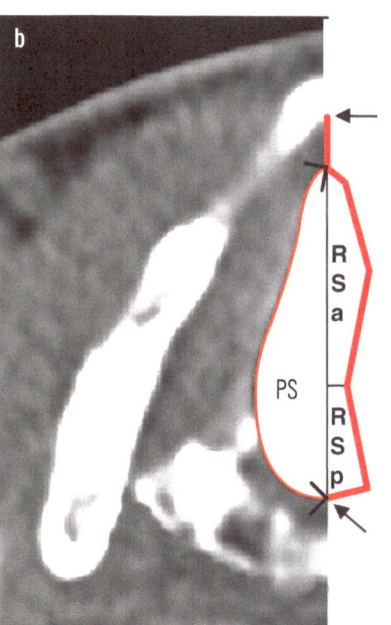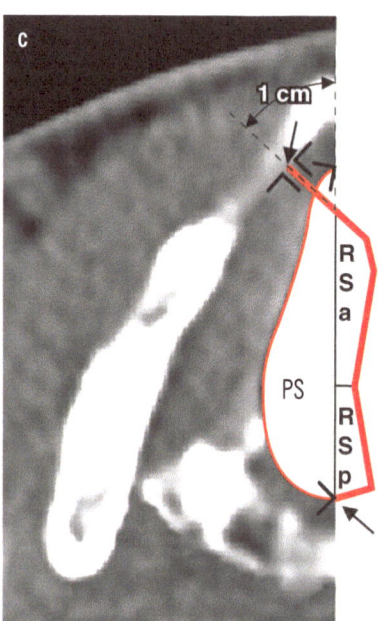

Figure 4.36. Graphical model for 'optimal position' of tracheal transplant at glottic level.
a. Graphical model to find the 'optimal position'. Simulation of left hemilaryngectomy defect on preoperative CT scan. The 'optimal position' for the tracheal autotransplant is determined on the CT scan during quiet respiration. Measurements are made on the intact (right=R) hemilarynx.
Point A=26 % of distance RM; A-I=8°; A-IV=8° abduction related to sagittal plane.
Line 1-2-I follows the anterior site of the right vocal fold.
Line I-A-IV follows the lines I-A and A-IV.
Line IV-3 follows the posterior site of the right vocal fold.
Line 1-2-I-A-IV-3 is reflected to the left side. The reflec-

tion line 1-2'-I'-A'-IV'-3 forms the 'optimal position' for the reconstructive tissue at the tumor side.
The anterior-posterior midline (dotted line) and the line that circumscribes the thyroid and cricoid cartilage posteriorly (dotted line) will be used to match the pre- and postoperative images and to compare the optimal position with the actual position after operation.
b. Model with anterior section line in anterior commissure.
Thick red line indicates the 'optimal position' for the tracheal transplant. The mean length of the intact vocal fold between anterior and posterior commissure (between open arrows) is 25.4 mm (SD=1.1 mm). The mean length of the tracheal autotransplant measured

between the anterior and the posterior section line (between full arrow) is 28.2 mm (SD=1.4 mm). RSa= surface area of resected side anteriorly; RSp= surface area of resected side posteriorly; PS=surface area of preserved side.

c. Model with resection of anterior commissure.

Thick red line indicates 'optimal position' for tracheal patch after resection of anterior commissure. A segment of 1 cm of the contralateral thyroid cartilage is resected with the anterior commissure. The line placed perpendicular to the thyroid cartilage at the place of resection forms the anterior boundary of the glottic gap. The mean length of the intact vocal fold between anterior and posterior commissure (between open arrows) is 25.4 mm (SD=1.1 mm). The mean length of the tracheal autotransplant measured between the anterior and the posterior section line (between full arrow) is 27.3 mm (SD=1.5 mm). RSa= surface area of resected side anteriorly; RSp = surface area of resected side posteriorly; PS=surface area of preserved side.

Figure 4.36 b shows the calculated 'optimal position' for the reconstructive tissue with the anterior section line placed in the anterior commissure (for glottic tumors with posterior localization or for pyriform sinus tumors). The mean length of the calculated reconstruction between anterior and posterior section line is 28.2 mm. The glottic gap is

divided in a preserved side and a reconstructed side by the anterior-posterior midline. The reconstructed side is divided in an anterior and in a posterior part by the line M-B. To approach the optimal position, it will be necessary to include a tracheal patch with the same length between the anterior and the posterior section margin. The position of the tracheal patch is visible as a green line in figure 4.37 a. A tracheal transplant with the optimal length will give a RSp value nearly similar to the RSp value of the calculated 'optimal position' (red line) while the RSa value will be larger than the RSa value of the calculated 'optimal position' due to the curvature of the trachea (Fig. 4.37 a).

Figure 4.36 c shows the calculated 'optimal position' for the reconstructive tissue for cases with inclusion of the anterior commissure in the resection (for glottic tumors reaching the anterior commissure). A segment of 1 cm of the contralateral thyroid cartilage and vocal fold is resected with the tumor. The line perpendicular on the thyroid cartilage forms the anterior margin of the glottic gap after reconstruction. The mean length of the

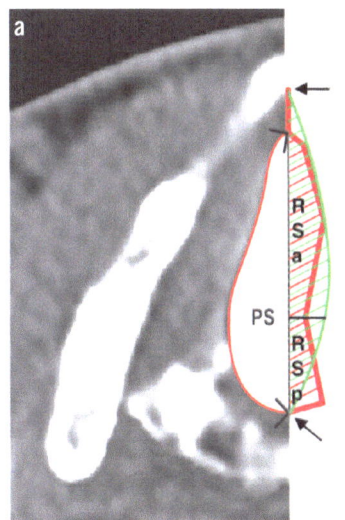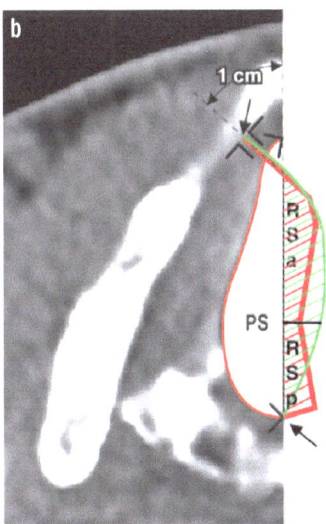

Figure 4.37. Tracheal autotransplant with optimal length at glottic level- Case of glottic competence.

a. Section line in anterior commissure. The tracheal patch has a length of 28.2 mm (similar as calculated reconstruction). The RSp value of the tracheal patch (green line) is similar to the RSp value of the optimal position (red line). The RSa value of the tracheal patch (green line) is larger than the RSa value of the optimal position (red line).

b. Section with inclusion of anterior commissure. The tracheal patch has a length of 27.3 mm (similar as calculated reconstruction). The RSp value of the tracheal patch (green line) is similar to the RSp value of the optimal position (red line). The RSa value of the tracheal patch (green line) is larger than the RSa value of the optimal position (red line).

calculated reconstruction between anterior and posterior section line is 27.3 mm. The glottic gap is divided in a preserved side and a reconstructed side by the anterior-posterior midline. The reconstructed side is divided in an anterior and in a posterior part by the line M-B.

To approach the optimal position, it will be necessary to include a tracheal patch with the same length between the anterior and the posterior section margin. The position of the tracheal patch is visible as a green line in figure 4.37 b. A tracheal transplant with the optimal length will give a RSp value nearly similar to the RSp value of the calculated 'optimal position' (red line) while the RSa value will be larger than the RSa value of the calculated 'optimal position' due to the curvature of the trachea. After reconstruction, the glottic gap may be divided in a 'preserved side=PS' and in a 'reconstructed side=RS'. The reconstructed side may be divided in an anterior (RSa) and in a posterior (RSp) part. The surface areas of the calculated 'optimal situation' (determined on the CTscan at the glottic level before operation-indicated by red line) may be compared with the surface areas of the actual situation visible on the CT scan after operation at the same axial level (indicated by green line). The reconstruction is evaluated as being **glottic competent** if the surface area of the posterior glottic gap, visible at the reconstructed side, is similar or smaller than the surface area of the glottic gap (RSp) in the calculated 'optimal situation' (Fig. 4.37). The recon-

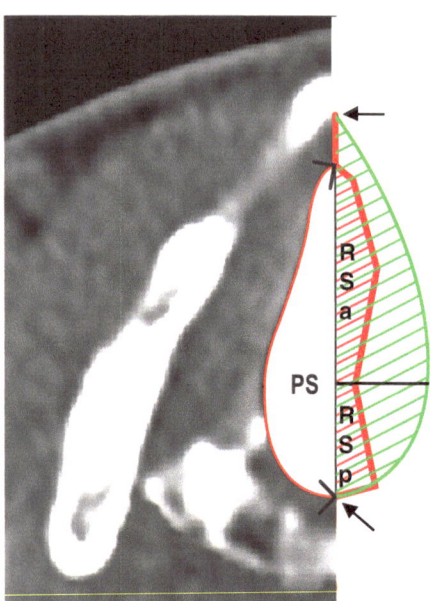
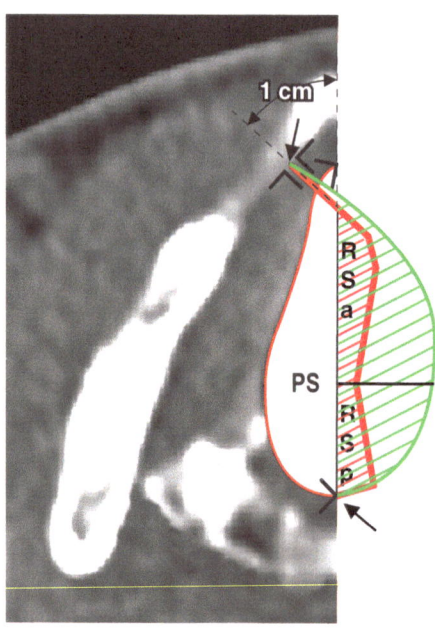

Figure 4.38.
Tracheal autotransplant that is too long at glottic level- Case of glottic incompetence.

a. Section line in anterior commissure. The tracheal patch is longer than the length of the calculated reconstruction (28.2 mm). The RSp value of the tracheal patch (green line) is larger than the RSp value of the optimal position (red line). The RSa value of the tracheal patch (green line) is larger than the RSa value of the optimal position (red line).

b. Section with inclusion of anterior commissure. The tracheal patch is longer than the length of the calculated reconstruction (27.3 mm). The RSp value of the tracheal patch (green line) is larger than the RSp value of the optimal position (red line). The RSa value of the tracheal patch (green line) is larger than the RSa value of the optimal position (red line).

struction is evaluated as being '**glottic incompetent**' if the surface area of the posterior, reconstructed side is larger than the posterior reconstructed side (RSp) in the calculated 'optimal situation' (Fig. 4.38). The glottic gap is divided in an anterior and in a posterior part because a posterior glottic gap is more detrimental for the

> **Table 4.3. Determination of optimal position for reconstructive tissue after extended hemilaryngectomy**
>
> - On preoperative CT scan during quiet respiration.
> - On hemilarynx opposite to the tumor.
> - Position of arytenoid point during phonation: 74 % medialized compared to arytenoid point during respiration.
> - Slope of glottic gap during phonation starting from most medialized point: 8° abduction.

sphincteric function than an anterior glottic gap. This graphical model can be constructed on the preoperative CT scan of each individual patient and the optimal reconstruction can be compared with the actual situation after projection within the postreconstructive CT scan at the same axial level (Table 4.3).

2. F.3. Morphometrical and functional evaluation of initial patient series

In the initial patient series, the radiological morphology of the reconstruction was compared with the optimal image-based model and was compared to the level of laryngeal functioning of each patient. Morphometry of the reconstruction could be assessed on the CTscan of 32 patients. Eight patients could not be evaluated (early tumor recurrence, definitive tracheostomy).

On a morphometrical and functional base, the postoperative situation was divided into 3 groups (Table 4.4):

-Laryngeal competence (N=11).

-Laryngeal incompetence with compensation (N=17). In this group, patients succeeded in swallowing of solids and liquids.

-Laryngeal incompetence-without compensation (N=4). In this group, patients had problems with swallowing of solids or liquids.

Table 4.4. Morphometrical data of initial patient series

Group	Length Vocal Fold (mm) (±SD)	Length Patch (mm) (±SD) Glottic Level	Length Patch (mm) (±SD) Subglottic Level	RSa (%Calculated Preoperative) Quiet Respiration (±SD)	RSp (%Calculated Preoperative) Quiet Respiration (±SD)
1. Competent N=11	28.4 (1.2)	25.4 (2.6)	40.6 (3.4)	112.7 (31.2)	52.6 (30.3)
2. Incompetent - Compensated N=17	27.2 (1.0)	32.8 (1.5)	41.5 (1.7)	382.5 (56.0)	139.5 (25.9)
3. Incompetent - Not Compensated N=4	27.4 (1.4)	34.3 (3.2)	42.2 (0.8)	371.0 (40.4)	151.7 (18.5)

The most extensive surface area augmentation in the groups with an incompetent reconstruction is for the RSa value.

2.F.3.a. Laryngeal competence

Morphometrical data of this patient group were characterized by:

-A patch length comparable to the optimal length at the glottic level.

-An anterior glottic gap (RSa) comparable to the calculated value in the optimal model.

-A posterior glottic gap (RSp) which is similar or smaller than the calculated value in the optimal model.

Morphometrical characteristics of a patient with glottic competence is visible in Fig. 4.39.

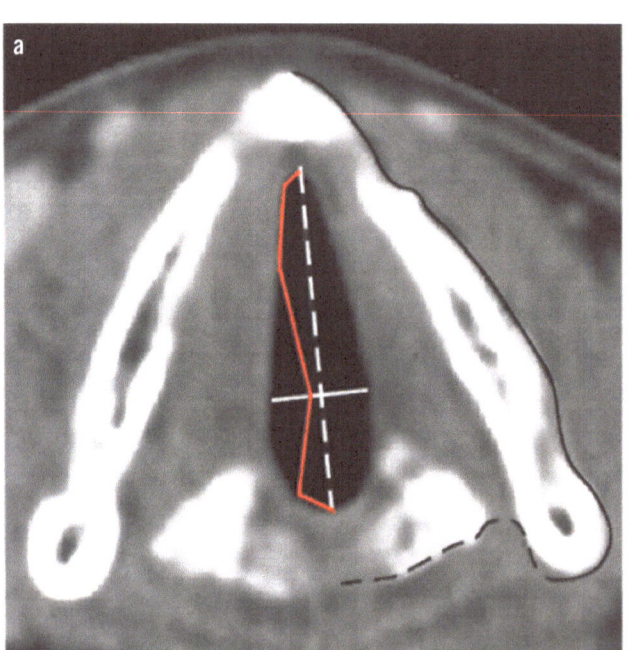

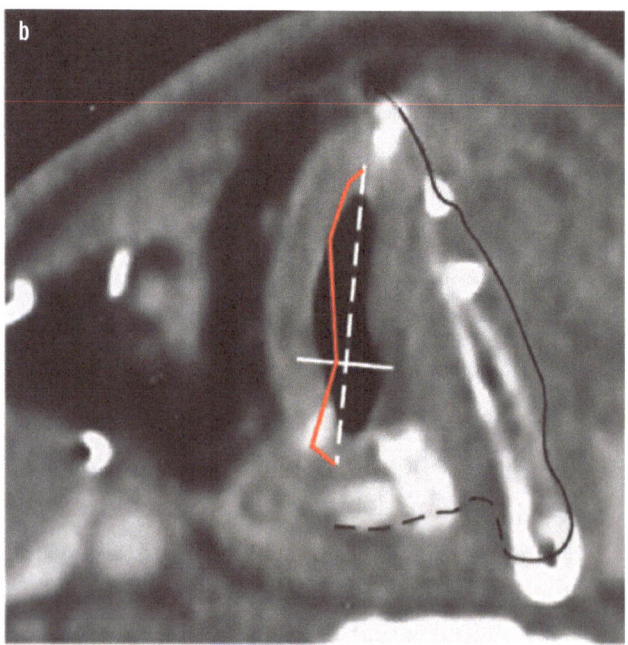

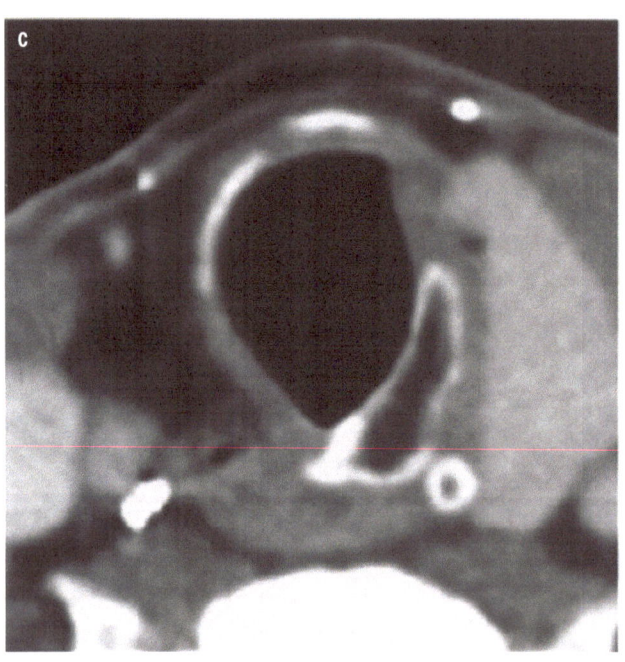

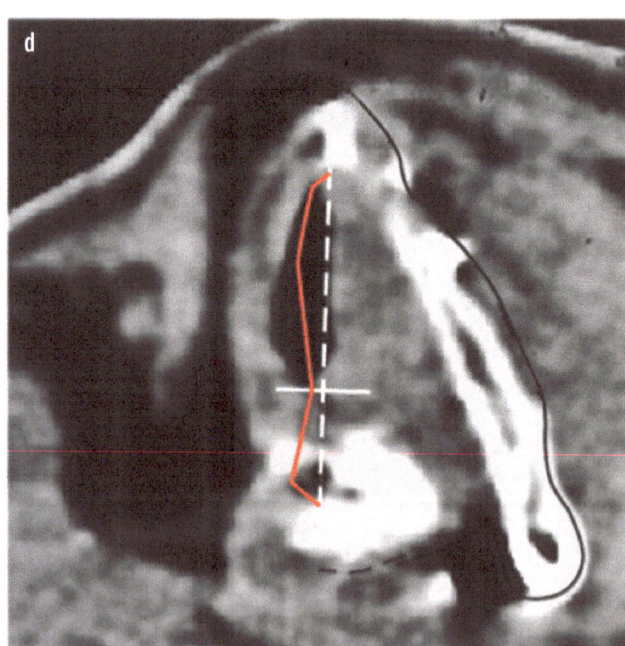

Figure 4.39. Morphometrical evaluation of larynx reconstruction-Case of glottic competence.
a.Axial CT scan at glottic level before operation. Extended hemilaryngectomy with placement of the anterior section line in the anterior commissure (tumor without extension to the anterior site of the vocal fold). The 'optimal position' for the tracheal transplant is indicated with a red line. The 'optimal position' will be projected on the postoperative CT scan at the same axial level. The anterior-posterior midline (white dotted line) and the line that circumscribes the thyroid and cricoid cartilage posteriorly (black dotted line) are used to match the pre- and postoperative CT images.
b.Axial CT scan (during quiet respiration) at glottic level after operation. The 'optimal position' is projected. The anterior-posterior midline (white dotted line) and the line that circumscribes the thyroid and cricoid cartilage posteriorly (black dotted line) are used to match the pre- and postoperative CT images. The length of the patch between anterior and posterior commissure= 27.2 mm.
c. Axial CT scan at subglottic level after operation. A tracheal segment with a length of 37 mm (full amount of cartilage ring) is included to optimally restore the subglottic airway lumen.
d. Axial CT scan (during phonation) at glottic level after operation. The 'optimal position' is projected. The anterior-posterior midline (white dotted line) and the line that circumscribes the thyroid and cricoid cartilage posteriorly (black dotted line) are used to match the pre- and postoperative CT images. The arytenoid shows a medial rotation with complete obliteration of the RSp and PS surface areas.

Within the group of laryngeal competence, the mean length of the reconstructive tissue at the glottic level was 25.4 mm (SD=2.6).

Reconstructions in this group were evaluated as being 'glottic competent' because the surface area of the glottic gap at the posterior part of the reconstructed side (RSp) was similar or smaller than the calculated 'optimal value'. Patients within this group showed good phonation and swallowing measures. Their voice could be described as 'mild

dysphonia' and they all had full oral feeding without weight loss.

The majority (21) of the patients were evaluated as morphologically 'incompetent'. The reason of the high number of glottic incompetency can be found in the low degree of elasticity of most of the tracheas and in the difference between patch length and upper mucosal section line of the laryngeal remnant (Fig. 4.40).

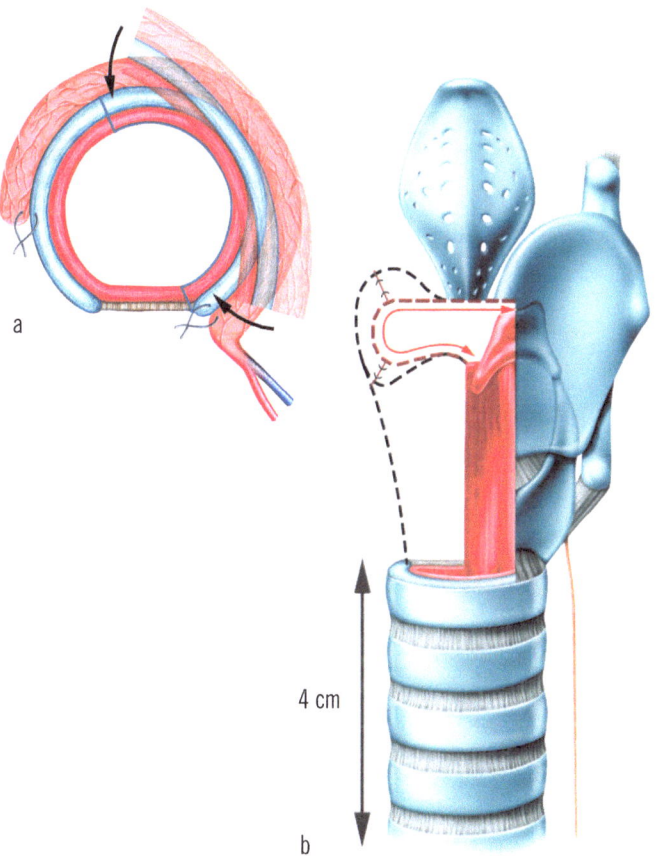

Figure 4.40.
Reason for high number of 'incompetency' after reconstruction.
a. The lower the elasticity of the trachea the more difficult it can be brought in a stretched position. The stretched patch has the tendency to retake the original shape (arrow).
b. The upper mucosal section line (between double arrow) measures between 5 and 6 cm. This section line has to be sutured to the upper site of the tracheal patch (optimal length less than 3 cm).

2.F.3.b. Laryngeal incompetence with compensation

Twenty one patients were evaluated as being 'incompetent at glottic level' on CT scan. Of the 21 patients, 17 patients could swallow solids and liquids without clinical signs of aspiration (they were compensated at the functional level).

Morphometrical characteristics of a patient with glottic incompetence but with compensation at the functional level is visible in Fig. 4.41 and Fig. 4.42.

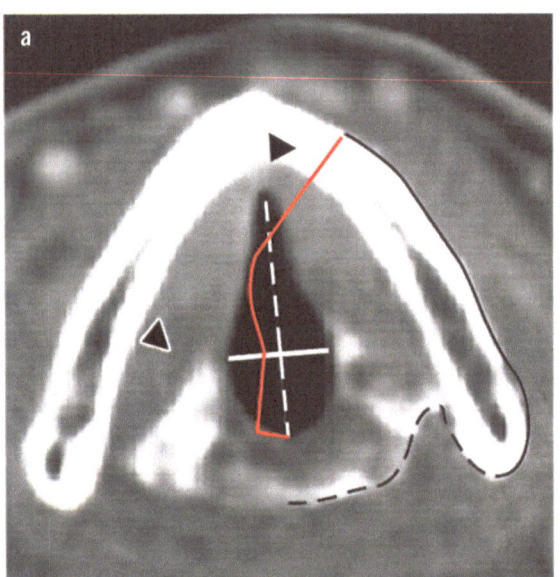
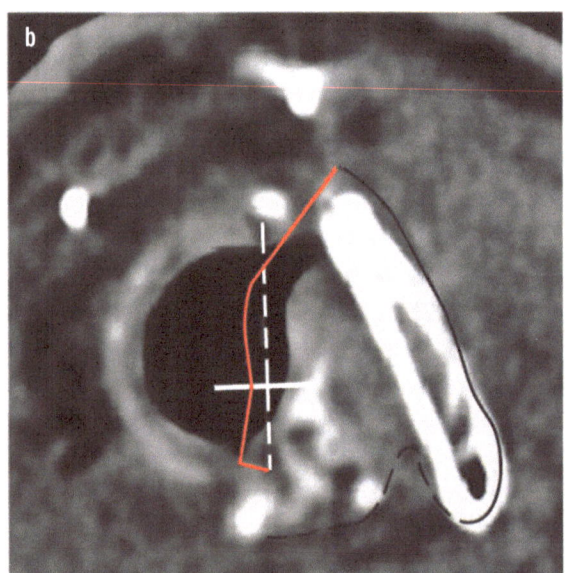
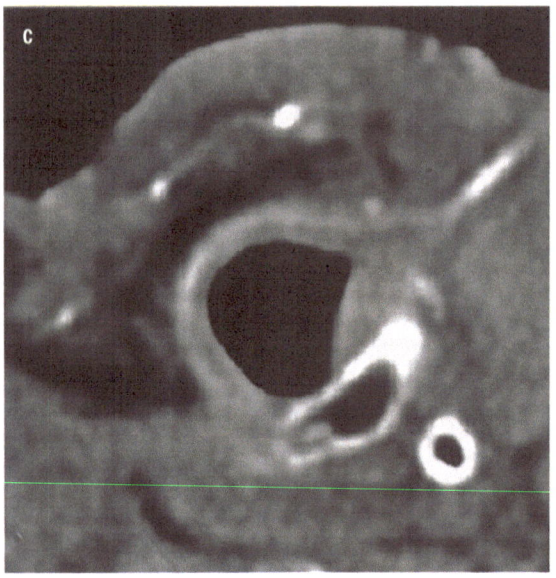
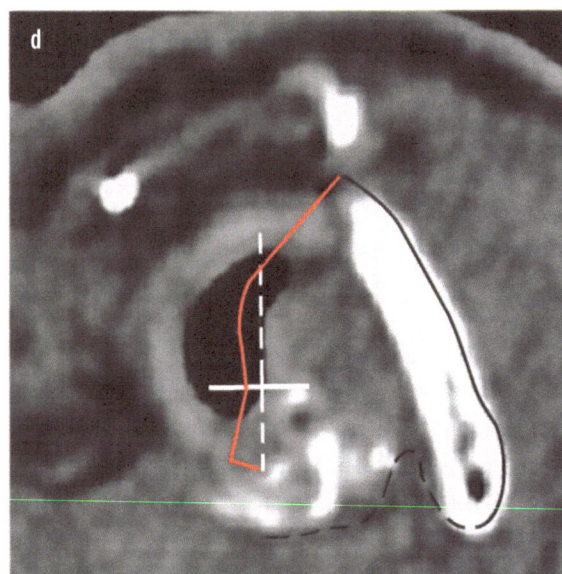

Figure 4.41.
Morphometrical evaluation of larynx reconstruction-Case 1 of glottic incompetence with compensation.
a. Axial CT scan at glottic level before operation. Tumor extension (between arrowheads) necessitated for a hemilaryngectomy with inclusion of the anterior commissure. The optimal patch position for the tracheal autotransplant is indicated with a red line. About 1 cm of the thyroid cartilage at the tumor site is resected together with the anterior commissure. The 'optimal position' will be projected on the postoperative CT scan at the same axial level. The anterior-posterior midline (white dotted line) and the line that circumscribes the thyroid and cricoid cartilage posteriorly (black dotted line) are used to match the pre- and postoperative CT images.
b. Axial CT scan (during quiet respiration) at glottic level after operation. The 'optimal position' is projected. The surface area of the glottic gap at the resected side posteriorly is larger than the preoperatively defined posterior gap (RSp). The length of the patch between anterior and posterior commissure= 32.5 mm.
c. Axial CT scan at subglottic level after operation. A tracheal segment with a length of 33 mm (full amount of cartilage ring) is included to optimally restore the subglottic airway lumen.
d. Axial CT scan (during phonation) at glottic level after operation. The 'optimal position' is projected. The arytenoid shows a medial rotation with a nearly complete obliteration of the RSp and PS surface areas. A gap remains anteriorly.

The patient presented in Fig. 4.41 is glottic incompetent because the RSp is larger than calculated. The patient showed a breathy voice and a swallowing function without clinical signs of aspiration (normal swallow for solids and liquids). Good compensatory closure at the posterior larynx (nearly complete obliteration of the RSp surface area) could explain the intact sphincteric function.

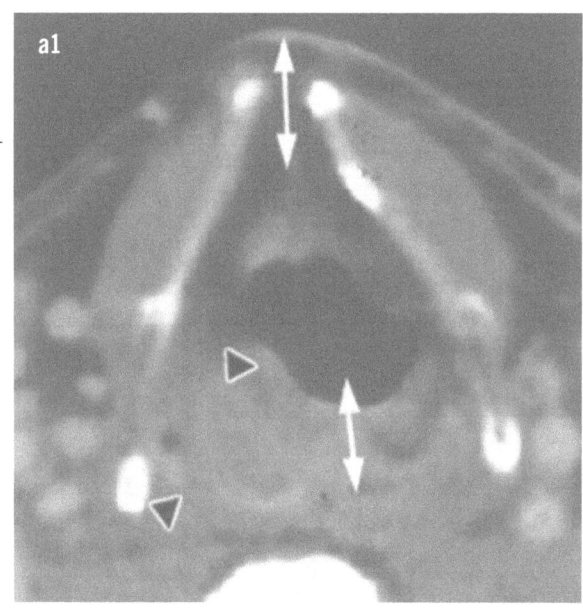

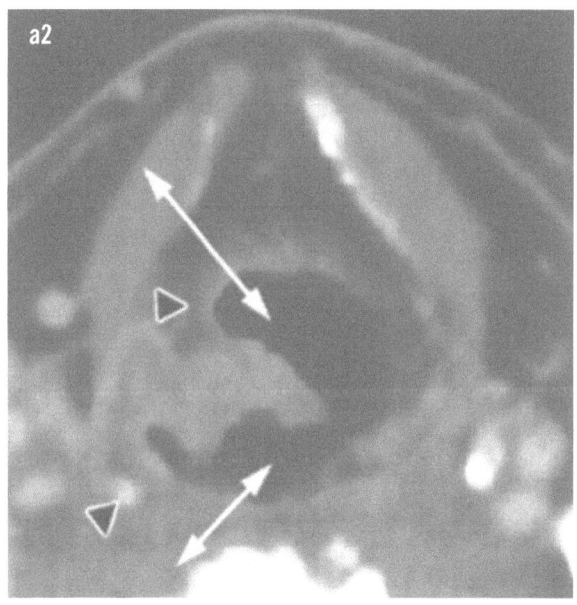

Figure 4.42.
Morphometrical evaluation of larynx reconstruction-Case 2 of glottic incompetence with compensation.
a. Axial CT scan before operation.
a1. Supraglottic level.
a.2. Supraglottic level.
Tumor extension (between arrowheads) in this patient necessitated for a hemilaryngectomy with inclusion of the right pyriform sinus.

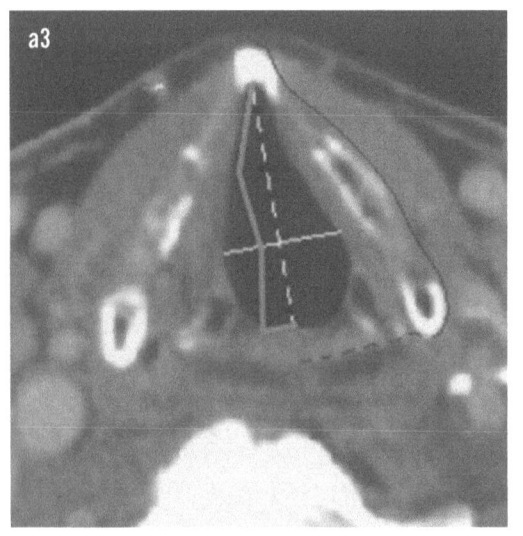
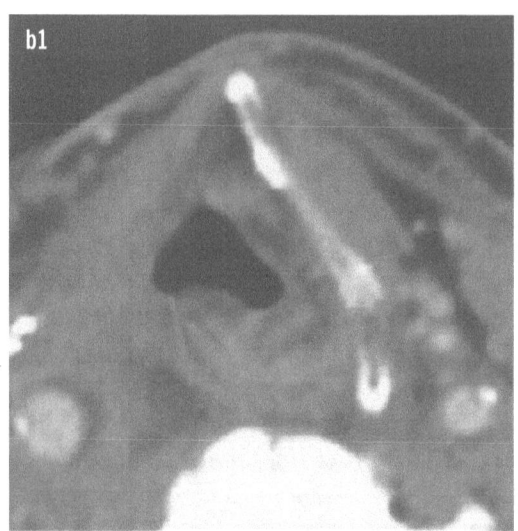
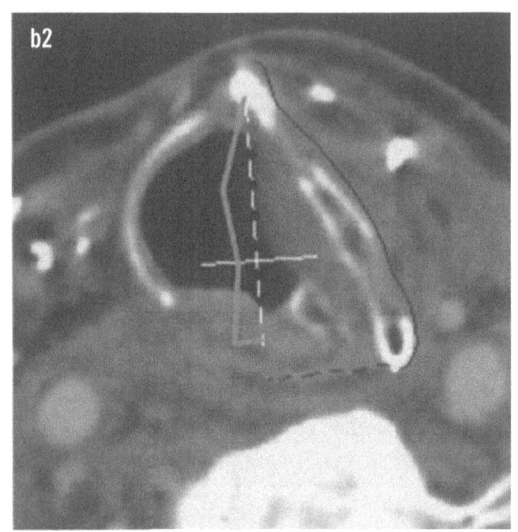
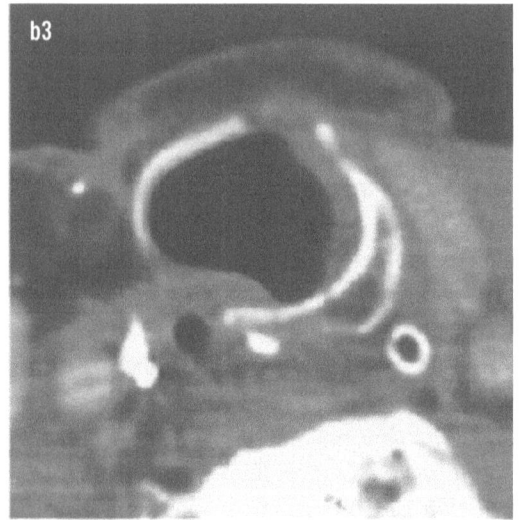
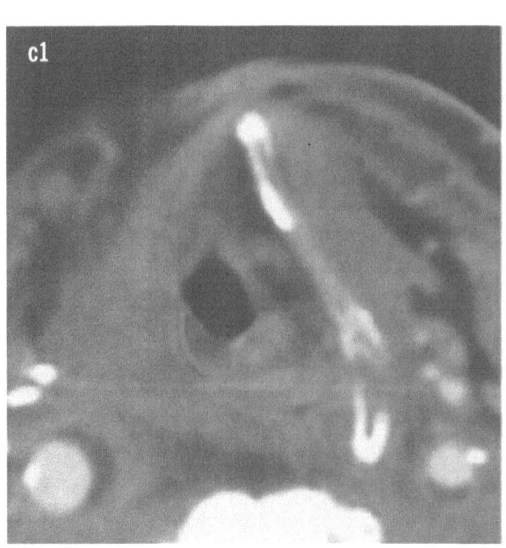
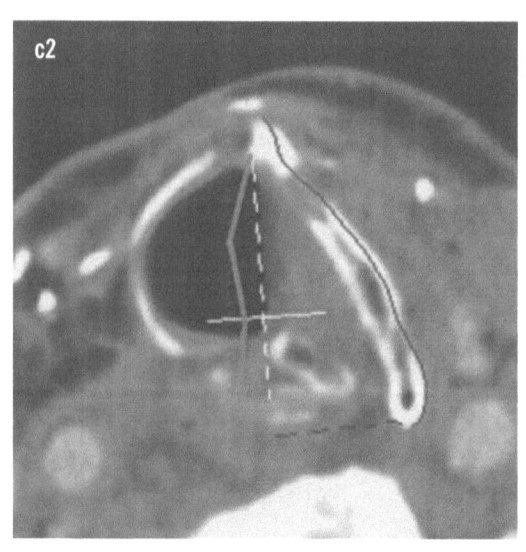

Figure 4.42.
Morphometrical evaluation of larynx reconstruction-Case 2 of glottic incompetence with compensation (continued).
a3. Glottic level. The optimal patch position for the tracheal autotransplant is indicated with a red line (a.3). The 'optimal position' will be projected on the postoperative CT scan at the same axial level.
b. Axial CT scan (during quiet respiration) after operation.
b1. Bulk (red line) in the region of the resected arytenoid is provided.
b2. Glottic level.
The 'optimal position' is projected. The surface area of the glottic gap at the resected side posteriorly is larger than the preoperatively defined posterior gap (RSp). The length of the patch between anterior and posterior commissure= 33.8 mm.
b3. Subglottic level. A tracheal segment with a length of 34 mm (full amount of cartilage ring) is included to optimally restore the subglottic airway lumen.
c. Axial CT scan during phonation after operation.
c1. Supraglottic level. The larynx is closed posteriorly (red line).
c2. Glottic level. The 'optimal position' is projected. The arytenoid shows a medial rotation with a nearly complete obliteration of the RSp and PS (preserved site) surface area. A gap remains at the reconstructed site anteriorly.

The patient presented in Fig. 4.42 is glottic incompetent because the RSp is larger than calculated. The patient showed a breathy-aphonic voice and a swallowing function without clinical signs of aspiration (normal swallow for solids and liquids). Good compensatory closure at the posterior larynx (nearly complete obliteration of the RSp surface area) could explain the intact sphincteric function. Compensatory closure is also seen at the supraglottic level (Fig. 4.42 c1).

Within the group of 'compensated laryngeal incompetence', the mean length of the reconstructive tissue at the glottic level was 32.8 mm (SD=1.5). All patients within this group had full oral feeding (solids and liquids) without weight loss and without pulmonary infection. The voice was characterized as 'mild dysphonia' in 5 patients; 12 patients showed an 'aphonic voice'. The reason for the difference between the morphometrical defined incompetency and the relatively intact sphincteric function may be found in compensatory closing mechanisms during speech and swallowing. Compensatory closure during phonation is seen at the glottic level posteriorly and at the supraglottic level. The gap at the reconstructed site anteriorly (RSa) needs protection by compensatory closing mechanisms at the supraglottic level. It is well known that glottic insufficiency with severe aspiration mostly results from a deficient closure of the posterior glottis (HABAL et al. 1972, MONTGOMERY 1975). Tolerance for anterior glottic insufficiency was also reported after reconstruction of anterior laryngeal defects with the epiglottic pull down technique (TUCKER et al. 1979).

2.F.3.c. Laryngeal incompetence without compensation

Of the 21 patients described as glottic incompetent, 4 patients showed no signs of compensatory closure of the glottic gap during speech and swallowing. These patients were unable to start oral feeding or they showed signs of aspiration pneumonia. Morphometrical characteristics of a patient with glottic incompetence without compensation at the functional level is visible in Fig. 4.43.

Functionally, the patient presented in Fig. 4.43 showed an aphonic voice and he displayed periods of aspiration pneumonia. The morphological difference with the patient presented in Fig. 4.42 is the presence of posterior bulk in the region of the resected arytenoid seen in the case with functional compensation (Fig 4.42).

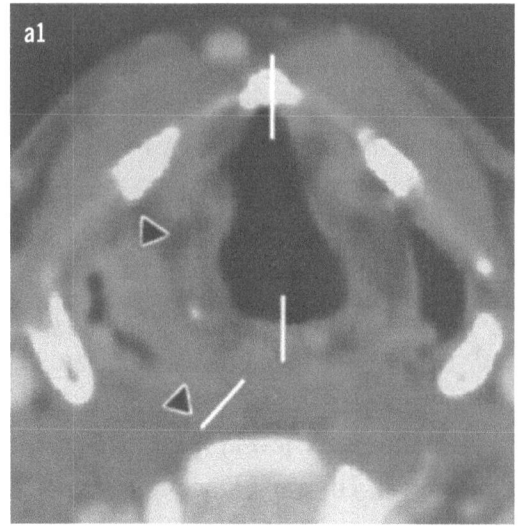

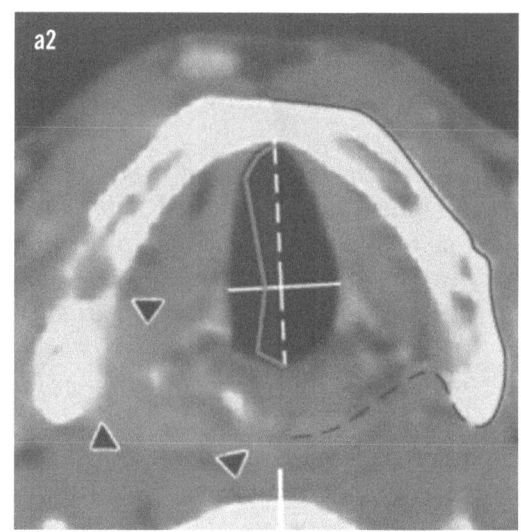

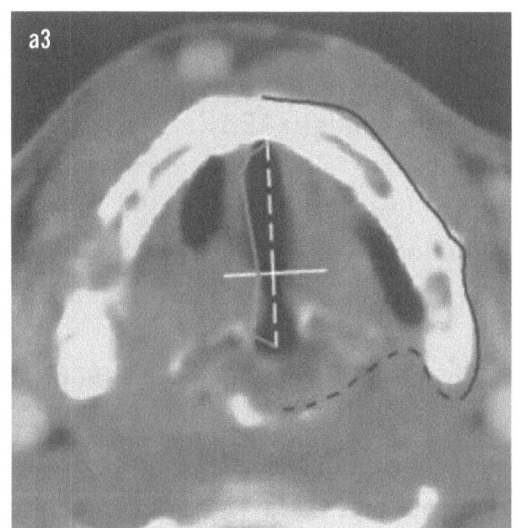

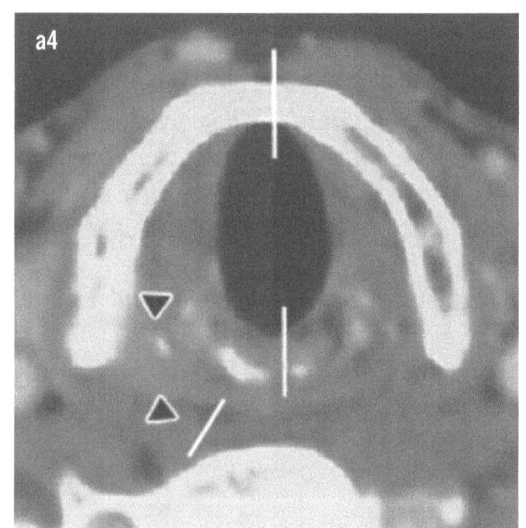

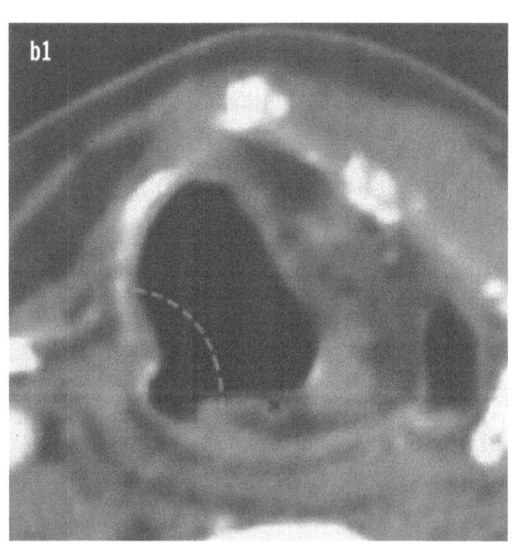

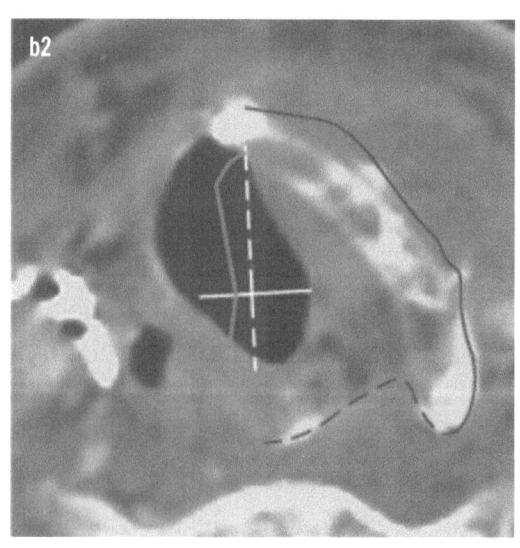

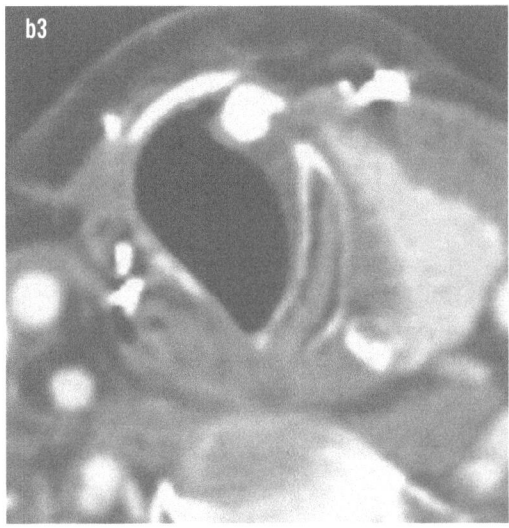

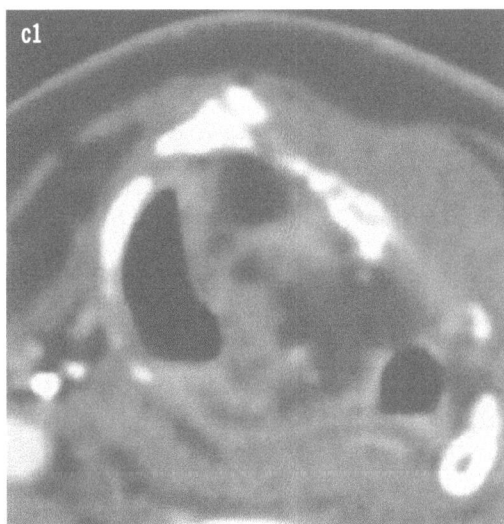

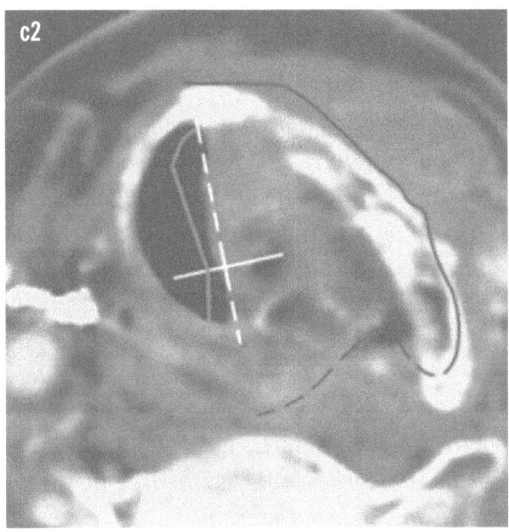

Figure 4.43.

Morphometrical evaluation of larynx reconstruction-Case of glottic incompetence without complete compensation.

a. Axial CT scan before operation.

a1. Supraglottic level.

a2. Glottic level quiet respiration.

a3. Glottic level phonation.

a4. Subglottic level.

Case with T2 cancer of pyriform sinus with extension into apex (between arrowheads). This tumor extension necessitates for a hemilaryngectomy with inclusion of the right pyriform sinus. The anterior section line is placed in the anterior commissure. The optimal patch position for the tracheal autotransplant is indicated with a red line. The 'optimal position' will be projected on the postoperative CT scan at the same axial level. The anterior-posterior midline (white dotted line) and the line that circumscribes the thyroid and cricoid cartilage posteriorly (black dotted line) are used to match the pre- and postoperative CT images. Image a.3 shows that the calculated optimal position corresponds to the free margin of the vocal fold on a phonation CT scan.

b.Axial CT scan (during quiet respiration) after operation.

b1. Supraglottic level. Absence of bulk posteriorly (desired 'bulk' is indicated by red dotted line).

b2. Glottic level. The 'optimal position' is projected. The surface area of the glottic gap at the resected side posteriorly is larger than the preoperatively defined posterior gap (RSp). The length of the patch between anterior and posterior commissure= 32.9 mm.

b.3. Subglottic level. A tracheal segment with a length of 34 mm is included to optimally restore the subglottic airway lumen.

c.Axial CT scan (during phonation) after operation.

c1. Supraglottic level.

c2. Glottic level.

The 'optimal position' is projected. The arytenoid shows a medial rotation with a complete obliteration of RS surface area. A gap remains both posteriorly (RSp) and anteriorly (RSa). This patient showed aspiration when using liquids. No posterior closure at supraglottic level.

A secondary correction was performed in 2 patients from the group without functional compensation. It was attempted to improve the sphincter function at the supraglottic level. This was done by creating bulk in the region of the resected arytenoid.

A medialization of the lateral wall at the supraglottic level was done with a small fasciocutaneous radial forearm flap taken at the remaining radial forearm donor site (Fig. 4.44, 4.45, 4.46).

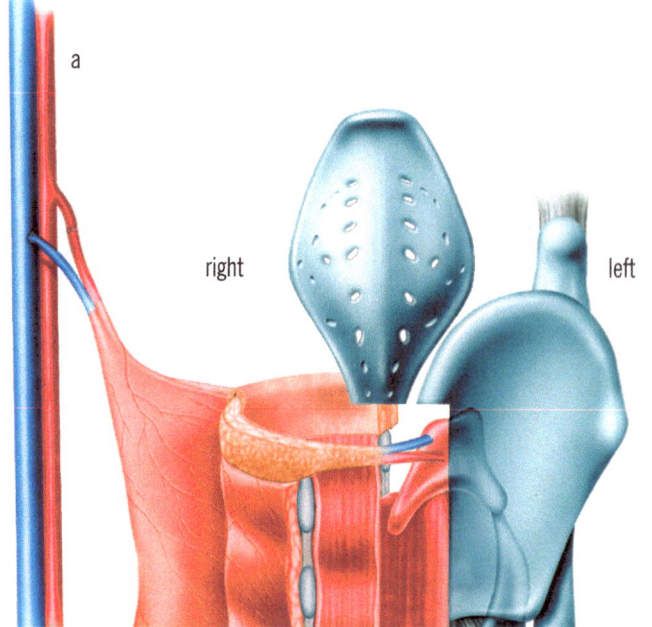

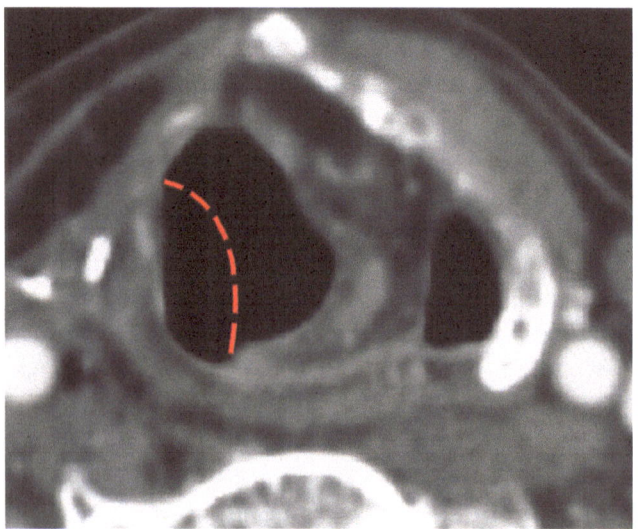

Figure 4.44.
Secondary correction by improvement of sphincteric function at supraglottic level.
CT scan at supraglottic level. Case of glottic incompetency without functional compensation. It was attempted to improve sphincteric closure at the supraglottic level by a medialization of the reconstructed lateral wall (dotted line).

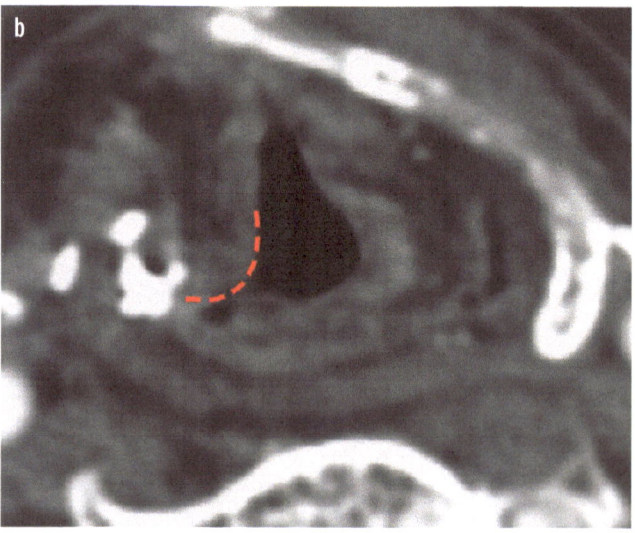

Figure 4.46.
Secondary correction by improvement of sphincteric function at supraglottic level.
a. The suture line between patch and epiglottis is reopened and a strip of radial forearm skin is inserted between patch and mucosal section line of the pyriform sinus and epiglottis. The skin flap restores the larynx at the supraglottic level. The blood vessels are anastomosed on the neck vessels opposite the reconstructed (left) site.
b. CT scan at supraglottic level. The radial forearm skin repares the supraglottic level in a position close to the midline. Posterior bulk in the area of the resected arytenoid is created (dotted line).

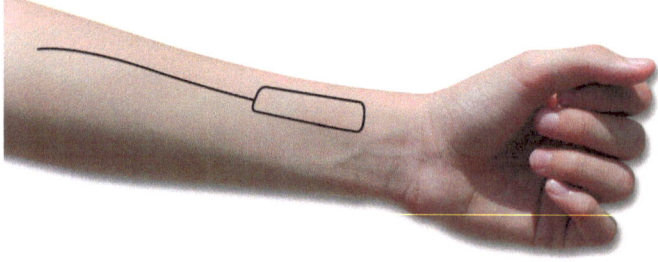

Figure 4.45.
Design of radial forearm flap for secondary correction.
A small fasciocutaneous flap (2 by 8 cm) is taken for insertion at the supraglottic level.

After secondary correction, the 2 patients were transformed from 'morphologic incompetent without compensation' into 'morphologic incompetent with compensation'.

Another possibilty in cases of glottic incompetency is to shorten the length of the patch at the glottic level and to bring the patient from group 2 into group 1 (glottic competence). This is however not always possible. Shortening of the tracheal patch may be jeopardized by a low degree of elasticity of the tracheal wall or by a long upper mucosal suture line (Fig. 4.40).

Two patients within the group of glottic incompetency without compensation were treated by shortening of the patch (Fig. 4.47). These 2 patients were unable to start oral feeding in the postoperative period after tracheal autotransplantation. Two patients were transformed into glottic competency with retake of normal oral feeding after secondary correction with shortening of the patch length.

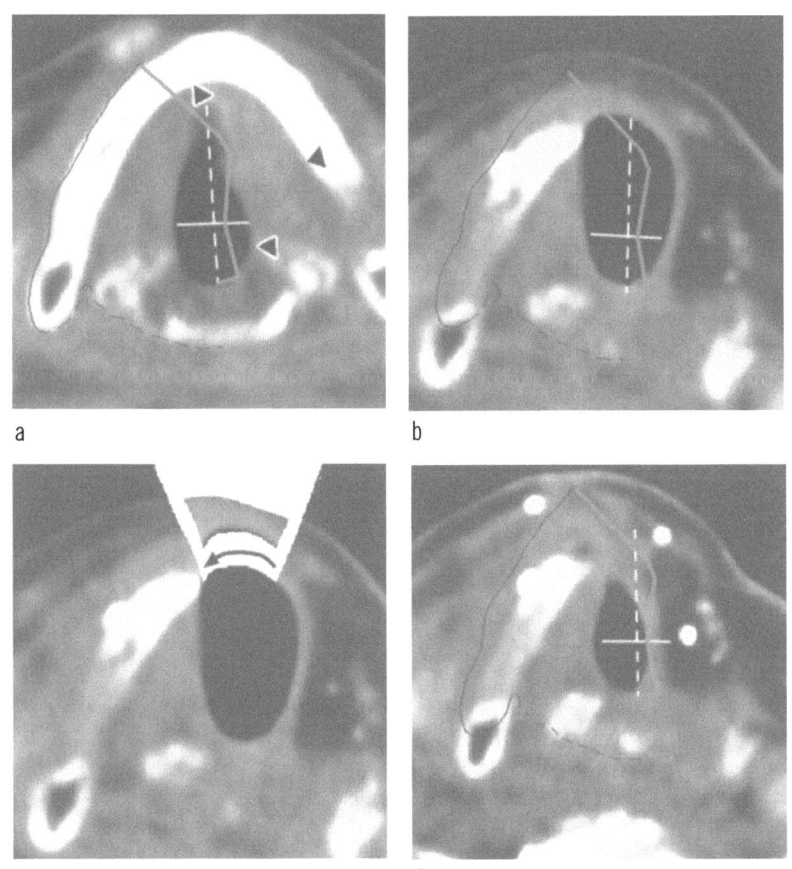

a

b

c

d

Figure 4.47.
Case of glottic incompetency with secondary correction.
a. Axial CT scan at glottic level before operation. Tumor extension (between arrowheads) in this patient necessitated for a hemilaryngectomy with inclusion of the anterior commissure. The optimal patch position for the tracheal autotransplant is indicated with a red line. About 1 cm of the thyroid cartilage at the tumor site is resected together with the anterior commissure. The 'optimal position' will be projected on the postoperative CT scan at the same axial level. The anterior-posterior midline (white dotted line) and the line that circumscribes the thyroid and cricoid cartilage posteriorly (black dotted line) are used to match the pre- and postoperative CT images.
b. Axial CT scan (during quiet respiration) at glottic level after operation. The 'optimal position' is projected. The surface area of the glottic gap at the resected side posteriorly is larger than the preoperatively defined posterior gap (RSp). The length of the patch between anterior and posterior commissure= 32.4 mm.
c. Axial CT scan (during quiet respiration) at glottic level after operation. The amount of patch that needs resection is indicated (7mm of anterior patch).
d. Axial CT scan (during quiet respiration) at glottic level after secondary correction.
The larynx reconstruction has become competent after shortening of the patch to a length of 25.4 mm.

2.F.4. Conclusion

The morphometrical and functional evaluation of the reconstructed larynges provided important information about the value of the revascularized trachea in repairing extended hemilaryngectomy defects (Table 4.5). The revascularized trachea is the ideal tissue to repair the subglottic larynx. The reconstruction can be improved in the area of the supraglottis and in the area of the glottis (Fig. 4.48). The convex shape of the trachea was too pronounced in the glottic area in 21 patients. The convexity of the tracheal patch at the glottic level resulted in a non-compensated incompetence in 4 patients because of absence of bulk in the area of the supraglottis.

Table 4.5. Morphologic and functional evaluation of reconstructed larynges	
MORPHOLOGY	FUNCTION
Competent (N = 11)	Mild dysphonia
	Full oral feeding (solids and liquids)
Incompetent-Compensated (N = 17)	Mild dysphonia (N = 5)-'breathy' voice (N = 12)
	Full oral feeding (solids and liquids)
Incompetent-Not compensated (N = 4)	'Breathy' voice-aphonia
	Aspiration for liquids
	Aspiration for solids (N = 2)

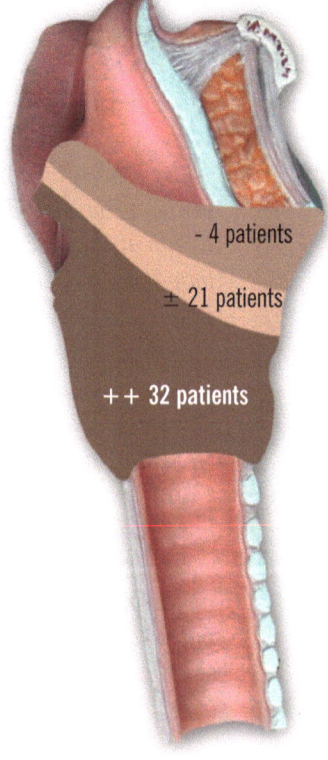

- 4 patients

± 21 patients

++ 32 patients

Figure 4.48.
Schematic presentation of reconstruction with tracheal autotransplant.
A tracheal autotransplant provides the optimal tissue to repair the larynx subglottically. More bulk in the region of the supraglottis was desired in 4 patients of our series. The glottis was not optimally repaired (convexity too pronounced) in 21 patients.

2.G. Tracheal autotransplantation after resection of transglottic cancer

Selected, unilateral transglottic cancer defined as lesions with surface presentation both above and below the entrance to the ventricle and with a fixed vocal fold may qualify for a conservation laryngectomy with tracheal autotransplantation.

In these cases, an extended hemilaryngectomy has to be combined with a supraglottic laryngectomy. Restoration of the larynx means tracheal auto-transplantation into the hemilaryngectomy defect, suspension of the reconstructed larynx to the hyoid bone, and closure between the reconstructed larynx and the mediastinal trachea (Fig. 4.49, 4.50).

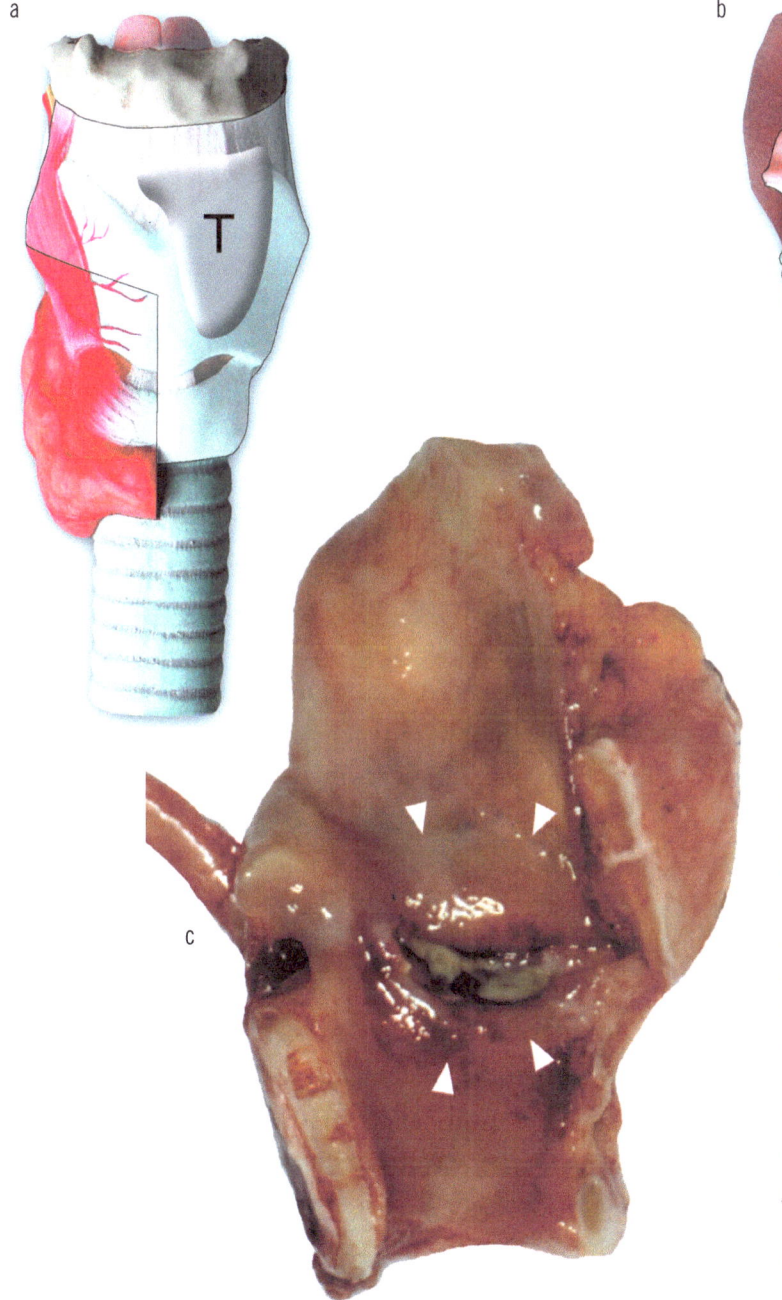

Figure 4.49.
Extent of resection for unilateral transglottic cancer.
a. Laryngeal model-anterior view. Midline sagittal section of cricoid cartilage. Combination of supraglottic laryngectomy and extended hemilaryngectomy is necessary to remove transglottic tumor (T).
b. Longitudinally incised laryngeal model showing the extent of resection. Internal view after midsagittal incision. Model showing left hemilaryngectomy defect in combination with a supraglottic laryngectomy.
c. Resection specimen after hemilaryngectomy for unilateral transglottic cancer.
Previously untreated transglottic cancer that originates in the ventricle with extension to supraglottic and subglottic (arrowheads) area.

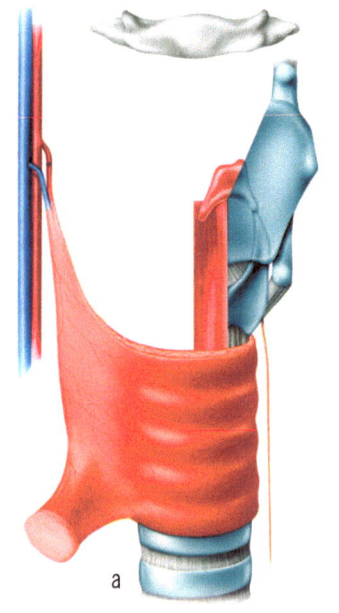
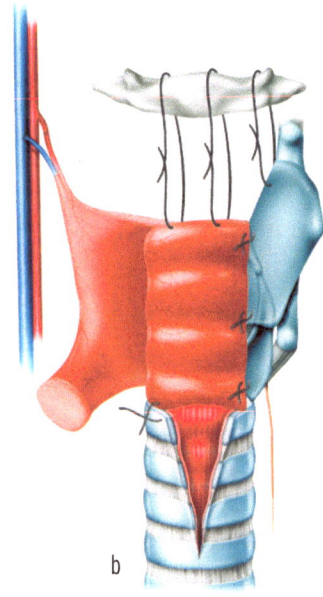

Figure 4.50.
Schematic presentation of reconstruction.
a. Situation after resection. Combination of supraglottic laryngectomy and extended hemilaryngectomy.
b. Situation after reconstruction. Closure between reconstructed larynx and hyoid bone and between reconstructed larynx and mediastinal trachea.

Resection for a transglottic cancer involves a hemilaryngectomy in combination with a supraglottic laryngectomy. The intervention results in the resection of the ipsilateral thyroid, cricoid and paraglottic space in combination with the whole epiglottis and pre-epiglottic space.

The tracheal transplant transforms the laryngeal remnant into a situation which is comparable to a classic supraglottic laryngectomy with one hemilarynx immobilized close to the midline. The closure is performed by creating a pexy between reconstructed laryngeal remnant and hyoid bone superiorly. Closure between reconstructed larynx and mediastinal trachea is similar as for the other tracheal transplantation indications (Fig. 4.50).

Two patients with a previously untreated unilateral transglottic cancer were treated with tracheal autotransplantation.

A combination of a supraglottic laryngectomy with a hemicricolaryngectomy is utilized for lateralized transglottic carcinoma with fixation and with subglottic extension. For this combined resection, the patient needs a good pulmonary reserve because the postoperative course is comparable to a supraglottic laryngectomy. The post-operative course of the 2 patients was similar. The reconstruction was evaluated as being morphometrical competent (Fig. 4.51). The patients had minor problems when swallowing solids but complained of aspiration when using liquids. Their voice was aphonic. The discrepancy between morphometry and patient function is due to the absence of supraglottic structures and hence to the absence of compensatory closure at the supraglottic level. Although technical possible, this combined resection of supraglottic laryngectomy and extended hemilaryngectomy has to be evaluated as '1 step too far'. Closure of the glottic gap at the anterior glottic level during speech and swallowing is not complete after tracheal transplantation. Compensatory closing at the supraglottic level is mandatory to compensate for the anterior glottic gap and to obtain good sphincteric function during speech and swallowing. The compensatory closure will not occur after supraglottic resection and aspiration will be unavoidable. After the small experience on 2 patients, transglottic cancers were no longer considered as indications for tracheal autotransplantation.

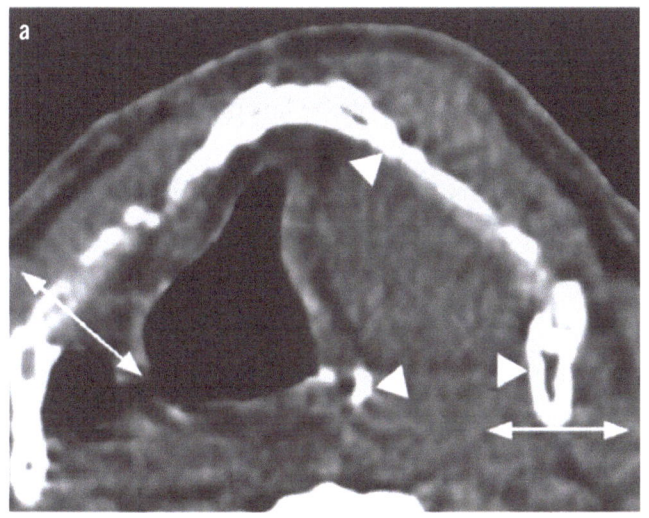

Figure 4.51.
Clinical example of tracheal autotransplantation for transglottic cancer.
a.Axial CT scan at supraglottic level before operation. Tumor extension is indicated by arrowheads. Resection includes a supraglottic laryngectomy in combination with a left-sided extended hemilaryngectomy.

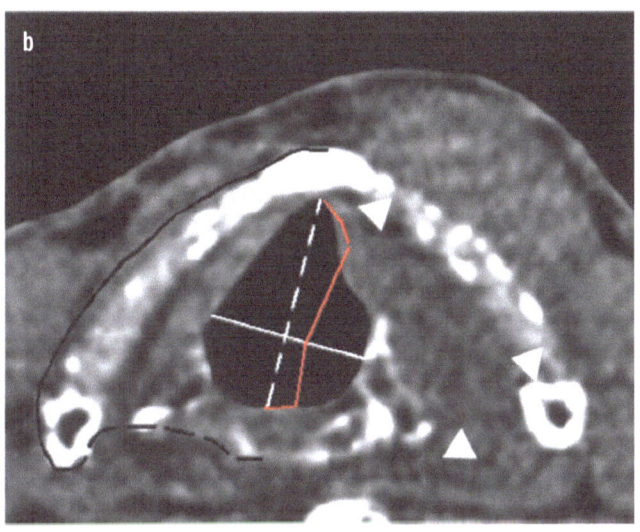

b. Axial CT scan at glottic level before operation. Hemilaryngectomy with placement of the anterior section line in the anterior commissure. The 'optimal position' for the tracheal transplant is indicated with red line. The 'optimal position' will be projected on the postoperative CT scan at the same axial level. The anterior-posterior midline (white dotted line) and the line that circumscribes the thyroid and cricoid cartilage posteriorly (black dotted line) are used to match the pre- and postoperative CT images. Tumor extension is indicated by arrowheads.

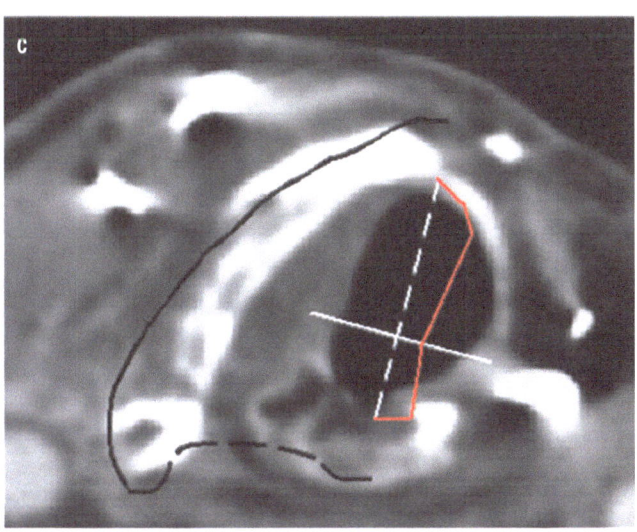

c.Axial CT scan (during quiet respiration) at glottic level after operation. The 'optimal position' is projected. The anterior-posterior midline (white dotted line) and the line that circumscribes the thyroid and cricoid cartilage posteriorly (black dotted line) are used to match the pre- and postoperative CT images. The surface area of the resected side posteriorly is similar to the preoperatively defined surface area of the posterior gap (RSp) (="glottic competency"). The length of the patch between anterior and posterior commissure= 31.2 mm.

2.H. Oncological evaluation of tracheal autotransplantation-initial concept

The major drawback of the initial concept of tracheal autotransplantation is that resection of the primary tumor is done during the second operation. Two disadvantages may be linked to this approach:

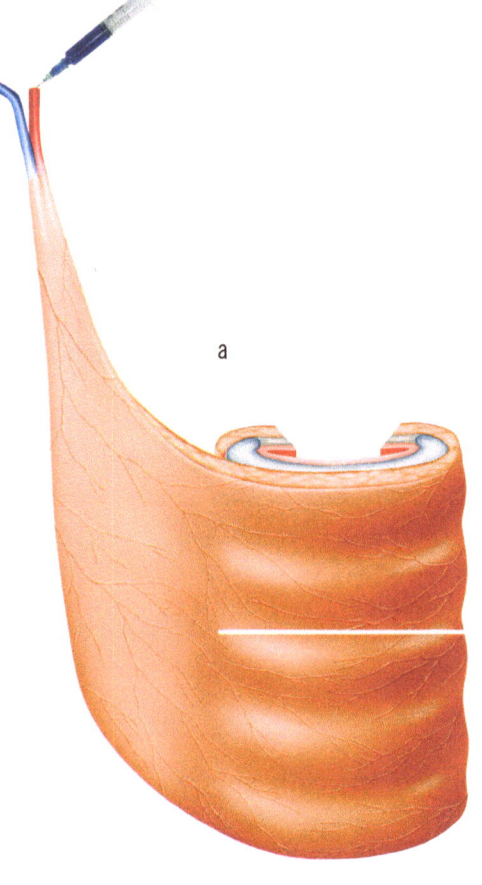

-Tumor beyond the resection margins of an extended hemilaryngectomy. This may become visible after opening of the larynx during the second operation.

-Locoregional recurrences after tracheal autotransplantation.

2.H.1. Total laryngectomy during second operation

Figure 4.52.
Tracheal revascularization-documentation in a patient undergoing total laryngectomy.

a. The revascularized trachea is isolated and the radial artery is injected with blue silicone after removal of the membranous trachea.
b. Macroscopy of revascularization process. Axial section through cartilage ring with fascial flap wrapping the trachea. The blue silicone, injected in the vascular pedicle of the fascia flap, colors the blood vessels of the fascia flap and of the submucosal layer.
c. Microscopy of revascularization process. Blood vessels are stained with silicone (Arrows point to yellow colored substance - color change from blue to yellow is due to fixation with formaldehyde - inside vessel lumen) on both sides of the tracheal cartilage. The fascia flap is well attached to the outer side of the cartilage ring. The blood supply of the mucosal component originates from the radial vascular pedicle reaching the mucosa through the intercartilaginous ligaments (H.&E. original magnification x 10). F=fascia flap.

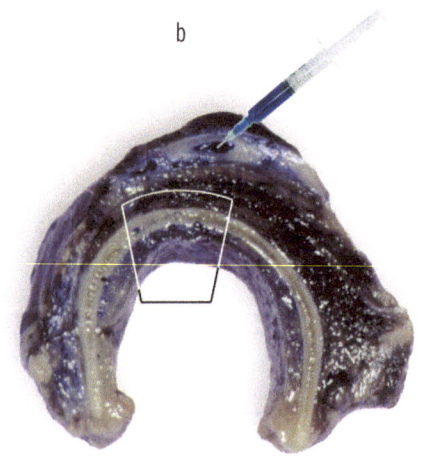

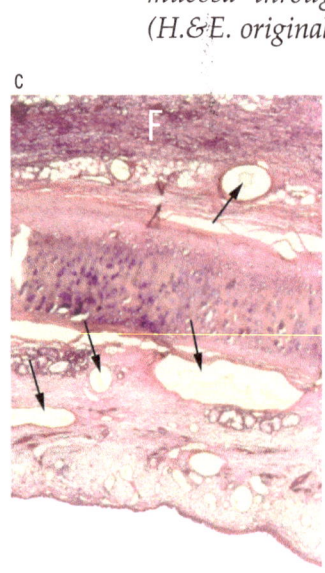

Two patients in the initial series underwent total laryngectomy during the second operation because the tumor extension was too close to the posterior midline to allow for an extended hemilaryngectomy. The posterior tumor extension was more advanced than expected on CTscan and during laryngoscopy.

In 1 patient, we used the revascularized trachea for documentation of the revascularization state after 2 weeks of fascial wrapping. At the time of the total laryngectomy, the upper 4 rings of cervical trachea, wrapped by vascularized fascia, were completely isolated from the airway with disruption of the intrinsic, mucosal vascularization. The vascular pedicle of the radial forearm flap was sectioned after removal of the membranous part of the isolated trachea. The radial artery was flushed with 10 mL of heparinized, normal saline solution (10 IU heparin/mL) followed by 5 mL of silicone dye (Microfil, Canton Bio-Medical Products, Inc., Boulder, CO). This material formed a cast of the vascular architecture of the fascia flap and the established vascular connections with the tracheal patch. After injection, the patch was inspected macroscopically. To document the amount of revascularization of a tracheal patch after 2 weeks of fascial wrapping, the patch was cut axially and embedded in paraffin and 4-μm-thick sections were cut and stained with hematoxylin-eosin.The amount of revascularization could be documented both macroscopically and histologically (Fig. 4.52).

In the second patient undergoing total laryngectomy, the cervical trachea was unwrapped and the fascia flap was preserved with intact vascular pedicle. The vascularized fascia flap was used to cover and protect the neopharyngeal closure line (Fig. 4.53).

The total laryngectomy was performed in the usual way with inclusion of 2 to 3 cervical tracheal rings. Secondary placement of a voice prosthesis was done in both patients. A primary tracheo-esophageal puncture may be problematic in these cases because the tracheal stump is incompletely attached to the esophagus at its upper end due to the tracheal mobilization during the first operation.

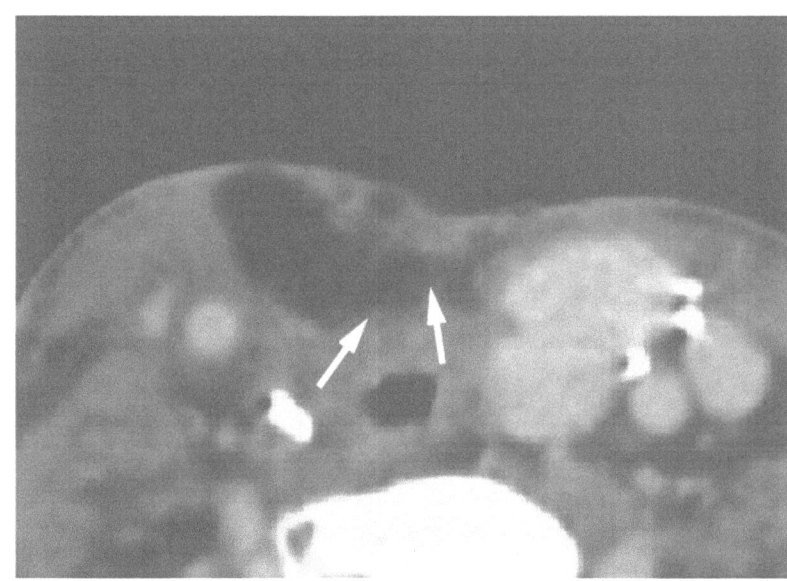

Figure 4.53.
CT scan after second stage total laryngectomy. The vascularized fascial flap (arrows) covers the neopharyngeal suture line.

2.H.2. Locoregional recurrence

Twelve locoregional tumor recurrences were seen in the initial patient series (after a mean follow-up period of 2.5 years) although all the margins of the hemilaryngectomy resection specimen were reported as tumor free.

Two different kind of locoregional recurrences could be distinguished:

1. 'Early recurrences' diagnosed between 5 and 8 months after tracheal transplantation. These recurrences had a bad prognosis: 1 patient could be salvaged by a total laryngectomy; the 7 other patients died of their desease.

2. 'Late recurrences' diagnosed 1 year or more after tracheal autotransplantation. Four patients showed a tumor recurrence on the preserved hemilarynx and they could all be salvaged by a total laryngectomy.

2.H.2.a Early recurrences

One patient showed a tumor recurrence at the supraglottic region and 7 patients showed a tumor recurrence at the glottic level with extension into the soft tissues of the neck. The patient with a tumor recurrence at the supraglottic region was the only one who could be salvaged by a total laryngectomy (Fig. 4.54, 4.55).

Tumor recurrence was diagnosed 5 months after operation on a routine CT scan. The patient could be cured with a total laryngectomy. Postfactum, this patient was not a good candidate for a hemilaryngectomy because of tumor involvement of the paraglottic space. Although the margins of the resection specimen were reported as being free of tumor, section margins at the supraglottic level were not safe for a tumor with involvement of the paraglottic space.

Seven patients showed an early tumor recurrence at the glottic-subglottic region. At the time of diagnosis, the patients also had tumor extension into the soft tissues of the neck and they all died of their disease. Two examples are presented in figure 4.56 and figure 4.57.

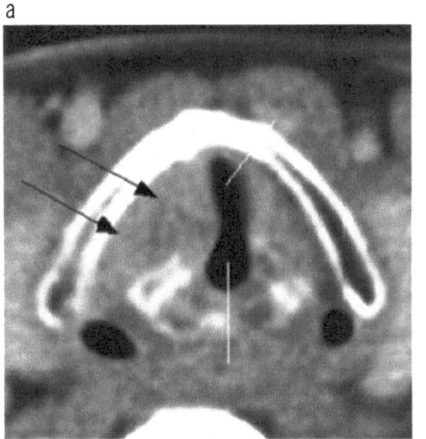 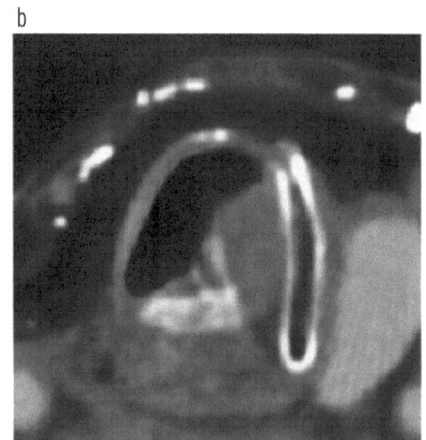 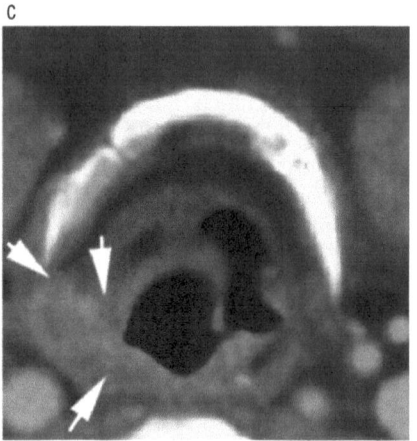

Figure 4.54. Tumor recurrence at supraglottic level.
a. Preoperative CT scan of T3 glottic cancer with indication of resection margins. Paraglottic tumor involvement is indicated by arrows.

b. Postoperative CT scan glottic level. Laryngeal remnant with tracheal transplant.
c. Postoperative CT scan at supraglottic level 5 months postoperatively. Tumor recurrence visible in right supraglottic area (arrows).

a

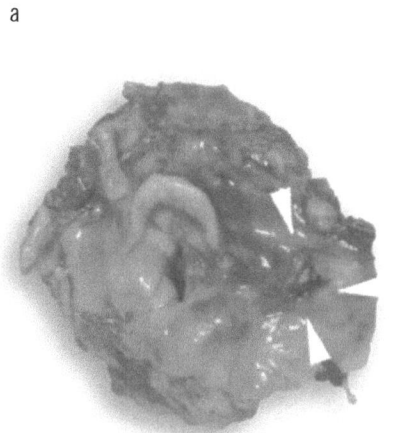

b

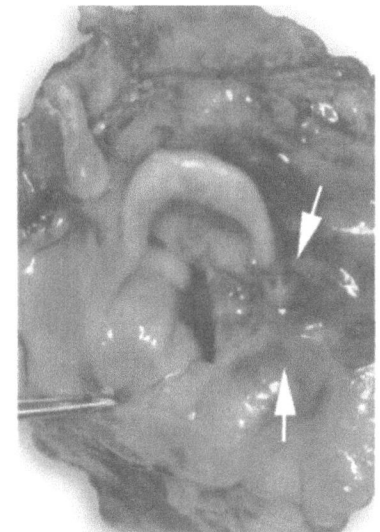

c

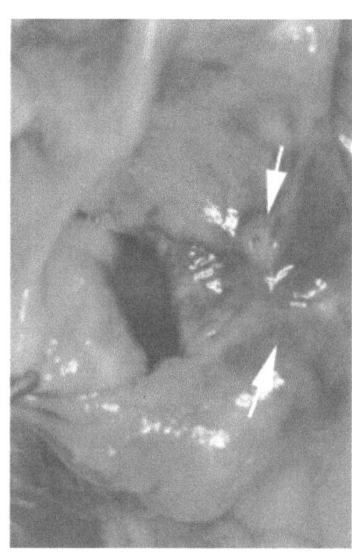

Figure 4.55. Tumor recurrence at supraglottic level-resection specimen (same patient as in Fig. 4.54).
The vascular pedicle of the radial forearm flap was injected with blue Microfil® to better delineate the tracheal patch. The patch is placed in a paramedial posi-tion at the glottic level, resembling the situation of a unilateral paralysis in the midline. Tumoral recurrence is indicated by arrows.

The patient's history showed that the tumor presented in figure 4.56 was not a good indication for hemilaryngectomy because of the extensive subglottic infiltration. Postirradiation, extensive subglottic infiltration in the direction of the posterior midline forms a contraindication for hemilaryn-gectomy because submucosal tumor extension within the conus elasticus is unpredictable. The margins of this resection specimen were reported as being free of tumor but extensive nerve and vessel involvement was mentioned in the pathol-ogy report.

a

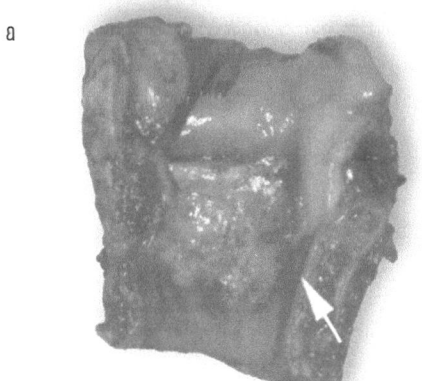

b

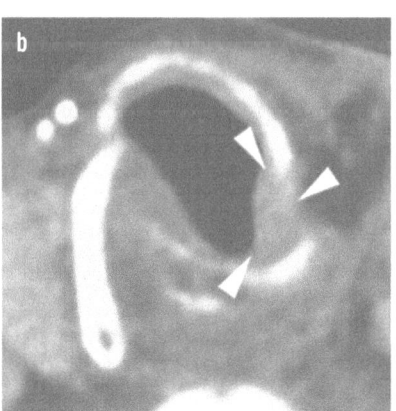

c

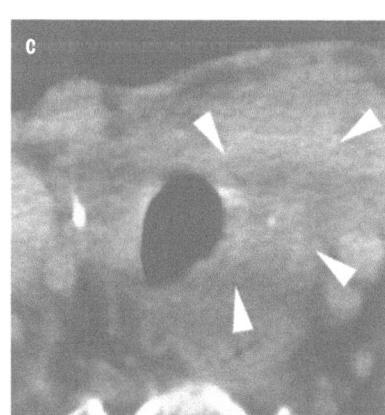

Figure 4.56. Tumor recurrence in glottic-subglottic area; Case 1.
a. Resection specimen of glottic T2 tumor with exten-sive subglottic extension after previous irradiation. Tumor extension close to posterior midline (arrow).
b. CT scan 5 months after tracheal autotransplanta-tion. Reconstructed larynx at subglottic level. There is a recurrence visible at the anastomosis between posterior patch and posterior site of preserved cricoid (arrow-heads).
c. CT scan 5 months after tracheal transplantation at the lower neck level. Tumor extension into soft tissue of the neck is indicated by arrowheads.

The most dramatic tumor recurrence within the initial patient series is presented in figure 4.57. The patient displayed a T3N0 glottic tumor with subglottic invasion. A radical resection was reported on the hemilaryngectomy specimen and no lymph nodes were found in the neck dissection specimen (area 2 to 5). Postoperative radiotherapy was started 3 weeks after tracheal autotransplantation. A massive locoregional tumor recurrence became apparent during the radiotherapeutic treatment and the patient died shortly after diagnosis of the recurrent tumor.

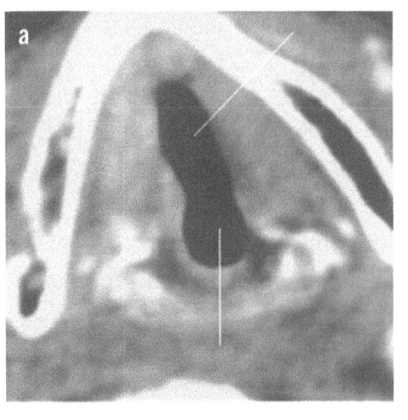
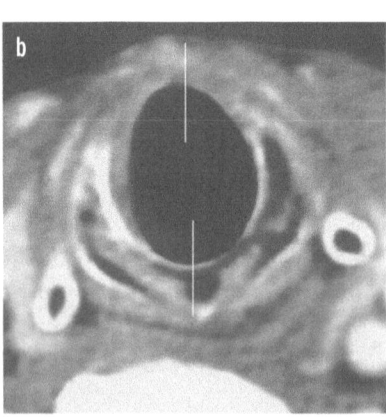
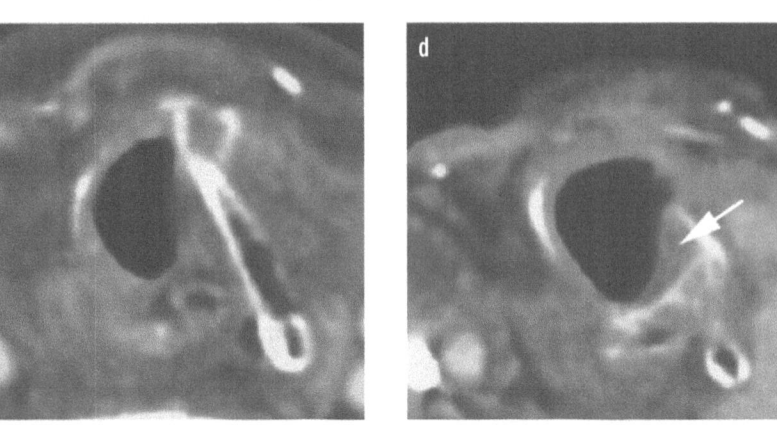
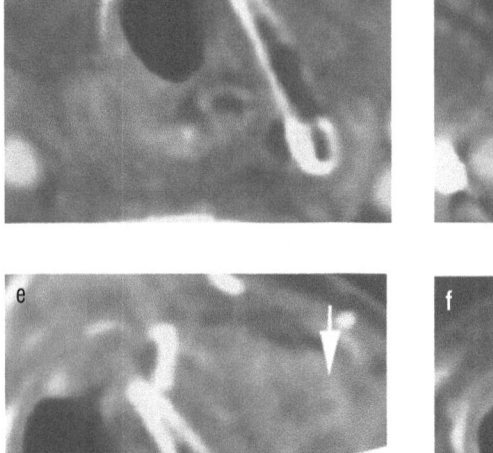
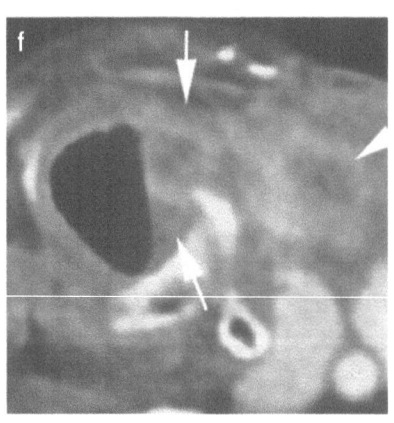

Figure 4.57.
Tumor recurrence in glottic-subglottic area; Case 2.
a. Preoperative CT scan at glottic level. Resection margins for extended hemilaryngectomy are shown.
b. Preoperative CT scan at subglottic level. Resection margins for hemilaryngectomy are shown.
c. Postoperative CT scan at glottic level 2 weeks after tracheal transplantation.
d. Postoperative CT scan at subglottic level 2 weeks after tracheal transplantation. Some thickening of the mucosa over the remaining cricoid is visible (arrow).
e. Postoperative CT scan at glottic level 5 weeks after tracheal transplantation. Recurrent tumor inside and outside the laryngeal remnant is indicated by arrows.
f. Postoperative CT scan at subglottic level 5 weeks after tracheal transplantation. Recurrent tumor inside and outside the laryngeal remnant is indicated by arrows.

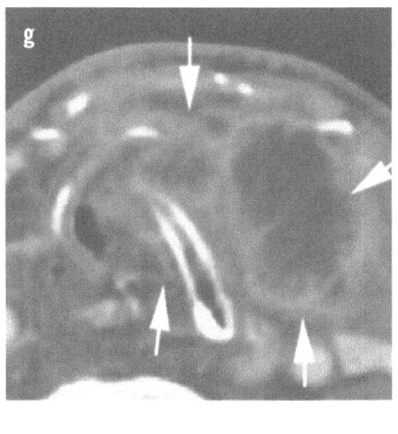

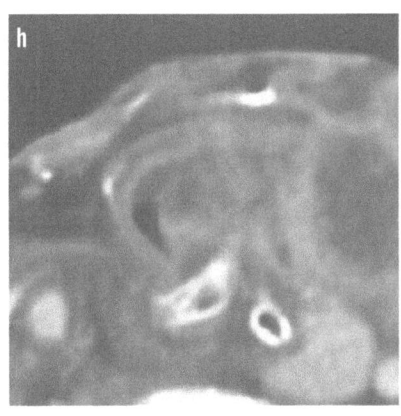

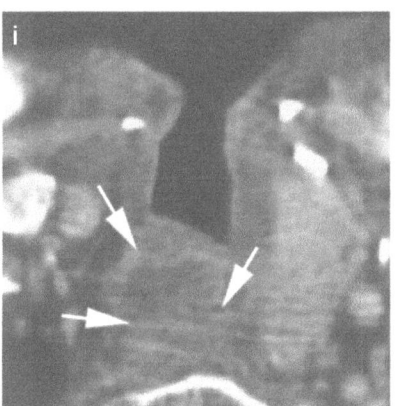

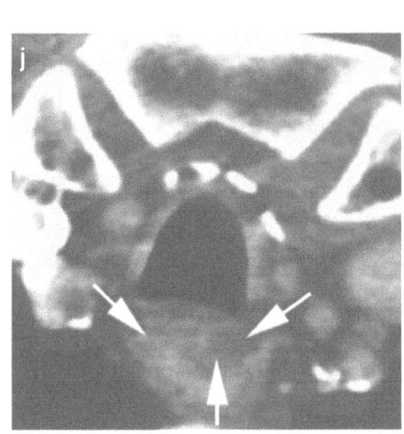

Figure 4.57.
Tumor recurrence in glottic-subglottic area; Case 2 (continued).
g. Postoperative CT scan at glottic level 8 weeks after tracheal transplantation. Recurrent tumor inside and outside the laryngeal remnant is indicated by arrows.
h. Postoperative CT scan at subglottic level 8 weeks after tracheal transplantation.
i. Postoperative CT scan 8 weeks after tracheal transplantation-level of tracheostomy. Tumor involvement of esophagus is indicated by arrows.
j. Postoperative CT scan 8 weeks after tracheal transplantation-level of mediastinal trachea. Tumor involvement of esophagus is indicated by arrows.

2.H.2.b New primary tumor

Four patients showed a recurrence after more than 1 year. The tumor occurred on the preserved vocal fold as a 'new primary tumor'. All 4 patients were successfully salvaged by performing a total laryngectomy (Fig. 4.58, 4.59).

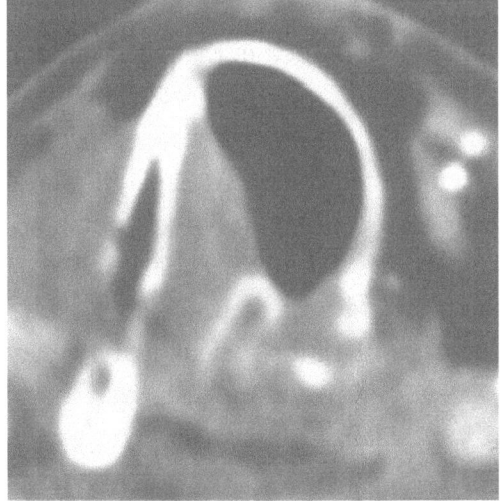

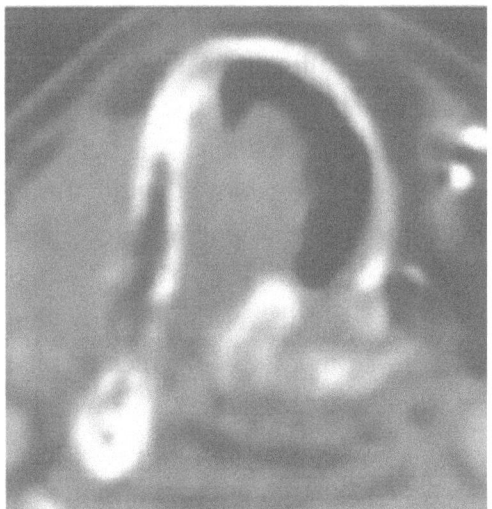

Figure 4.58. Tumor recurrence as 'new primary tumor'.
a. CT scan at glottic level. Hemilaryngectomy for T2 glottic cancer at the left side.

b. CT scan at glottic level 15 months later. Tumor recurrence on vocal fold remnant at right side.

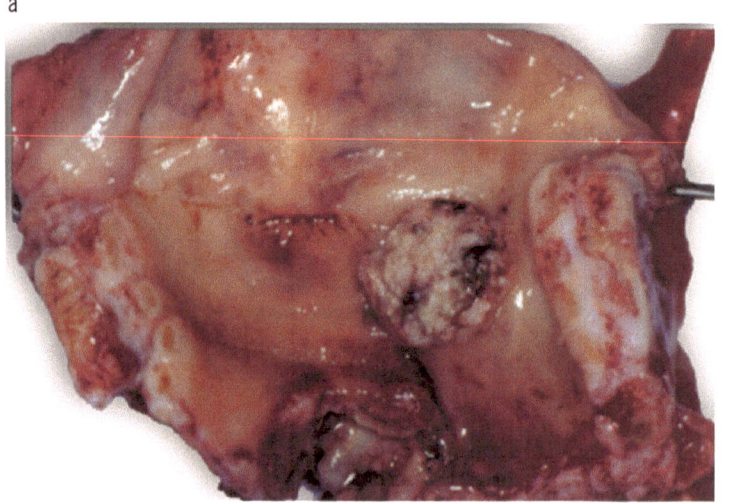

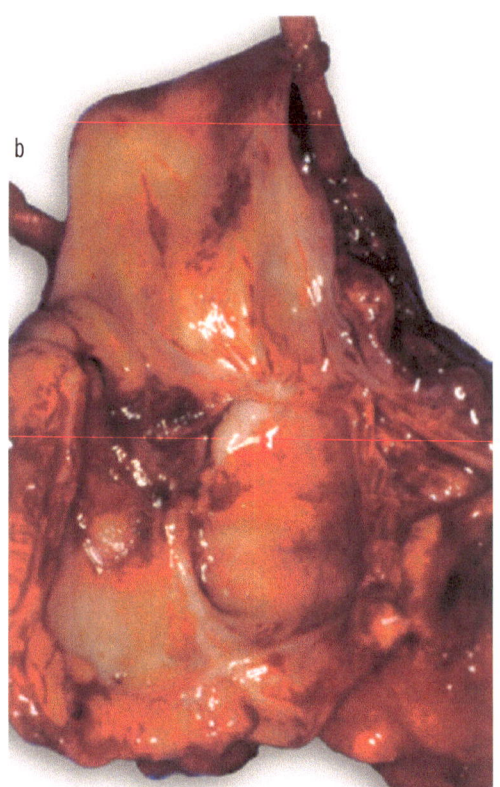

Figure 4.59. Salvage total laryngectomy specimen.
a. Recurrence on remaining right vocal fold. This resection specimen corresponds with the tumor recurrence seen in Fig. 4.58.

b. Recurrence on remaining left vocal fold in another patient.

The most important objection against the initial concept of tracheal autotransplantation is the low reliability of the procedure from an oncological viewpoint:

-The first operation is done without direct view on the tumor and without full security that the tumor will be suitable for the conservation procedure. Owing to the 2-stage resection approach, the first operation and transfer of the radial forearm flap becomes unnecessary in cases in which a total laryngectomy is indicated.

-The order reversal (neck dissection 2 weeks before resection of primary tumor) goes against "good oncological practice", which requires either that the tumor be removed en bloc with the cervical nodes, or that the tumor be removed before dissection of the neck. It is unlikely that the 2 step-resection approach is fully responsible for all the local recurrences encountered in the initial patient series. Local recurrences were reported for most partial laryngectomy procedures and even after near-total laryngectomy, recurrences with bad prognosis did occur in the laryngeal remnant (DeSANTO et al. 1989, PEARSON at al. 1998). After conservation laryngectomy, local recurrences leading to death of the patient are however difficult to accept because these cases may have been cured if a total laryngectomy was performed as the initial surgical treatment. The tracheal autotransplantation concept was modified to make the procedure more reliable from an oncological viewpoint.

BIBLIOGRAPHY

Burkey BB, Hoffman HT, Thornton AF, McClatchey KD. Chondrosarcoma of the head and neck. Laryngoscope 1990;100:1301-5.

DeSanto LW, Pearson BW, Olsen KD. Utility of near-total laryngectomy for supraglottic, pharyngeal, base-of-tongue, and other cancers. Ann Otol Rhinol Laryngol 1989;98:2-7.

Ferlito A, Nicolai P, Montaguti A, Cecchetto A, Pennelli M. Chondrosarcoma of the larynx: review of the literature and report of three cases. Am J Otolaryngol 1984;5:530-9.

Habal MB, Murray JE. Surgical treatment of life-endangering chronic aspiration pneumonia: Use of an epiglottic flap to the arytenoids. Plast Reconstr Surg 1972;59:305-11.

Hicks JN, Walker EE, Moor EE. Diagnosis and conservative surgical management of chondrosarcoma of the larynx. Ann Otol Rhinol Laryngol 1982;91:389-91.

Kozelsky T, Bonner J, Foot R, et al. Laryngeal chondrosarcomas : the Mayo Clinic experience. J Surg Oncol 1997;65:269-73.

Montgomery WW. Surgery to prevent aspiration. Arch Otolaryngol 1975;101:679-82.

Nikolai P, Ferlito A, Sasaki CT, Kirchner JA. Laryngeal chondrosarcoma: incidence, pathology, biological behavior, and treatment. Ann Otol Rhinol Laryngol 1990;99:515-23.

Pearson B, DeSanto L, Olsen K, Salassa J. The results of near-total laryngectomy. Ann Otol Rhinol Laryngol 1998;107:820-5.

Randestad A, Lindholm CE, Fabian P. Dimensions of the cricoid cartilage and the trachea. Laryngoscope 2000;110:1957-61.

Tucker HM, Wood BG, Levine II, et al. Glottic reconstruction after near total laryngectomy. Laryngoscope 1979;89:608-18.

CHAPTER 5

Modification of Tracheal Autotransplantation Concept:

Towards optimal reconstruction of extended hemilaryngectomy defects

1. Introduction

A reconstruction technique for the larynx after removal of a malignant tumor must be reliable from a reconstructive viewpoint, must lead to predictable and good functional results, and may not interfere with the oncological safety of the surgical treatment. The tracheal autotransplantation technique was modified in an attempt to improve the reliability of the procedure from an oncological viewpoint. After 38 patients, the reconstructive concept was modified in 2001. Attempts were made to improve the initial concept (Table 5.1).

Table 5.1. Factors that could be improved in the initial autotransplantation concept

-Tumor resection during second operation.

-Early local tumor recurrences with bad prognosis.

-Incompetent reconstruction at supraglottic and glottic level.

-Absence of tracheostomy during tracheal revascularization.

The main modification was towards a 1-stage resection procedure with delayed tracheal auto-transplantation (Fig. 5.1, Table 5.2). Since 2001 all patients were treated by the modified concept and tumor resection with neck dissection was performed during the first operation.

Evolution to the modified concept was made possible by the experience obtained from the initial series and was based on the following 2 assumptions: 1/ Temporary closure of the laryngeal defect with simultaneous tracheal revascularization might be done with 1 radial forearm flap. Therefore, the radial forearm flap needs a distal island of fascia (for revascularization) and a proximal island of skin (for temporary closure), and 2/ The 'tracheostomy' that will be necessary during tracheal revascularization might be introduced at the distal end of the temporarily repaired larynx.

In the modified concept, complete tumor resection (primary tumor and neck nodes) is done during the first operation. Tracheal revascularization and temporary reconstruction of the hemilaryngectomy defect is perfomed with 1 radial forearm flap (Fig. 5.2).

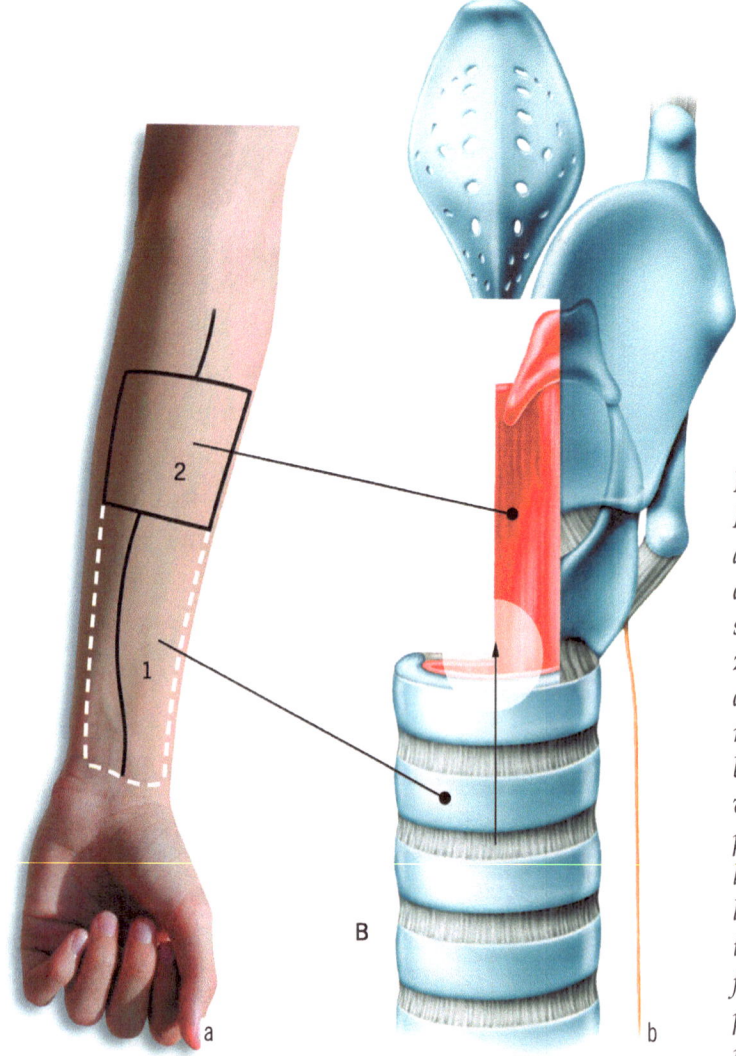

Figure 5.1.
Modified tracheal autotransplantation concept.
a. The radial forearm flap is designed with a paddle consisting of fascia and a paddle consisting of skin. The fascial paddle will serve for revascularization of the cervical trachea (1) and the skin paddle will serve as temporary closure for the hemilaryngectomy defect (2).
b. Situation after extended hemilaryngectomy with inclusion of the anterior commissure. The posterior incision is located in the posterior midline; the anterior incision is located at the contralateral side. One cm of contralateral thyroid cartilage is resected. The skin paddle of the radial forearm flap cannot restore the airway and the placement of a stomy (arrow) for breathing will be necessary.

Table 5.2. Tumor resection during first or second operation-surgical steps		
	Second stage tumor resection **Initial concept**	**First stage tumor resection** **Modified concept**
Stage 1	°Neck dissection °Tracheal revascularization	°Neck dissection °Tumor resection °Tracheal revascularization °Temporary closure laryngeal defect °Tracheostomy
Stage 2	After 2 weeks °Tumor resection °Tracheal autotransplantation °Tracheostomy	After 4 months °Removal skin flap (except upper site) °Tracheal autotransplantation °Tracheostomy
Stage 3	°Closure of tracheostomy (LA)	° Closure of tracheostomy (LA)

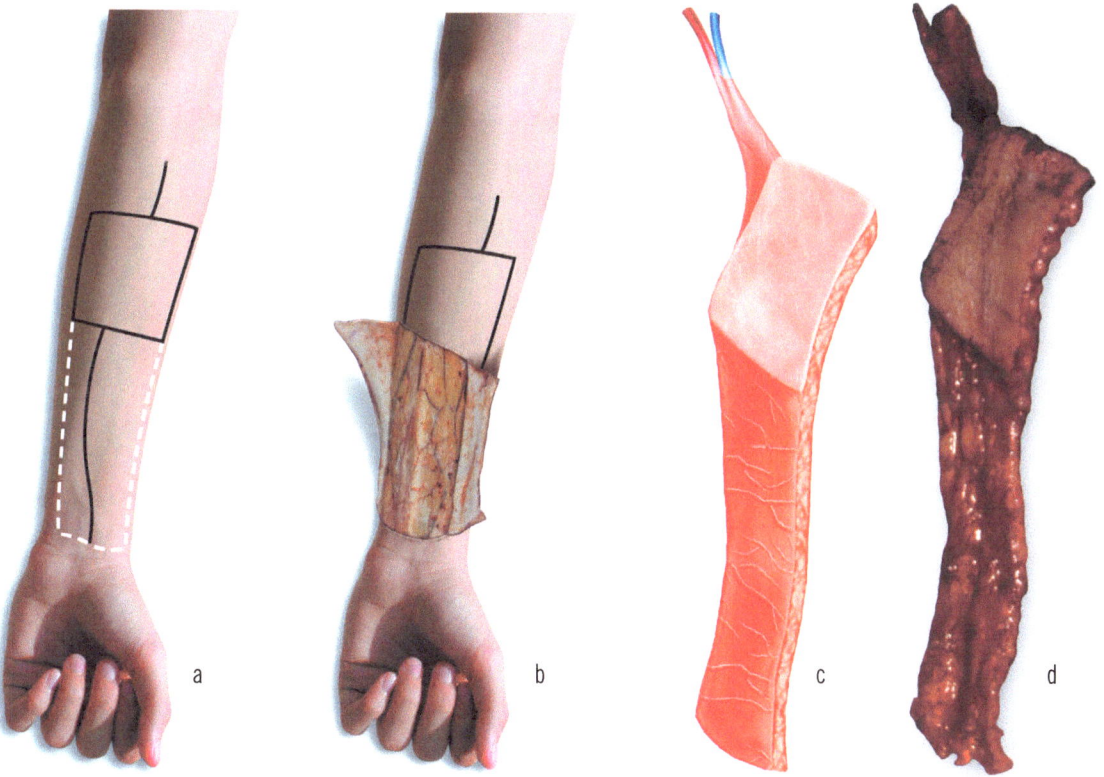

Figure 5.2. Design of radial forearm flap in modified tracheal autotransplantation concept.
a. Outlining of flap. Black lines show skin incisions. White dotted lines show extent of fascial dissection.
b. The skin is elevated from the underlyng subcutaneous tissue and fascia.

c. Drawing of dissected flap with distal fascial paddle, proximal skin paddle, and radial artery and vein.
d. Dissected radial forearm flap.

The objective was to repair the laryngeal sphincter function with the skin paddle and to wait for 4 months before the autotransplantation of the trachea. By this approach it is possible to have a 'second look' that allows for a re-evaluation of the section margins. In this setting, the fascia can revascularize the trachea during a longer time interval and therefore, circumferential tracheal wrapping is no longer necessary. Only the amount of trachea that will be used for laryngeal repair will undergo wrapping with fascia (Fig. 5.3).

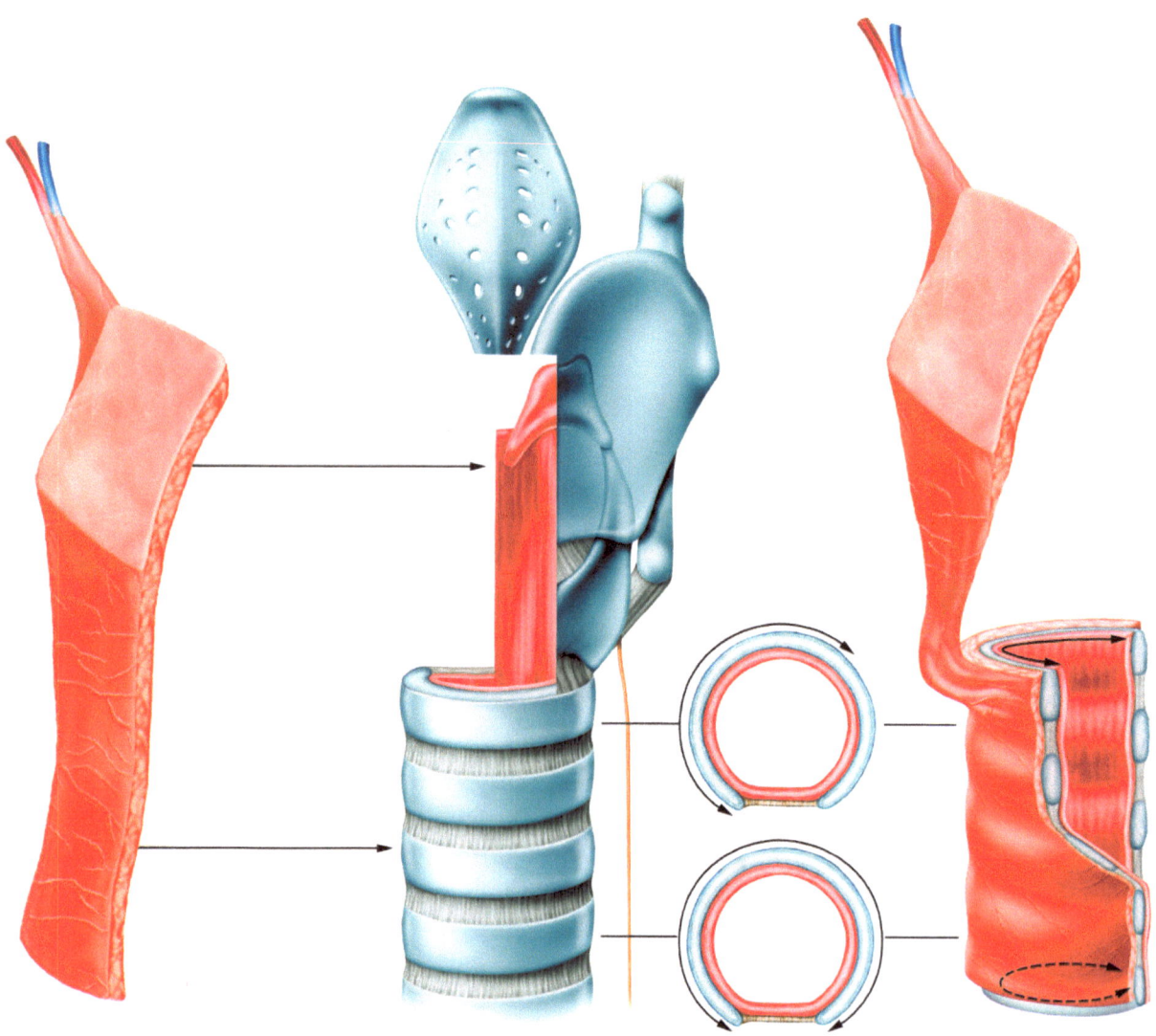

Figure 5.3. Principle of modified tracheal revascularization concept.
The amount of trachea that will be used for larynx reconstruction will be wrapped with fascia. The upper site of the trachea will reconstruct the larynx at the glottic level. A competent larynx is obtained by using a patch between 2.5 and 3.0 cm. Three cm of trachea will be wrapped at the upper site. A safe airway lumen is obtained at the subglottic level with a patch containing the full amount of cartilage ring. The full amount of cartilage ring (without membranous trachea) will be wrapped at the lower site.

Within the modified concept, it was attempted to optimize the definitive reconstruction of the laryngeal defect. The morphometrical evaluation of the reconstructed larynges within the initial concept showed that the tracheal autotransplant provides for the optimal tissue to repair the larynx subglottically. More bulk in the region of the supraglottis was desired in 4 patients of the initial series and the glottis was not optimally repaired in 21 patients. In the modified concept, we wanted to improve the reconstruction by using the trachea for reconstruction at the glottic-subglottic level and by using the forearm skin for reconstruction at the supraglottic level (Fig. 5.4).

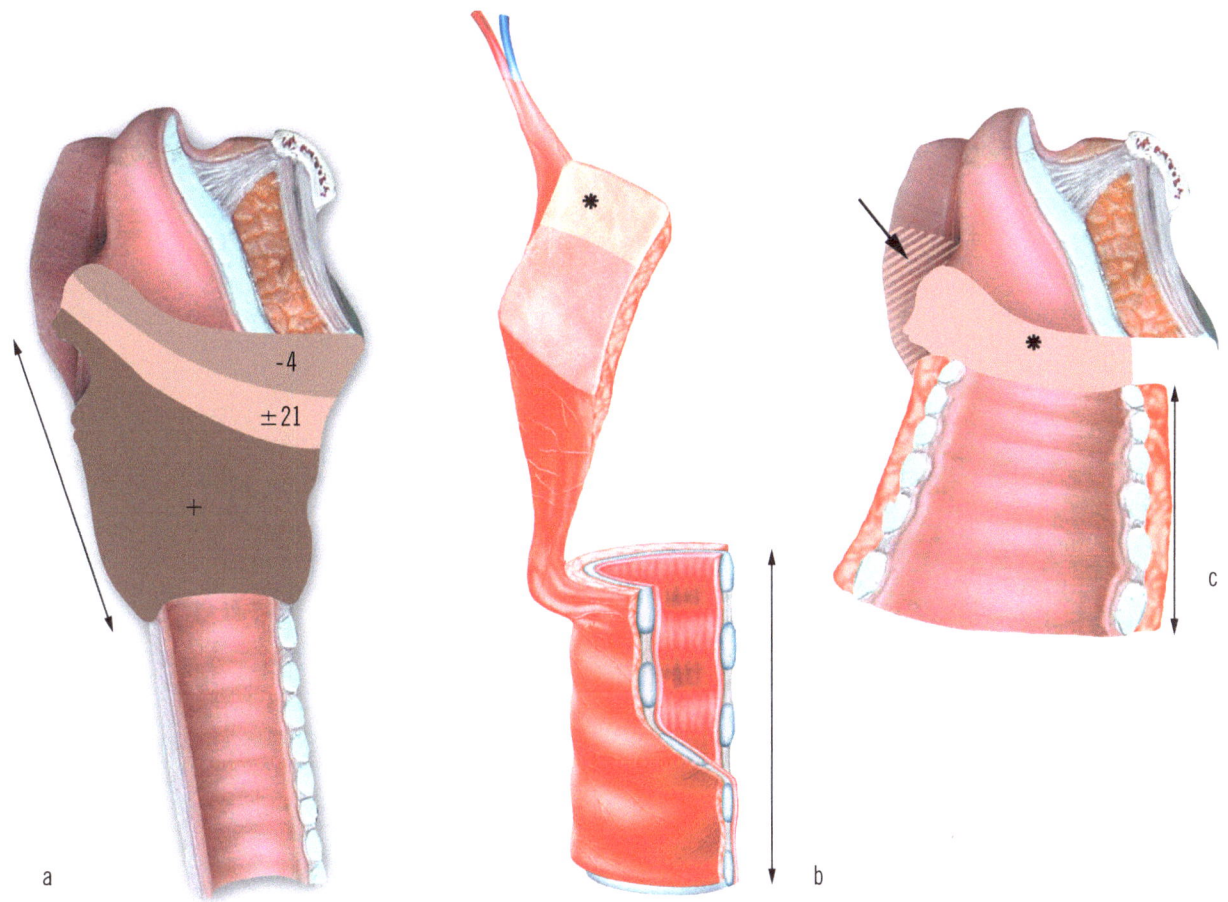

Figure 5.4. Principle of modified tracheal autotransplantation concept.

a. A tracheal autotransplant provides for the optimal tissue to repair the larynx subglottically. More bulk in the region of the supraglottis was desired in 4 patients and the convexity of the glottic reconstruction was too pronounced in 21 patients of the initial series.

b. The tracheal patch with a length of 4 cm will be used to reconstruct the larynx at the glottic-subglottic level. The upper part of the radial forearm skin (asterisk) will be used for repair of the supraglottic level.

c. Schematic situation after reconstruction. The tracheal patch repairs the subglottic larynx. Three cm (2.5 cm in females) is used at the glottic level while the full amount of cartilage ring is used to reconstruct the lower end of the larynx.

The forearm skin repairs the larynx at the supraglottic level (asterisk). The pyriform sinus (lined area) can be removed when dealing with hypopharyngeal cancer.

The blood supply to the reconstructive tissue is based on vascular induction (Fig. 5.5). The blood supply to the reconstructive tissue will be reliable because of the 4 months time interval between tracheal wrapping and tracheal autotransplantation. It takes 4 months before the forearm skin (at supraglottic level) is separated from its vascular pedicle.

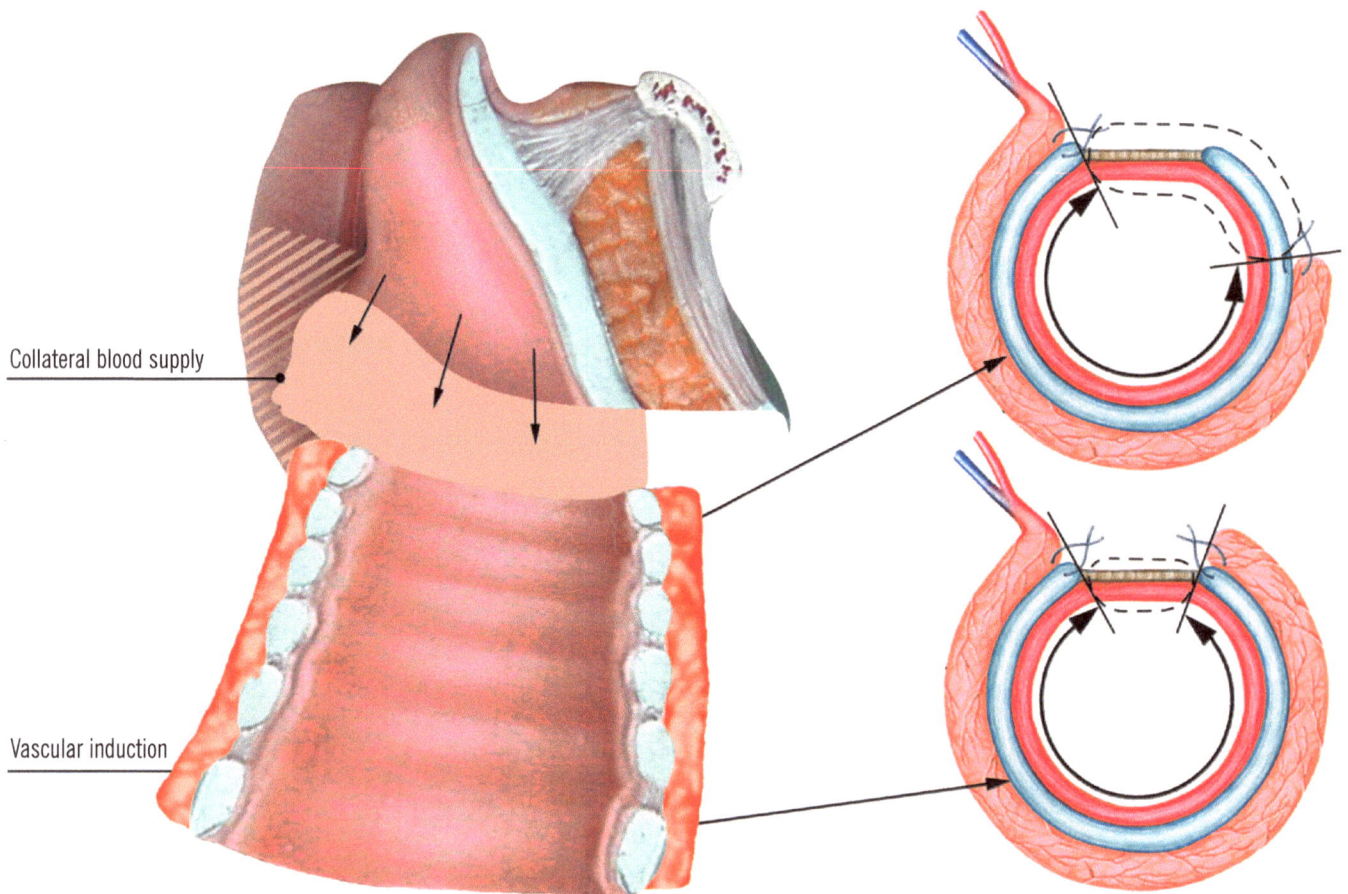

Collateral blood supply

Vascular induction

Figure 5.5. Vascular supply of reconstructed larynx in modified concept.
After tracheal autotransplantation, the survival of the forearm skin at the supraglottic and glottic level is based on blood supply from the surrounding laryngeal tissues (arrows). Survival of the trachea is based on vascular induction from the fascia flap. Because of the long time interval between fascial wrapping and autotransplantation, only the amount of trachea needed for reconstruction is removed. The areas indicated by dotted lines are left in situ.

2. Optimal larynx reconstruction with the modified concept-learning curve

2.A. First patients

2.A.1. Operative procedure
2.A.1.a. Patient 1

A 73-year-old male patient had a carcinoma of one hemilarynx. He failed treatment after initial radio-therapy (6600 cGy) for a T1N0 tumor (American Joint Committee on Cancer classification). At the time of tumor recurrence, the patient showed tumor recurrence on the vocal fold with impaired mobility but without crossing of the anterior or posterior commissure and without involvement of the supraglottis and pre-epiglottic space (Fig. 5.6).

Figure 5.6.
Patient 1. Tumor extension and extend of resection.
a. Overview of tumor extension on right vocal fold with extend of resection. The anterior commissure is included in the resection.
b. CT scan of tumor resection.
b1: supraglottic level; b2: glottic level; b3, b4, b5: subglottic level.
Tumor extension is indicated with arrows.
Extend of resection is indicated with dotted lines. The ipsilateral thyroid gland (asterisk) will be removed during tumor resection.

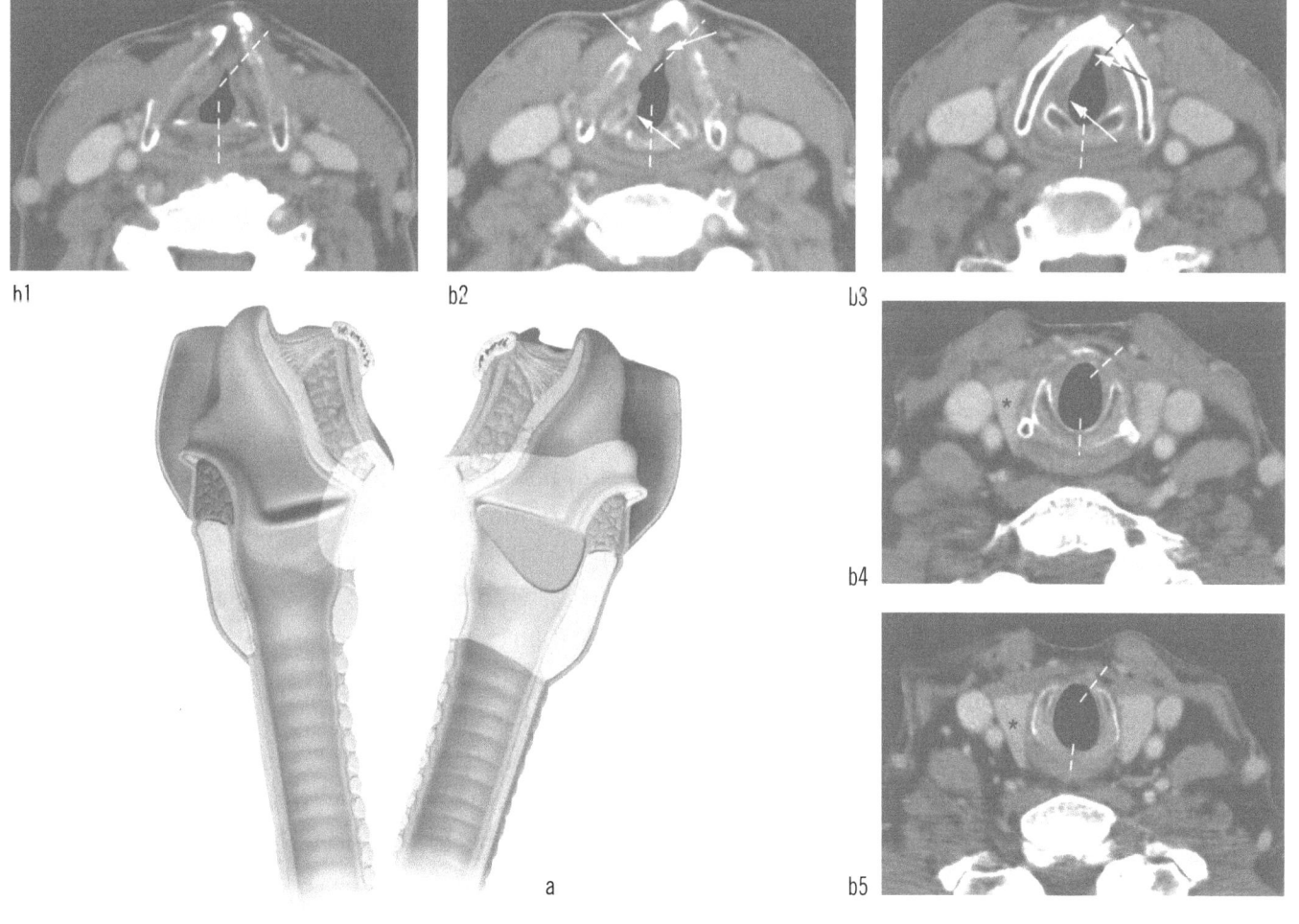

Tumor resection. For tumor resection, a standard apron incision is placed at the level of the second tracheal ring. The operation is started with a selective lateral neck dissection. An ipsilateral neck dissection of levels 2 to 4 is performed. The ipsilateral thyroid gland and the tracheoesophageal lymph nodes are removed. After neck dissection, the cricotracheal ligament is incised at the tumor side and the intubation tube is placed in this incision. The primary tumor is removed by performing a hemilaryngectomy with inclusion of half of the cricoid cartilage. The larynx is incised anteriorly (cartilage cut) with inclusion of 1 cm of the contralateral side. The thyroepiglottic ligament is incised and the epiglottic petiole is sectioned. The larynx is opened superiorly so that the anterior mucosal cut can be placed under direct vision. The posterior cut is placed in the midline to complete the resection.

The extended hemilaryngectomy includes the thyroid cartilage, the paraglottic space, the cricoid and arytenoid cartilage, and the true and false vocal folds at the tumor side. One centimeter of the contralateral thyroid cartilage with 1 cm of the contralateral membranous vocal fold is resected because the tumor reaches the anterior site of the vocal fold without crossing of the anterior commissure.

Dissection of radial forearm flap. The reconstruction is started after obtaining a negative report of the frozen sections taken at the anterior and posterior section margins. A left-sided (right arm was dominant) radial forearm flap is elevated under tourniquet. The radial forearm fascial flap consists of a distal, 4 x 9-cm patch of fascia and of a proximal, 4 x 8-cm patch of skin. The donor defect is closed with a split-thickness or full-thickness skin graft.

Tracheal revascularization. The forearm fascia flap is wrapped around the 4-cm segment of cervical trachea. The upper surface of the fascia is lying against the tracheal wall. The fascia is sutured to the trachea following the pattern shown in figure 4.7. Only the amount of trachea that is necessary for larynx reconstruction is wrapped by fascia. An expanded polytetrafluoroethylene (ePTFE) membrane (Preclude Pericardial Membrane, 0.1 mm, W.L. Gore and Associates, Inc. Flagstaff, AZ) is applied over the fascia flap and between fascia and neck vessels. The ePTFE prevents adhesions between flap and surrounding tissue and facilitates dissection during the second operation.

Temporary reconstruction. The skin island of the radial forearm flap is placed into the laryngeal defect (Fig. 5.7). The laryngeal defect is not completely closed by the radial forearm skin flap. A 'tracheostomy' is left at the caudal part of the reconstructed larynx. The fascial flap is revascularized by anastomosis of the radial artery to the superior thyroid artery (end-to-end) and by anastomosis of the radial vein to the internal jugular vein (end-to-side) at the same side as the laryngeal tumor. Ipsilateral revascularization is necessary to allow for transfer of the trachea to the larynx without manipulation of the vascular pedicle during the second operation. At the subglottic level, the skin flap succeeds in closing of the defect but the airway lumen is not sufficient to allow for restoration of the respiratory function. The neck skin is closed with formation of a 'tracheostomy' at the distal larynx. The tracheostomy is formed by the caudal part of the cricoid cartilage and by the caudal part of the radial forearm skin flap (Fig. 5.8). The patient receives tube feeding (PEG tube is placed during first operation) after the operation and attempts to start oral feeding are made after 6 days.

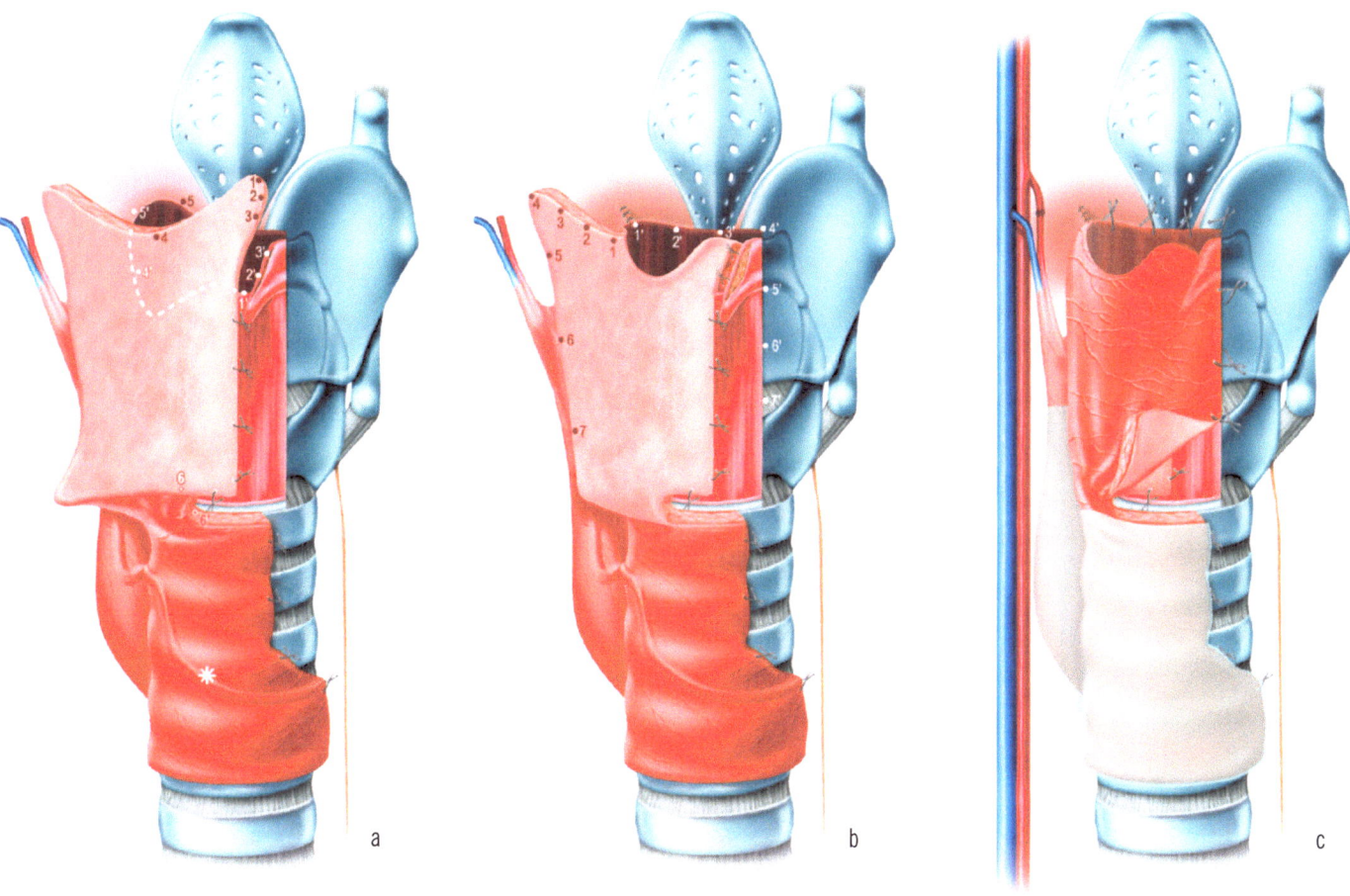

Figure 5.7. Overview of first operative procedure.

a. The upper 4 cm of trachea is wrapped by fascia. The upper surface of the fascia is lying against the tracheal wall. The vascular pedicle is located outside (asterisk). The fascia is attached to the cartilage with several (Dexon 2-0) sutures. The lateral side of the skin flap is sutured to the posterior laryngeal section margin of the cricoid cartilage from inferior to superior. The lower side of the skin flap is sutured to the upper tracheal cartilage ring (6 to 6'). The mucosal lining over the preserved arytenoid is incised at the medial site, and a pharyngeal and laryngeal layer is developed. The radial forearm skin is sutured to the pharyngeal mucosal layer (1-2-3 to 1'-2'-3') and to the section line of the ipsilateral pyriform sinus (4 to 4'). The superior edge of the pharyngeal defect is closed primarily (5 to 5').

b. The upper side of skin flap is sutured to the upper mucosal section line formed by the caudal end of the epiglottis (respectively, 1-2-3-4 to 1'-2'-3'-4'). The lateral side of the skin flap is sutured to the anterior section line of the thyroid cartilage from superior to inferior until the upper side of the cricoid cartilage is reached (respectively, 5-6-7 to 5'-6'-7').

c. The free, lower edge of the radial skin is not sutured into the laryngeal defect, and an opening is left at the caudal larynx. An expanded polytetrafluoroethylene membrane (Pericardial membrane, 8x16 cm/0.1 mm) is placed over the fascial enwrapped trachea and between the trachea and the internal jugular vein in the caudal neck area.

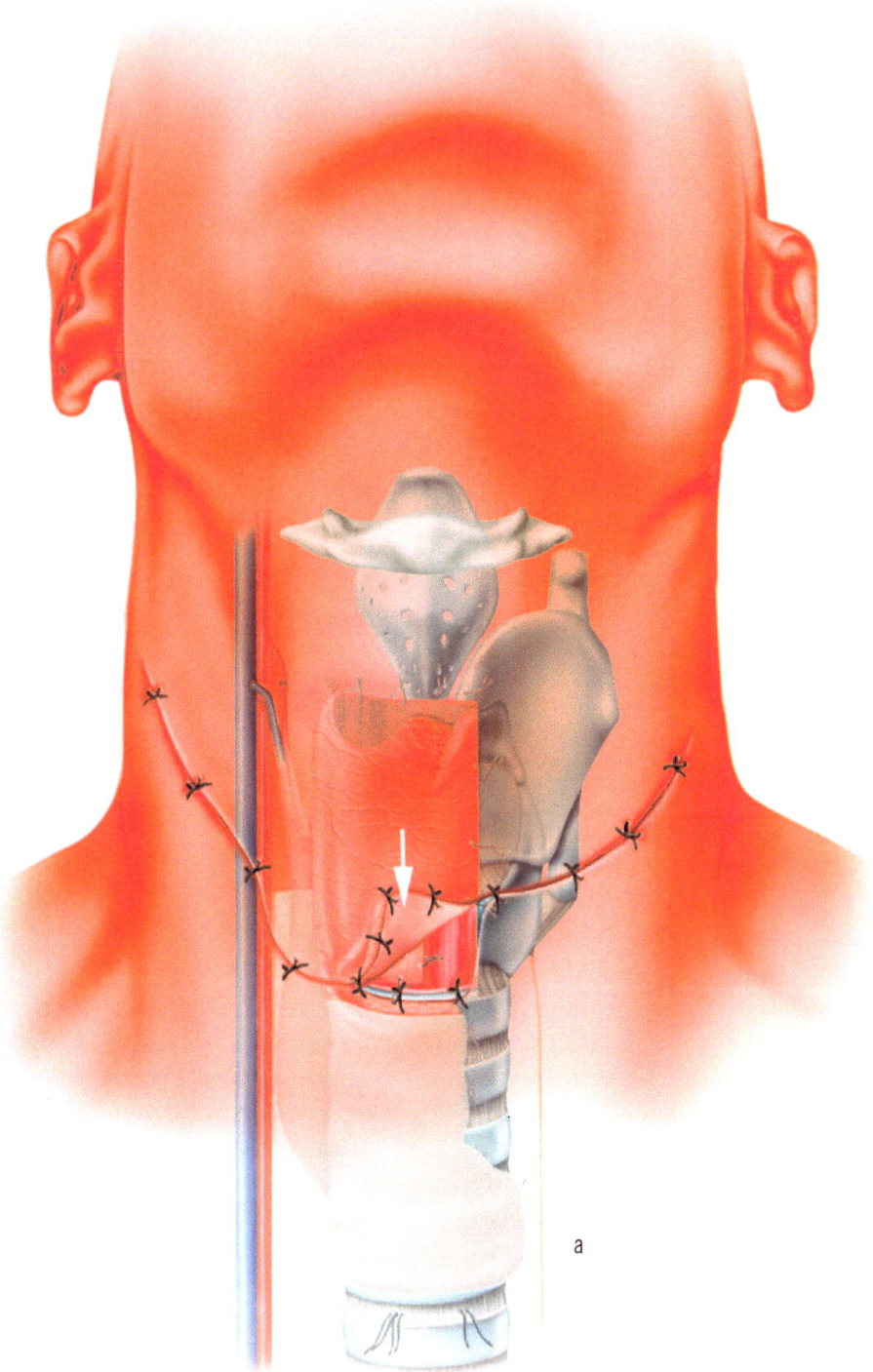

Figure 5.8. Situation after first operation.
a. Schematic presentation.
The upper neck skin flap is attached to the superior side of the 'tracheostome' and the lower neck skin flap is *attached to the inferior side of the tracheostome. The lower edge of the radial skin (arrow) serves as an external monitor for the radial forearm flap.*

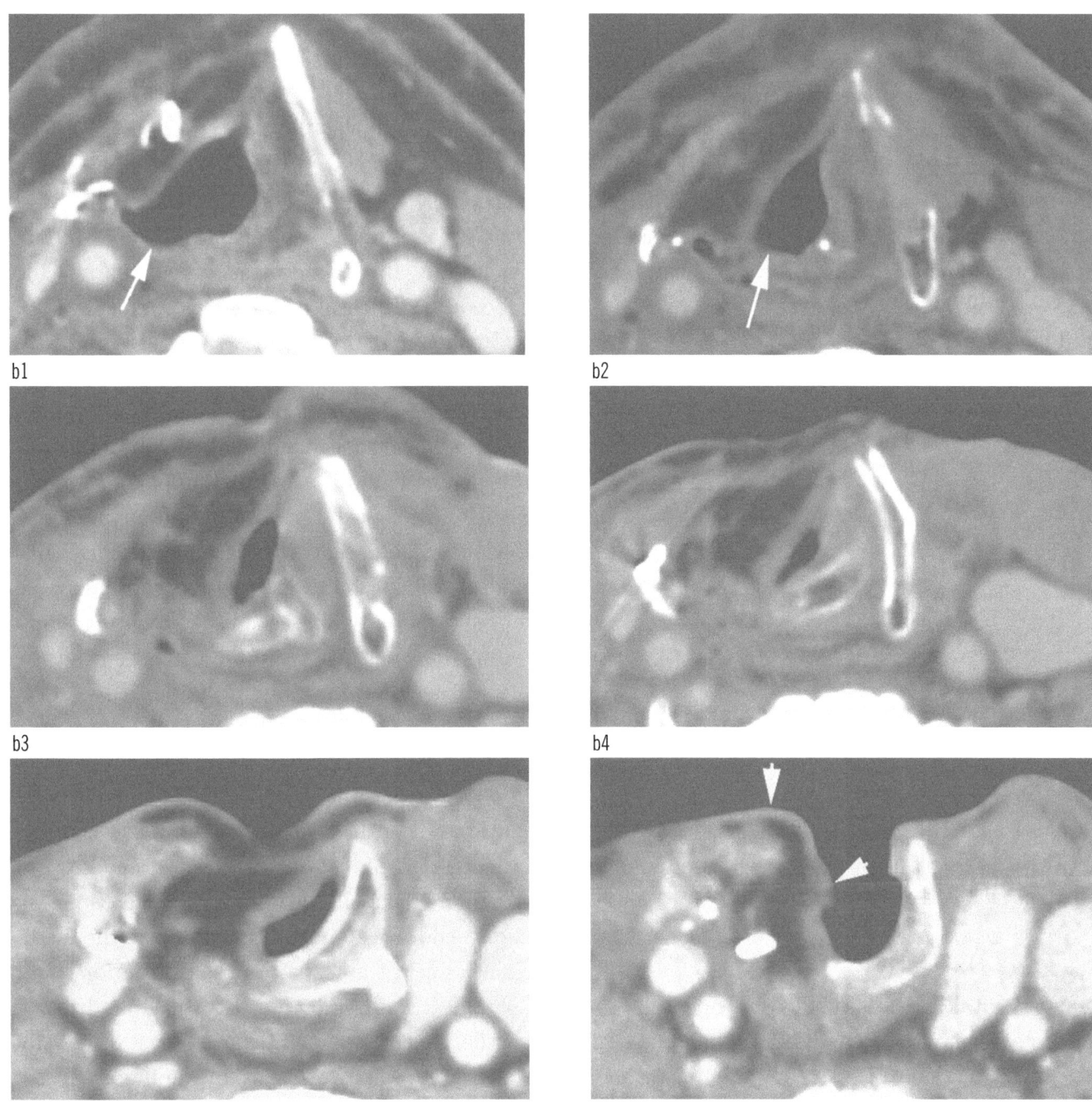

b1

b2

b3

b4

b5

b6

Figure 5.8. Situation after first operation (continued).
b. *CT scan after first operation.*
b.1., b.2. *Supraglottic larynx. The bulk provided by the radial forearm skin in the posterior larynx (arrow) is not sufficient. This results in aspiration for liquids.*
b.3. *Glottic larynx. Radial skin flap is located close to the midline.*
b.4. *Subglottic level.*
b.5. *Subglottic level. Levels 4 and 5 are axial sections*

cranial from the 'tracheostomy'. Restoration of the airway lumen is not sufficient to allow for decannulation.
b.6. *Subglottic larynx at the level of the tracheostomy. One side of the tracheostomy is formed by cricoid cartilage; the other side by radial forearm skin. The lower edge of the radial forearm skin (arrowheads) is exteriorized and serves as an external monitor. Usually, the tracheostomy is self sustaining.*

Antibiotics (Metronidazole 3x500 mg/d and Cefadroxil 3x1 g/d) are administered to avoid infection of the tracheostomy during the first week. With a viable radial forearm flap, no wound healing problems will be encountered after the first operation. In some patients, the lower neck skin flap may show dehiscence at the lower site of the tracheostome so that the Gore-tex membrane becomes visible. This is however well tolerated until the second operation (Fig. 5.9).

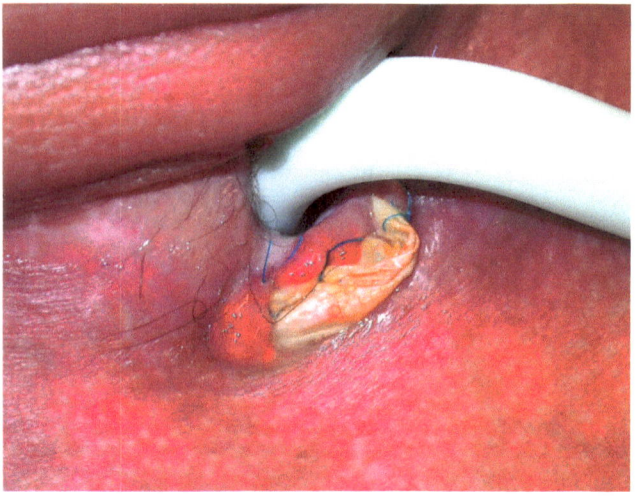

Figure 5.9. Tracheostomy before second operation. Patient is intubated before start of second operation. ePTFE membrane is visible at lower site of tracheostomy.

Removal of skin flap. The second operation is performed 4 months after the first operation. At that time, neck skin flaps are elevated using the same skin incision. The anterior suture line between laryngeal remnant and radial forearm skin is identified, and the suture line is opened except for the upper 2 cm. The radial forearm skin flap is removed except for a strip of radial forearm skin that remained at the supraglottic level (Fig. 5.10). The definitive reconstruction is started after obtaining a negative report of the frozen sections taken at the original anterior and posterior section margins.

Mobilization of trachea. The fascia wapping the cervical trachea is identified. The ePTFE membrane around the fascia allows for easy identification. The fascia is well attached to the underlying trachea. The fascial-enwrapped part of cervical trachea is excised as visible in Fig. 5.10.b. Technically, this is the most difficult part of the procedure. Tracheal mobilization can be facilitated by the ePTFE membrane as visible in Fig. 5.16.

Tracheal autotransplantation. The isolated fascial-enwrapped part of cervical trachea is brought up into the laryngeal defect. The tracheal patch is transferred without manipulation of the vascular pedicle. Inset of the tracheal autotransplant into the laryngeal defect occurs as shown in Fig. 5.10.

End-to end anastomosis. After reconstruction, the airway continuity is re-established by bringing up the mediastinal trachea to the caudal end of the reconstructed larynx. A blunt finger dissection is performed to release the tracheal wall down into the mediastinum. After tracheal autotransplantation the mediastinal trachea is still in continuity with the reconstructed larynx through the membranous part of cervical trachea. A small rim of membranous trachea is removed to allow for easy end-to-end anastomosis. The stump of the mediastinal trachea is reanastomosed posteriorly and laterally towards the cricoid cartilage and to the hemilaryngeal patch. A tracheostome is formed by suturing the skin towards the anterior airway defect (Fig. 5.11). The end-to-end anastomosis is performed without tension.

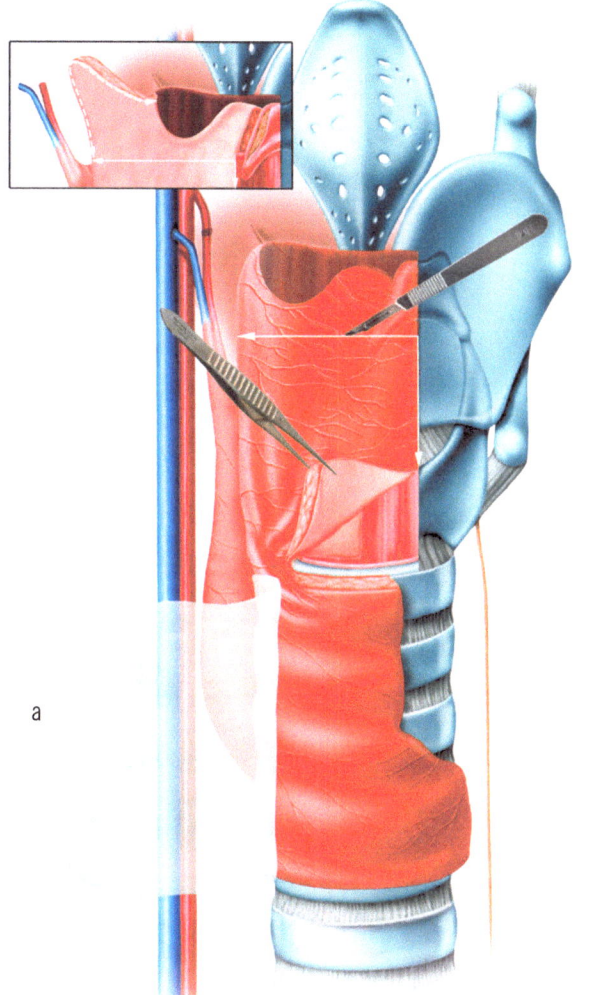

a

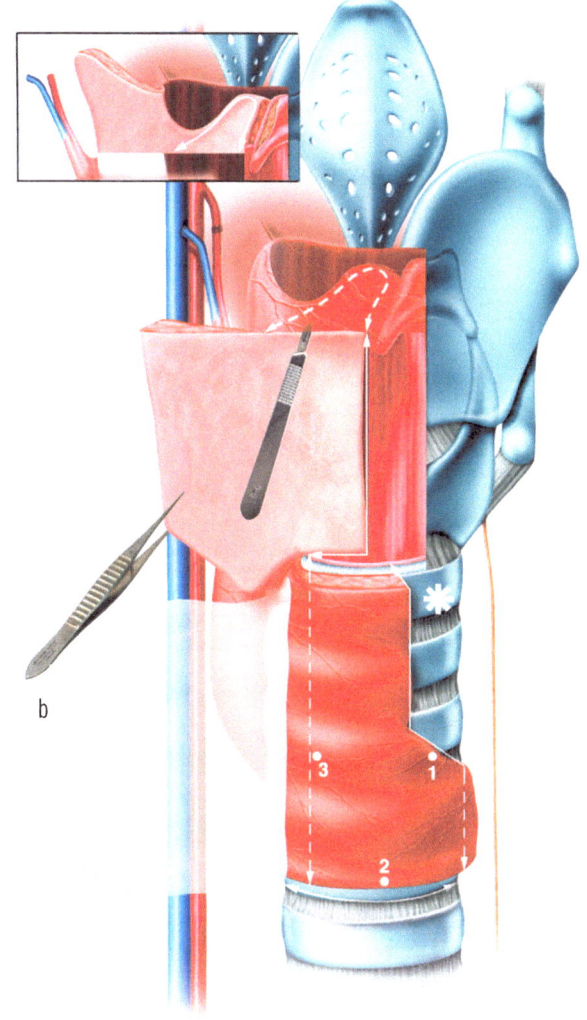

b

Figure 5.10. Overview of second operative procedure.
a. Situation after re-elevation of the neck skin flaps. The expanded polytetrafluoroethylene membrane is removed from the revascularized segment of trachea. The anterior suture line between radial forearm skin flap and laryngeal remnant is opened except for the upper 2 cm at the supraglottic level. The radial forearm skin flap is incised (double arrow) leaving a strip of skin attached to the mucosal section line formed by the pyriform sinus and the caudal border of the epiglottis.
Inset: View after opening of the anterior and superior suture line of the preserved skin flap (white dotted double arrow).
b. The radial forearm skin flap is completely separated from the laryngeal remnant except for the cranial strip of skin, which remains attached to the laryngeal and

pharyngeal mucosal suture line. The skin flap is completely separated from the superior skin strip and is pulled outwards. The fascial enwrapped portion of trachea is isolated. At the tumor side the trachea is incised over a height of 4 cm between the cartilage ring and the membranous trachea (3). At the side opposite the tumor, the trachea is incised over a height of 4 cm following the pattern of fascial wrapping (1). Below the 4 cm segment, the trachea is incised in an axial plane with preservation of the membranous trachea (2). At the side opposite the tumor, a part of cartilaginous trachea (asterisk) will stay in place. Inset: View of skin incision after opening of the anterior and superior suture line of the preserved skin flap.

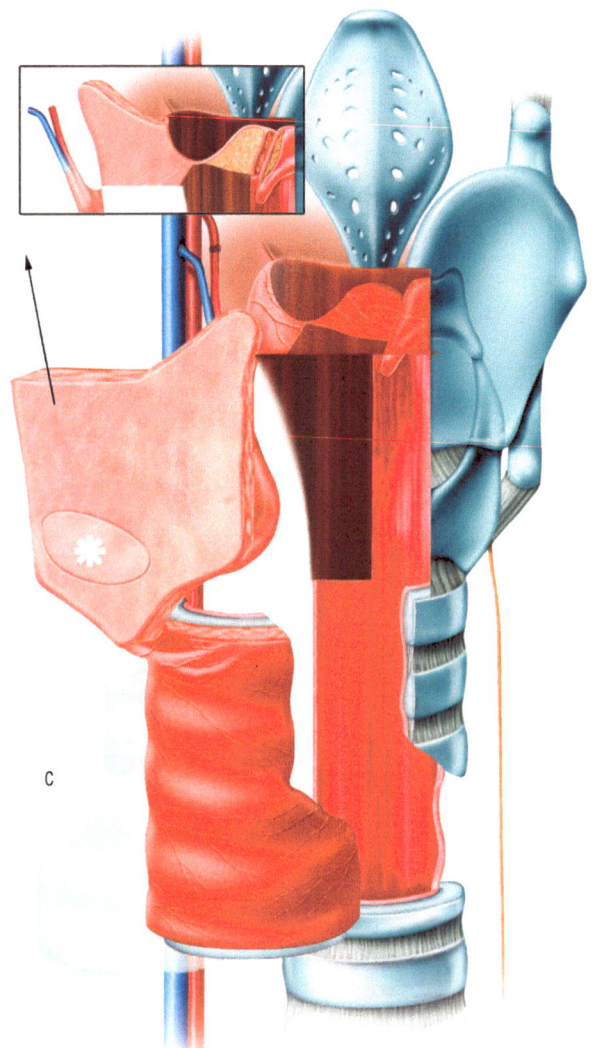

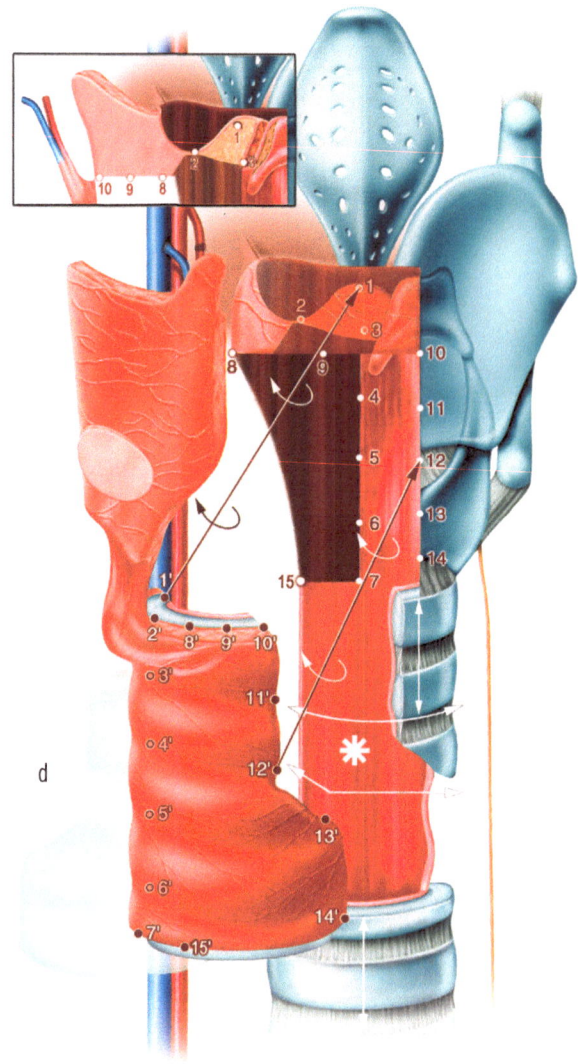

Figure 5.10. Overview of second operative procedure (continued).

c. *The skin island of the radial forearm flap and the fascial enwrapped trachea are completely isolated. The skin flap is moved upward and outside (arrow) and the epithelium will be removed except for a small island (asterisk) that is placed in the neck skin incision (serving as an external monitor).*

Inset: View after opening of the anterior and superior suture line of the preserved skin flap.

d. *The patch of revascularized trachea is moved upwards and will be rotated in a clockwise direction (arrow) towards the laryngeal defect. The posterior glottic bulk is restored by suturing the patch to the radial forearm skin (1'-2'-3' to 1-2-3). The posterior*

site of the tracheal patch (4' to 7') is sutured to the posterior section line of the cricoid cartilage (4 to 7) from superior to inferior. The upper site of the tracheal patch (8' to 10') is sutured to the cranially located strip of radial forearm skin (8 to 10). The anterior site of the tracheal patch (11' to 14') is sutured to the anterior laryngeal section line (11 to 14) from superior to inferior. A small part of the membranous trachea is resected (asterisk) to allow for easy end-to-end anastomosis between reconstructed larynx and mediastinal trachea. The upper 2 rings of mediastinal trachea are incised anteriorly. Inset: View after opening of the anterior and superior suture line of the preserved skin flap.

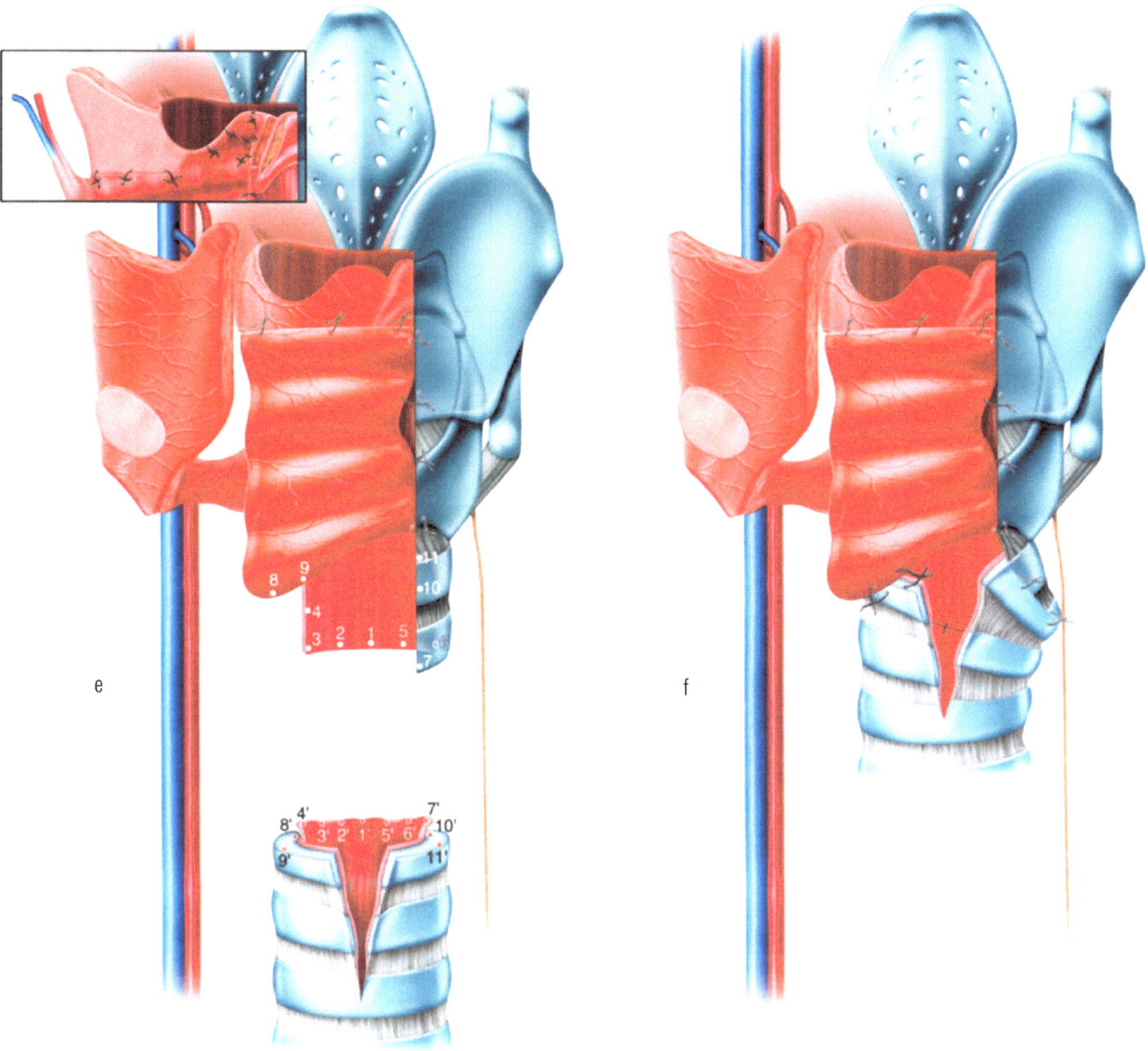

e

f

Figure 5.10. Overview of second operative procedure (continued).

e. After insetting of the patch, the mediastinal trachea can be mobilized superiorly and sutured to the reconstructed larynx. The trachea is mobilized by blunt finger dissection. The trachea (1'-11') is sutured to the laryngeal remnant (1-11).

Inset: View after opening of the anterior and superior suture line of the preserved skin flap.

f. Situation after tracheal autotransplantation and end-to-end anastomosis of mediastinal trachea.

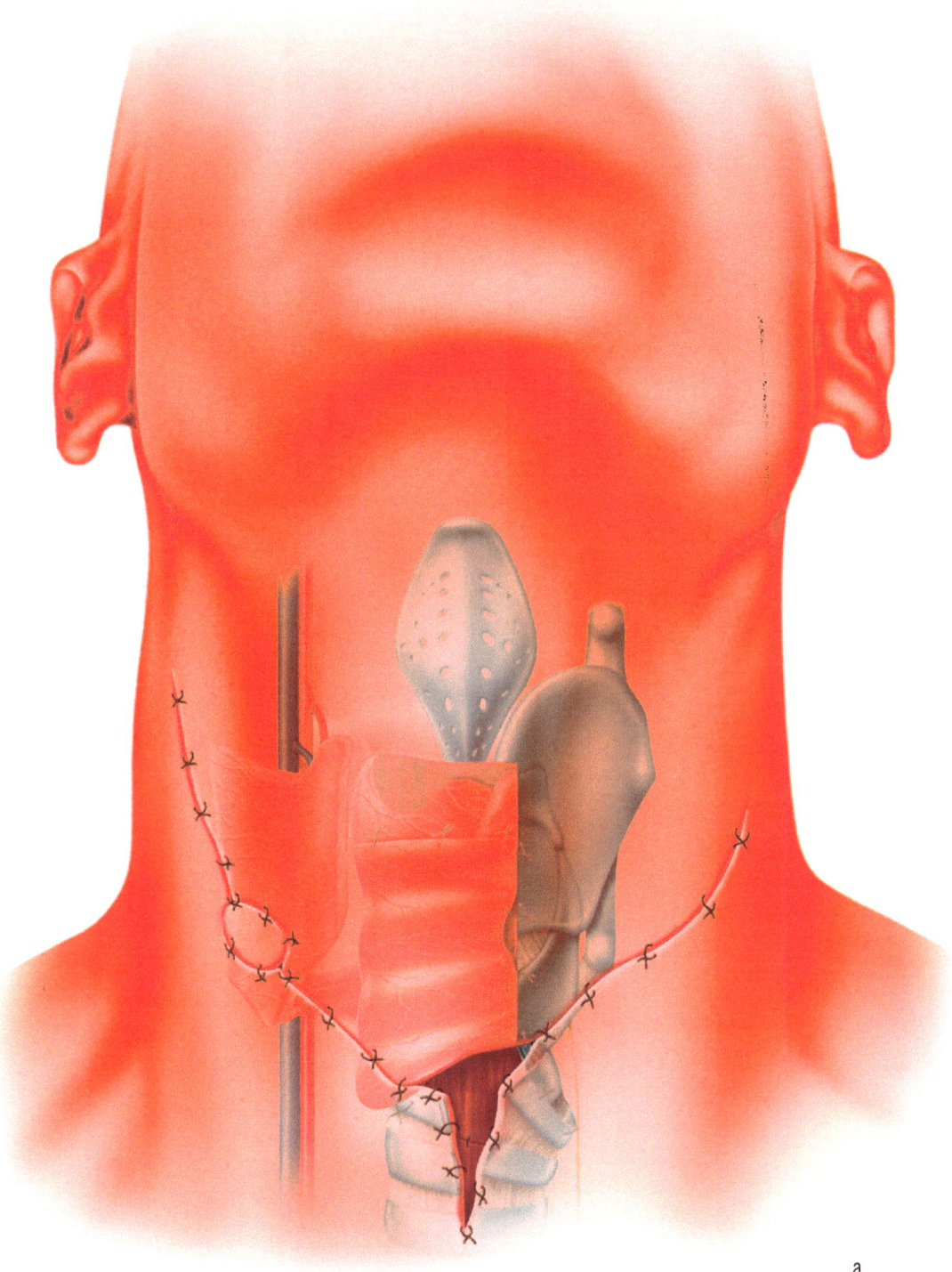

a

Figure 5.11. Situation after second operation.
a. Overview. The upper neck skin flap is sutured to the reconstructed larynx and the lower neck skin flap is sutured to the incised trachea anteriorly. A tracheosto- *my is created. The small skin paddle of the radial forearm flap is placed in the neck incision and serves as a monitor.*

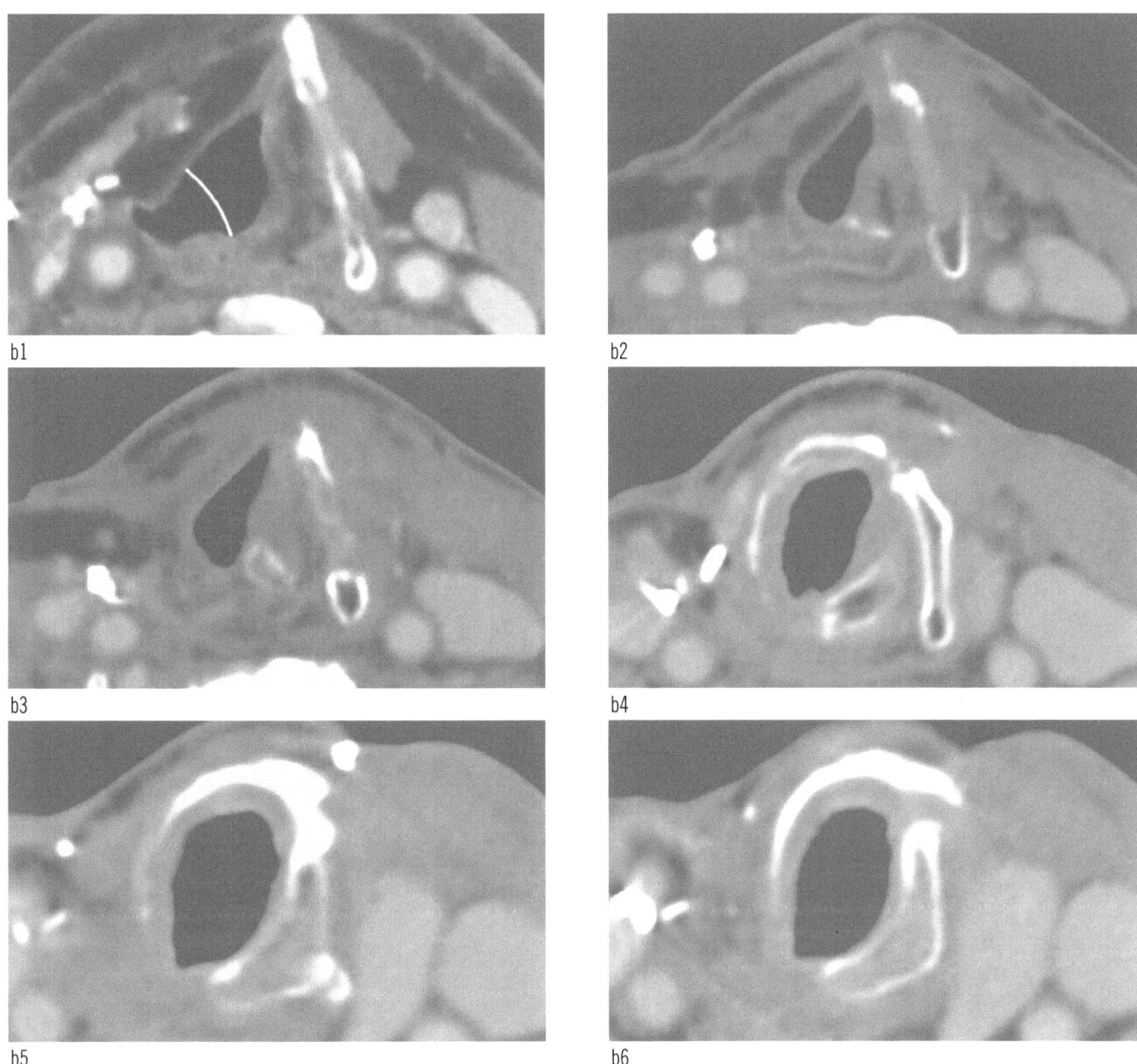

Figure 5.11.
Situation after second operation (continued).
b. Computer tomography images after second operation
b.1. Supraglottic larynx 1. Absence of posterior bulk (desired bulk indicated by white line) at supraglottic level.
b.2. Supraglottic larynx 2.
b.3. Glottic larynx.
A strip of radial forearm skin is preserved anteriorly at the supraglottic and glottic level. After 4 months, the
strip of skin is sufficiently perfused by collateral supply from the laryngeal and pharyngeal suture line. The posterior larynx is restored by the tracheal transplant.
b.4. Subglottic level 1.
b.5. Subglottic level 2.
b.6. Subglottic level 3.
The subglottic airway lumen is fully restored to allow for decannulation. The full amount of cartilage ring repairs the larynx at the subglottic level.

2.A.1.b. Patient 2

A 54-year-old male patient presented with a liposarcoma of the right hemilarynx and the right pyriform sinus. He was treated before by several endoscopical resections and 1 external approach. A temporary tracheotomy had to be placed after 1 of his endocopical resections 4 years before his actual presentation. At the time of tumor recurrence, the patient showed a submucosal mass at the right vocal folds with impaired mobility but without crossing of the anterior or posterior commissure. There was involvement of the supraglottis at the level of the false vocal fold (Fig. 5.12, 5.13).

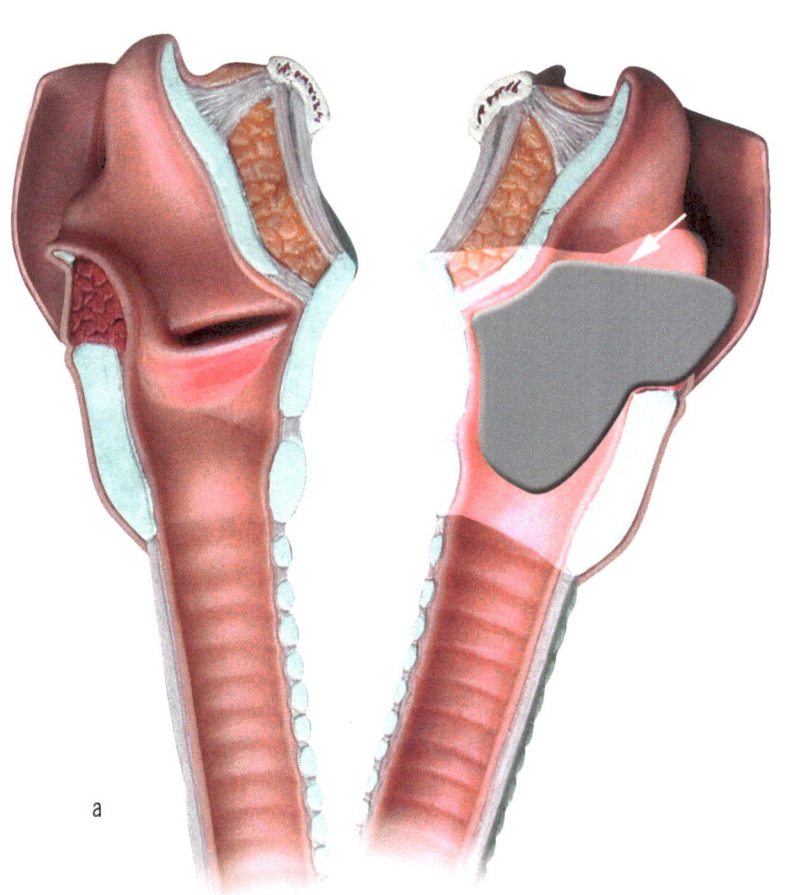
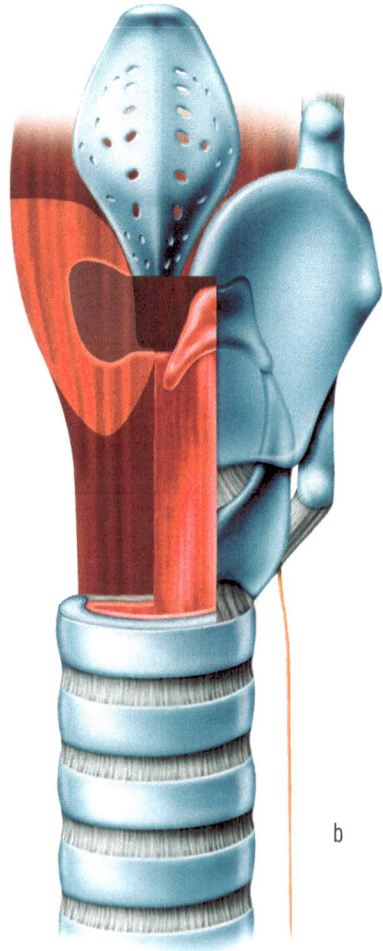

Figure 5.12. Patient 2. Tumor extension and extend of resection.
a. The tumor is resected by performing an extended hemilaryngectomy at the right side. Involvement of the supraglottis is a contraindication for tracheal transplantation. However, this low-grade liposarcoma can be removed completely at the superior section margin (arrow). The anterior section margin is located in the anterior commissure.

b. The right pyriform sinus mucosa is resected together with the tumor.

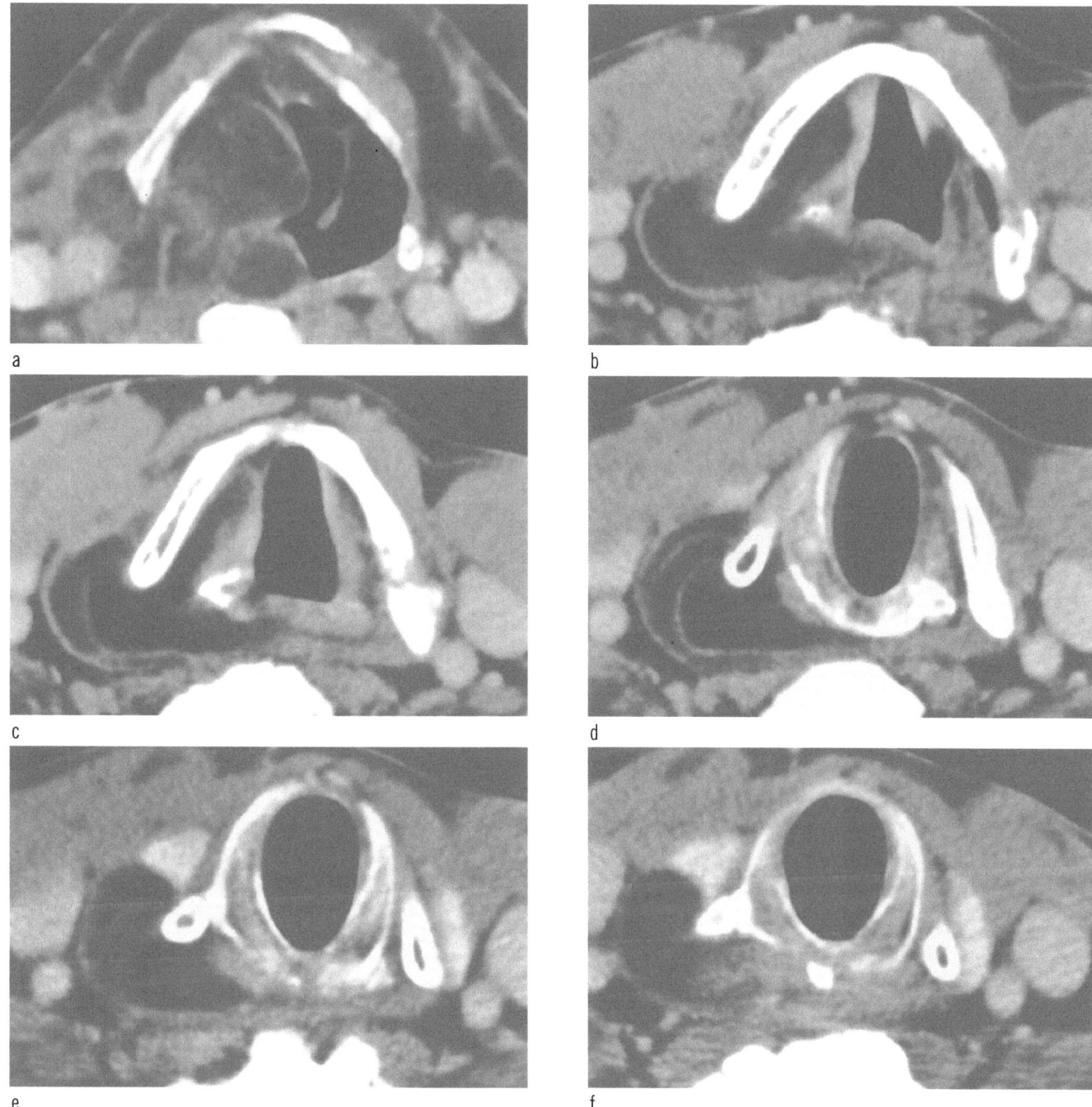

Figure 5.13. Tumor extension on CT scan.
a. Supraglottic level.
b. Supraglottic level.
c. Glottic level.
d. Subglottic level (high).
e. Subglottic level.
f. Subglottic level (low).

Tumor invades the supraglottis (level of the false vocal fold), paraglottic region, cricothyroid joint, and pyriform sinus region.

The patient was treated, similar to patient 1, with the modified autotransplantation concept. A time interval of 4 months existed between the 2 opera- tions. CT images after tracheal autotransplanta- tion are visible in Fig. 5.14.

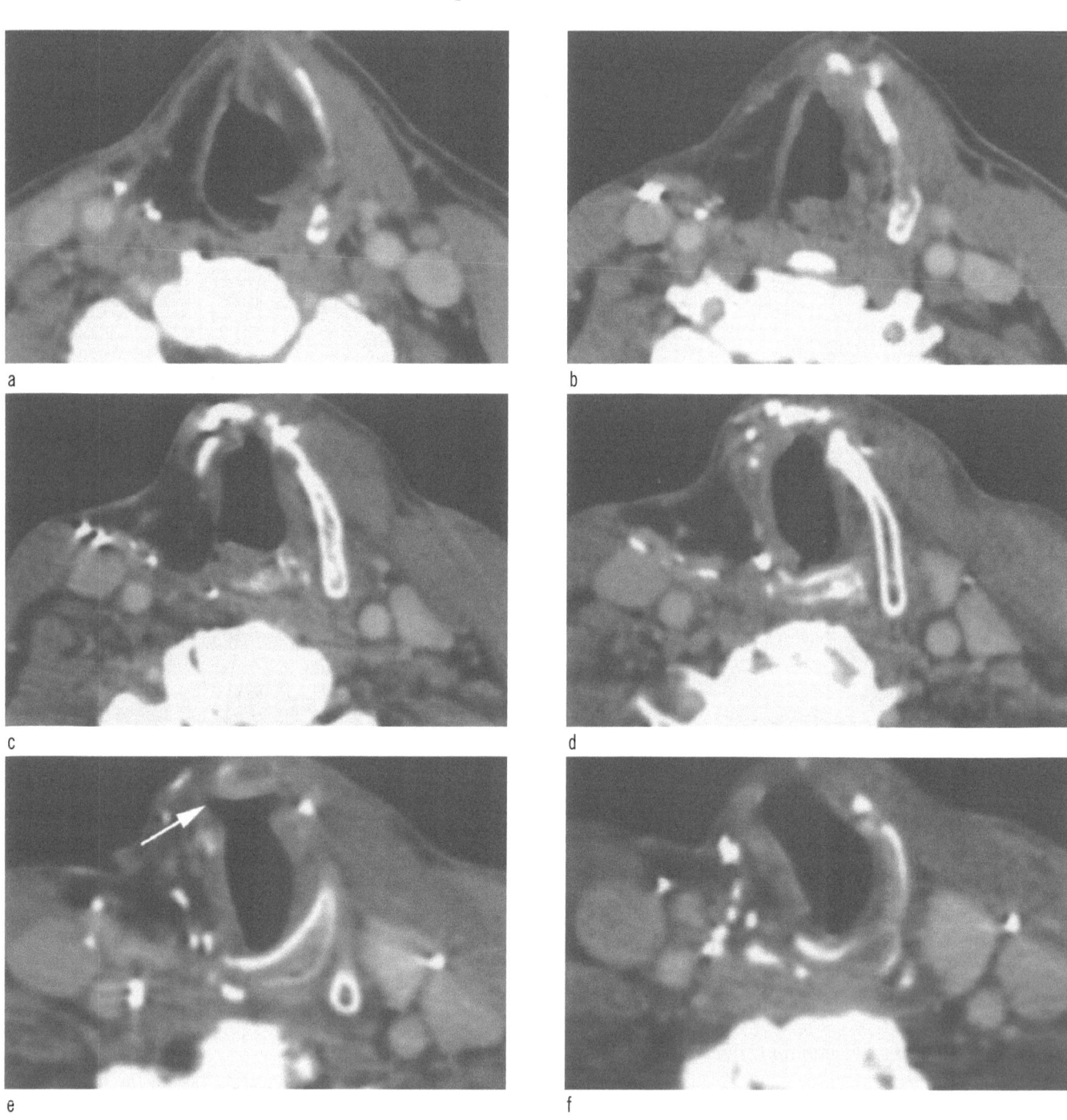

Figure 5.14. CT scan after reconstruction.
a. Supraglottic level.
b. Supraglottic level.
c. Glottic level.
d. Subglottic level (high).
e. Subglottic level.
f. Subglottic (low)
Arrow points to a weak point in the tracheal patch (pre- vious tracheotomy site).

With the modified approach, removal of the neck nodes and resection of the primary tumor occur in the first operation and the fascial wrapping of the cervical trachea is performed after having full security about the indication for a conservation laryngectomy. In the modified concept, tracheal autotransplantation serves as a "second-look" procedure at the critical time period (4 months) to detect local recurrences. Other advantages when using the modified concept are the presence of a "tracheostomy" after the first operation and the fact that the second operation is easier to perform from a technical viewpoint. With the initial concept, in approximately 10% of the patients extubation could not be performed after the first operation, and these patients remained in the intensive care unit for the 2-week revascularization period. The presence of a tracheostomy allows for a fast recovery of the laryngeal functions and for a relatively short hospital admission time. Technically, the most challenging parts of the procedure in the initial concept were the complete mobilization of the circumferentially wrapped cervical trachea and the restoration of the airway continuity after tracheal autotransplantation. In the modified concept, only that part of the cervical cartilaginous trachea that is necessary for reconstruction is wrapped by fascia. Mobilization of the enwrapped part of trachea without dissection of the membranous trachea is much easier than the circumferential mobilization necessary with the initial concept. Furthermore, the preserved posterior part of cervical trachea allows for an easy, tension-free, end-to-end anastomosis between the mediastinal trachea and the reconstructed larynx. A disadvantage of the 4-month delay period between the two operations is that the tissue adhesions may be more pronounced than after a 14-day revascularization period. The disadvantage of difficult dissection can be overcome by the proper placement of an ePTFE membrane. The membrane consists of expanded polytetrafluoroethylene, one of the most chemically inert and biocompatible materials known. The membrane thickness is 0.1 mm with a pore size of less than 1 µm. This small pore size excludes tissue ingrowth, thereby limiting attachment between the membrane and adjacent structures. The ePTFE membrane allows for a relatively easy upwards mobilization of the revascularized trachea (Fig. 5.15, 5.16). Using a ePTFE membrane to wrap the forearm fascia dramatically reduces adhesions and facilitates tracheal isolation and transplantation.

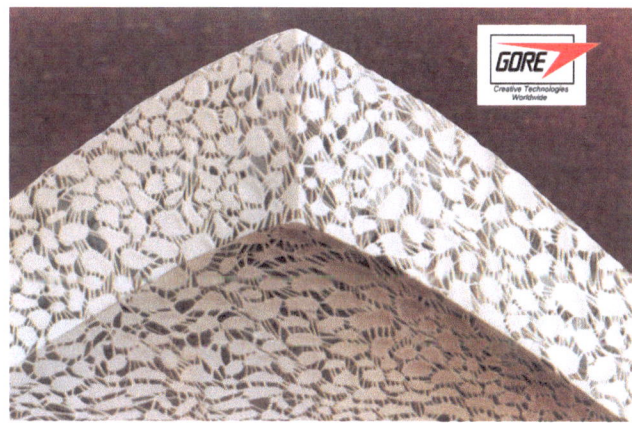

Figure 5.15. Ultrastructure of ePTFE membrane.
The tight microstructure of the ePTFE surface is effective at minimizing tissue attachment. With an average porosity of less than one micron, the microstructure prevents penetration by fibroblasts and other mesenchymal cells and thus minimizes dense fibrous ingrowth. After three to four months in vivo, the membrane becomes translucent. This occurs through a wetting process in which air molecules within the ePTFE structure diffuse into the surrounding aqueous environment. As body fluid displaces the gas molecules, the material becomes translucent because of the similar index of refraction of the fluid end the ePTFE.

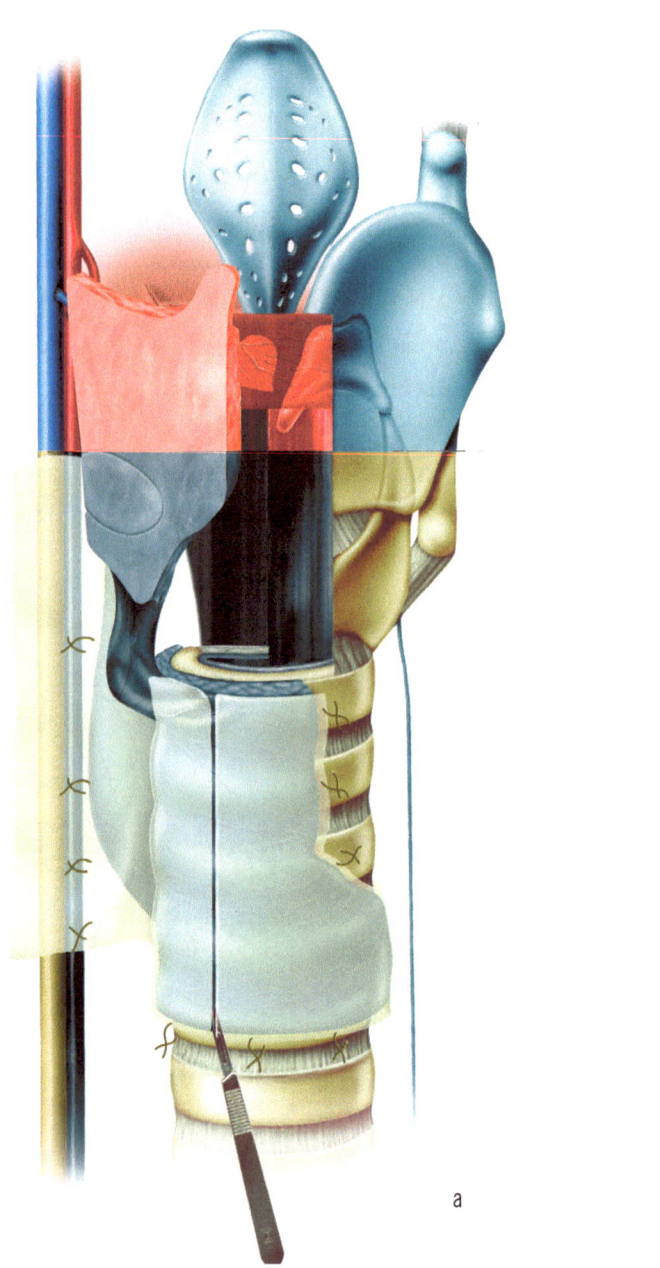

a

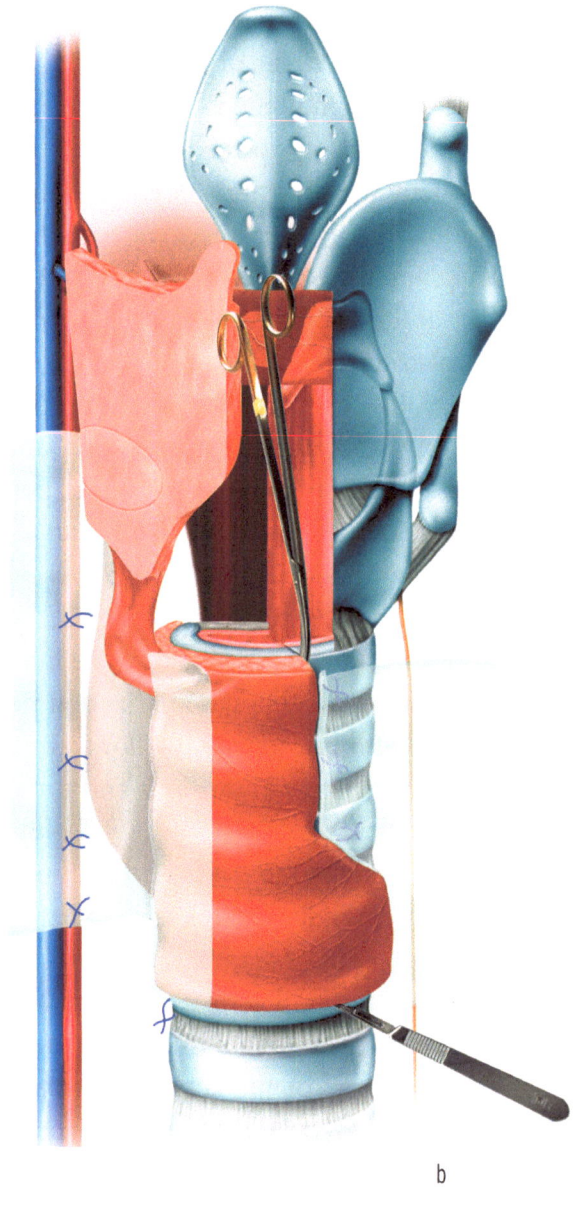

b

Figure 5.16. Mobilization of revascularized segment of trachea with the help of the ePTFE membrane.

a. One side (distal end) of the expanded polytetrafluo-roethylene (ePTFE) membrane (Preclude Pericardial Membrane, 8 x 16 cm/0.1 mm) is sutured to the trachea using interrupted 4-0 Prolene sutures. The membrane is carefully sutured to the tracheal cartilage between the distal end of the fascia flap and the preserved recurrent nerve. The membrane is also attached to the trachea caudal from the fascial enwrapped part. The fascia wrapping the trachea is completely separated from the surrounding tissues by the ePTFE membrane. At the tumor site the membrane is sutured to the prevertebral fascia medial from the common carotid artery

and internal jugular vein. The distal end of the membrane covers the carotid artery and jugular vein.

During the second operation the ePTFE membrane is incised in the midline.

b. The distal part of the membrane is turned to the site of the preserved hemilarynx and protects the recurrent nerve during tracheal isolation. The trachea can be incised safely in the sleeve between the distal end of the ePTFE membrane and the distal end of the fascia flap. Another tracheal incision is placed caudal from the fascial enwrapped trachea.

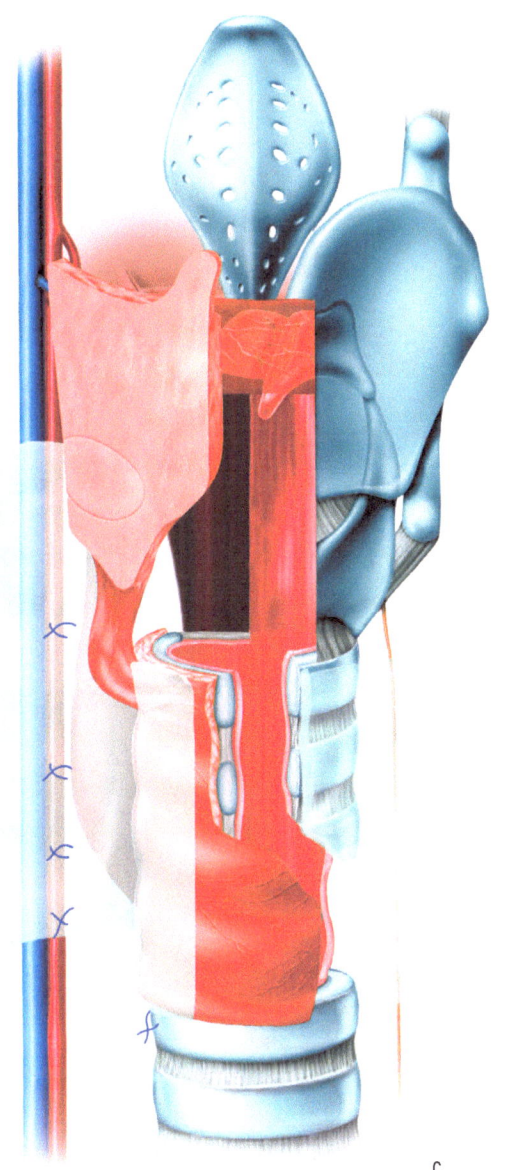

c

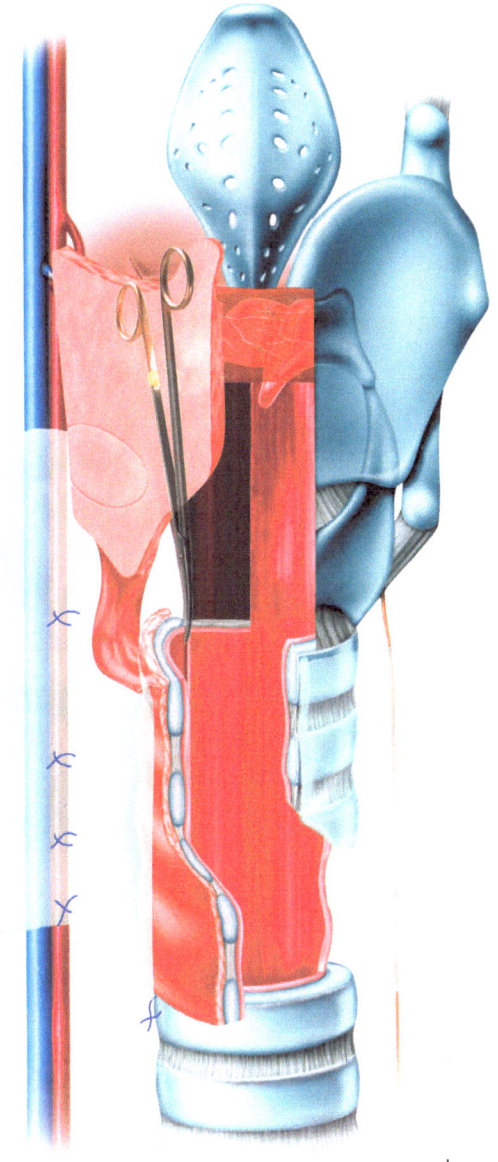

d

Figure 5.16. Mobilization of revascularized segment of trachea (continued).
c. The trachea is rotated to the site of the hemilaryngectomy.

d. After rotation, the tracheal incision can be placed between the cartilaginous ring and the membranous trachea. The part of the ePTFE membrane that wraps the neck vessels allows for an easy upwards mobilization of the revascularized trachea.

The donor defect of the radial forearm donor site is visible in Fig. 5.17.

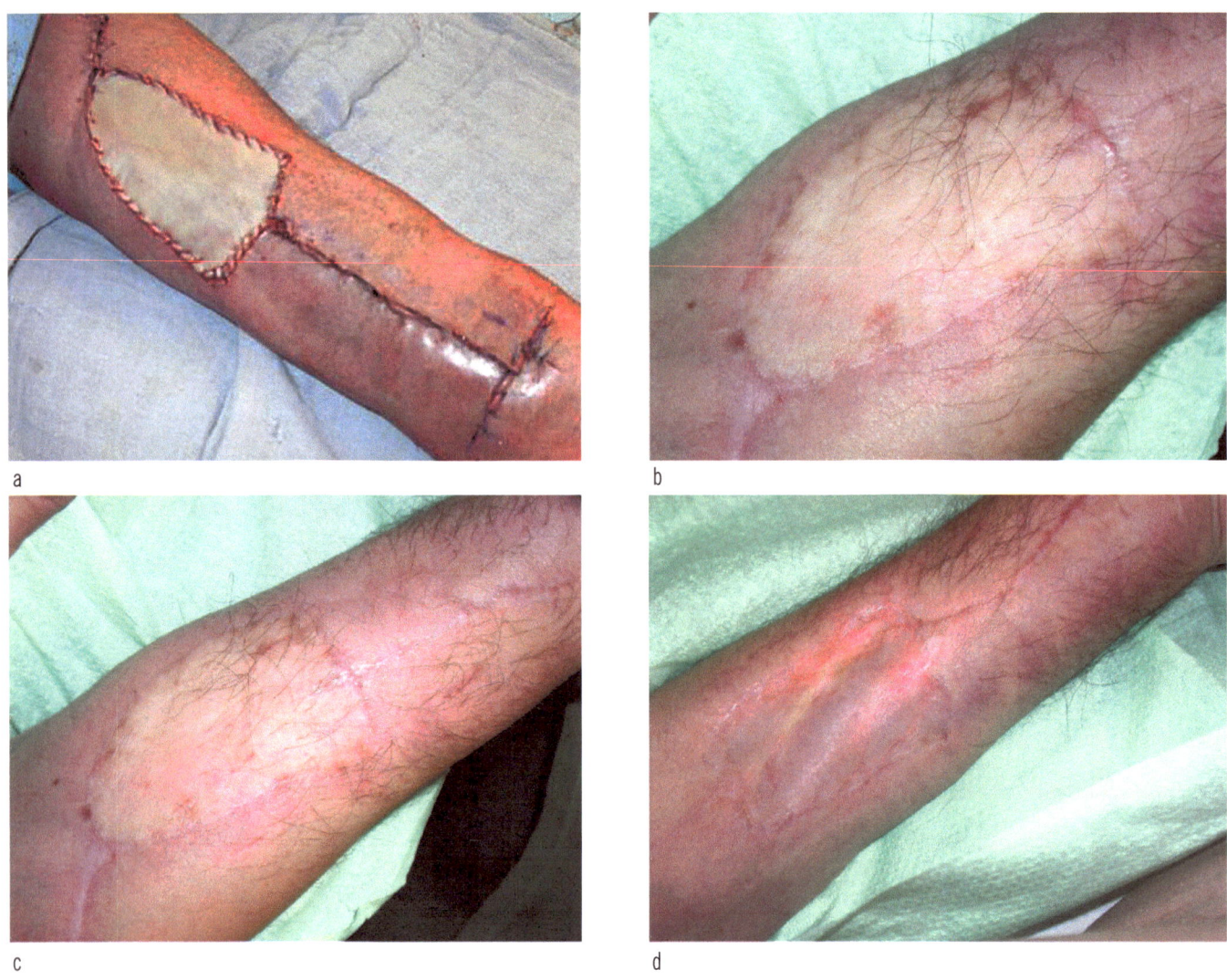

a

b

c

d

Figure 5.17. Radial forearm donor site.
a. Donor defect immediately after first operation. The defect of the skin paddle is repaired with a full-thickness skin graft (from groin area). The donor defect of the fascial paddle is closed primarily.

b. and c. Same defect as under a at the time of the second operation.
d. Donor defect 4 months postoperatively. Skin defect is closed with split-thickness skin graft (from thigh).

2.A.2. Functional results

2.A.2.a. After first operation

The tracheostomy was self-sustaining in the 2 patients. The patients could produce voice when the cannula or tracheostomy was closed during expiration (Fig. 5.18).

Figure 5.18. Function after first operation.
a. A cuffed Shiley cannula is inserted. A cannula without cuff is placed 3 days after the operation to allow for speaking during closure of the cannula.
b. The 'tracheostomy' is self-sustaining and the patient can produce voice when the tracheostomy is closed during expiration.

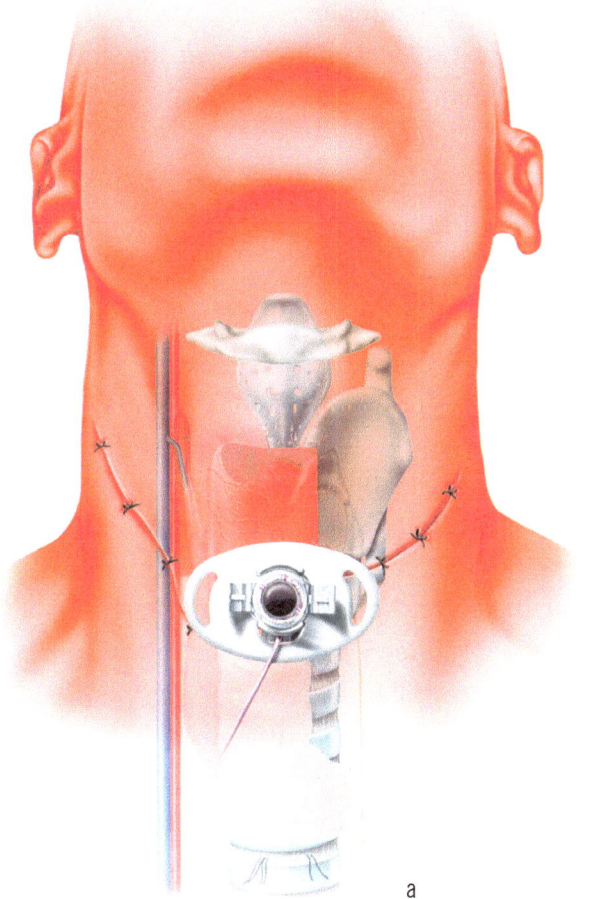

a

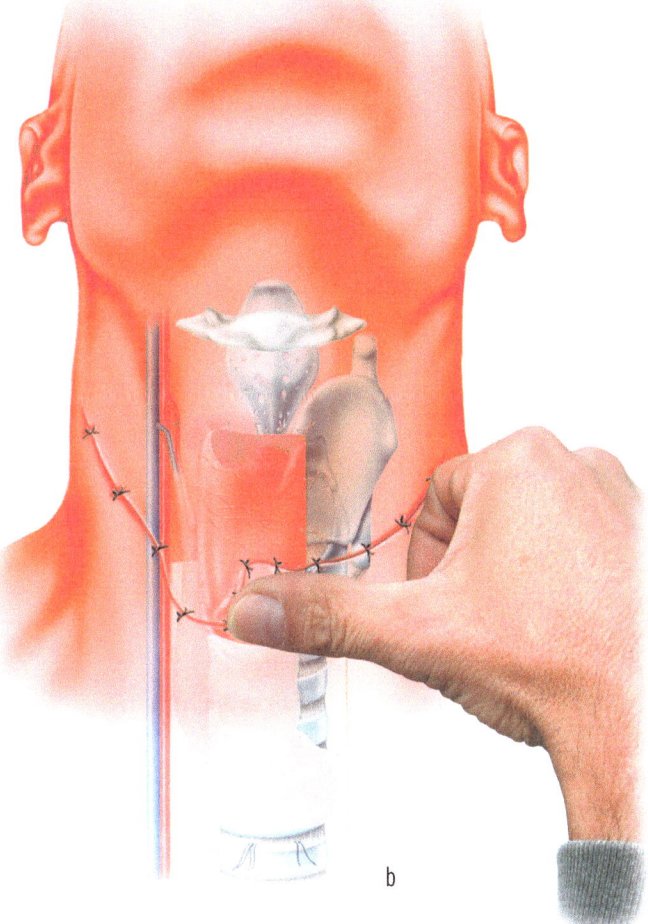

b

The sphincteric function was partially restored by the skin paddle of the radial forearm flap. Oral intake of solids was possible after 1 week. The 2 patients showed aspiration for liquids, and they used the gastrostomy for supplemental intake of liquids. The reason for the aspiration of liquids can be seen on the axial CT scan (Fig. 5.19.a). How to improve function in subsequent patients is shown in Fig 5.19.b.

2.A.2.b. After second operation

No recurrent tumor was detected on analysis of the frozen sections taken at the margins after removal of the skin paddle. Complete mobilization of the fascial-enwrapped trachea was the most difficult part of the procedure, because of adhesions with the surrounding tissues. Proper placement of the ePTFE membrane facilitated the procedure considerably (Fig. 5.16). The tracheostomy was self-sustaining in the 2 patients. The patients could produce voice when the cannula or tracheostomy was closed during expiration (Fig. 5.20). The patients received tube feeding after operation and attempts to start oral feeding were made after 1 week.

The tracheostomy can be closed (under local or general anesthesia) 4 to 6 weeks after tracheal autotransplantation. After tracheostomy closure, antibiotics are administered and the patient receives tube feeding during 5 days to prevent infection. The PEG tube can be removed 1 week after tracheostomy closure (Fig. 5.21).

After the second operation, oral intake of solids was possible after 8 days. It took however several weeks before oral intake of liquids without aspiration was possible. The reason of the long-term aspiration for liquids and saliva is the insufficient bulk in the region of the resected arytenoid. After closure of the tracheostomy, the voice remained 'breathy'. The voice could be improved by exercising some pressure over the reconstructed laryngeal side (Fig. 5.22).

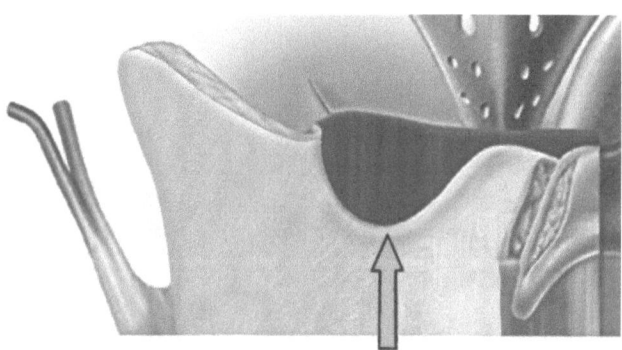

Figure 5.19.
How to improve function after first operation?
a. CT scan at glottic level. The posterior gap between arytenoid and forearm skin flap (arrow) results in aspiration for liquids.
b. There is too much skin included in the anterior glottic and supraglottic area. The gap (arrow) between the tissue bulk provided in the posterior larynx and the anterior skin flap has to be avoided.

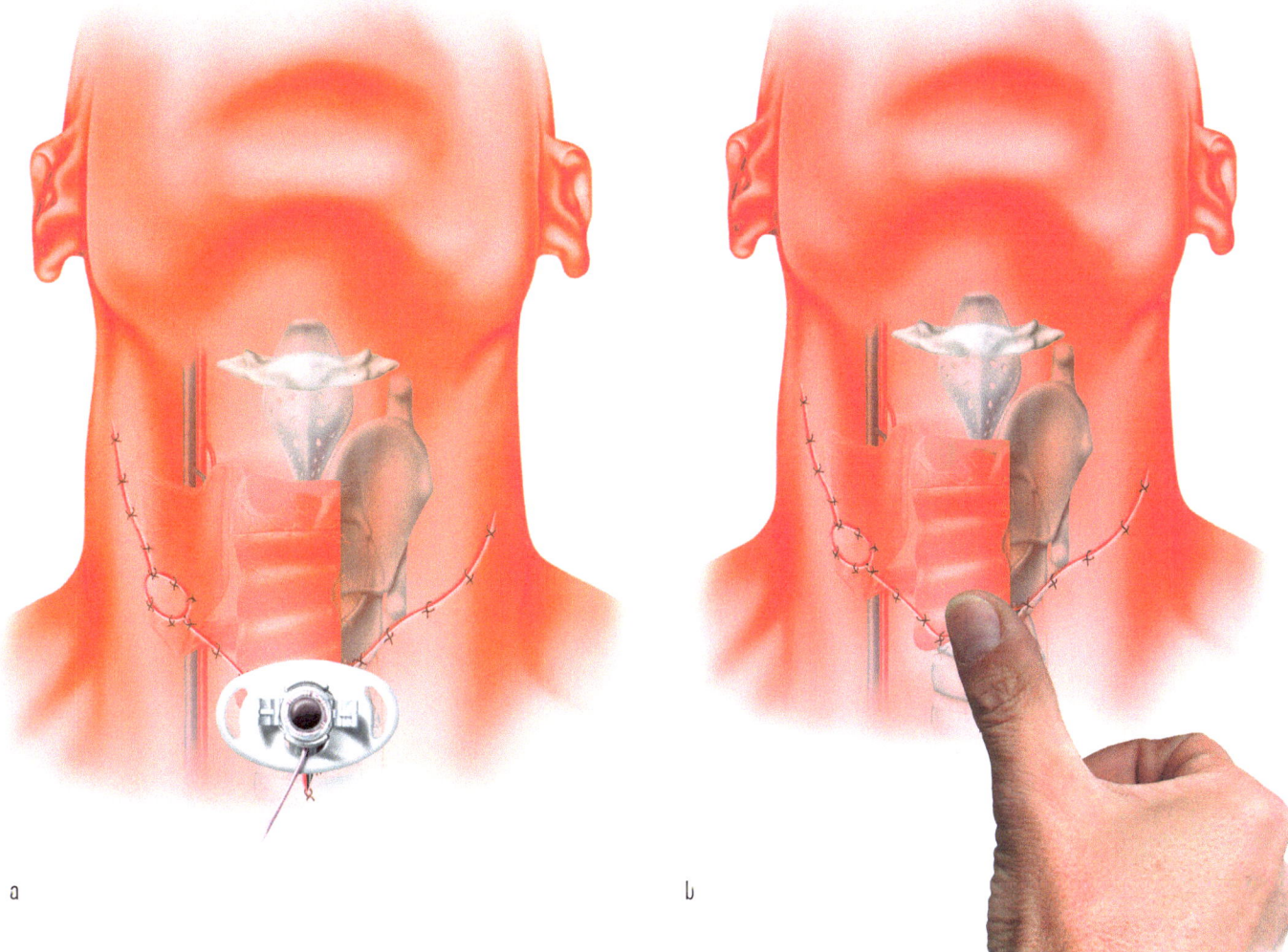

a   b

Figure 5.20.
Function after second operation.
a. A cuffed Shiley cannula is placed in the tracheostome.
b. The cannula is removed 3 days after operation to allow
for speaking during closure of the tracheostome.

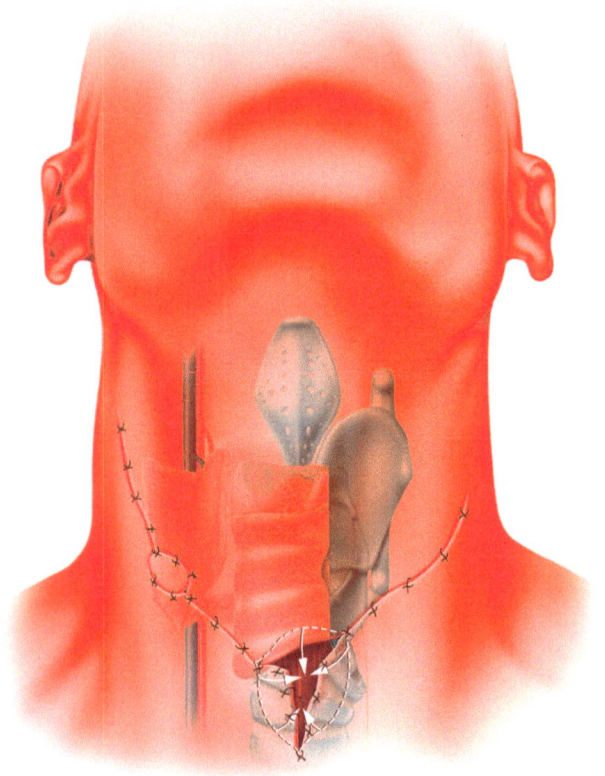

a

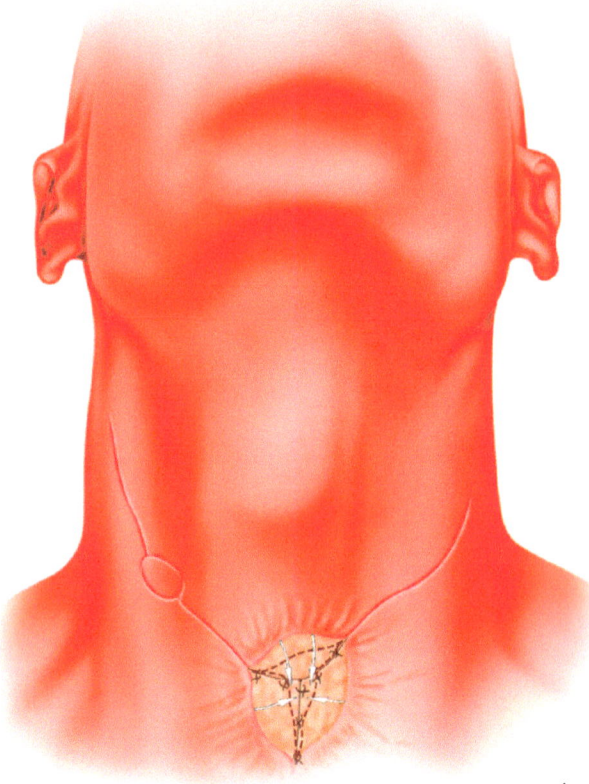

b

Figure 5.21. Closure of tracheostomy.
The tracheostomy is closed 6 weeks after the definitive
reconstruction. The tracheostomy is closed by (a) inci-
sion and (b) inversion of the skin around the tracheo-
stome. The upper and lower neck skin flap are under-
mined and closed (c).

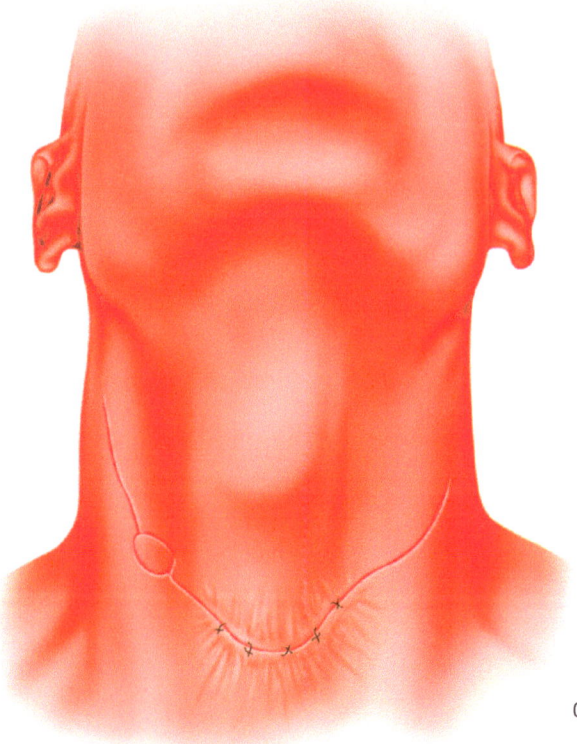

c

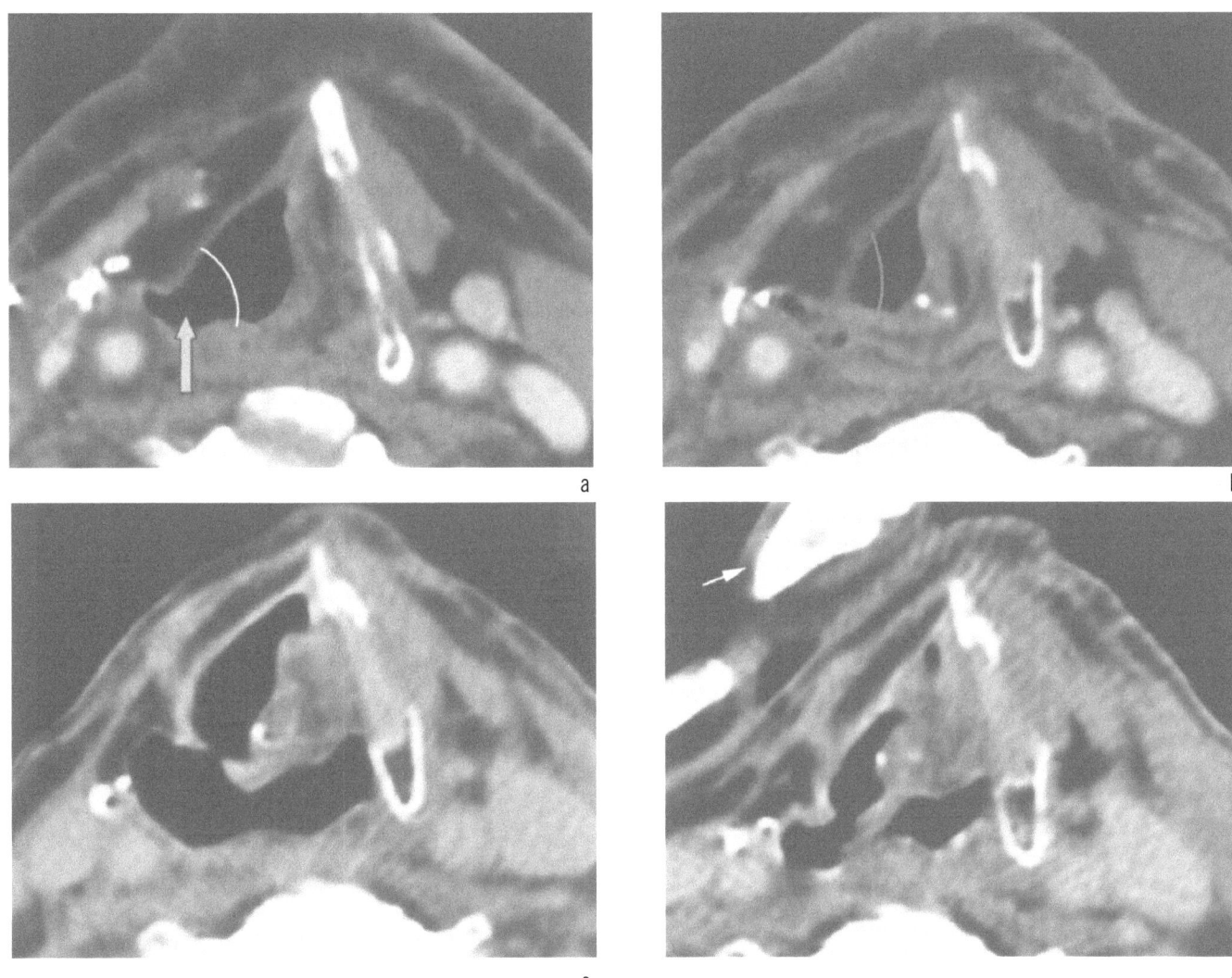

Figure 5.22. Functional results after second operation.
a. CT scan supraglottic level. The gap (arrow) between the top of the arytenoid and the skin flap results in aspiration for liquids. The desired posterior bulk is indicated by a white line.
b. CT scan glottic level. The bulk in the region of the posterior larynx is insufficient. The desired posterior bulk is indicated by a red line.

c. CT scan glottic level during phonation. Posterior insufficiency results in an aphonic voice during phonation and in aspiration for liquids.
d. CT scan glottic level during phonation and during finger pressure. The voice can be improved by external pressure exercised on the neck skin at the side of reconstruction. Arrow indicates finger over reconstructed larynx.

How to improve function after tracheal autotransplantation in subsequent patients is shown in Fig 5.23.

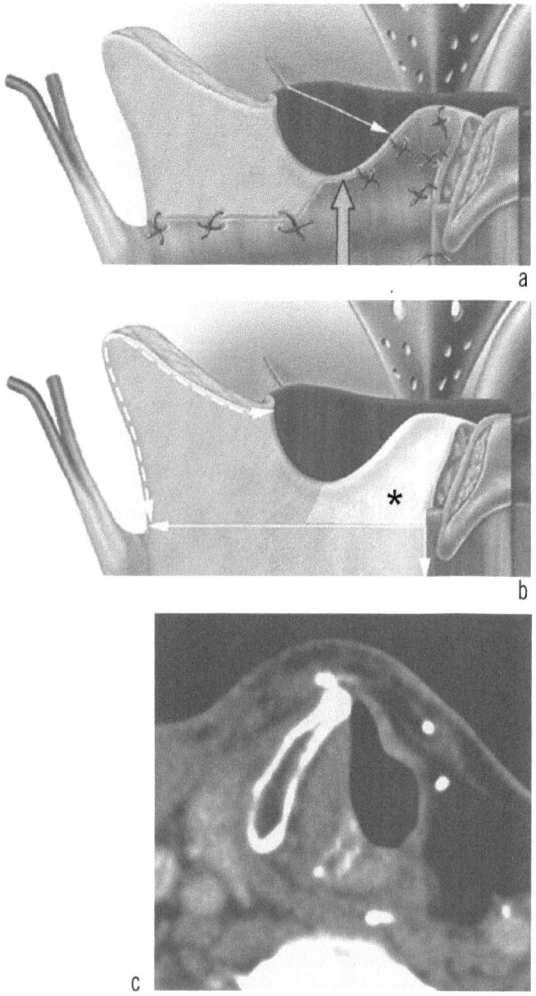

Figure 5.23. *How to improve function after second operation?*
a. Posterior bulk can be improved by removal of the skin flap in the anterior supraglottic and glottic larynx. The gap lateral of the reconstructed arytenoid (green arrow) has to be avoided. The aryepiglottic fold has to be sutured to the upper side of the tracheal patch (white arrow). Function may be improved by preserving the skin posteriorly (more bulk) and by resecting the skin anteriorly (contrary to situation in b and c).
b. Situation during second operation: anterior skin flap is preserved; posterior skin (asterisk) is removed.
c. Axial CT scan. Preserved skin flap is visible anteriorly and tracheal patch is visible posteriorly. Morphology leading to insufficiency.

2.B. *Optimal reconstruction of extended hemilaryngectomy defects*

From the functional results obtained in the first 2 patients, guidelines were set forward to improve speech and swallowing function after tracheal autotransplantation (Fig. 5.19 and 5.23). The optimal reconstruction after extended hemilaryngectomy was defined on the coronal CT scan of a normal larynx taken during quiet respiration and during phonation (Fig. 5.24, 5.25).

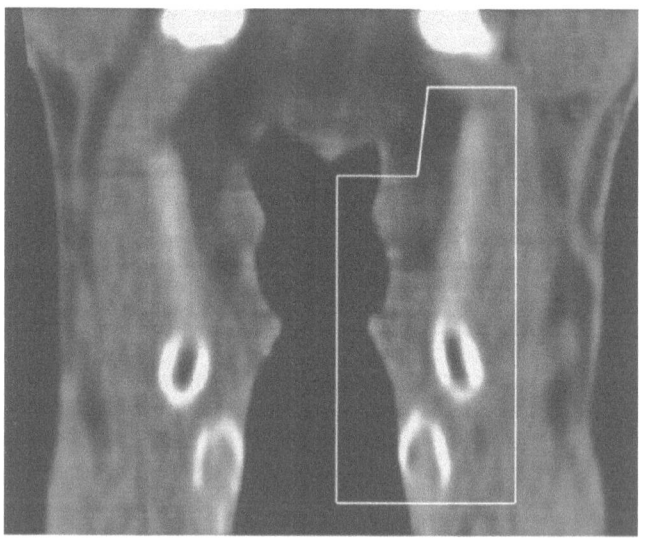

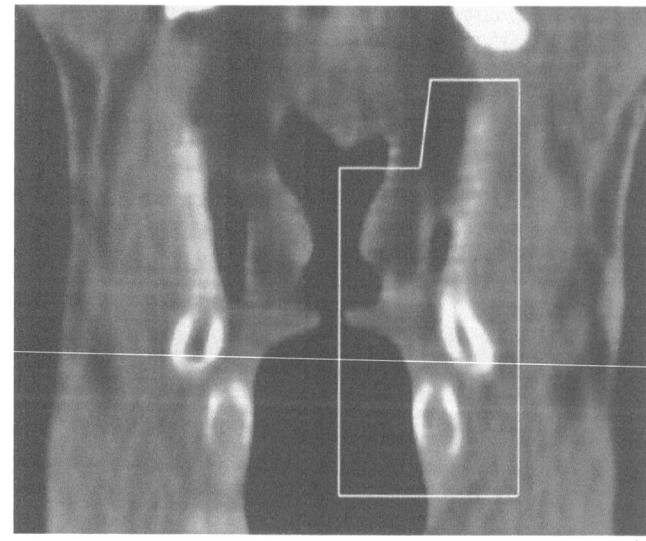

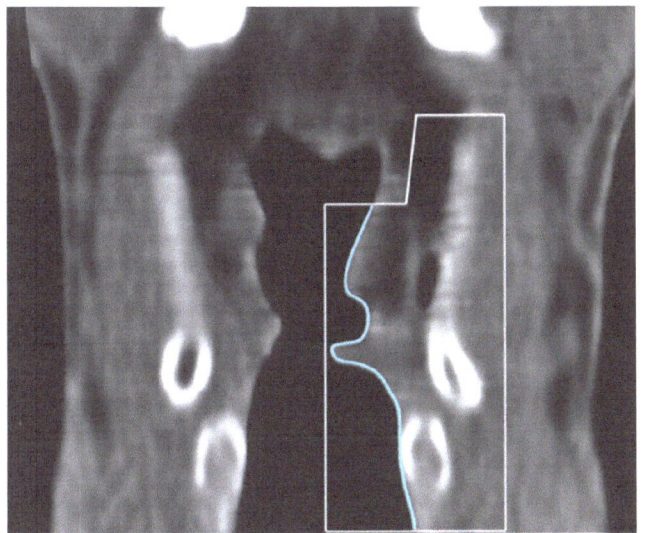

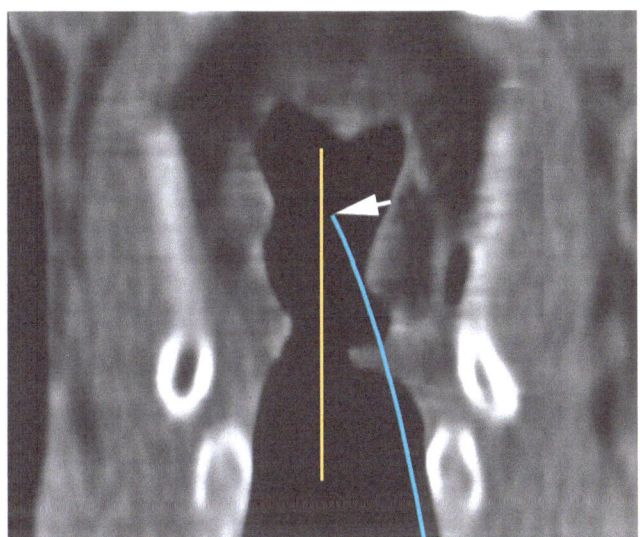

during quiet respiration (right) with CT scan during phonation (left). During the first operation, the radial forearm flap (yellow line) is placed in the midline. The optimal position of the tracheal patch is indicated with a blue line. No skin is preserved during the definitive reconstruction in the anterior larynx and the tracheal patch is sutured to the aryepiglottic fold (arrow). The glottic gap can not be closed during phonation. After reconstruction, the anterior larynx serves as 'respiratory larynx'.

A definition of the morphologic characteristics of an optimal reconstruction after extended hemilaryngectomy was made using morphometrical data from normal and reconstructed larynges. The normal larynx was studied morphologically by Hirano et al. in 1986. This study concluded that in the normal larynx, the anterior glottic plays the most important role for phonation while the posterior glottis plays an equally important role in respiration. The epithelium in the posterior glottis is a respiratory epithelium, whereas it is stratified squamous epithelium in the anterior glottis. Diseases of the anterior glottis usually cause voice problems. They disturb respiration only when they present a very large obstruction to the airway. Diseases of the posterior glottis result in respiratory distress. They do not affect phonation until they become very extensive and inhibit vocal fold closure. In the normal situation, the posterior glottis is a respiratory glottis, while the anterior glottis is a phonatory glottis (HIRANO et al., 1986).

The morphological situation is different after reconstruction of extended hemilaryngectomy defects. The theoretical optimal position of the reconstructive tissue is comparable to the position of the hemilarynx during phonation. Morphometric evaluation of reconstructed larynges showed a difference between the posterior and anterior larynx. Closure of the posterior larynx is important for swallowing without aspiration.

Figure 5.24. Definition of optimal reconstruction-Coronal reformation of anterior larynx.
a. Images during quiet respiration. Extended hemilaryngectomy defect is outlined.
b. Images during phonation. Extended hemilaryngectomy defect is outlined-vocal folds are in adduction.
c. Theoretical optimal position of reconstructive tissue after extended hemilaryngectomy. Combination of CT scan during quiet respiration (right) with CT scan during phonation (left). The optimal reconstruction of an extended hemilaryngectomy defect is provided by a reconstruction comparable to the position of a hemilarynx during phonation (blue line).
d. Optimal position of reconstructive tissue during tracheal autotransplantation. Combination of CT scan

Endoscopic evaluation showed that contact areas between the intact and the reconstructed hemilarynx during phonation are situated posteriorly. After extended hemilaryngectomy, voice production is situated in the posterior glottic and supraglottic area. Restoration of the posterior bulk is extremely important for obtaining a functioning laryngeal remnant. After extended hemilaryngectomy, the posterior larynx becomes a 'sphincteric larynx'. The posterior, respiratory glottis is partially lost after reconstruction of the tissue bulk posteriorly (Fig. 5.25). The anterior, phonatory glottis is also lost after reconstruction. Even with the tracheal patch in a paramedian position, the mucosal vibration pattern between anterior vocal fold and tracheal patch will not occur. After reconstruction the phonatory glottis is moved from anterior to posterior. After reconstruction, the anterior glottis is less important for speech and swallowing and it may be transformed from phonatory into respiratory (Fig. 5.24). With the tracheal patch in a position between paramedial and lateral, the amount of airway lumen that is lost in the posterior larynx will be gained anteriorly.

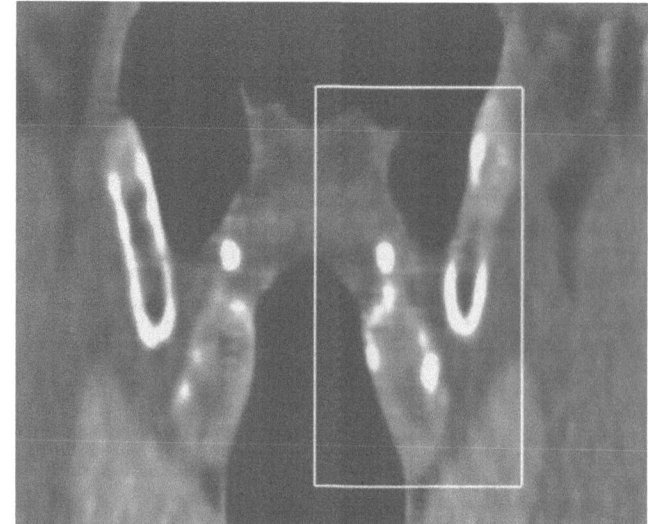

b

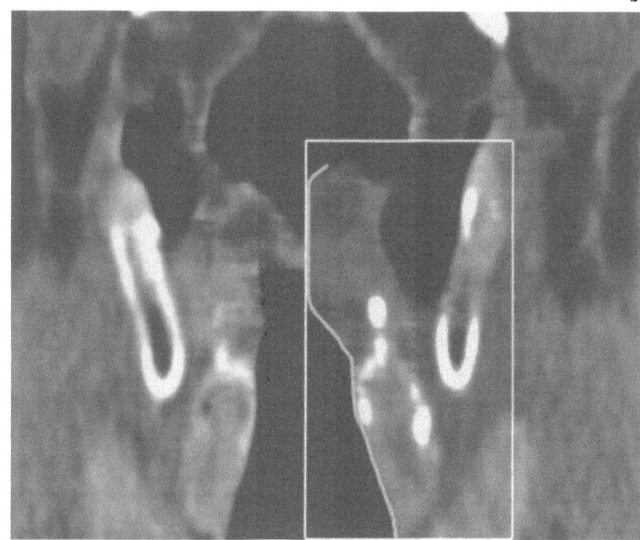

c

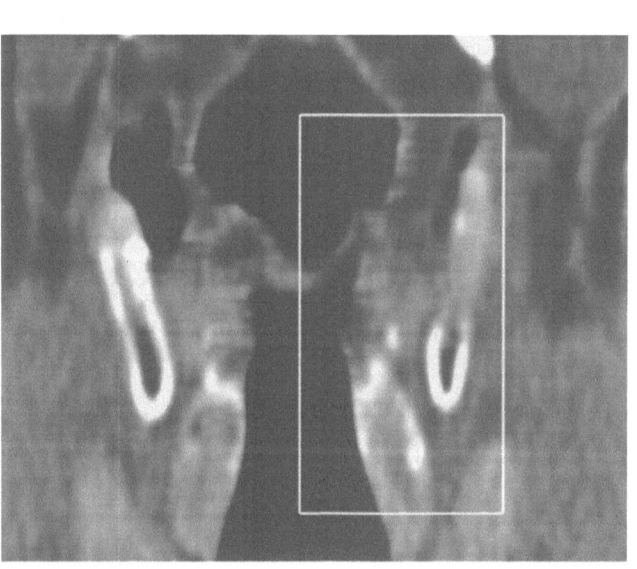

a

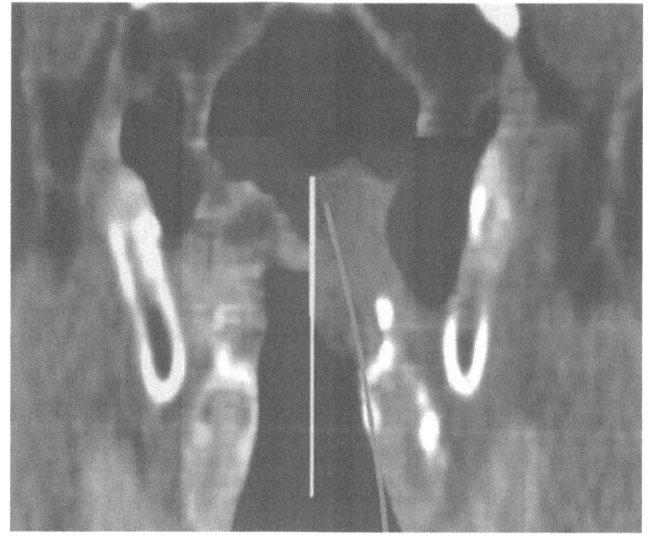

d

Figure 5.25. Definition of optimal reconstruction-Coronal reformation of posterior larynx.
a. Images during quiet respiration. Extended hemilaryngectomy defect is outlined.
b. Images during phonation. Extended hemilaryngectomy defect is outlined-arytenoids are in adduction.
c. Theoretical optimal position of reconstructive tissue after extended hemilaryngectomy. Combination of CT scan during quiet respiration (right) with CT scan during phonation (left). The optimal reconstruction of an extended hemilaryngectomy defect is provided by a reconstruction comparable to the position of a hemilarynx during phonation (blue line).
d. Optimal position of reconstructive tissue during tracheal autotransplantation. Combination of CT scan during quiet respiration (right) with CT scan during phonation (left). During the first operation, the radial forearm flap (small yellow line) is placed in the midline. A piece of radial forearm skin is preserved during the definitive reconstruction in the posterior larynx to improve the bulk in the area of the resected arytenoid (thick yellow line). The tracheal transplant position is indicated with a blue line. The glottic gap is completely closed posteriorly. Respiration is difficult in the posterior larynx. After reconstruction, the posterior larynx serves as 'sphincteric larynx'.

All subsequent patients were reconstructed following the pattern shown in Fig 5.24.d and 5.25.d.

Table 5.3. Optimal reconstruction of extended hemilaryngectomy defects revisited
ANTERIOR LARYNX: - tracheal patch in paramedial or in lateral position. - Anterior larynx is 'respiratory larynx'.
POSTERIOR LARYNX: - full restoration of height of resected arytenoid. - tracheal patch in midline position. - bulk is improved with preserved strip of radial forearm skin. - posterior larynx is important for speech and swallowing. - posterior larynx is 'sphincteric larynx'.

The optimal reconstructive design of the modified transplantation concept is illustrated on a laryngeal model which is incised in the sagittal midline (Fig. 5.26, 5.27). The morphological result after reconstruction is illustrated on CT scan while the functional results are shown on DVD during endoscopy.

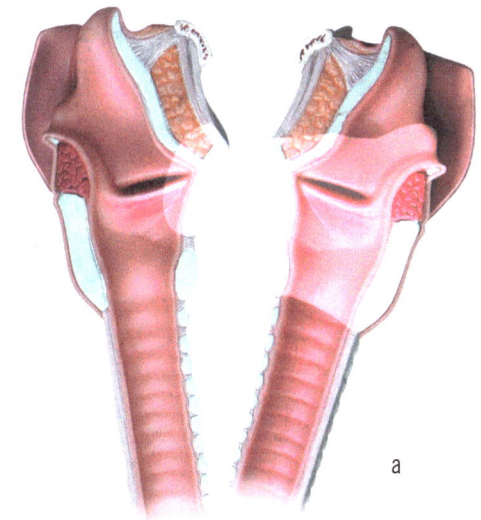

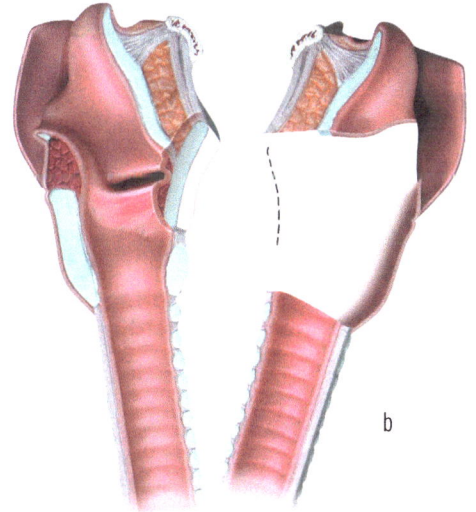

Figure 5.26.
Optimal reconstructive design-tumor resection.
a. Outlining of resection. Amount of resection for a unilateral glottic tumor is shown. The anterior commissure is included in the resection.
b. Extended hemilaryngectomy defect. Defect after extended hemilaryngectomy with inclusion of the anterior commissure.

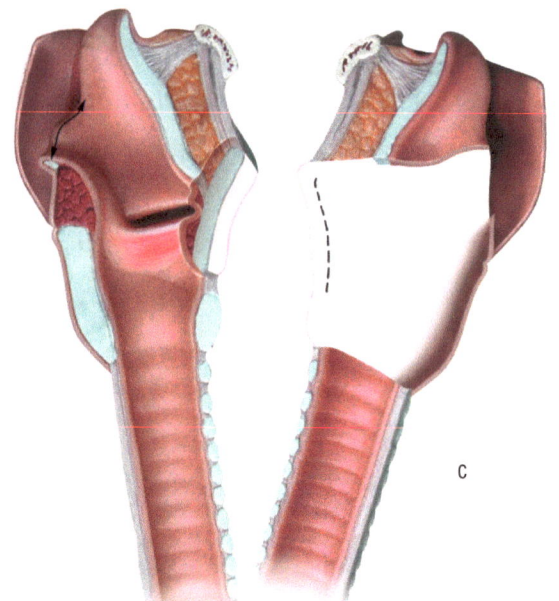

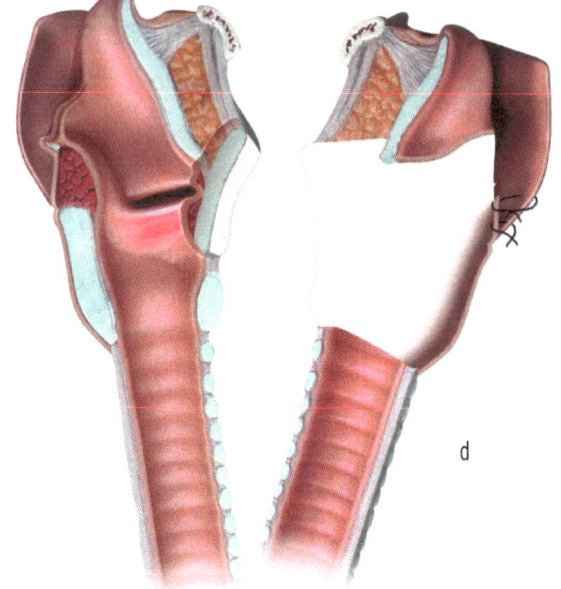

Figure 5.26. Optimal reconstructive design-tumor resection (continued).

c. Incision of mucosa over preserved arytenoid. The mucosa over the preserved arytenoid is incised and a pharyngeal and laryngeal layer is developed.

d. Primary closure of pyriform sinus. The pyriform sinus at the side of the resection is closed primarily.

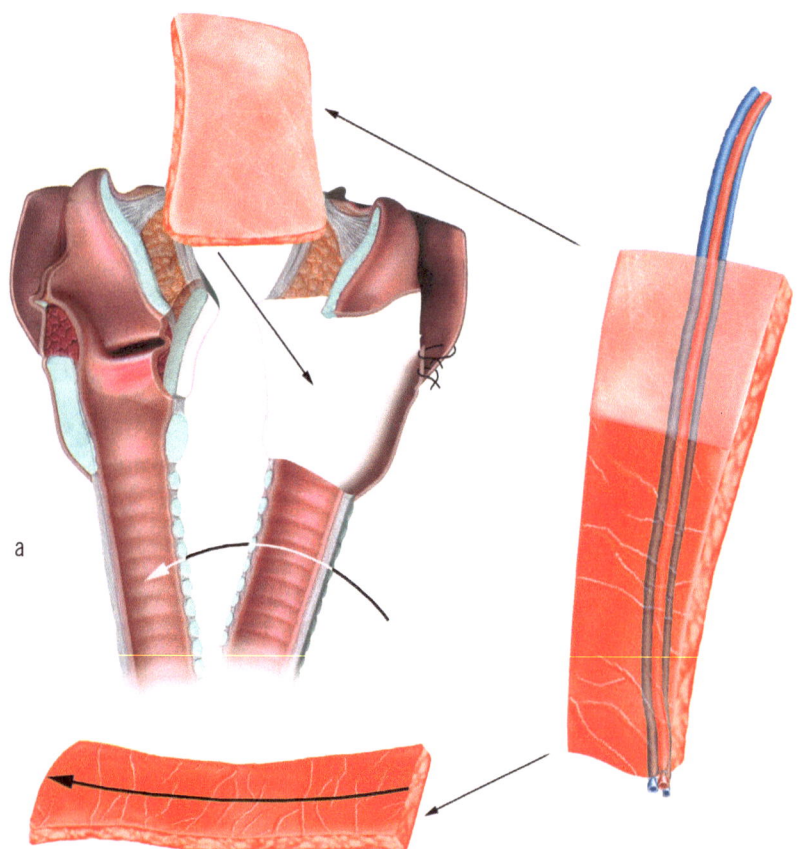

Figure 5.27.
Optimal reconstructive design-temporary reconstruction.
a. The skin paddle of the radial forearm flap is introduced into the laryngeal defect and the fascia flap is wrapped around the trachea.

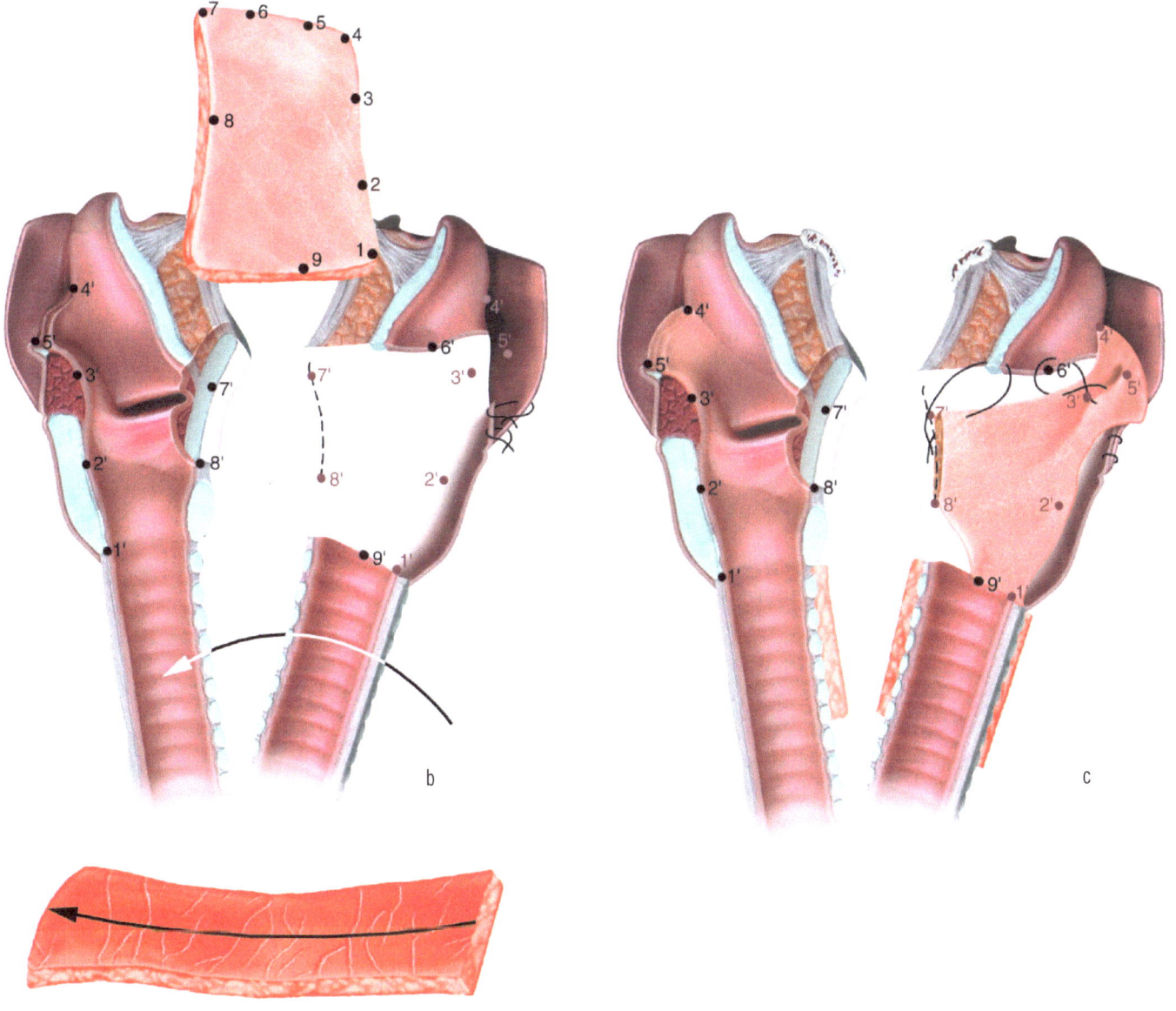

Figure 5.27. Optimal reconstructive design-temporary reconstruction (continued).
b. *The skin flap is sutured into the defect by suturing points 1-9 to points 1'-9' respectively. Important is to restore the bulk at the site of the resected arytenoid. This can be done by suturing the skin flap to the pharyngeal and laryngeal layer after mucosal incision of the preserved arytenoid. Point 3-4-5 are sutured to points 3'-4'-5' to create this bulk.*

c. *The radial forearm skin flap is placed in the midline position at the supraglottic and glottic level. A midline position is obtained by using a flap with a width between 2.5 cm (females) and 3 cm (males). An opening is left that serves as a 'tracheostome' (between 8' and 9').*

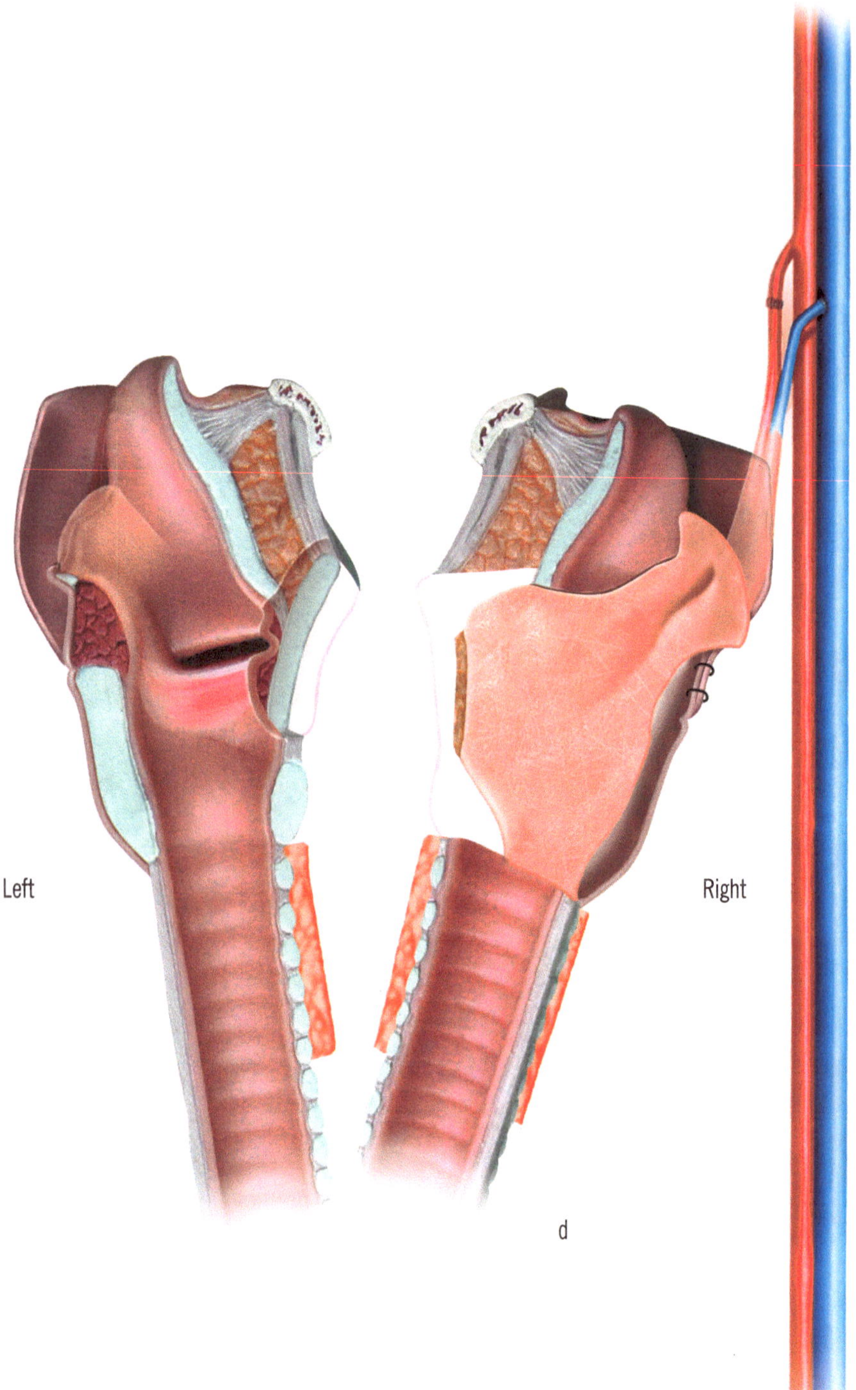

Left

Right

d

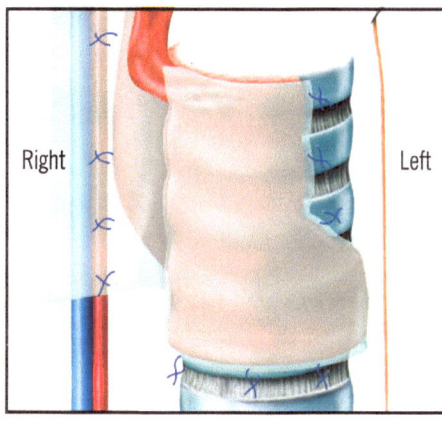

Right

Left

Figure 5.27. Optimal reconstructive design-temporary reconstruction (continued).
d. Situation after the first operation. The radial forearm flap is revascularized by suturing the flap vessels to the neck vessels at the same side as the laryngeal tumor. The radial forearm skin holds a midline position at the glottic level. The fascia is wrapped around the upper segment of trachea. The thyroid gland is preserved at the uninvolved side. The skin flap succeeds in repairing

of the sphincteric function.
Inset: Anterior view of fascia-enwrapped trachea. An expanded polytetrafluoroethylene (ePTFE) membrane is applied over the fascia flap to prevent adhesions with the surrounding tissues and to facilitate tracheal mobilization.

The morphology of the temporary reconstructed larynx can be evaluated on CT scan (Fig. 5.28, 5.29).

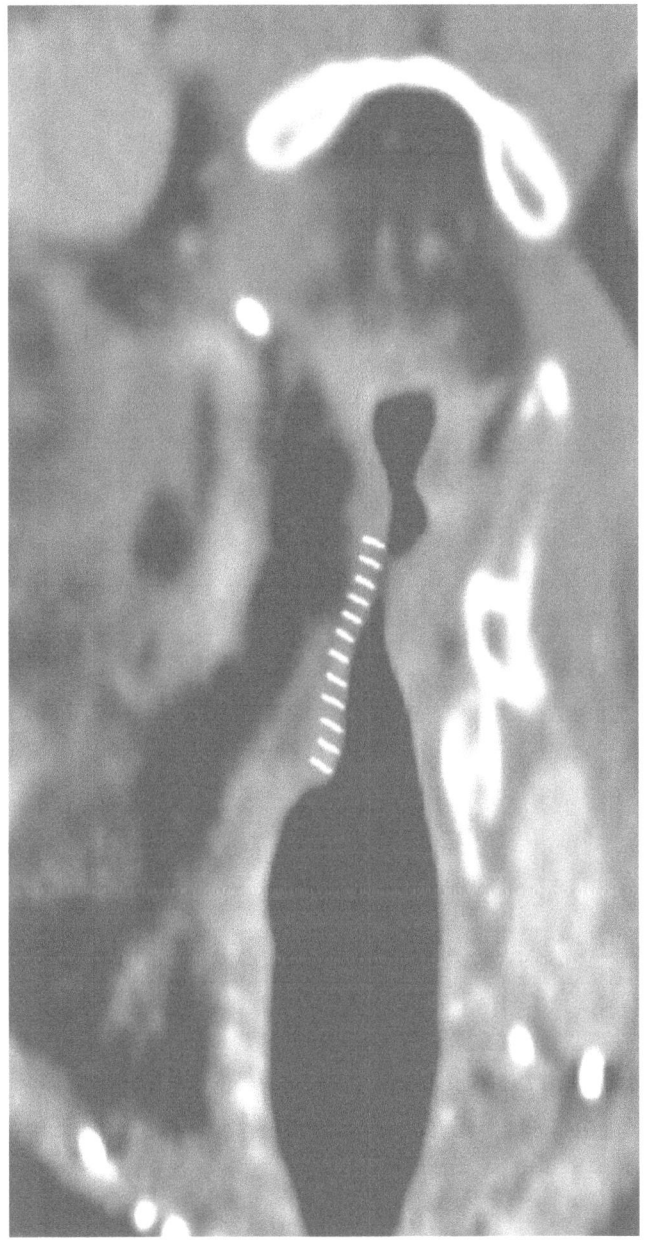 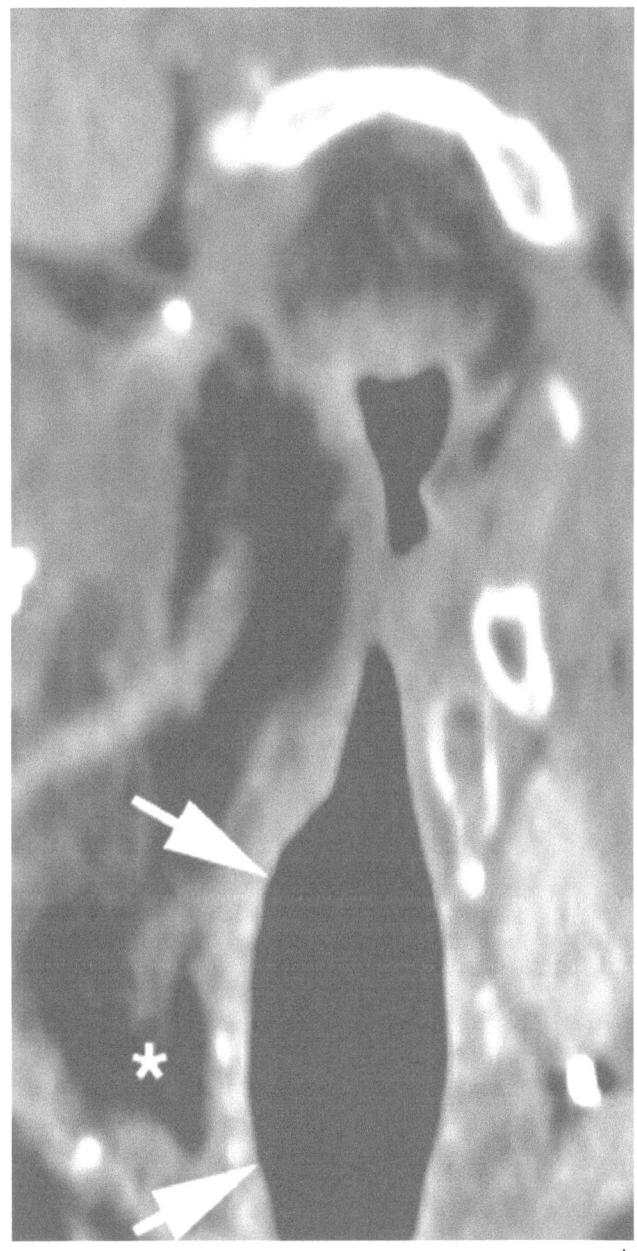

a

b

Figure 5.28. CT scan after first operation-coronal reformation.
a. The skin paddle is placed in the midline position. The forearm skin is in contact with the true vocal fold. The glottic and subglottic airway is not restored. The amount of skin removed during the second operation is indicated.

b. The upper 4 cm of cervical trachea (between arrows) is wrapped by fascia (asterisk).

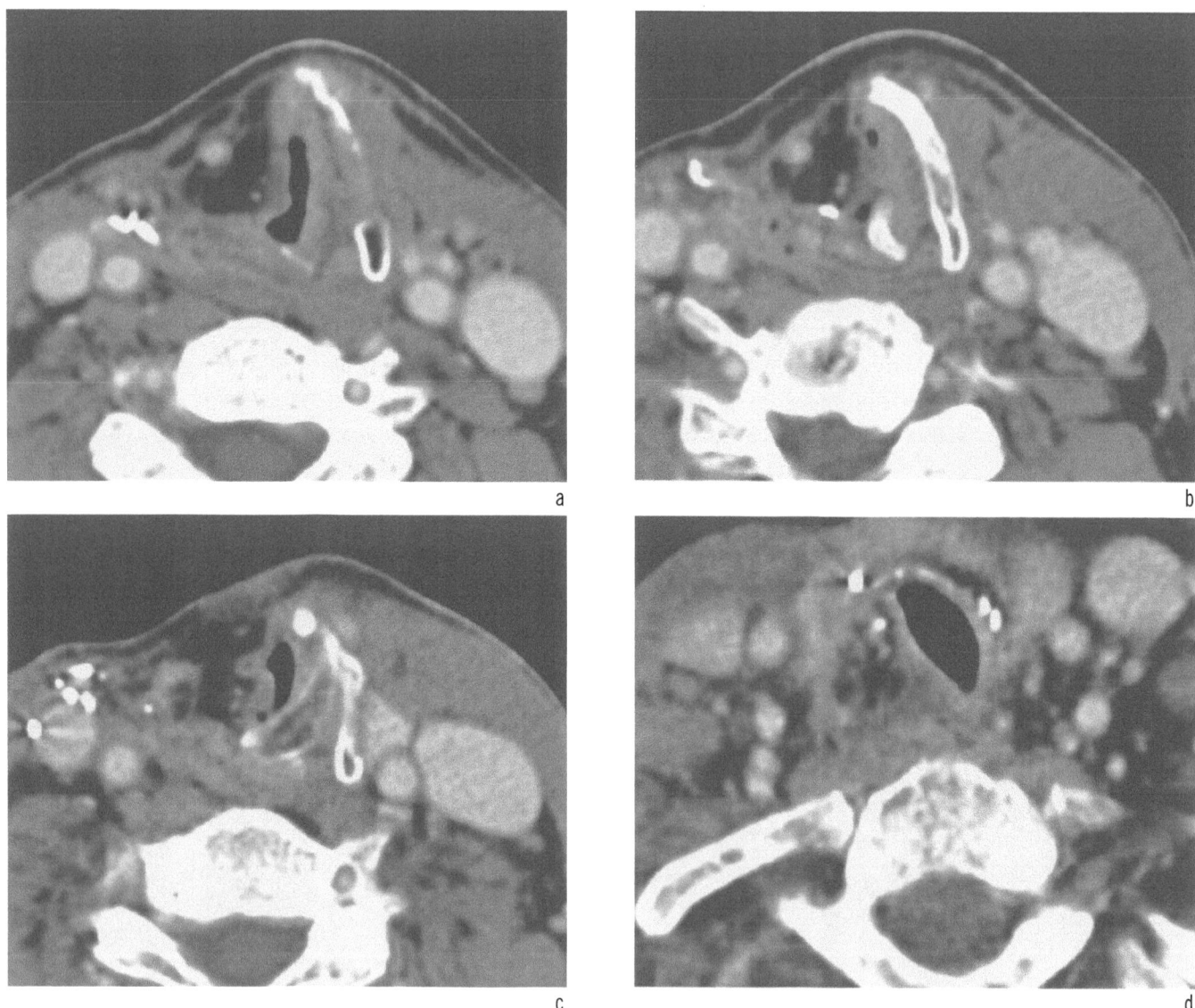

Figure 5.29. CT scan after first operation-axial section. a. Supraglottic level. b. Glottic level. The skin paddle is placed in the midline position with restoration of the sphincteric function.

c. Subglottic level. The airway lumen is not restored. d. Tracheal level. The fascia flap is wrapping the cervical trachea.

The definitive reconstruction with tracheal auto-transplantation is shown in Fig. 5.30, Fig. 5.31 and Fig. 5.32.

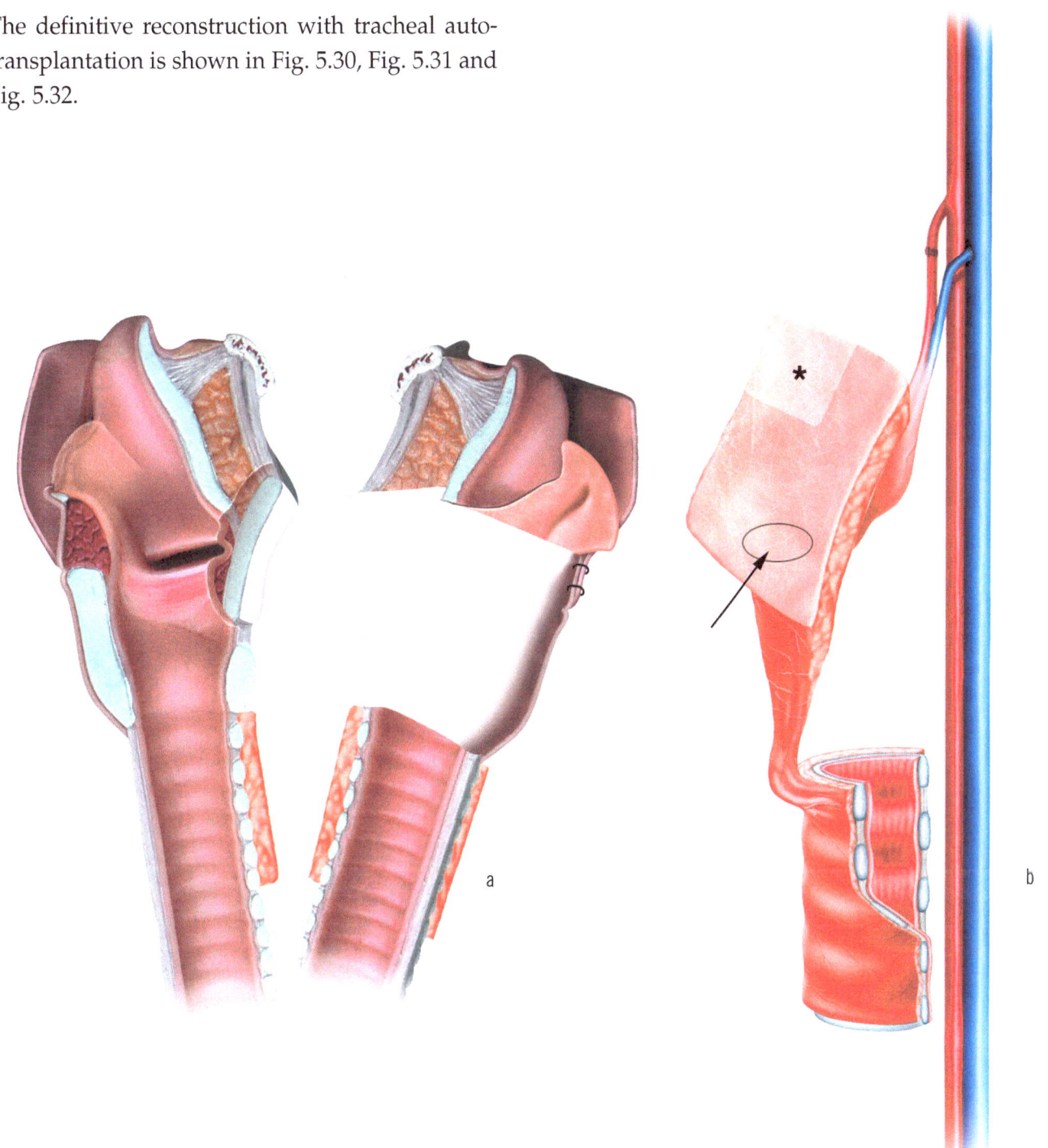

Figure 5.30. Optimal reconstructive design-definitive reconstruction with removal of skin flap.

a. During the second operation, the skin paddle is removed except for a piece of skin at the side of the resected arytenoid. This piece of skin survives on the collateral supply from the surrounding laryngeal mucosa. The collateral blood supply to the skin is sufficiently developed after 4 months.

b. The fascial enwrapped segment of trachea is isolated and will be sutured into the laryngeal defect. The amount of skin that remains in the defect is outlined (asterisk). The skin flap will be desepithelialized except for a small piece of skin (arrow) that will be placed in the neck incision (monitor).

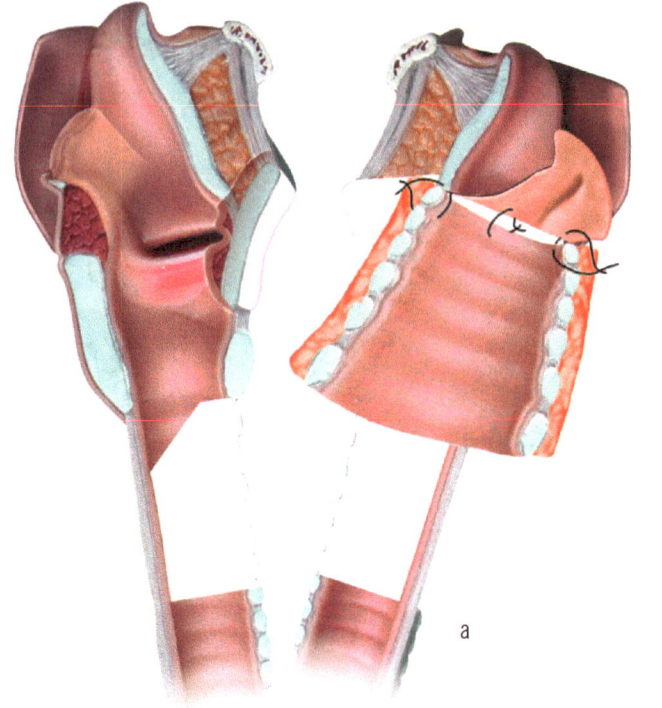
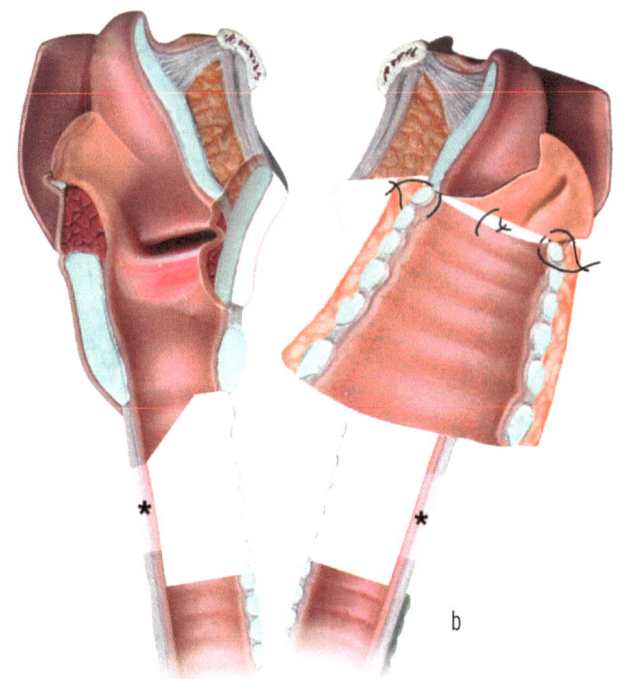

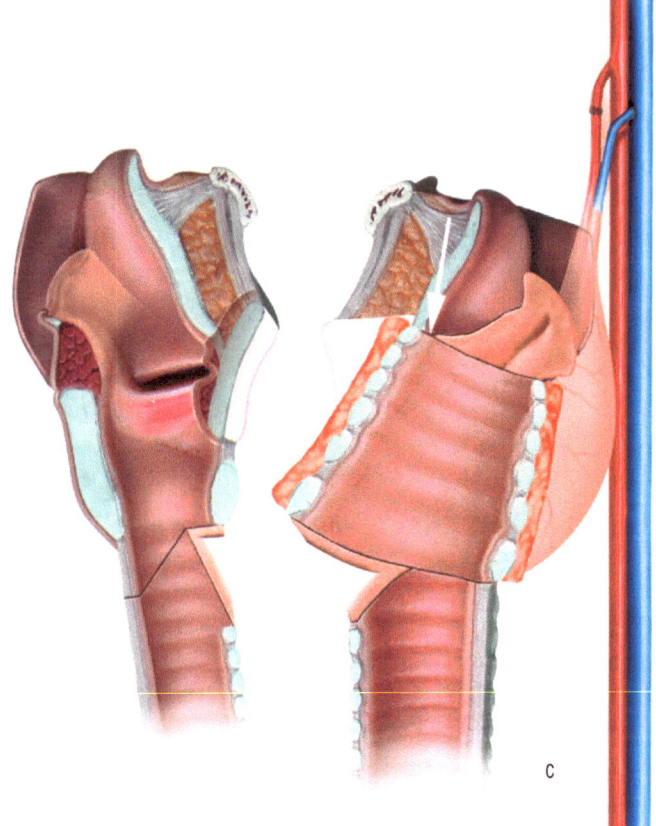

Figure 5.31.

Optimal reconstructive design-definitive reconstruction with tracheal autotransplantation and end-to-end anastomosis.

a. The tracheal patch is sutured into the laryngeal defect. The superior margin of the transplant is sutured to the epiglottis anteriorly and to the forearm skin posteriorly. The tracheal transplant remains vascularized as visible in 5.31.c. The vascular anastomosis remains untouched during the second operation.

b. A part of the membranous trachea (asterisks) is resected to allow for anastomosis of the mediastinal trachea to the reconstructed larynx.

c. Situation after autotransplantation and end-to-end anastomosis. The neck skin flaps are sutured to the tracheostome. For good speech and swallowing function, it is important to suture the tracheal patch to the epiglottic remnant (arrow). No skin is preserved anteriorly.

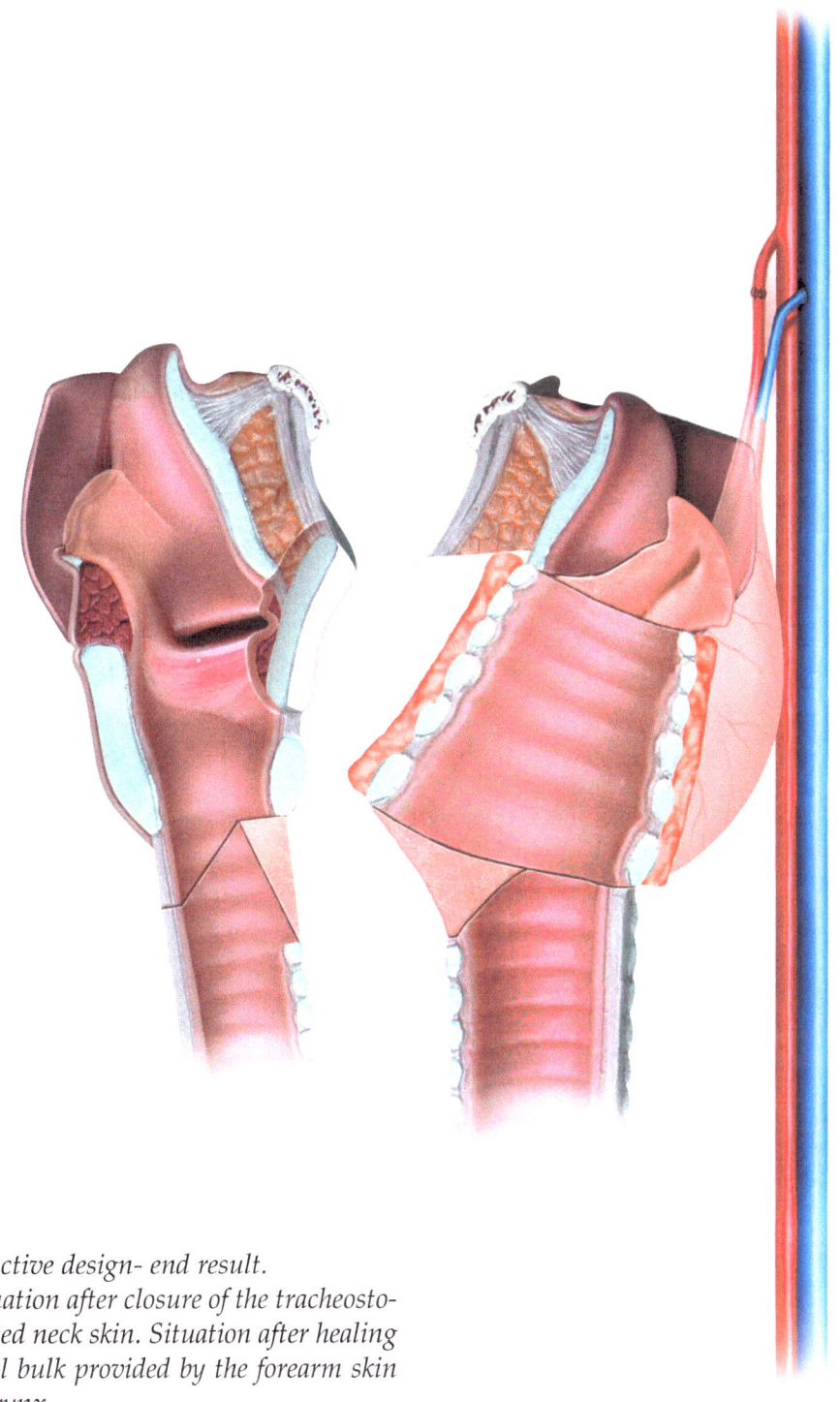

Figure 5.32.
Optimal reconstructive design- end result.
Internal view. Situation after closure of the tracheosto-
my with the inverted neck skin. Situation after healing
with the additional bulk provided by the forearm skin
in the posterior larynx.

The morphology of the reconstructed larynx can be evaluated on CT scan (Fig. 5.33).

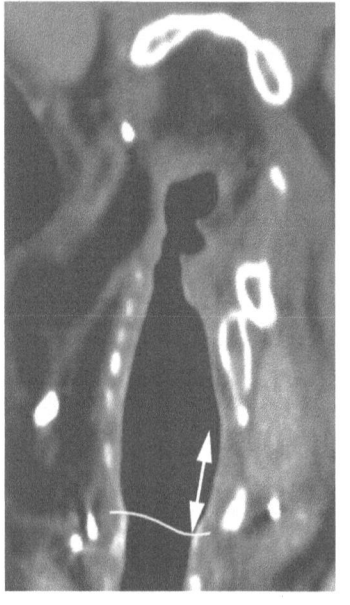

a

Figure 5.33. CT scan after second operation.
a. coronal reformation.
The tracheal patch is placed in the paramedial position at the glottic level.
The subglottic larynx shows a sufficient airway lumen. The anastomosis between mediastinal trachea and reconstructed larynx is indicated with a white line. At the side of the intact hemilarynx, a segment of native trachea remains attached to the larynx (double arrow). This segment of trachea protects the important recurrent nerve.
b. axial section.
b.1. Supraglottic level. Posterior bulk at the site of the resected arytenoid is provided.
b.2, b.3. Glottic level. Tracheal patch is in a paramedial position. The posterior larynx serves as the sphincteric larynx; the anterior larynx is the respiratory larynx.
b.4. Subglottic level. The subglottic airway is fully restored.

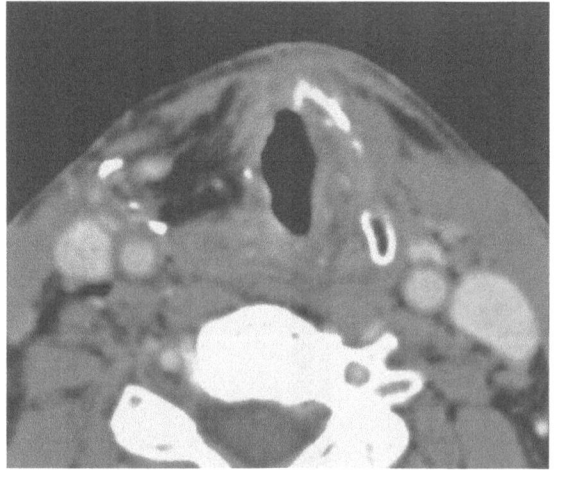

b1

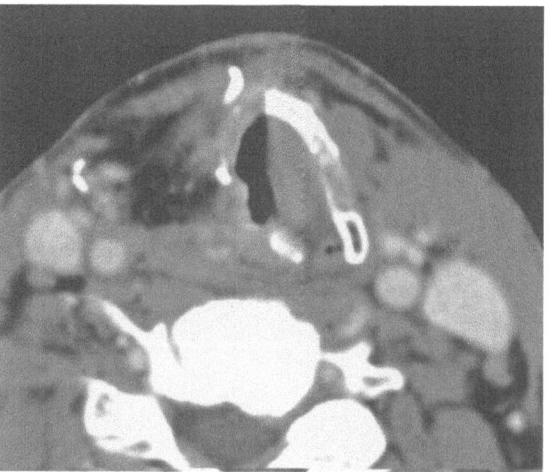

b2

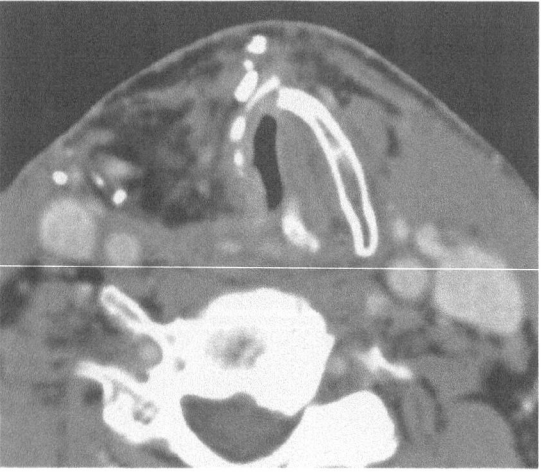

b3

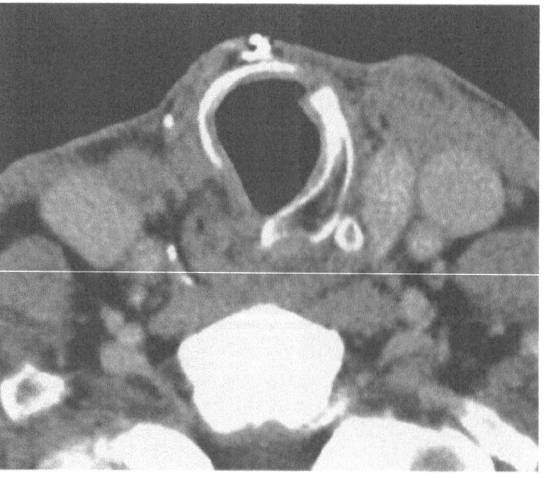

b4

The modified tracheal autotransplantation concept used for reconstruction of extended hemilaryngectomy defects has a unique place within the armentarium of reconstructive surgery. It is an example of how the needs for obtaining an optimal reconstruction and the needs for adequate tumor removal with no or minimal risk to diminish the oncologic safety work synergistically. The extended hemilaryngectomy allows for a complete removal of a suitable tumor, neck dissection, hemithyroidectomy and removal of the ipsilateral tracheoesophageal lymph nodes. The reconstruction is a combination of immediate reconstruction with a fasciocutaneous free flap and of flap prefabrication with the fascial part of the same fasciocutaneous free flap. The flap prefabrication during a 4 month time interval will lead to optimal reconstructive results and will lead to the possibility of a second look with re-examination of the section margins of the hemilaryngectomy defect. The 4 months prefabrication period allows for laryngeal repair with a well vascularized trachea in combination with forearm skin that is perfused through the mucosal suture line. After removal of the skin paddle during the second intervention the small piece of skin that remains inside shows a sufficient marginal blood perfusion. The definitive reconstruction has some plasticity because the bulk provided by the remaining skin paddle can be reduced (laser) or augmented (injection technique) as shown in Fig. 5.34, 5.35. The 4 months time delay between the tumor resection and the definitive reconstruction allows for a 'second look' with control of the resection margins. A total laryngectomy can be performed during the second procedure in cases of local recurrence.

Untill now, twelve patients were treated with the modified concept (Table 5.4). After a mean follow-up period of 1 year, no locoregional recurrences were encountered in this series. Larger patient numbers with longer follow-up will be necessary to evaluate the importance of a second look in the detection of locoregional recurrences.

Table 5.4. Patient series treated with the modified concept

Gender	Age	Tumor	Stage	RT	Tracheostomy	Status
1. Male	77	Carcinome	T3N0	Yes	No	NED
2. Male	75	Carcinome	T2bN0	Yes	No	NED
3. Male	57	Liposarcome	T3N0	No	No	NED
4. Male	68	Carcinome	T3N0	No	No	NED
5. Male	75	Carcinome	T3N0	No	No	NED
6. Male	53	Carcinome	T2bN0	No	No	NED
7. Male	67	Chondrosarc	-	No	No	NED
8. Male	65	Chondrosarc	-	No	No	NED
9. Male	77	Carcinome	T2bN0	Yes	Yes	NED
10. Male	43	Carcinome	T3N0	No	No	NED
11. Male	55	Chondrosarc	-	No	No	NED
12. Male	65	Carcinome	T2bN0	No	No	NED

RT= radiotherapy. The 3 irradiated patients failed radiation treatment as initial procedure (66 Gray). NED=no evidence of desease.

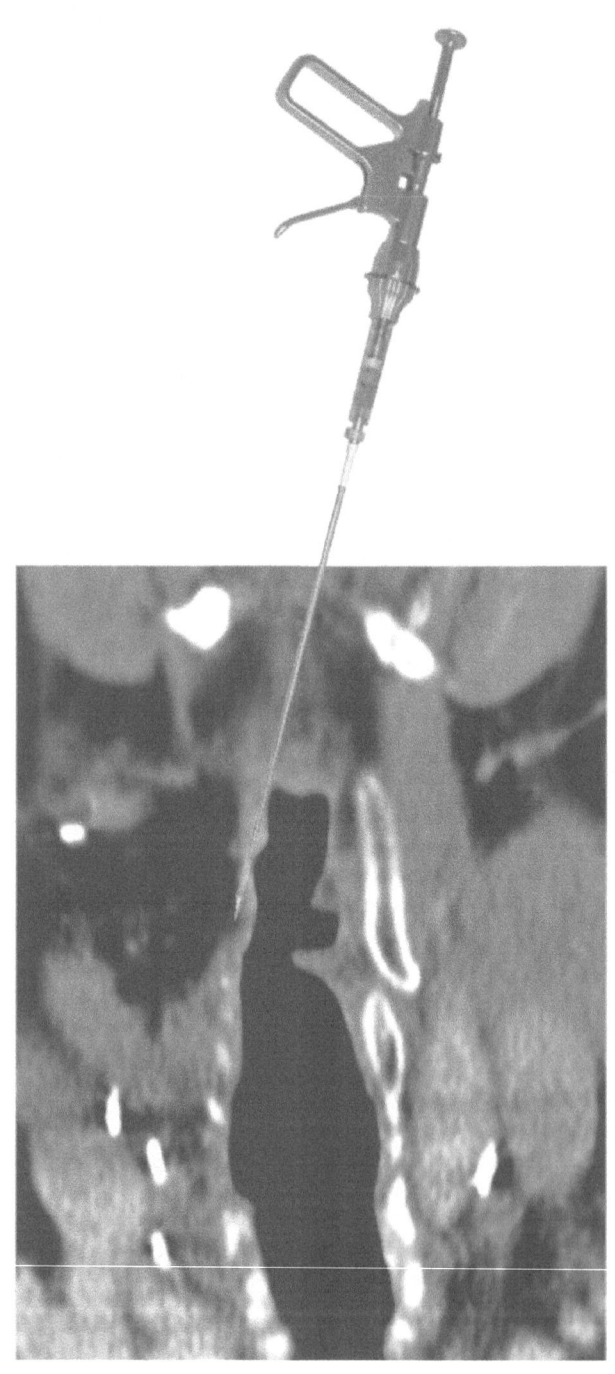

Figure 5.34.
Plasticity of reconstructive concept.
a. The preserved piece of forearm skin allows for correction of the glottic gap. Laser debulking (1) can be done in cases of substenosis; silicone particles (VOX implant) can be injected in cases of glottic insufficiency.
b. Coronal CT reformation. Situation after tracheal autotransplantation. Patient showed no aspiration for solids and liquids. His voice was breathy and silicone particles were injected in an attempt to improve his voice.

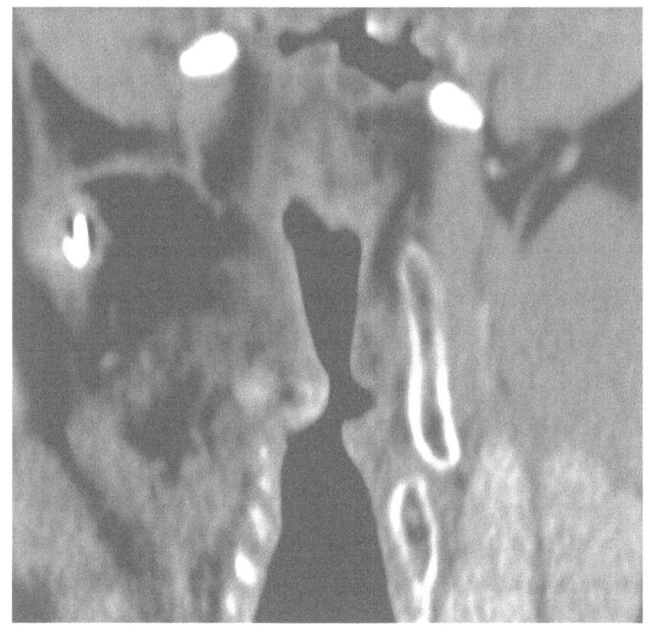

a

Figure 5.35. Augmentation of reconstructed side with silicone particles.
a. Coronal reformation after injection. Medial displacement of radial forarm skin by silicone implant.
b. Axial section at supraglottic level before injection.
c. Axial section at supraglottic level after injection. The reconstructed side is medialized posteriorly by silicone implant.

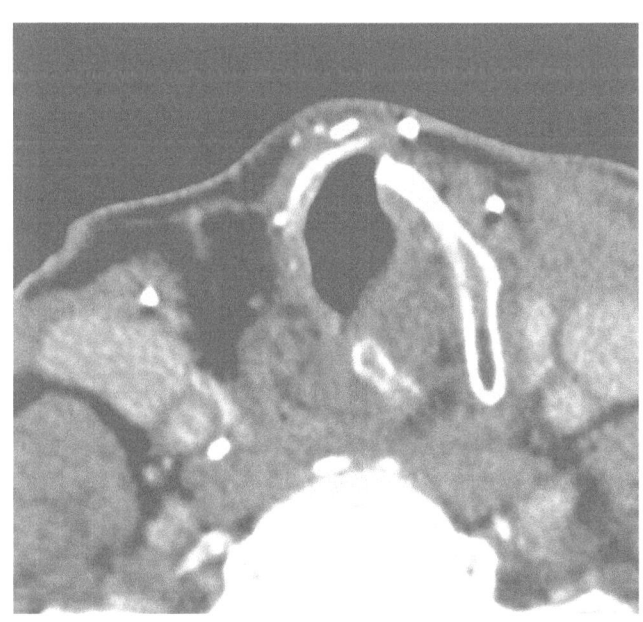

b

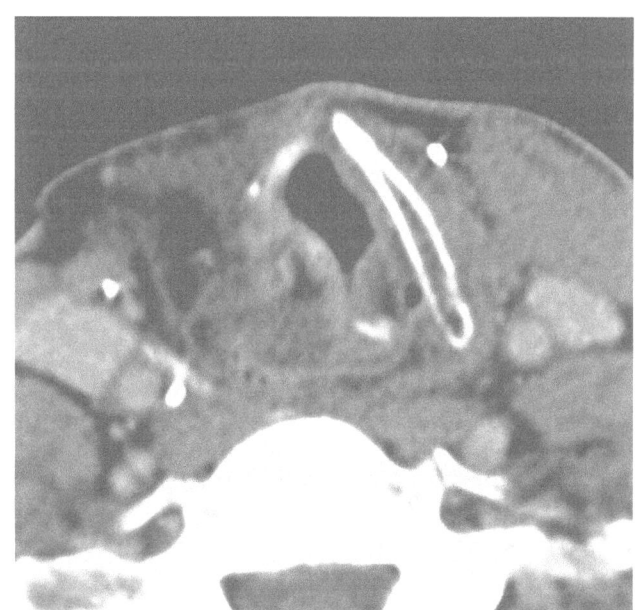

c

3. Indications

3.A. Glottic cancer

Tracheal autotransplantation allows for conservation laryngectomy for unilateral glottic tumors with arytenoid cartilage fixation and infraglottic tumor extension reaching the upper border of the cricoid cartilage, two major contraindications for all 'classical' conservation procedures. An extended hemilaryngectomy may be utilized for unilateral T2-T3 glottic cancers with posterior glottic extension greather than 5 mm but without extension into the ventricle. The resection can be extended towards the anterior third of the contralateral vocal fold for tumors reaching the anterior commissure (Fig. 5.36).

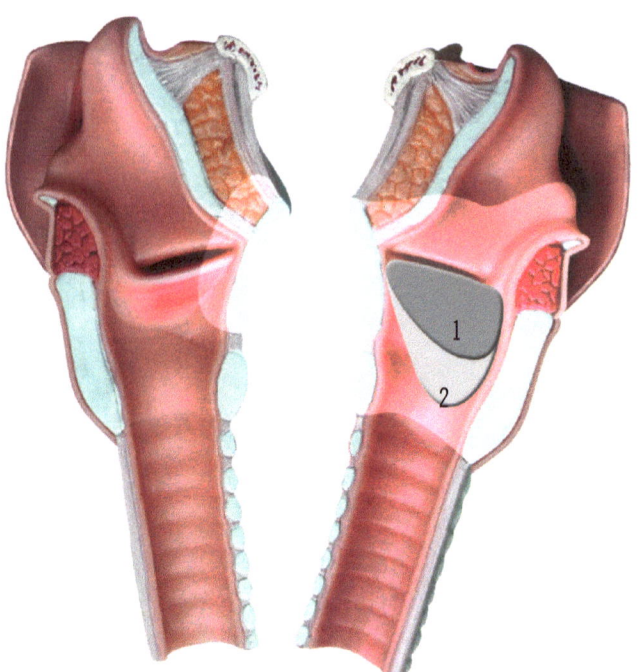

Figure 5.36. Extent of tumor extension.
1. Glottic tumor with subglottic extension. The tumor can reach the anterior commissure but the posterior midline and the supraglottis has to be free of any tumor.
2. This extensive subglottic tumor extension is an indication in non irradiated patients but is too risky in irradiation failures (submucosal tumor spread).

The unilateral glottic tumor with fixation of the vocal fold is a good indication for tracheal autotransplantation. Currently, these tumors are treated with radiotherapy with or without chemotherapy with an average chance for local control of about 50 %. Surgical treatment for the recurrent or persistent tumor means total laryngectomy. This treatment policy may change when a function and organ saving surgical procedure becomes available. For unilateral glottic tumors, tracheal autotransplantation allows for a resection with margins comparable to a total laryngectomy and with a predictable good function.

The unilateral T2, T3 glottic cancer (Fig. 5.37) forms an indication when all other partial laryngectomies (with inclusion of the supracricoid partial laryngectomy) are contraindicated:

1. Tumors of the glottis with fixation of the arytenoid cartilage.
2. Tumors of the glottis with subglottic extent reaching the upper border of the cricoid cartilage or invading the cricoid cartilage.

Oncologic contraindications for a tracheal autotransplantation include the following:
1. Tumors originating in the ventricle or the anterior commissure, since they have a propensity for early invasion of the preepiglottic space.
2. Tumors of the glottis invading the posterior commissure.
3. Bilateral mucosal invasion of the arytenoid cartilage.
4. Tumor involvement of both vocal folds.

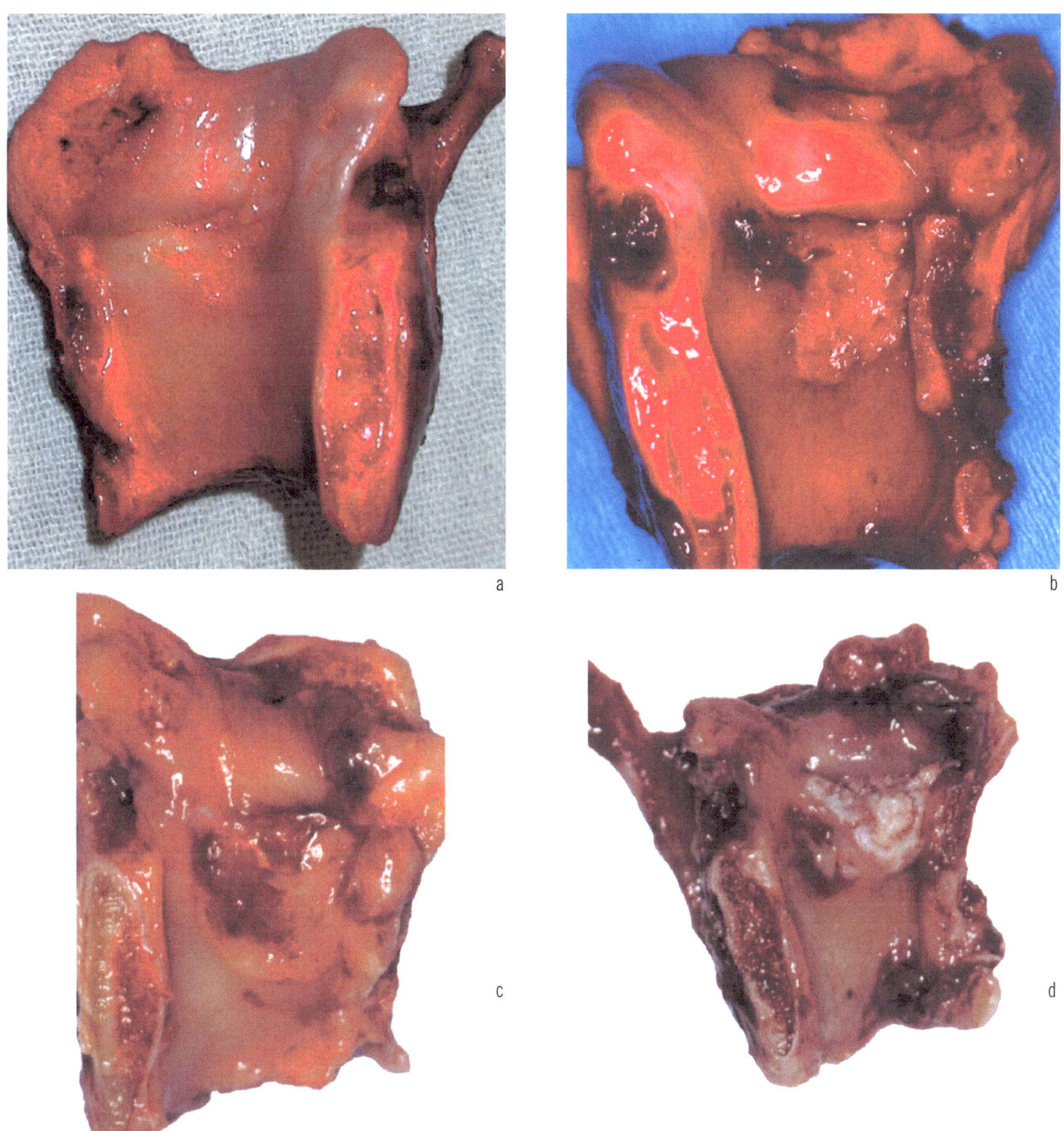

Figure 5.37. Resection specimen after extended hemilaryngectomy for T2-T3 glottic cancer.
a. Tumor of the vocal fold with posterior subglottic extension.
b., c., d. Tumor of the vocal fold with subglottic extension. The anterior commissure is included in the resection.

The tumor extension visible in a., b., c. and d. is suitable for extended hemilaryngectomy in both non-irradiated and irradiated cases.

The maximal amount of tumor extension allowed in non-irradiated cases is visible in Fig. 5.38.

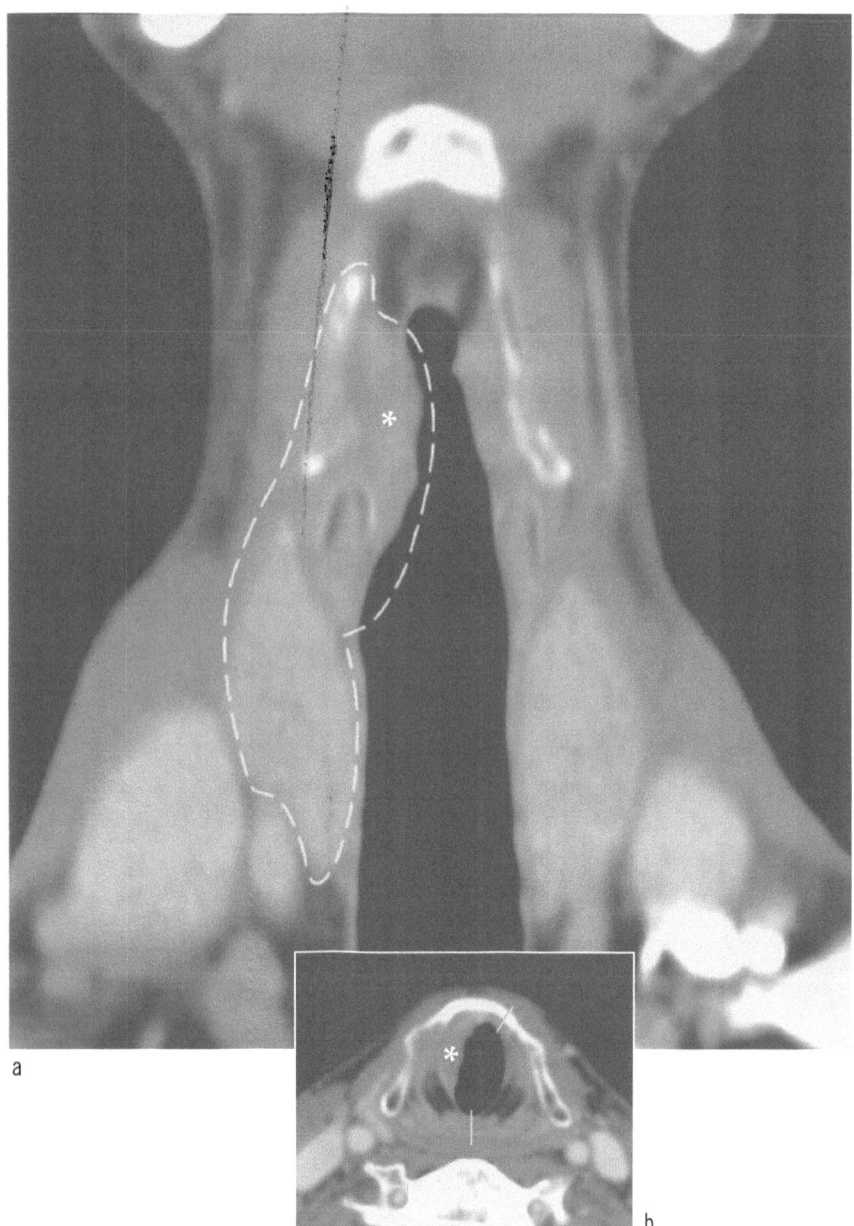

a

b

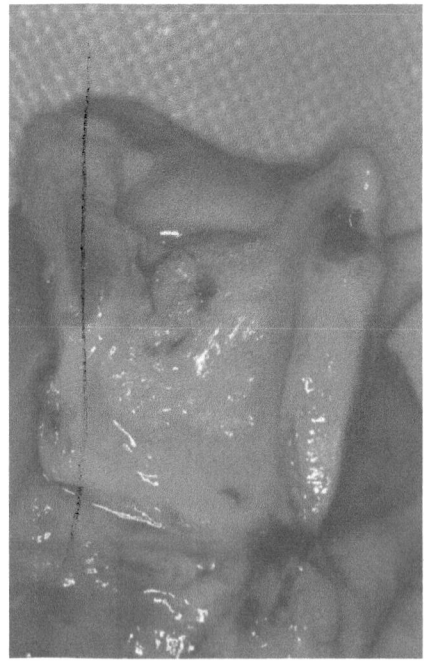

c

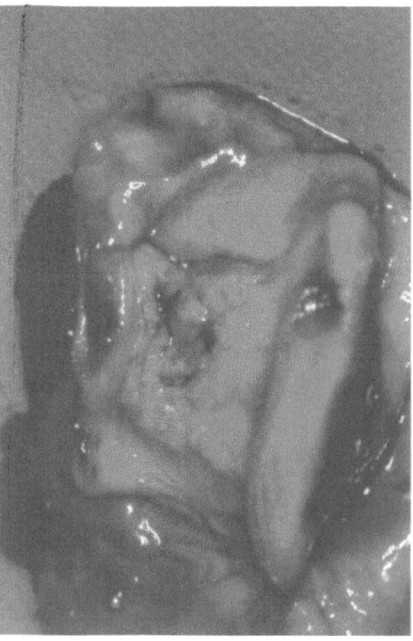

d

Figure 5.38. Maximal amount of tumor resection.
a. Contrast-enhanced CT. Coronal reformatted view shows the tumor (star) with subglottic extension. Amount of resection is indicated. Ipsilateral thyroid gland and tracheoesophageal lymph nodes are removed.
b. Axial CT scan at subglottic level shows the tumor
(star). Amount of resection is indicated.
c. Resection specimen. Anterior commissure is included in the resection.
d. Resection specimen. Posterior commissure is free of tumor.

After irradiation, the unilateral T2-T3 glottic cancer without extension to the ventricle and without extension to the posterior midline may be treated with this technique.

The different operative steps are summarized in Fig. 5.39, 5.40, 5.41, 5.42, 5.43, 5.44, 5.45 for a unilateral T2-3N0 glottic cancer at the right side.

Table 5.5.
Tracheal autotransplantation-Indications glottic cancer

T2-T3 glottic cancer with unilateral localization
Contraindications: -Involvement of ventricle
                     -Posterior commissure involvement
                     -Involvement of both vocal folds

Figure 5.39. Neck skin incision.
The incision is placed 2 to 3 cm above the sternal notch. After the first operation, the lower neck skin flap will be sutured to the first tracheal ring (arrow) without tension. The neck incision will be extended to the mastoid at the tumor side.

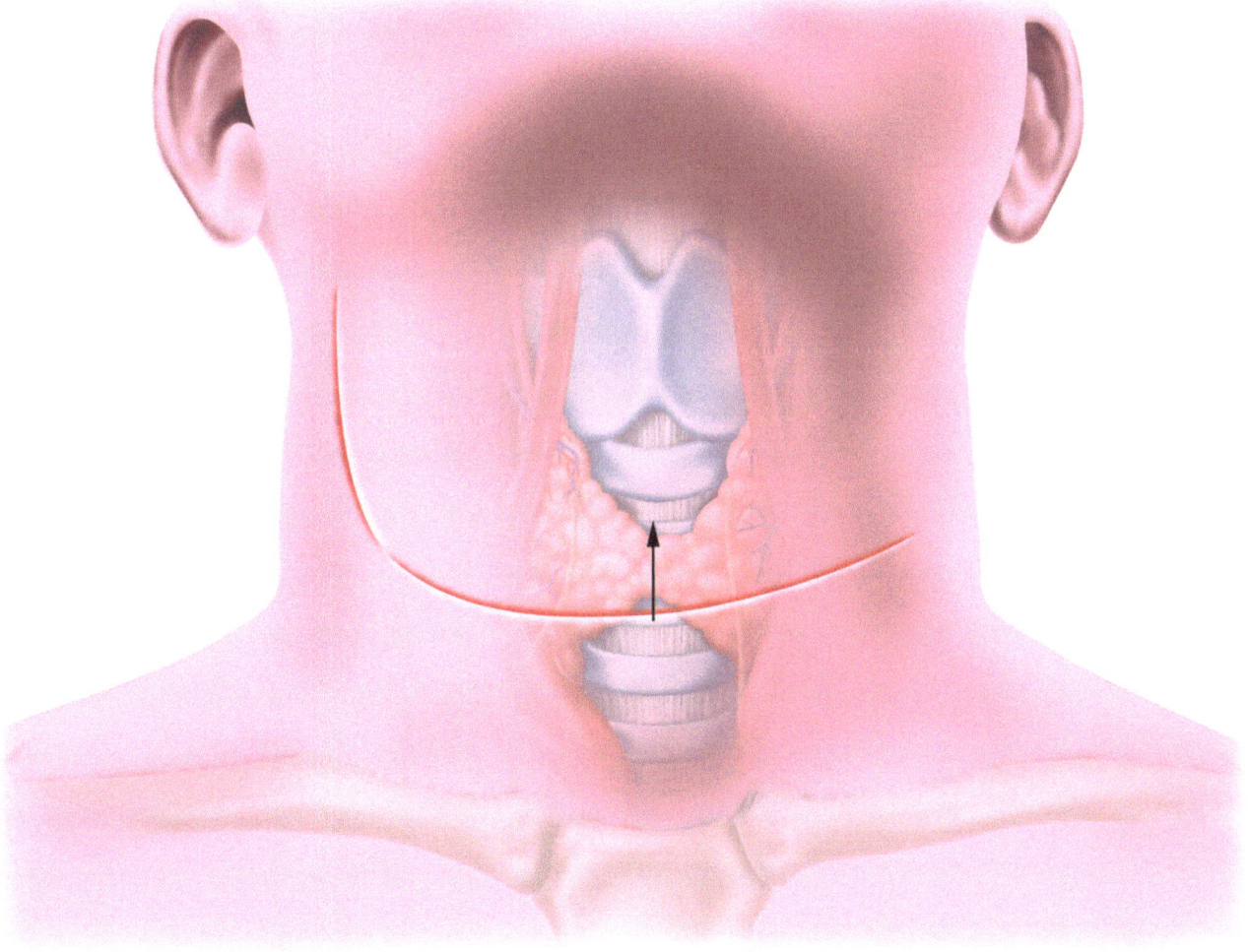

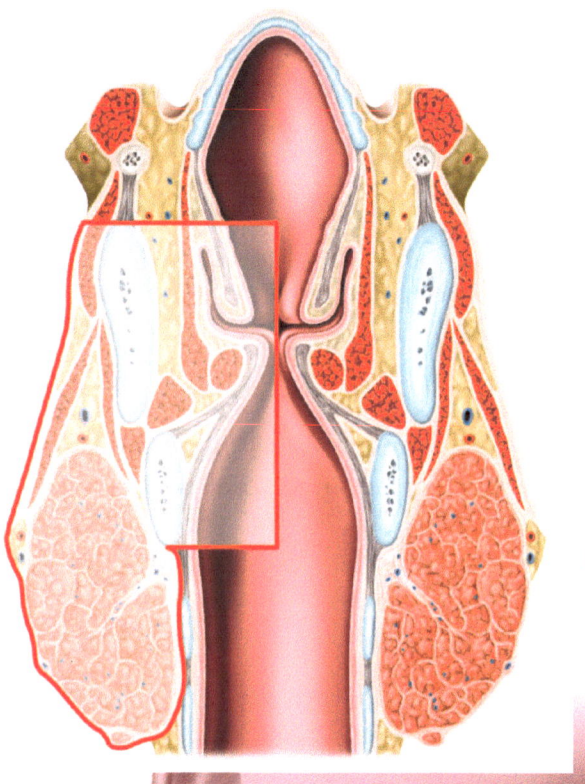

b

Figure 5.40.
Amount of resection for a unilateral T2-3N0 glottic cancer at the right side.
a. Overview. The amount of larynx included in the resection is indicated. One cm of the contralateral thyroid cartilage is included in the resection. An anterolateral (levels II, III, IV) neck dissection will be done. The ipsilateral thyroid gland, recurrent nerve, and tracheoesophageal lymph nodes will be removed.
b. Frontal section.

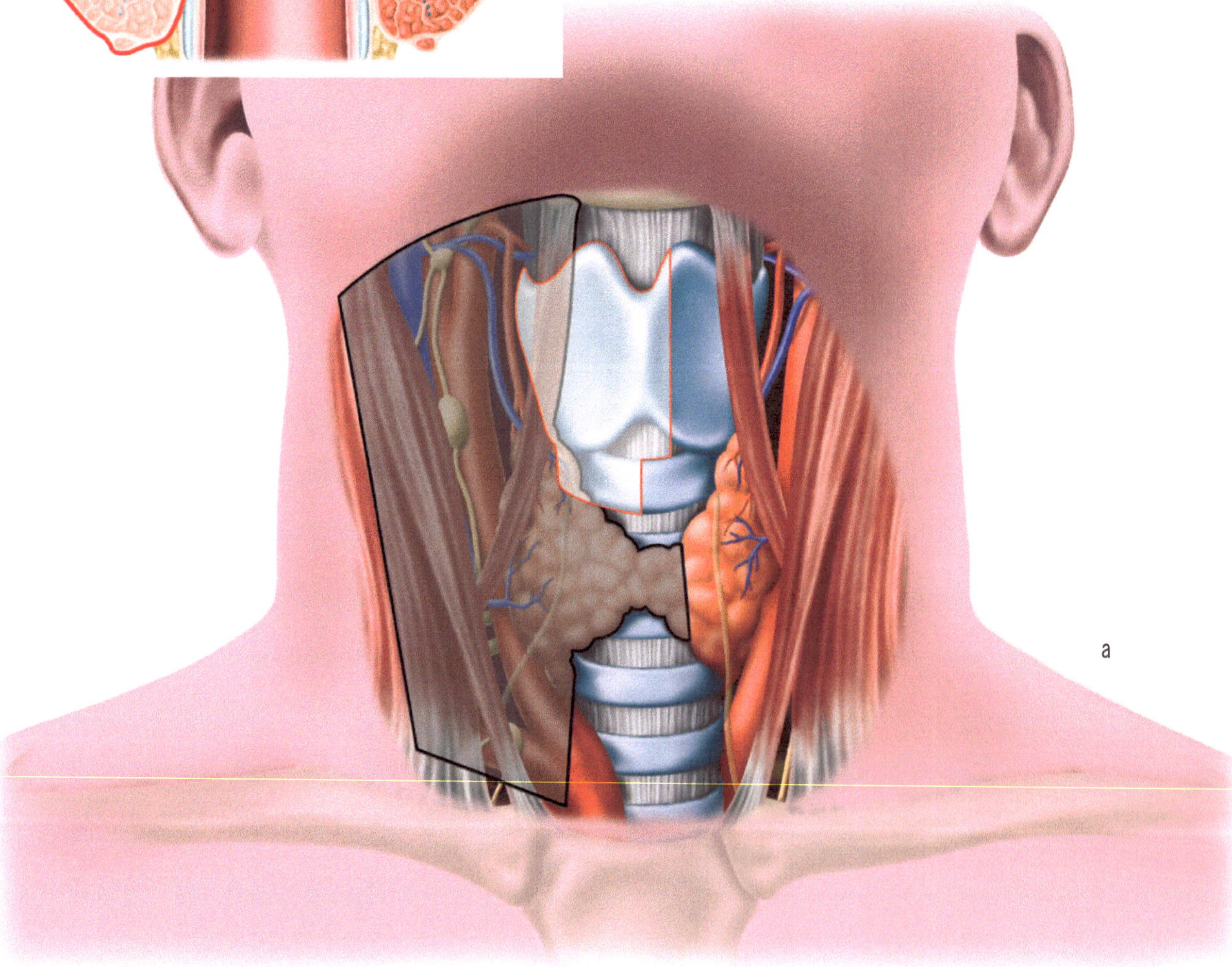

a

Figure 5.41. First operation.
a. Situation after tracheal wrapping, temporary larynx reconstruction, and suturing of the radial vessels to the superior thyroid vessels. The contralateral recurrent nerve is identified in the caudal neck. Full dissection of the contralateral recurrent nerve until it enters the larynx is not necessary. The contralateral thyroid lobe can be dissected from the trachea without danger for damage to the recurrent nerve.

b. Radial forearm flap used for reconstruction. The fascial paddle measures 4 x 10 cm. The skin paddle measures 4 by 8 cm. Between 2.5 and 3 cm of the skin flap is included at the glottic level. The skin flap is somewhat larger than strickly needed and the excessive amount of skin paddle (bright area) can be desepithelialized during inset of the flap.

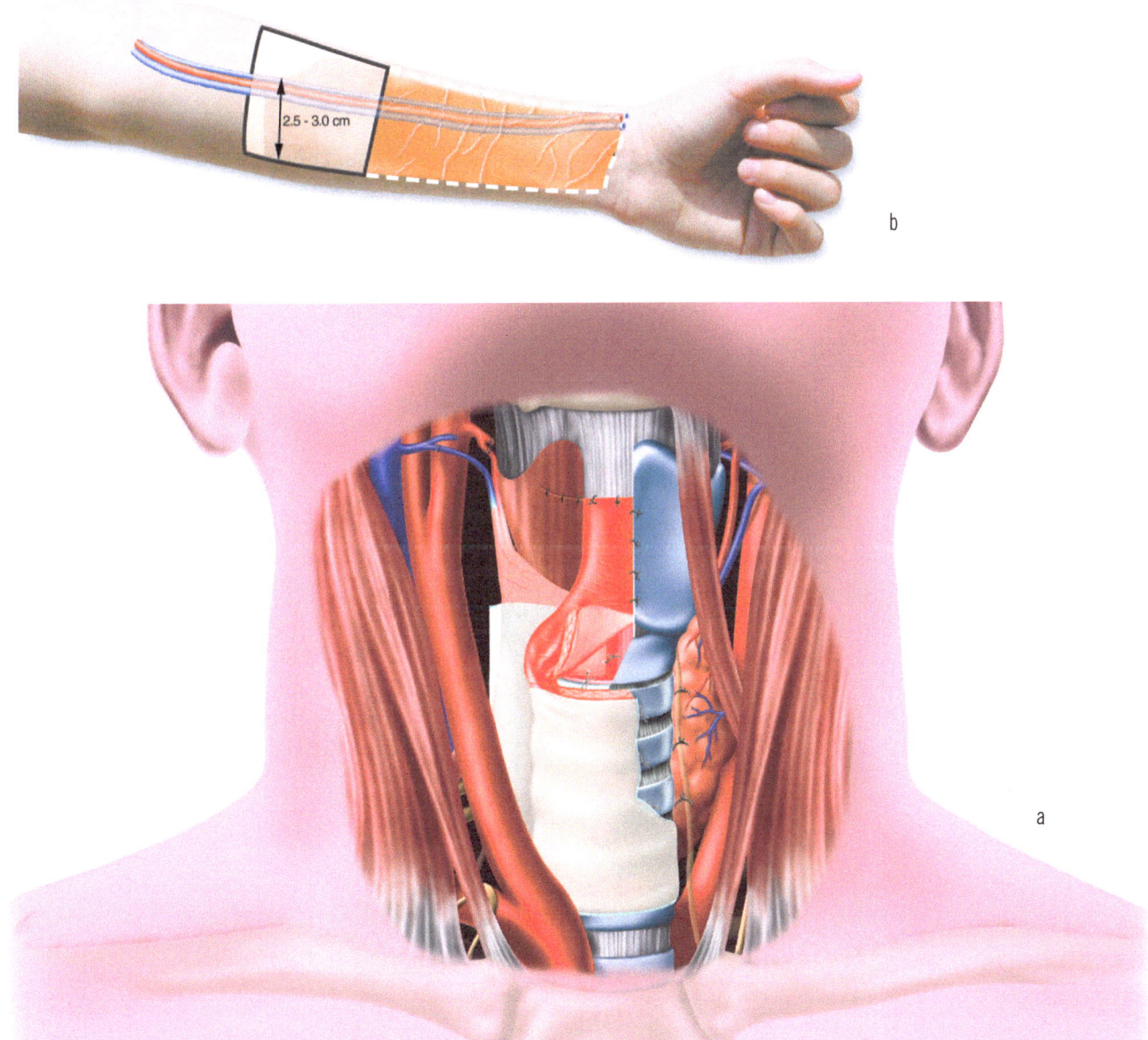

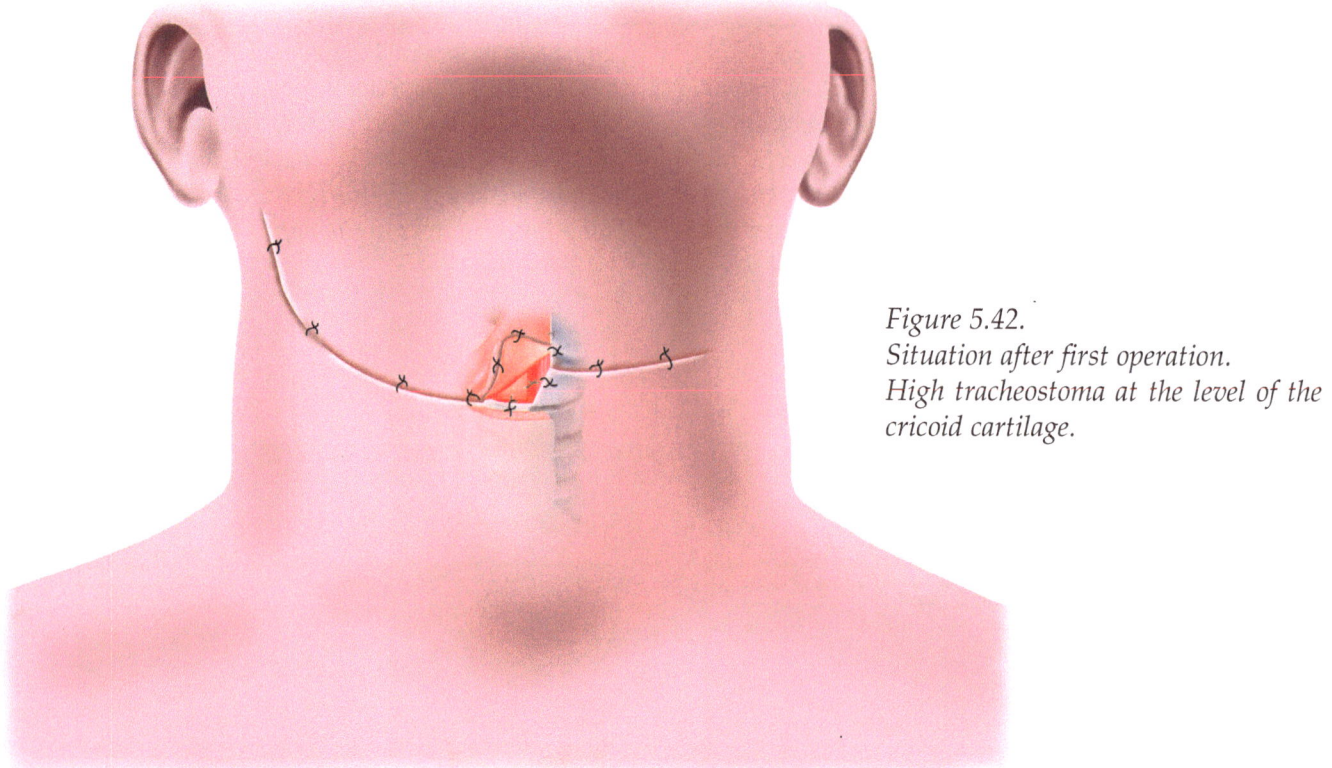

Figure 5.42.
Situation after first operation.
High tracheostoma at the level of the
cricoid cartilage.

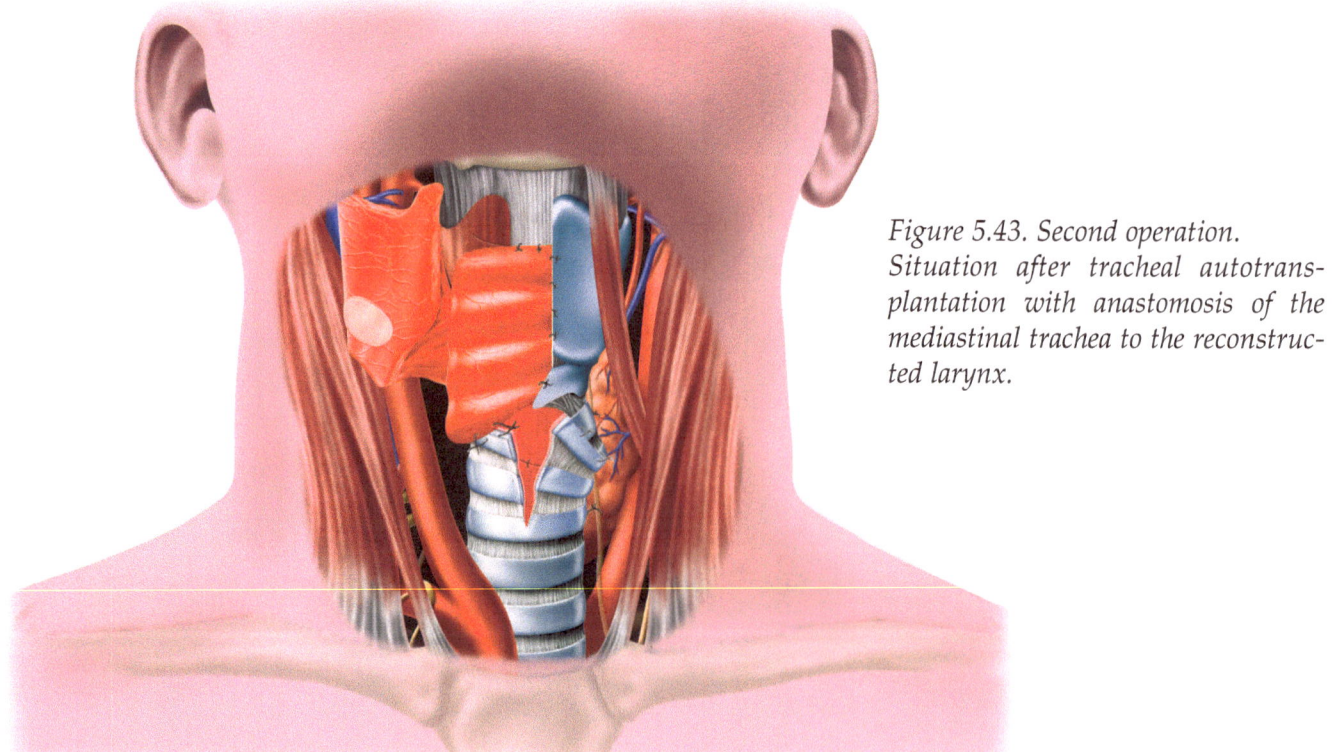

Figure 5.43. Second operation.
Situation after tracheal autotrans-
plantation with anastomosis of the
mediastinal trachea to the reconstruc-
ted larynx.

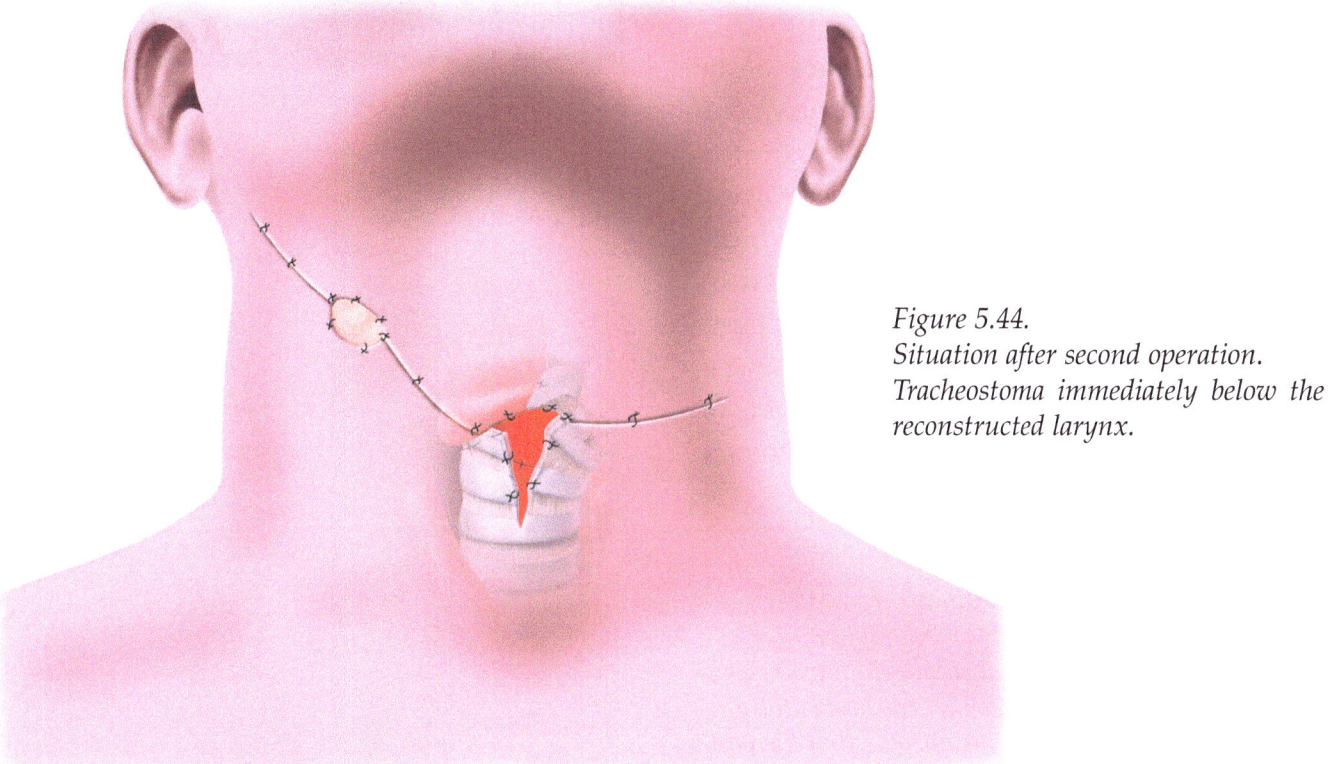

Figure 5.44.
Situation after second operation.
Tracheostoma immediately below the
reconstructed larynx.

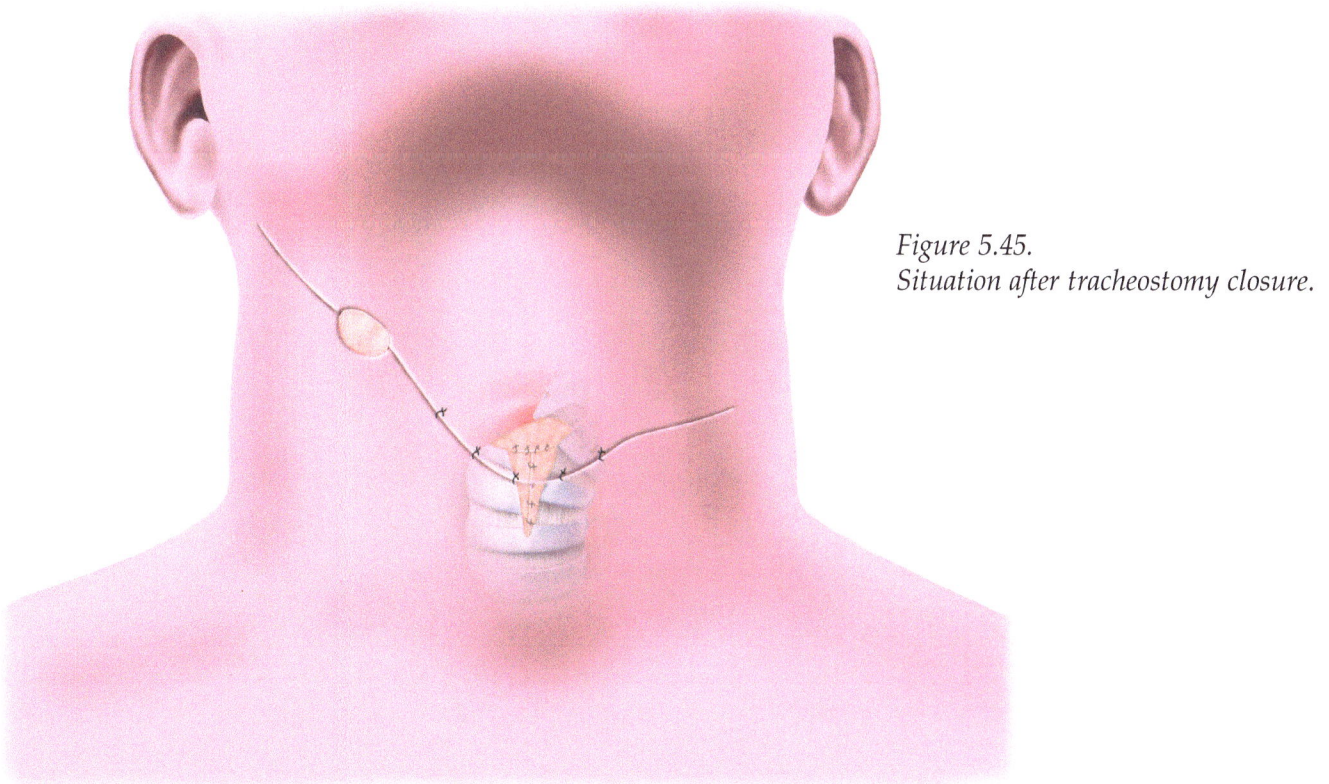

Figure 5.45.
Situation after tracheostomy closure.

B. Hypopharyngeal cancer

Hypopharyngeal cancer can be an indication in very selected cases (Fig 5.46). Four patients in our series (initial and modified concept) were treated for hypopharyngeal cancers. Two patients were treated for a carcinoma and 2 patients were treated for a sarcoma (1 liposarcoma and 1 fibrosarcoma). The 2 carcinoma patients underwent postoperative irradiation; the 2 sarcoma patients were not irradiated. The 4 patients or free of tumor (2 to 6 years postoperatively) and all tracheostomies were closed.

Figure 5.46. Hypopharyngeal cancer.
a. Indication for tracheal autotransplantation.
A small tumor of the pyriform sinus with involvement of the apex may be an indication for tracheal autotransplantation. The section margins are placed in the posterior and anterior commissure. The hypopharyngeal defect is closed primarily.
b. Extend of resection. The anterior laryngeal section line is located in the midline. Neck dissections in patients with clinically negative necks should include lymph node levels II, III, and IV because of the low risk of metastatic disease in the submandibular triangle (level I) and posterior triangle (level V). The ipsilateral thyroid gland, recurrent nerve, and tracheoesophageal lymph nodes will be removed.

Table 5.6.
Tracheal autotransplantaton-Indications hypopharynx

T2-3 pyriform sinus tumor with infiltration in apex
    -Tumor not beyond the midline
    -Primary closure of hypopharynx necessary

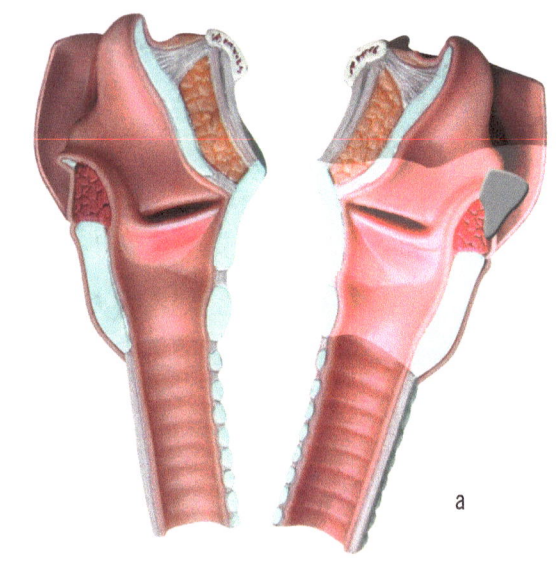

a

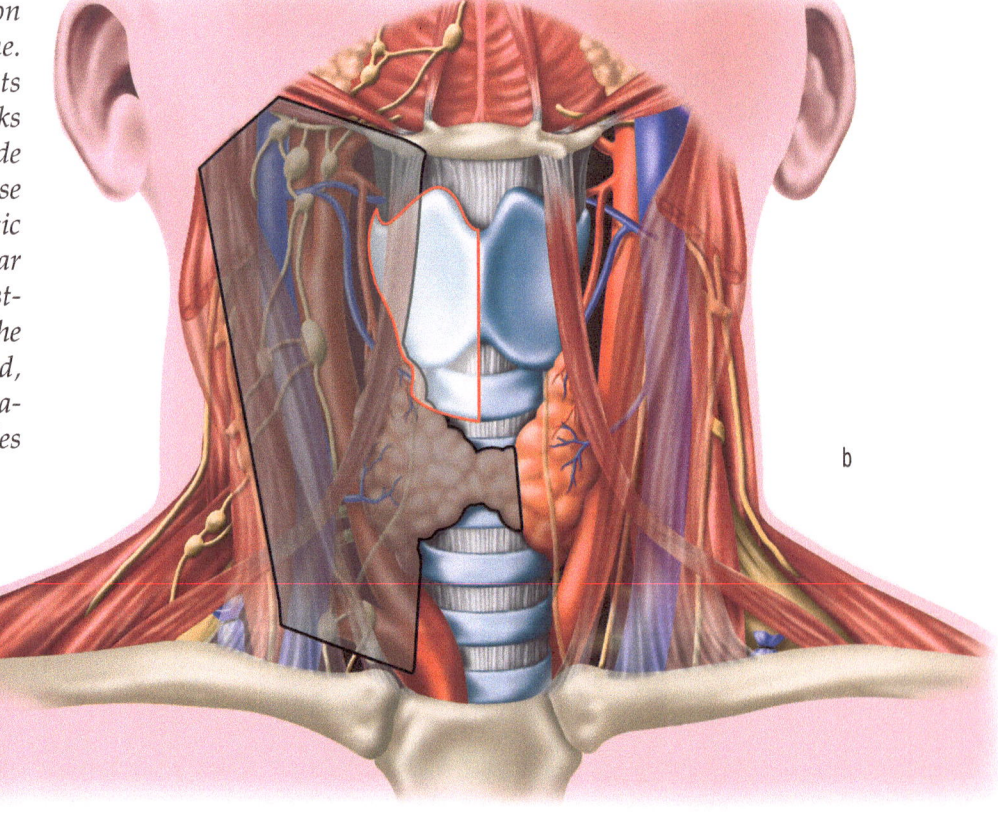

b

C. Chondrosarcoma

Lateralized chondrosarcomas of the cricoid cartilage form an excellent indication for tracheal autotransplantation. One chondrosarcoma was treated with the initial concept and three cases were treated with the modified concept. Of the three cases treated with the modified concept, 2 were considered large tumors while one, small tumor was treated differently.

C.1. Large tumor

Two cases with a chondrosarcoma showed extensive tumor extension. The tumors were lateralized in both cases and they could be treated successfully with the modified autotransplantation concept (Fig. 5.47, 5.48).

The tumor was resected during the first operation and the definitive reconstruction occurred 4 months after the first operation.

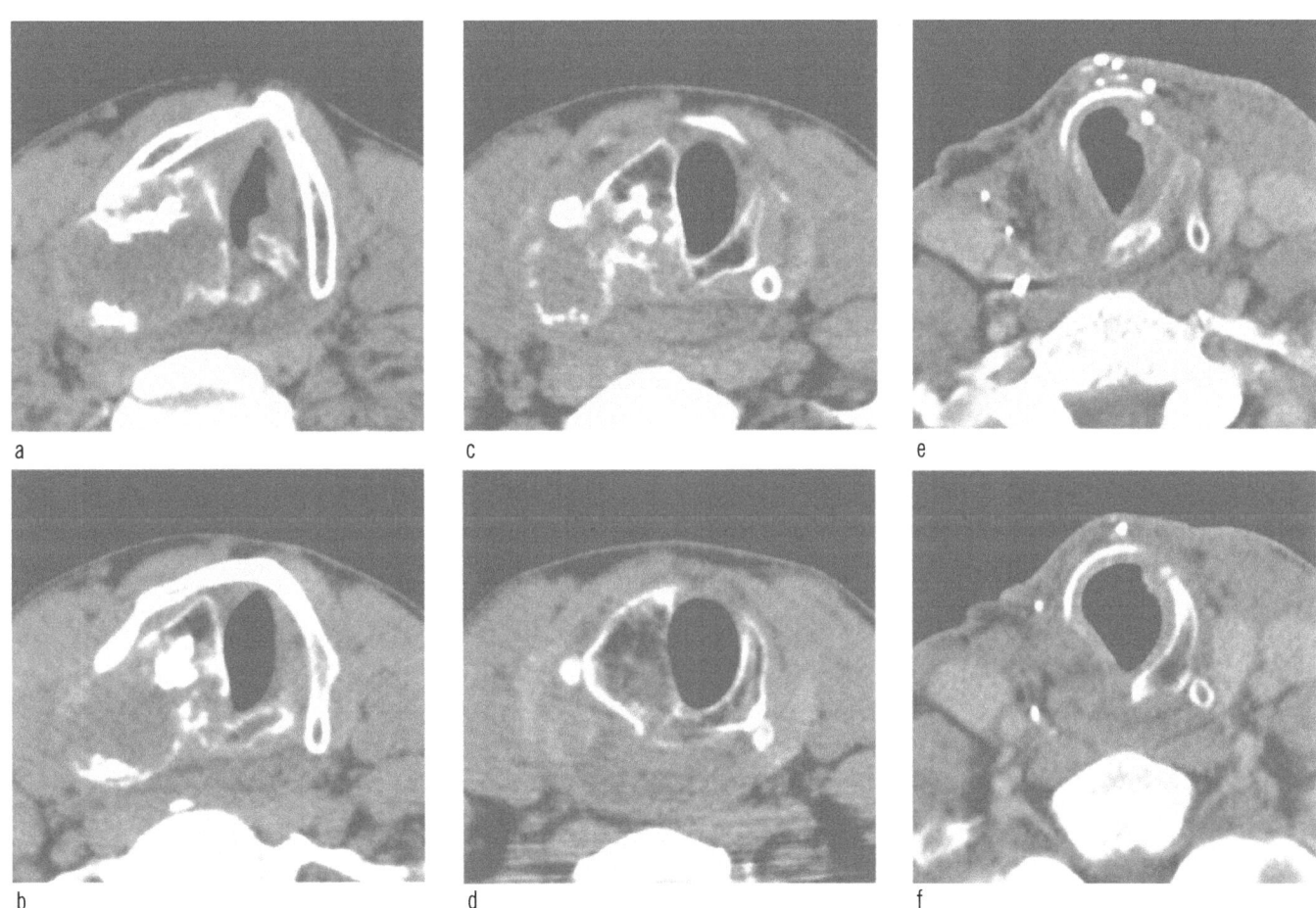

Figure 5.47. Chondrosarcoma-large tumor.
a. Preoperative glottic level.
b., c. and d. Preoperative subglottic level.
Lateralized chondrosarcoma of the subglottic area at the right side with involvement of the vocal fold.

e. and f. Postoperative situation after tracheal autotransplantation. The tumor was resected by performing and extended hemilaryngectomy with tracheal autotransplantation.

C.2. Small tumor

One patient treated with the modified concept showed a small tumor. He (65-year-old male) was referred with the diagnosis of a chondrosarcoma of the left cricoid cartilage (Fig. 5.49). The patient was asymptomatic and the diagnosis was made on a CT scan that was taken because of cervical arthrosis. It was decided to treat the patient differently because the vocal fold and arytenoid was not

Figure 5.48. Tracheal autotransplantation for large, unilateral chondrosarcoma.
No neck dissection is performed. The ipsilateral thyroid gland will be removed for access (wrapping of trachea) and not for oncological reasons.

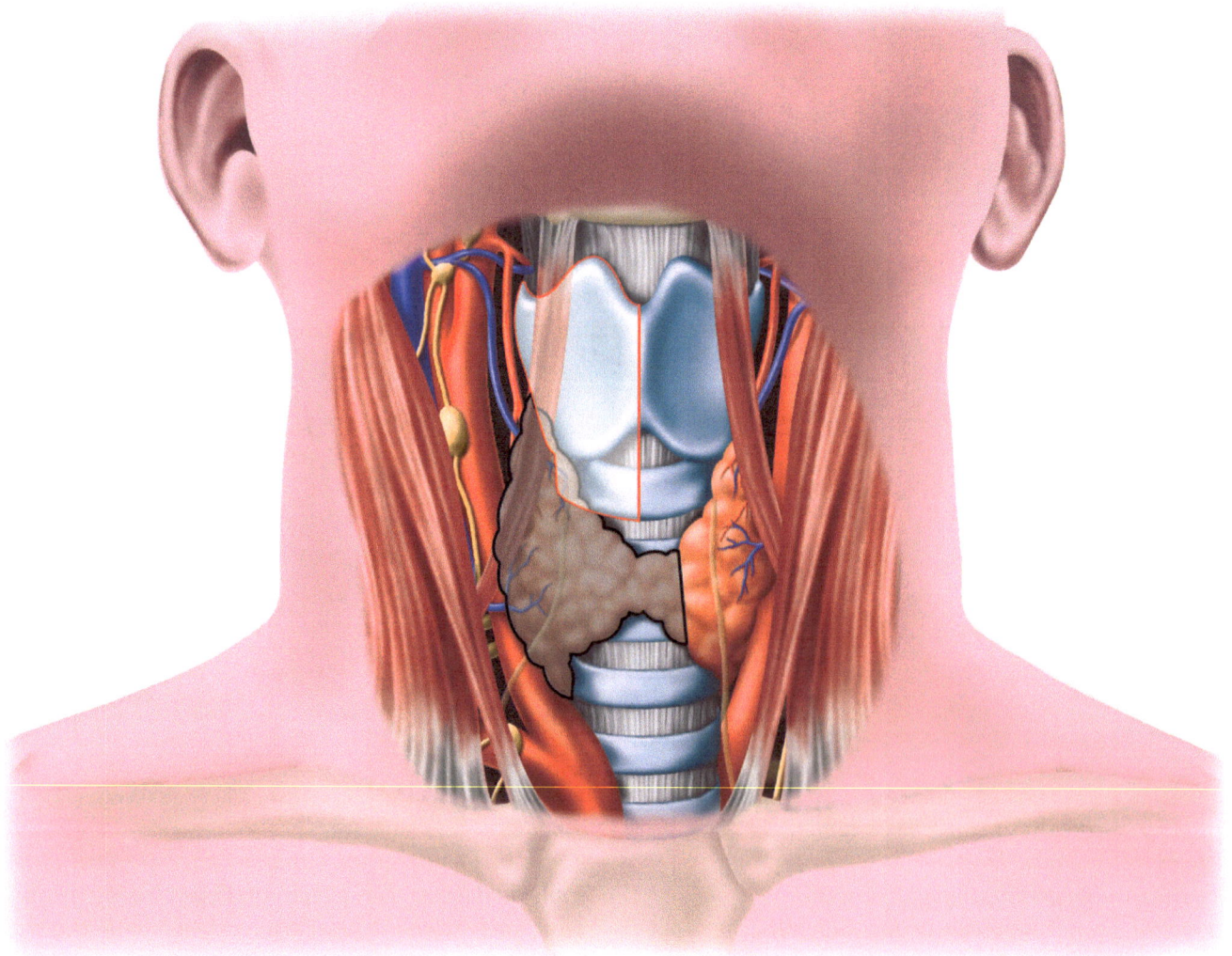

involved at the tumor side and because a laryngeal chondrosarcoma is usually low-grade with a very low tumor progression. In the first operation, the tumor was not resected. The cervical trachea was wrapped by fascia. Wrapping was done as in the modified concept and not circumferentially as in the initial concept (Fig. 5.50).

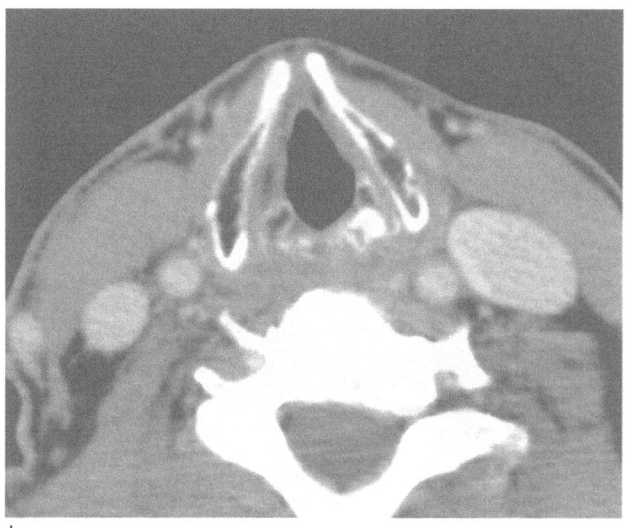
b

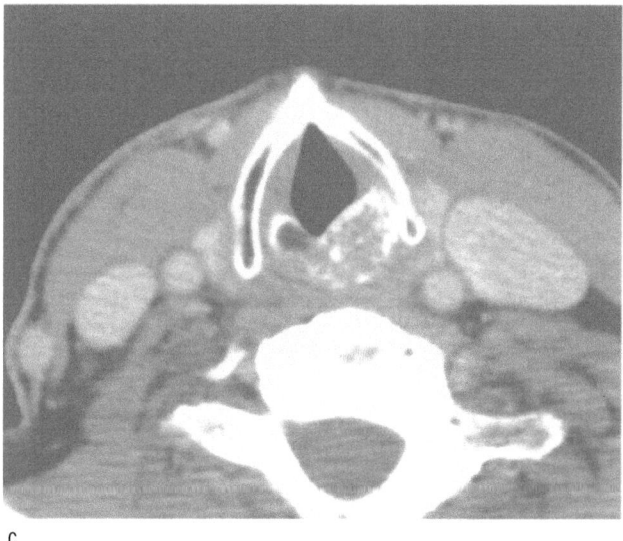
c

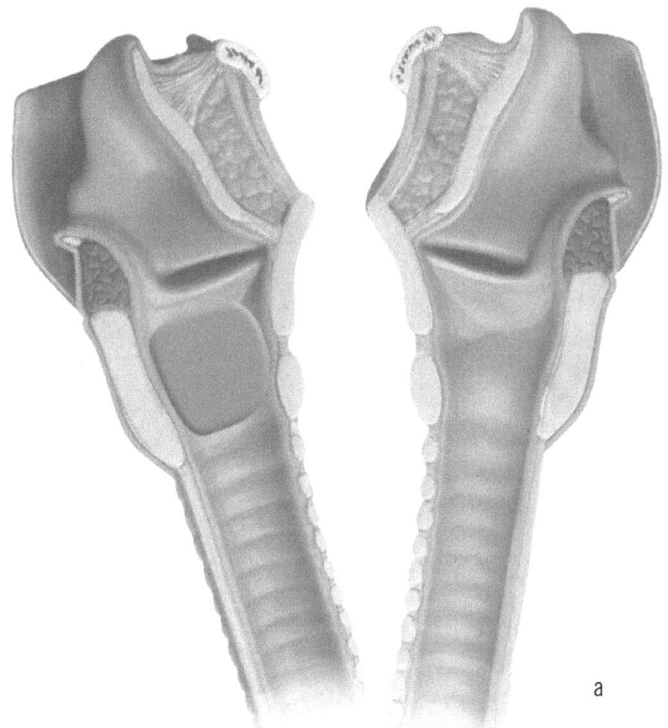
a

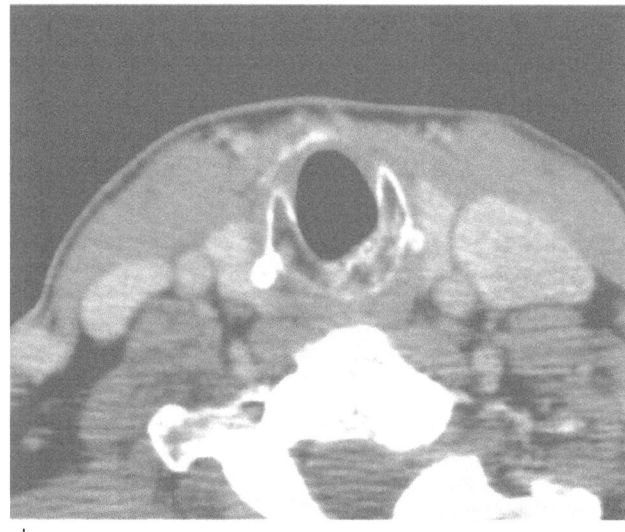
d

Figure 5.49.
Chondrosarcoma-small tumor.
a. Amount of submucosal tumor infiltration.
b., c., d. Axial CT scan showing extent of tumor.
The left side of the cricoid cartilage is involved.
The vocal fold and arytenoid are not involved.

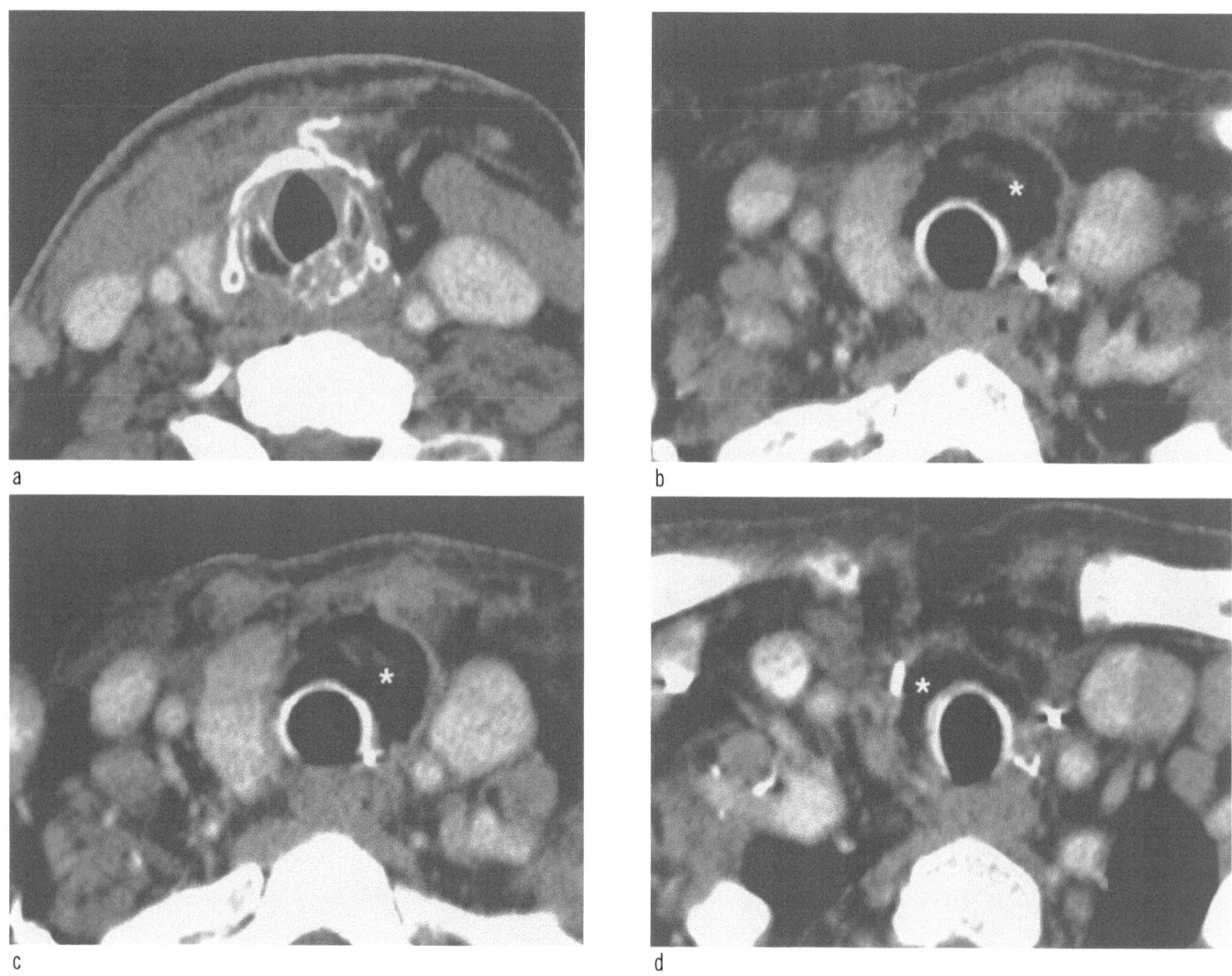

Figure 5.50. Small chondrosarcoma- Axial CT scan after first operation.
a. Cricoid level. The tumor is not resected during the first operation.
b., c. and d. Tracheal level (from high to low). The upper 4 cm of trachea is wrapped with fascia following the pattern of the modified concept: 3 cm of the circumference at the upper level and the full amount of cartilage ring at the lower level. Fascia is indicated by asterisks.

Tumor resection and tracheal autotransplantation occurred 4 months after the first operation. Tumor removal was delayed to avoid the tracheostomy during the 4 month time interval. The posterior forearm skin paddle necessary to create the posterior bulk was not warranted because the vocal fold and arytenoid was preserved at the tumor side (Fig. 5.51).

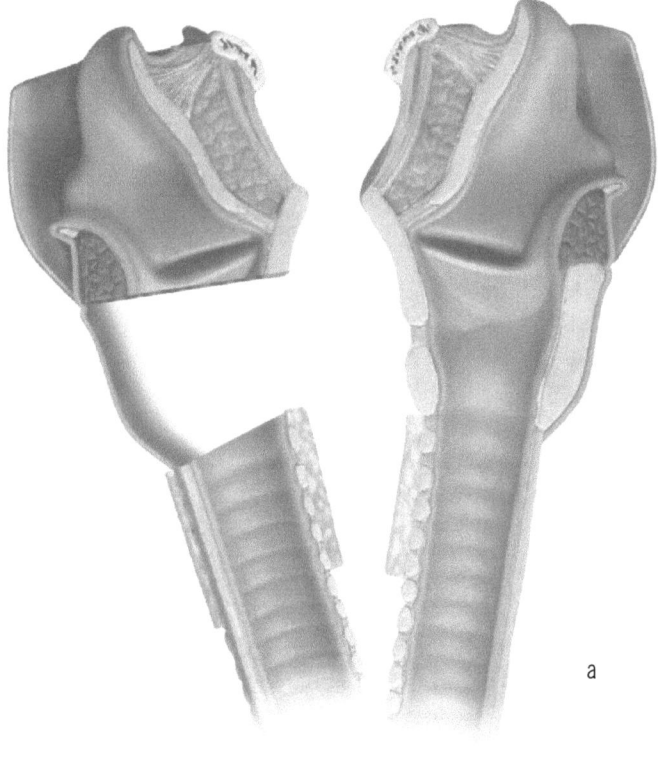

a

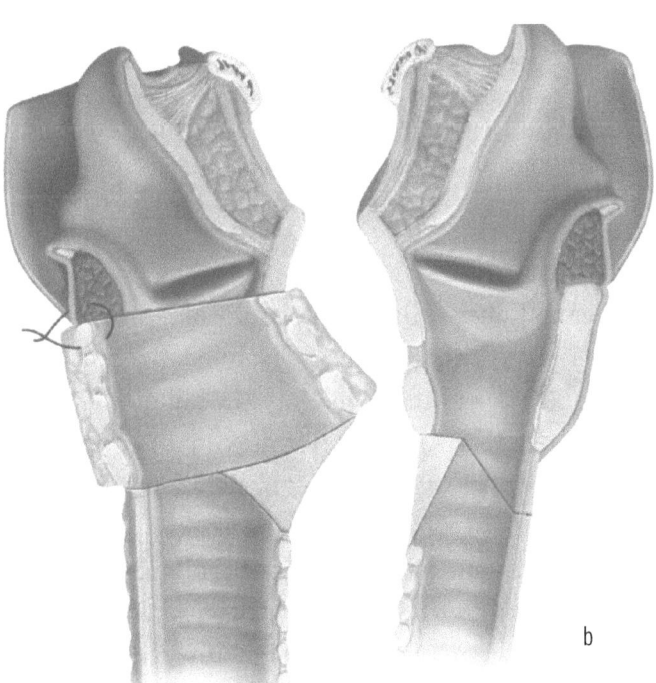

b

Figure 5.51.
Small chondrosarcoma- Second operation.
a. Amount of tumor resection.
b. Situation after tracheal autotransplantation and closure of the tracheostomy.
The vocal fold and arytenoid at the tumor side were sutured to the superior margin of the tracheal auto-transplant and they were placed in a midline position.

A tracheostomy was performed after the second operation and it was closed after 1 month under local anesthesia. Voice and swallowing function were excellent and comparable to a unilateral vocal fold paralysis in the midline position. Laryngeal morphology after reconstruction can be evaluated on the CT scan visible in Fig 5.52 and Fig. 5.53.

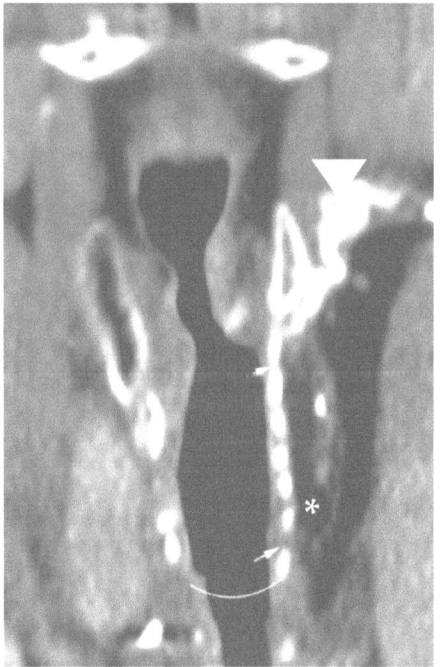

Figure 5.52.
Postoperative CT scan. The coronal reformation shows the tracheal autotransplant repairing the subglottic larynx (between arrows). Fascia flap is indicated by asterisk. Anastomosis between mediastinal trachea and reconstructed larynx is indicated with white line. The preserved vocal fold and arytenoid are visible on top of the tracheal transplant. Arrowhead points to ePTFE membrane that remained in place.

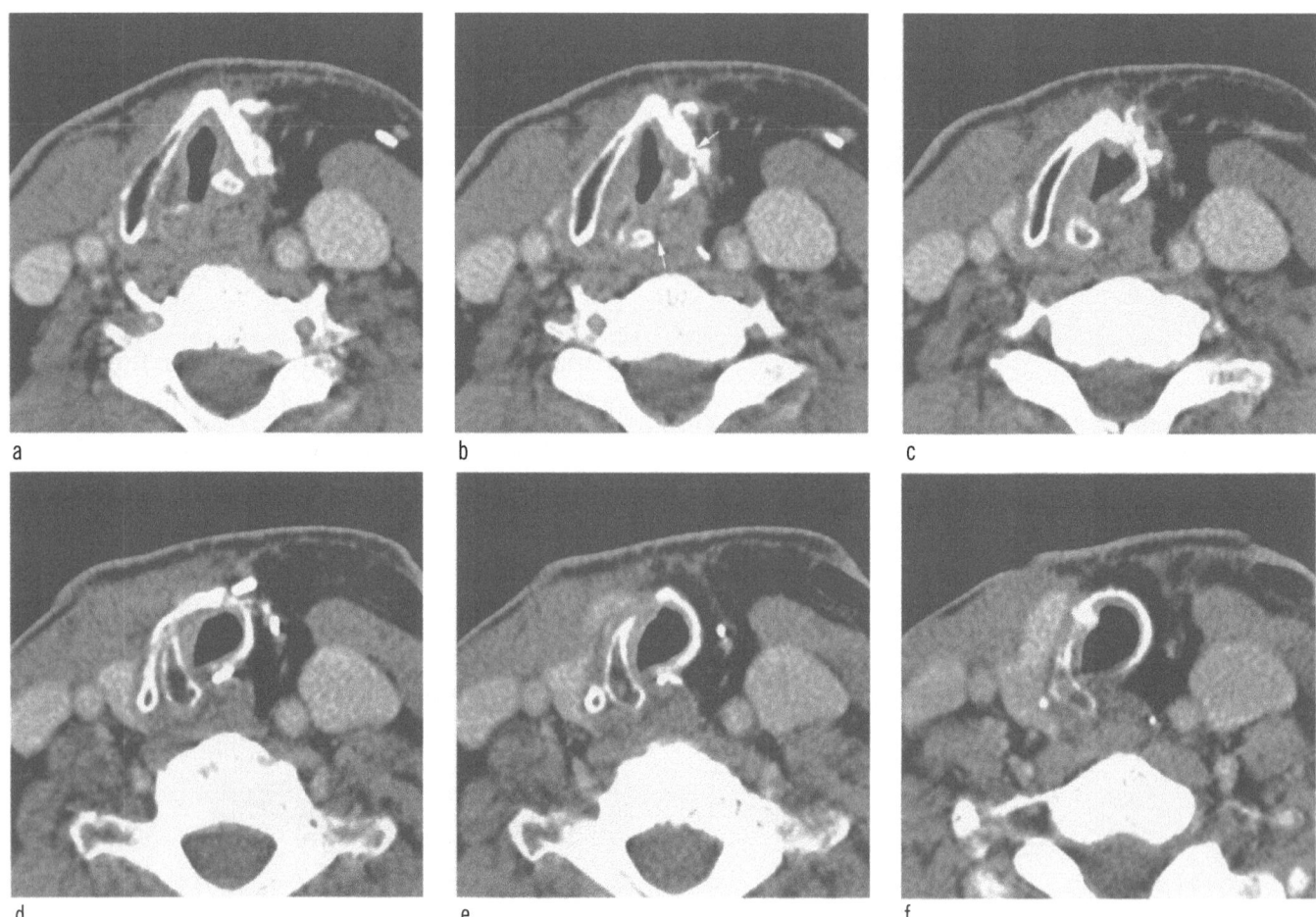

Figure 5.53. Postoperative CT scan-Axial sections.
a. Supraglottic level. Left vocal fold is immobilized in medial position. The preserved arytenoid has become sclerotic.
b. Glottic level. Tracheal transplant restores posterior site (between arrows).

c., d., e. and f. Subglottic level (from high to low). Hemicricoid defect is restored by revascularized trachea with full restoration of airway lumen.

Table 5.7.
Tracheal autotransplantaton-Indications chondrosarcoma
Large tumor lateralized
- Modified autotransplantation concept.
- Tumor resection during first operation.
Small tumor lateralized
- Modified autotransplantation concept (4 months time interval, no circumferential wrapping)
- Tumor resection during second operation with preservation of vocal fold and arytenoid.

The small chondrosarcome could also be treated in a 1-stage procedure as described by Zur and Urken (ZUR et al. 2003). Only the subglottic area needs reconstruction and this can be done by doing a direct tracheal autotransplantation with the transplant pedicled on the superior thyroid artery and vein. The transfer of the trachea, with the adjacent thyroid gland, has been accomplished in a single-stage because of the ability to move the thyroid gland in a cephalad direction without the need to interrupt the inferior and superior blood supplies. Tracheal autotransplantation on the thyroid artery and vein has the advantage of a 1-stage procedure but it is probably more risky than indirect revascularization. The tracheal transplant will be lost if the vascular supply through the superior thyroid vessels is interrupted. No second transplant can be taken, and the patient will become cannula dependent due to stenosis. Tracheal prefabrication is a safe procedure for preservation of the transplant viability. A second radial forearm flap can be taken in cases of flap failure during the first operation and the vascular pedicle needs no manipulation during the second intervention.

4. Conclusion

The key points of the optimal reconstructive technique are summarized in Table 4.8.

The radial forearm skin provides a midline reconstruction after the first operation with restoration of the sphincteric function.

The combination of the preserved radial forearm skin (at the posterior glottic and supraglottic level) with the tracheal patch provides for an optimal reconstruction after the second operation. (Fig. 5.54) with restoration of the sphincteric and respiratory function.

Table 5.8.
Optimal reconstruction of extended hemilaryngectomy defects-KEY POINTS

First operation
- Width of forearm flap at glottic level: 3 cm (between 2.5 and 3.0 cm in females).
- Restoration of posterior bulk (mucosal incision over preserved arytenoid).
- Epiglottis is sutured to skin flap anteriorly at level of false vocal fold (arrow).

Second operation
- Preservation of radial forearm skin posteriorly
- Width of tracheal patch at glottic level: 3 cm (between 2.5 and 3.0 cm in females).
- Full amount of tracheal patch is included inferiorly.
- Epiglottis is sutured to superior margin of tracheal patch anteriorly (no excessive forearm skin at supraglottic level anteriorly).

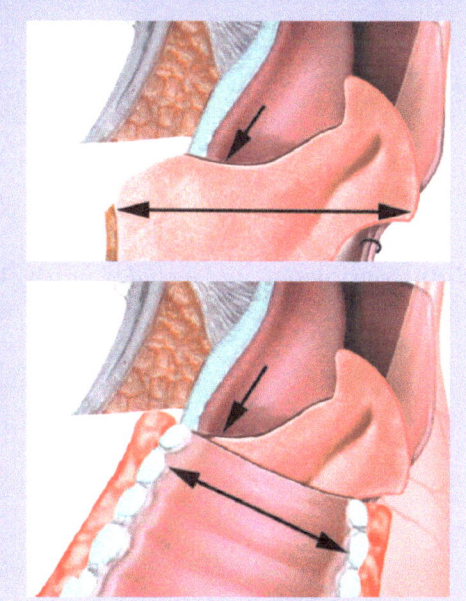

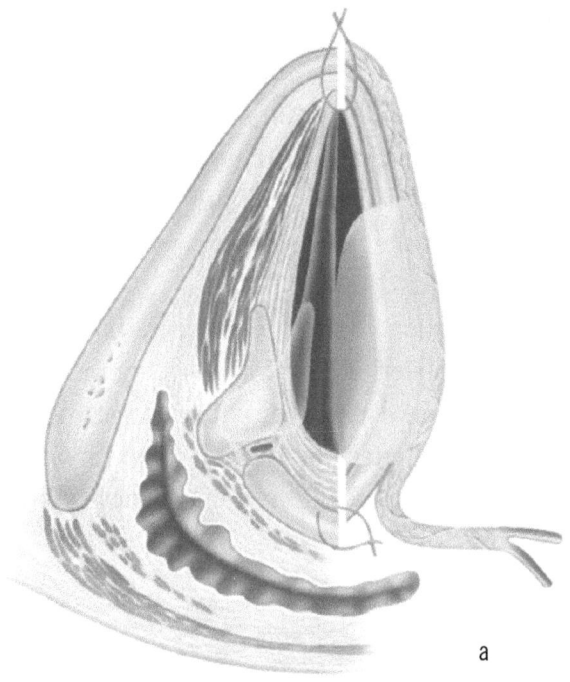
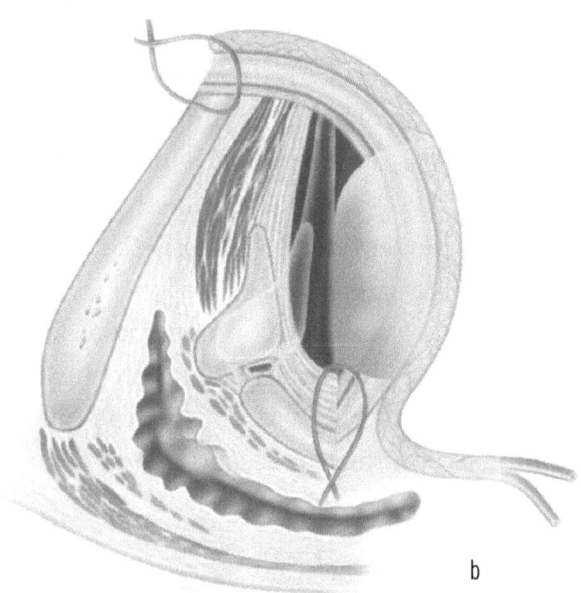

a

b

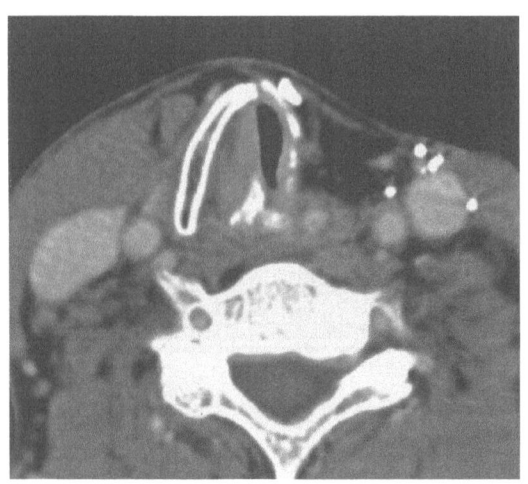
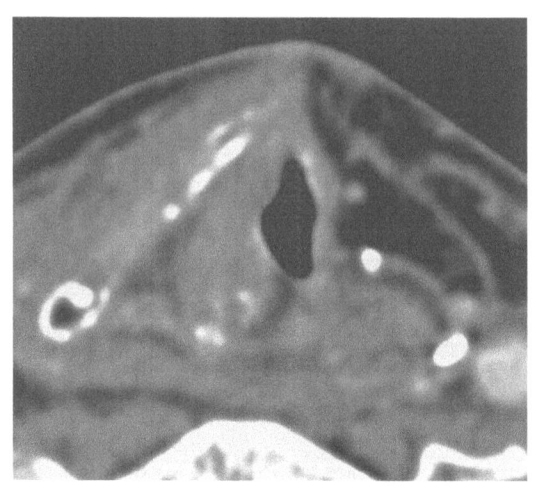

Figure 5.54. Optimal reconstruction at glottic level in modified concept.
a. Anterior section in midline.
b. Anterior commissure included in resection.
The combination of forearm skin and tracheal patch leads to an optimal morphology at the glottic level. The anterior larynx is the respiratory larynx; the posterior larynx is the sphincteric larynx.

BIBLIOGRAPHY

Hirano M, Kurita S, Kiyokawa K, Sato K. Posterior glottis. Morphological study in excised human larynges. Ann Otol Rhinol Laryngol 1986;95:576-81.

Zur K, Urken M. Vascularized hemitracheal autograft for laryngotracheal reconstruction: a new surgical technique based on the thyroid gland as a vascular carrier. Laryngoscope 2003;113:1494-8.

CHAPTER 6

From Wound Healing Research to Tracheal Reconstruction with Preformed, Composite Tissue

1. Etiology and treatment of laryngotracheal stenosis

Laryngotracheal stenosis usually involves the subglottic and/or tracheal area and can be congenital or acquired. Acquired stenosis is currently the most common form. An obstructed airway is most commonly due to sequelae following iatrogenic lesions caused by intubation, tracheotomy, and coniotomy (cricothyrotomy). Direct pressure by endotracheal tube cuffs to levels > 25-30 mm Hg induces mucosal ischemia (STAUFFER et al. 1981). Normal capillary pressure of tracheal mucosae is 20 to 30 mm Hg (NORDIN 1977). Mucosal ischemia leads to ulcerations, exposure of cartilaginous rings which may become infected by adjacent secretions. Long-term tracheostomy can also be a cause of tracheal stenosis (Fig. 6.1).

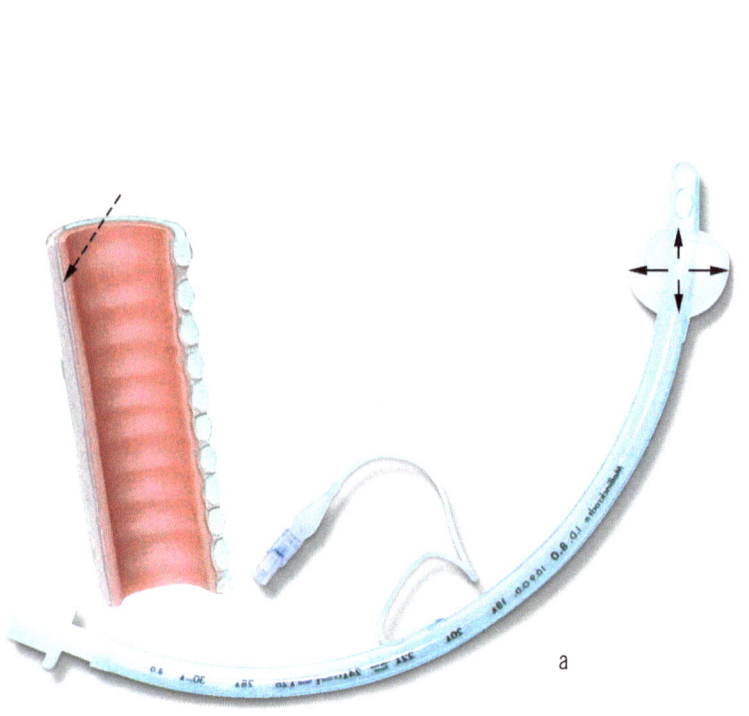

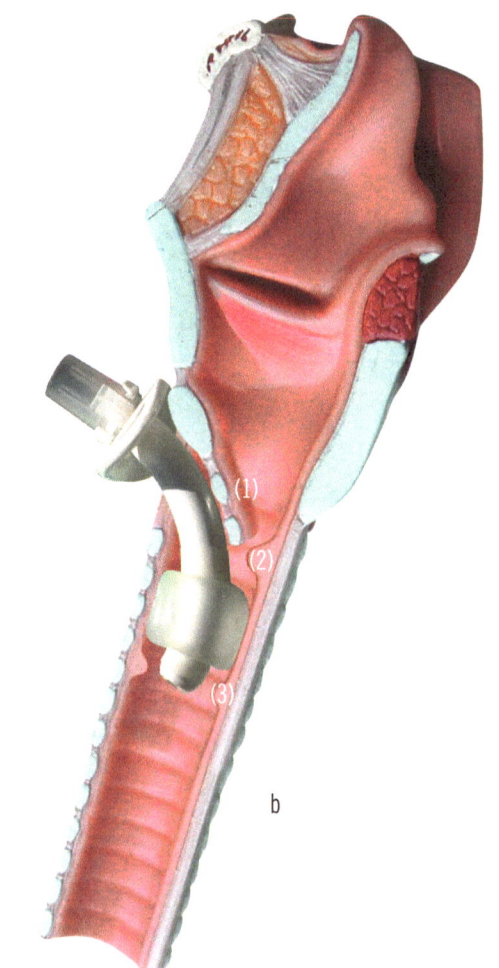

Figure 6.1. Causes of tracheal stenosis.
a. Excessive cuff pressure.
Endotracheal tubes with a cuff pressure above the capillary mucosal pressure will lead to mucosal necrosis and airway stenosis.

b. Common damaging effects of long-term tracheostomy.
Buckling of the anterior tracheal wall (1) under pressure of the curved tube. The inflammatory response may result in a stenotic shelf on the posterior tracheal wall (2) opposite the fenestra. If the tip of the tube abuts against the tracheal wall, circumferential stenosis (3) may result. Damage of the mucosa from overinflated cuffs is also a hazard.

Although subglottic or tracheal stenosis may occur after any intubation during a time period of any length, several factors are associated with an increased risk of developing stenosis. These factors include the utilization of a large endotracheal tube, laryngopharyngeal reflux, traumatic reintubation or emergent intubation, prolonged intubation and individual patient factors such as a narrow subglottic lumen, diabetes, sepsis (systemic infection), and immunodeficiency. Injury to the airway mucosa is the inciting event, regardless of the cause of the stenosis. Gastroesophageal reflux has been proposed as a medical condition which may exacerbate the pathogenesis of laryngotracheal stenosis (BAIN et al. 1983).

The methods available for treating postintubation stenosis fall into two categories: endoscopic and open surgical methods. Mild stenosis can be treated with endoscopic laser resection. Laser vaporization of tracheal strictures has been employed with variable success. Several different types of laser techniques have been described, and either the carbon dioxide or the Nd:YAG laser can be used with equal efficacy. Regardless of the laser technique used, it should only be used in select circumstances (Fig. 6.2). Poor results are guaranteed when there is circumferential scarring, the stenosis is greater than one centimeter in vertical dimension, there has been loss of cartilage, tracheomalacia is present, or when there is a history of tracheal infection secondary to a tracheotomy.

Mitomycin-C is an antineoplastic antibiotic that acts as an alkylating agent by inhibiting DNA and protein synthesis. It can inhibit cell division, protein synthesis, and fibroblast proliferation. Topical application of mitomycin-C (0.4-1.0 mg/mL) can be used as an adjuvant treatment in the endoscopic laser management of laryngeal and tracheal stenosis (RAHBAR et al. 2001).

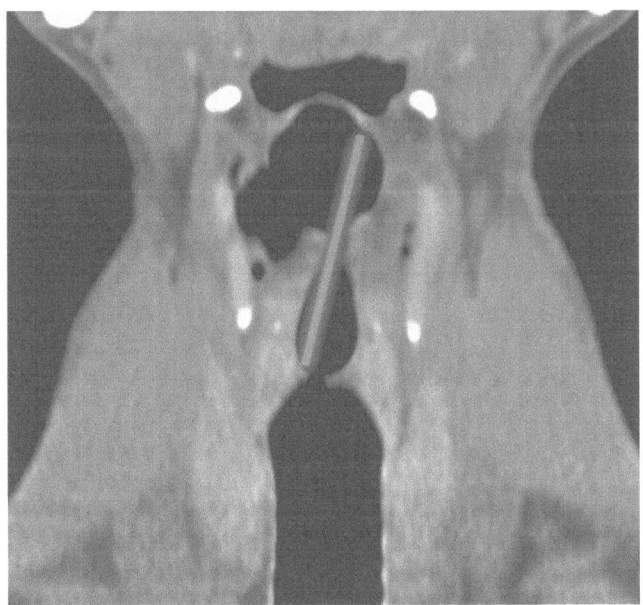

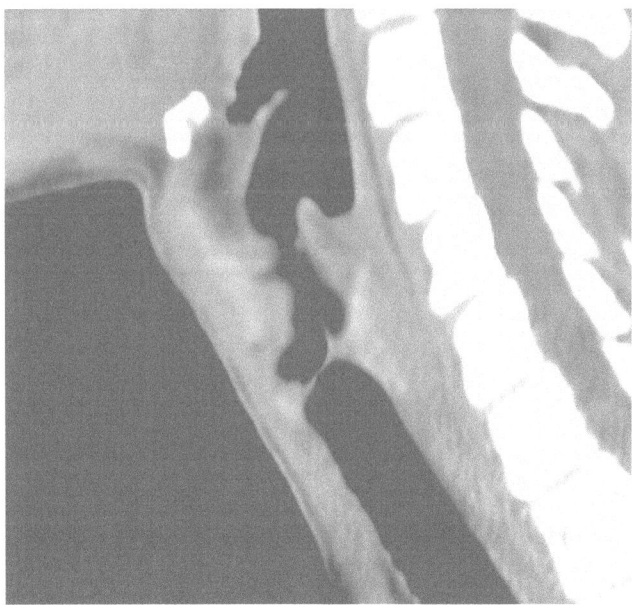

Figure 6.2. CT subglottic web.
a. Coronal reformation of subglottic web. The substenosis was treated by laser vaporization and topical (3 minutes) application of Mitomycin (1.0 mg/mL).

b. Sagittal reformation of subglottic web.

Most tracheal stenoses can be treated successfully by segmental resection and end-to-end anastomosis (GRILLO et al. 1995). Segmental resection can also be done when the cricoid cartilage is involved. Since the mid-1970s, cricotracheal resection (CTR) with anastomosis of the trachea to the thyroid cartilage (Fig. 6.3, 6.4) has become the treatment of choice for the cure of subglottic stenosis acquired after prolonged intubation or trauma (MONNIER at al. 1995, 1999, PEARSON et al. 1996).

CTR is performed as a single-stage operation with resection of the tracheostoma site. An exception to this rule includes cases in which the tracheostoma site is situated too far distally and unnecessarily requires the resection of a long segment of trachea.

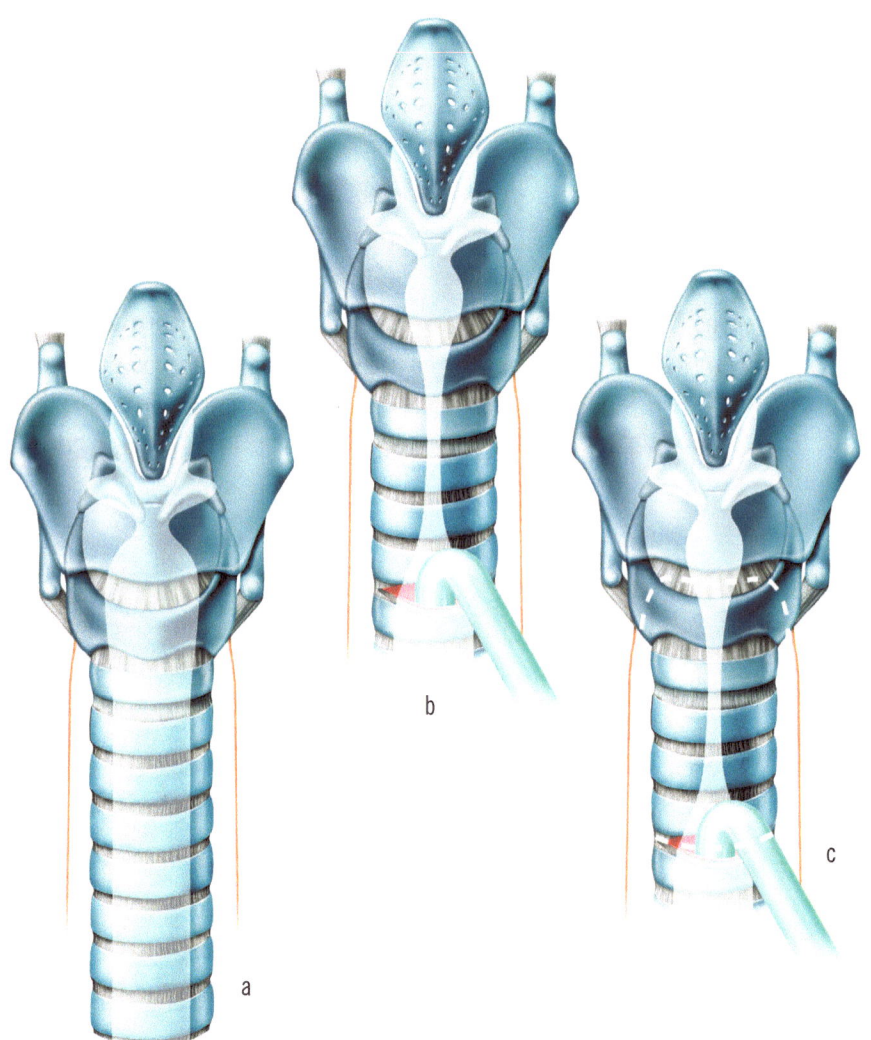

Figure 6.3. Cricotracheal resection for subglottic stenosis.
a. Larynx and trachea with normal airway lumen.
b. Larynx and trachea with stenosis of subglottis and upper trachea.

c. Cricotracheal resection. The inferior resection line is made at the superior border of the first normal tracheal ring. The superior resection line is made at the inferior border of the thyroid cartilage, and the lateral section of the cricoid arch is made just anterior to the cricothyroid joints.

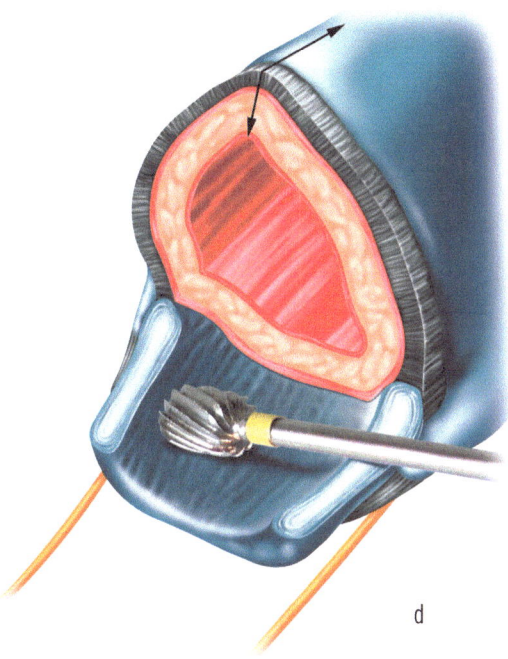

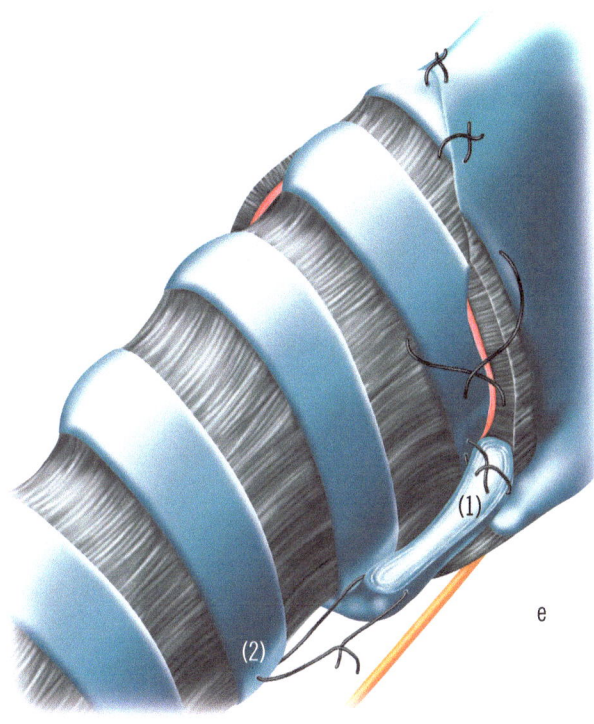

Figure 6.3. Cricotracheal resection for subglottic stenosis (continued).

d. Oblique view of the subglottis after resection of the stenotic cricotracheal segment. The uppermost posterior section of the mucosa is made just below the cricoarytenoid joints. A diamond burr is used to widen the denuded cricoid plate. An inferior midline thyrotomy (double arrow) up to the level of the anterior commissure of the larynx (but without transecting it) is performed.

e. Lateral view of the thyrotracheal anastomosis. The first (1) posterolateral stitch is passed between the first tracheal ring and the cricoid plate. The stitch should emerge in a subperichondrial plane from the outer surface of the cricoid plate to avoid any lesion to the recurrent laryngeal nerve. A second stitch (2), placed between the third tracheal ring and the inferior border of the cricoid plate, is used to release the tension at the site of the anastomosis.

During CTR, one should enlarge the subglottic lumen as much as possible without compromising voice quality. This is best achieved by widening the cricoid plate posteriorly and laterally with a diamond burr and by performing an inferior midline thyrotomy up to the level of the anterior commissure of the larynx. Interrupted Vicryl sutures are used for the posterior anastomosis, with the knots tied inside the lumen. Fibrin glue is used to secure the membranous trachea to the cricoid plate. Vicryl sutures with the knots tied outside the lumen are used for the anterior and lateral anastomosis.

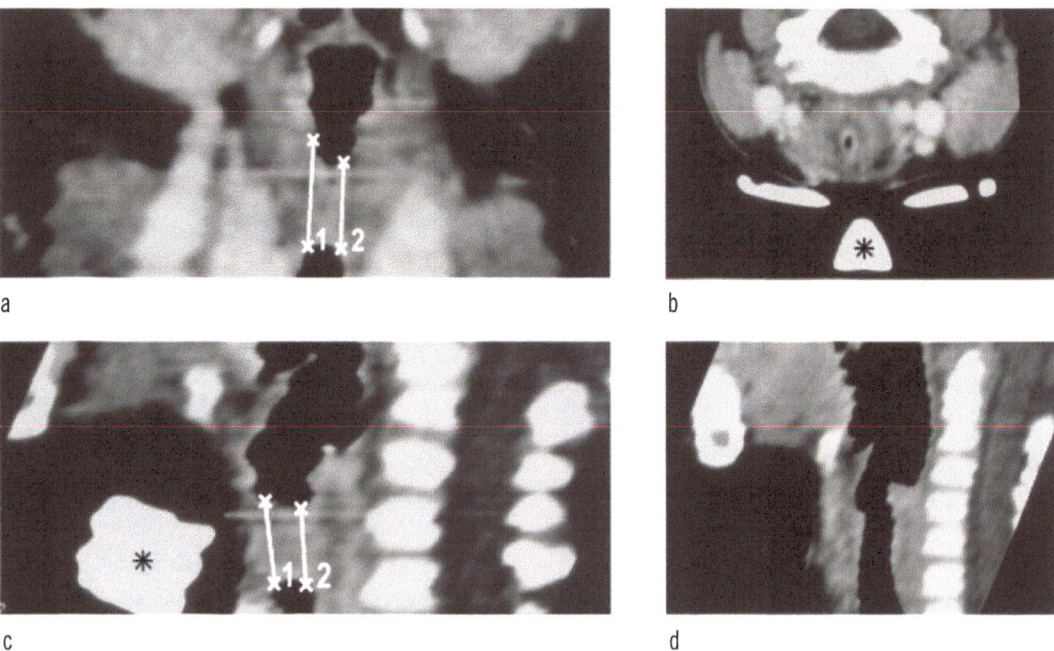

a

b

c

d

Figure 6.4. CT scan of subglottic stenosis treated with cricotracheal resection.
a. Preoperative frontal reformation.
b. Preoperative axial section.
c. Preoperative-sagittal reformation.
d. Postoperative-sagittal reformation.

Congenital subglottis stenosis. Asterisks indicate tracheostomy tube. The stenosis was treated with a cricotracheal resection with inclusion of the tracheotomy site.

Resection of the trachea with end-to-end anastomosis is the ideal procedure if less than 40% to 50% of the length of the trachea is involved in the stenosis.

Acquired posterior subglottic stenosis results from the chronic presence of an endotracheal tube in the upper airway. The endotracheal tube compresses the mucosa overlying the cartilage of the medial arytenoids and cricoid ring (Fig. 6.5). When the force of compression by the endotracheal tube exceeds the mucosal capillary perfusion pressure then ischemic necrosis of the mucosa will result. Mucosal ulceration will give a local tissue response of repair and regeneration that will result in granulation tissue proliferation, fibrosis and eventually stenosis.

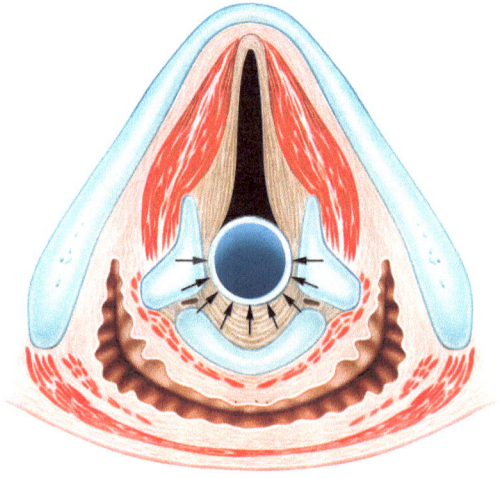

Figure 6.5. Posterior glottic stenosis-etiology.

The commonest reconstructive procedure for posterior subglottic stenosis involves harvesting rib cartilage which is sculptured and used as an autogenous graft to widen a posterior subglottic lumen (RETHI 1956). Surgical correction is usually necessary for posterior glottic stenosis with bilateral ankylosis of the arytenoids.

The stenotic scar tissue is divided but not resected. The cricoid cartilage is divided from upper to lower edge exactly in the midline to expose the inner mucoperichondrium of the postcricoid hypopharyngeal region. The two halves of the cricoid are retracted laterally and the cartilage graft is interposed between the medial edges of the incised cricoid (Fig. 6.6, 6.7). The most common graft is autologous rib cartilage harvested from the patient's submammary region, usually from the right side at the costochondral junction.

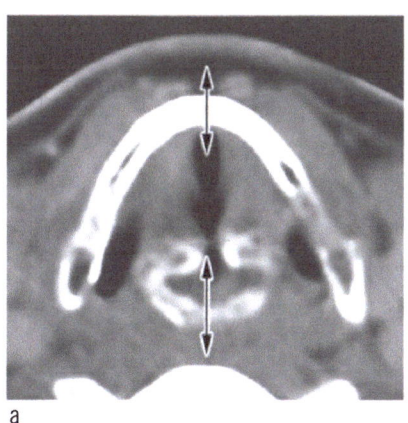

a

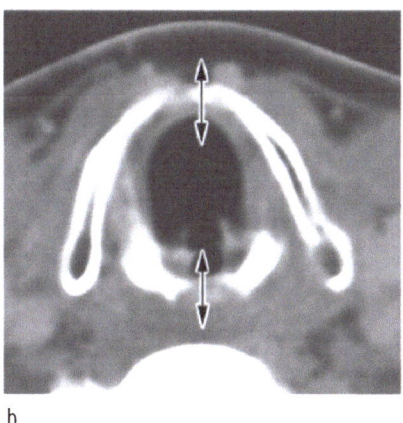

b

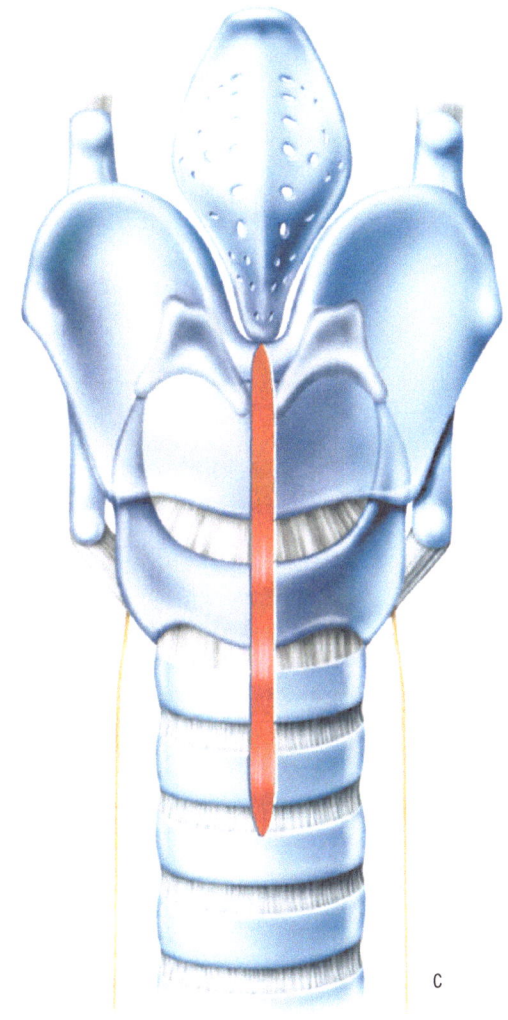

c

Figure 6.6. Posterior laryngeal stenosis-Surgical approach.
a. Posterior glottic stenosis with bilateral ankylosis of the arytenoids. The larynx is divided in the midline anteriorly and posteriorly (double arrows).

b. Posterior stenosis at subglottic level.
c. Laryngofissure is used to reach the posterior larynx. Following laryngofissure, the posterior cricoid cartilage is incised in the midline.

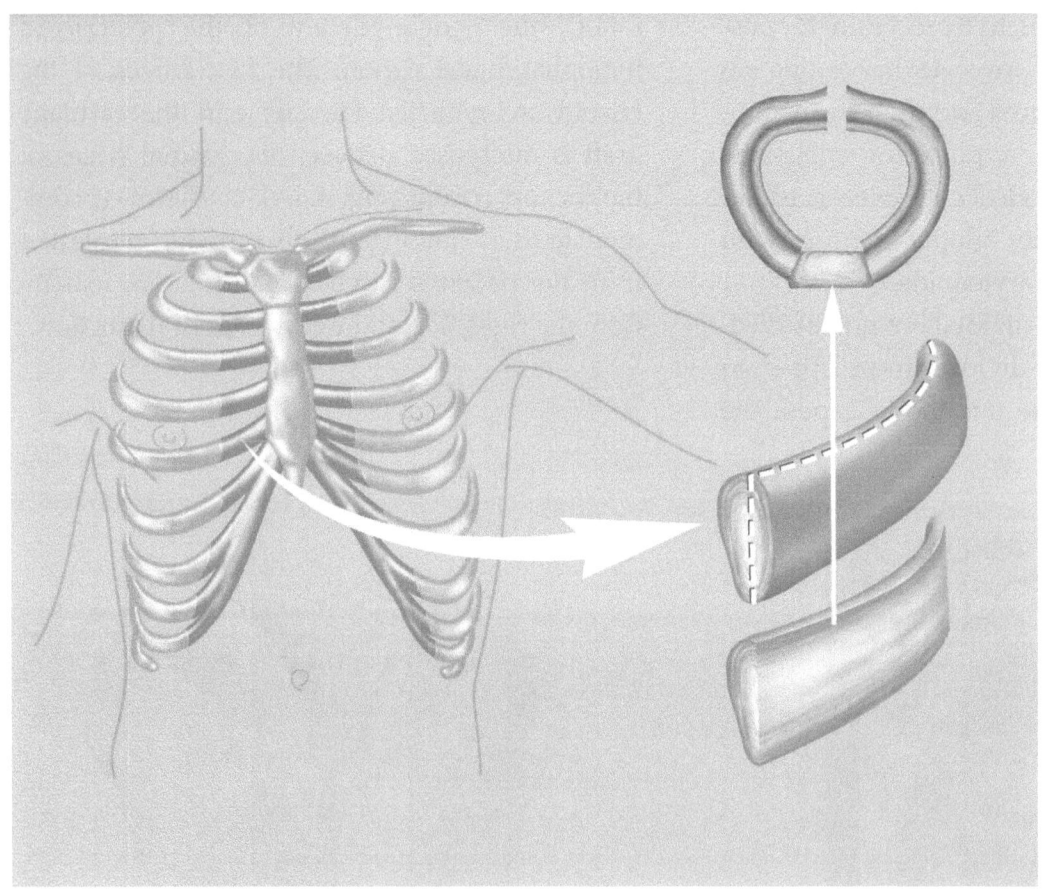

Figure 6.6. (continued).
d. Posterior laryngeal stenosis-Surgical approach.
A rib cartilage graft is placed in the posterior lamina of the cricoid cartilage.

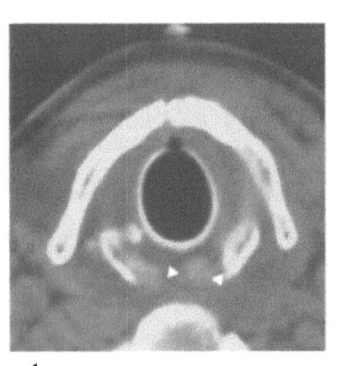

a 1

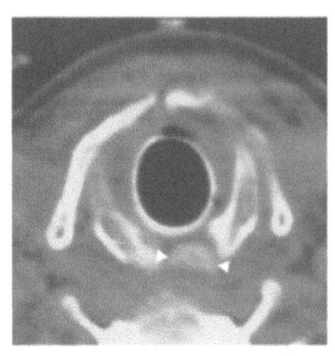

a 2

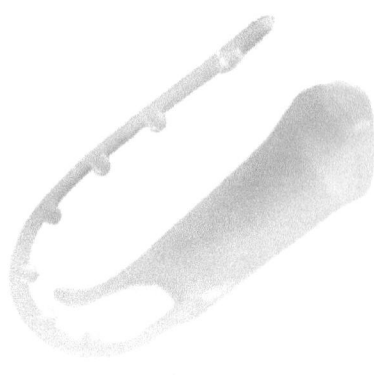

a 3

Figure 6.7. Posterior cartilage graft Postoperative.
a. Cartilage graft (between arrowheads) is placed between divided halfs of the cricoid lamina-situation with stent.
a.1. Axial CT-glottic level.

a.2. Axial CT-subglottic level.
a.3. Eliachar stent. This stent gives support to the cartilage graft during some (4-6) weeks.

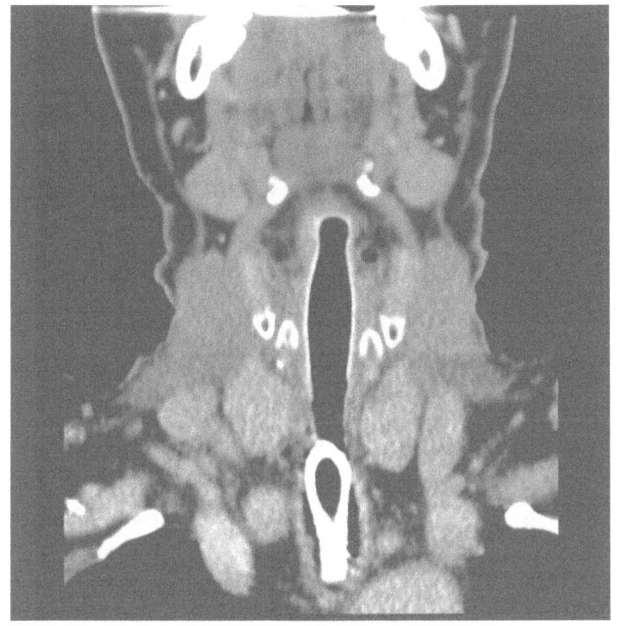

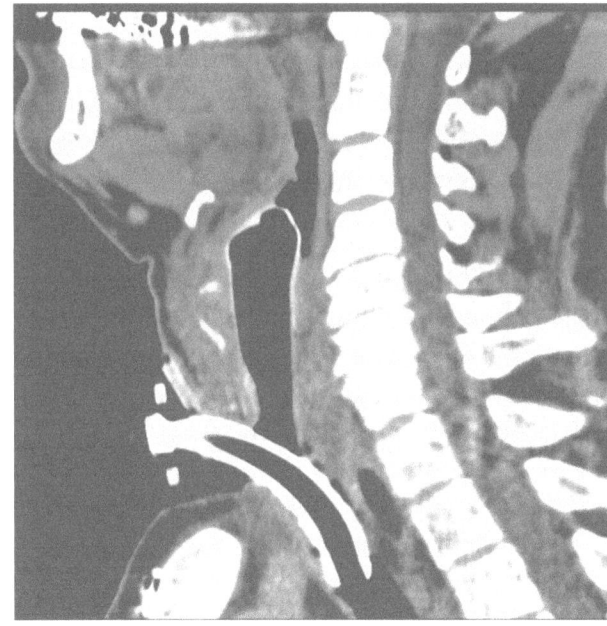

b1

b2

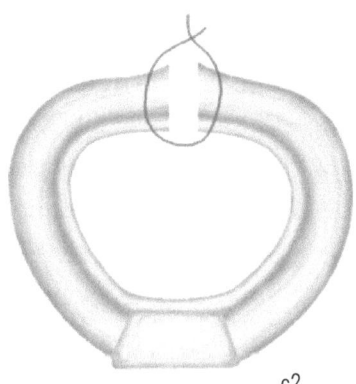

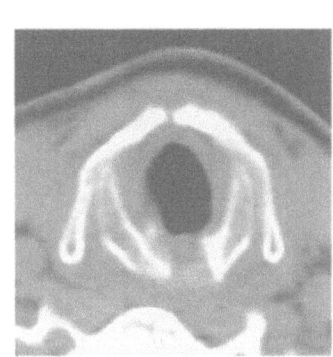

c1

c2

c3

Figure 6.7. Posterior cartilage graft Postoperative (continued).
b. Overview of postoperative situation with stent and tracheal cannula.
b.1. CT scan-coronal reformation.
b.2. CT scan-sagittal reformation.
c. Postoperative situation-without stent. Posterior glottic stenosis after correction.
c.1. Axial CT-glottic level.

c.2. Schematic drawing. The mucosal lining is growing over the cartilage graft.
c.3. Axial CT-subglottic level.

Free cartilage grafts undergo secondary healing with reepithelialization and revascularization induced from the margins of the defect. Grafts of cartilage do survive in the posterior larynx because relatively small grafts are used in a well vascularized area. Patients with both synchronous posterior glottic and subglottic stenosis present a major challenge in management. In these cases, functional reconstruction is best achieved combining a circumferential cricotracheal resection with placement of a cartilage graft in the posterior lar-

ynx (MONNIER et al. 1999). A costal cartilage graft is interposed in the midline after a posterior vertical cricoidotomy, and the expanded cricoid plate is covered by the membranous portion of the trachea advanced upwards to the posterior commissure of the larynx.

Congenital tracheal stenosis is usually caused by complete tracheal rings. Slide tracheoplasty (Fig. 6.8) may be a solution for a long segment tracheal stenosis in cases with complete tracheal rings. This procedure shortens the reconstructed stenotic segment by 50%, increases the reconstructed tracheal circumference by a factor of two, and increases the cross-sectional area by a factor of four. The trachea is thus repaired with tracheal wall containing native cartilages and is immediately lined with normal tracheal epithelium. Satisfactory subsequent growth has been demonstrated experimentally and clinically (GRILLO et al. 2002).

A slide tracheoplasty can bring a solution for congenital, long segment stenosis. Congenital long segment stenosis usually shows a normal consistency of the tracheal wall with a stenosis resulting from complete cartilaginous O rings without membranous ligament. Slide tracheoplasty is not usefull for acquired, long-segment stenoses.

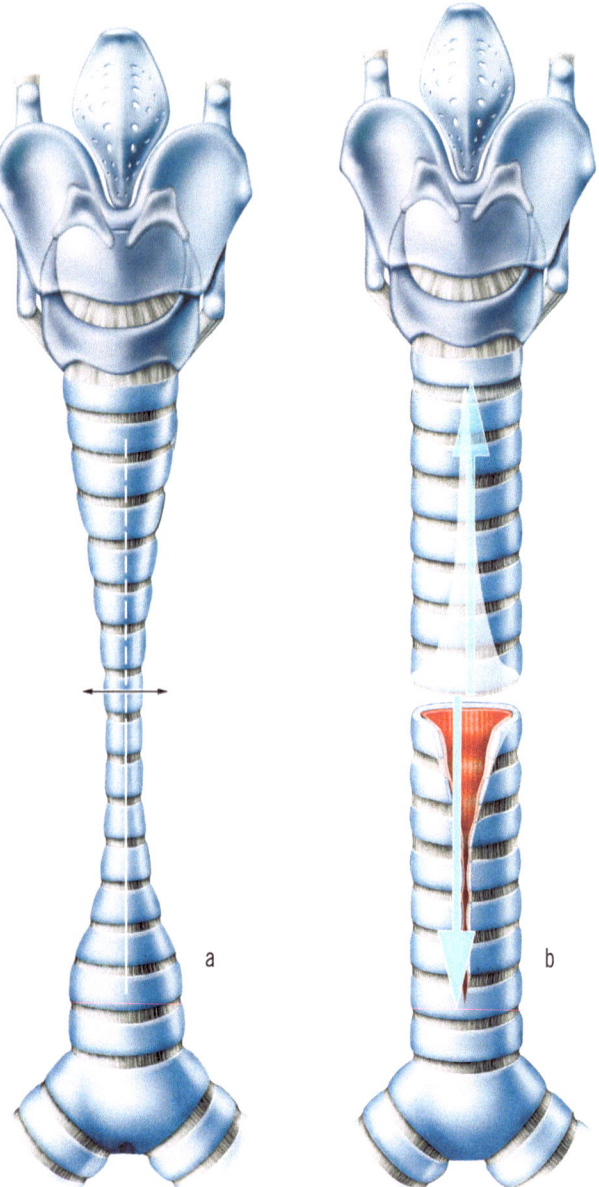

a

b

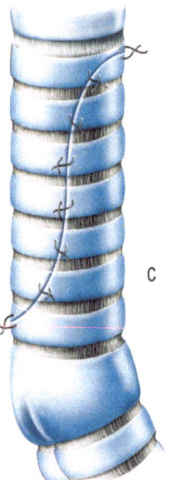

c

Figure 6.8.
Slide tracheoplasty.
(a)Trachea is transected at the mid point of the stenotic segment. (b) The posterior surface of the upper stenotic segment and the anterior surface of the lower segment are vertically incised. (c) The two ends are slide together and anastomosed.

2. New in vivo wound healing model

An important factor in the etiology of laryngotracheal stenosis is damage to the mucosal lining. The evolution of mucosal damage towards stenosis is not well understood. An important question during healing of mucosal airway defects is to what extend the wound will contract and to what extend the wound will re-epithelialize. We developed a wound healing model to quantify wound contraction and re-epithelialization.

Quantification of wound contraction and re-epithelialization is difficult in airway wound healing because most in vivo models are based on endoscopical approaches. The healing mechanism of full-thickness skin defects is better known because wound contraction and re-epithelialization can be evaluated on full-thickness excisional skin models that allow for direct observation. Full-thickness skin defects are wounds with complete removal of the epidermis and dermis. Wound healing is characterized by an involvement of all dermal layers and by a reepithelialization process that originates from the wound edges. Healing of full-thickness skin wounds occurs from the periphery of the wound. A fibrin clot is formed and is replaced initially by granulation tissue and later by migrating epithelium from the wound margins. This process is accelerated by wound contraction, in which wound fibroblasts assume some characteristics of smooth muscle cells, induce contraction of the granulation tissue, and result in a subsequent decrease in wound dimensions. Loose-skinned animals (rabbit, rat) close 90% of their wound area by contraction. In contrast, wound contraction contributes only 25-50% of total wound closure in humans (CATTY et al. 1965). A way to avoid wound contraction is to localize the wounds in an area with skin that is adherent to underlying structures. The rabbit ear wound model exhibits minimal wound contraction because the dermis on the inner surface of the rabbit ear is tightly adherent to the underlying cartilage. A full-thickness wound in this area heals greater than 90% by the production of granulation tissue and epithelial migration from the wound periphery. This model has been useful in consistently producing scars histologically similar to human hypertrophic scars. The delay in wound reepithelialization, as a result of limited wound contraction, results in excessive granulation tissue production and a hypertrophic scar after complete re-epithelialization (AHN et al, 1990).

We used an invasive, excisional wound healing model to quantify wound contraction and re-epithelialization for full-thickness mucosal defects inside the trachea. In contrast to endoscopical models, opening of the airway lumen allows for airway wounding to be performed in a controlled manner. The problem with an open approach however is the interferention with the airway's blood supply after anterior incision of the airway wall. An in vivo experimental model that interferes with the airway's vascularization is not acceptable because of the importance of an intact blood supply for normal tissue healing. Another problem after anterior incision of the airway wall is the interferention with the cartilaginous support that also may influence the healing process of mucosal wounds.

An invasive in vivo model was developed without interferention with the airway's blood supply and without interferention with the airway's cartilaginous support. The model consists of a complete isolation of tracheal segments after previous tracheal revascularization. With this model, the internal site of the trachea could be exteriorized and the trachea could be reimplanted after wounding without interferention with the blood supply or with the cartilaginous support. This model allowed us to study the mucosal healing of denuded segments of trachea (vascularized carti-lage rings and intercartilaginous ligaments) and allowed us to study the influence of mitomycine application on wound healing of full-thickness mucosal defects.

2.A. New in vivo wound healing model

This model allows for isolation and mucosal expo-sition of segments of trachea without interferen-tion with the blood supply and without interfer-ention with the cartilage support. The operative procedure consists of 2 operative stages:

2.A.1. Stage 1. Vascular induction through staged tracheal transfer

A staged vascular induction technique in the orthotopical position is used (Fig. 6.9).
The trachea is dissected from the underlying esophagus and cleared from most of the connec-tive tissue without incising the trachea. The tra-chea is still perfused in situ but is stripped of its connective tissue envelope containing part of the blood supply. The ischemic cervical trachea is wrapped over 2 cm by the transposed lateral tho-racic fascial flap. The lateral thoracic and cervical skin is closed with interrupted sutures.

Figure 6.9.
Revascularization of the rabbit trachea stage 1.
a. A 2 cm segment of cervical trachea (double arrow) is dissected from the surrounding tissue. The left lateral thoracic fascia flap is incised.
b. The left lateral thoracic fascial flap is dissected and transferred to the neck region. A 2 cm segment of cer-vical trachea is wrapped by the fascia flap.
c. The cervical skin of the neck is closed and the fascia is allowed to revascularize the cervical trachea during 2 weeks.

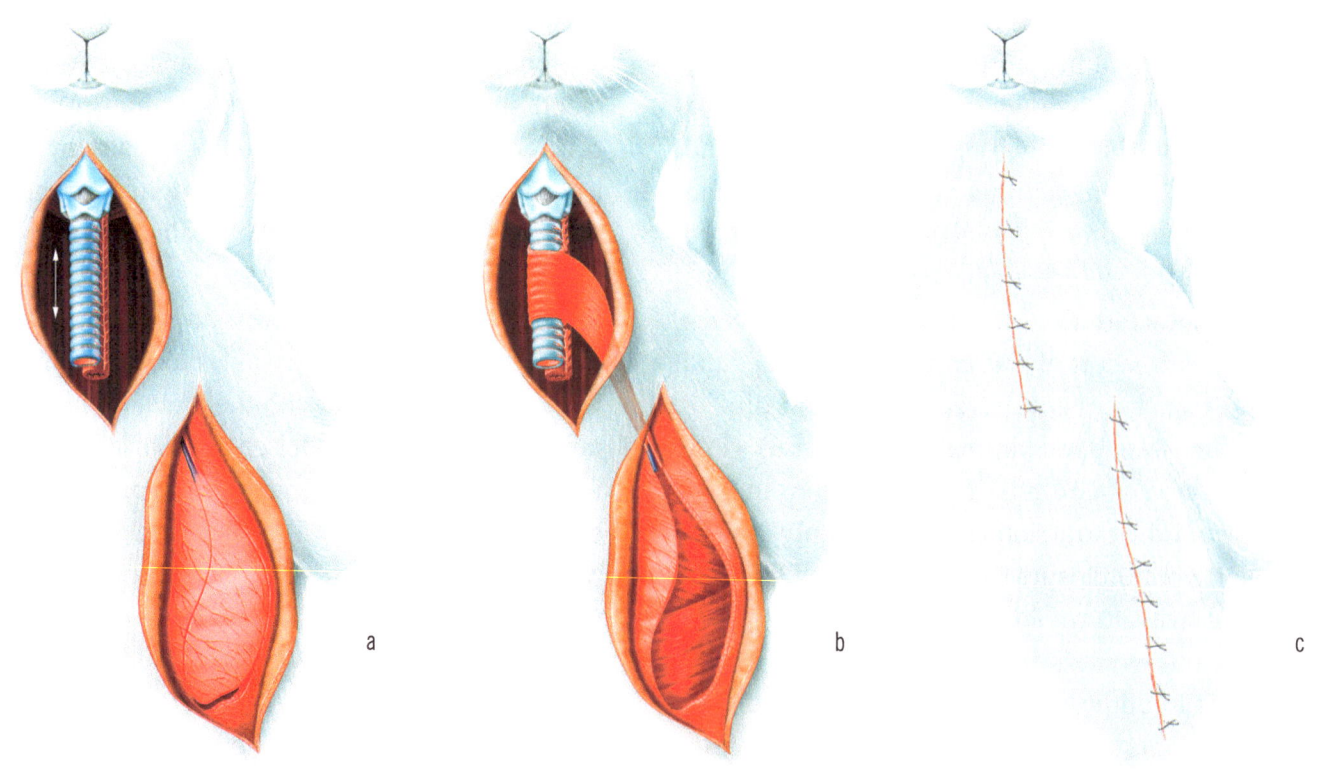

a   b   c

2.A.2. Stage 2. Tracheal isolation, exteriorization of luminal site, tracheal reimplantation

After 14 days, the trachea on its fascial vascular carrier becomes transferable by vascular induction. In a second stage, the neck is reopened and the cervical trachea with a length of 2 cm is dissected with its new, thin fascial envelope. The revascularized trachea is transformed into a patch after incision of the membranous trachea (Fig. 6.10). The isolated tracheal patch can be closed and reintroduced into the airway as visible in Fig. 6.11.

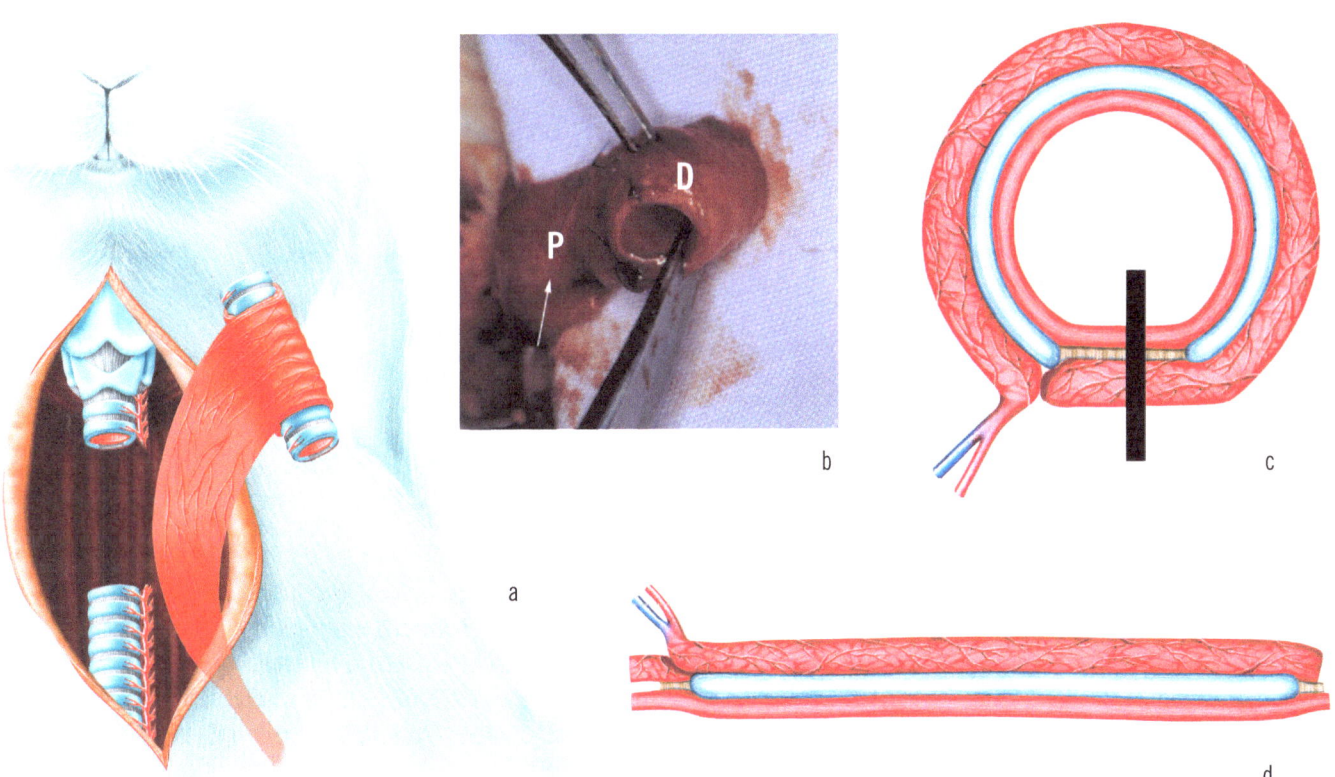

Figure 6. 10. Experimental model stage 2 - Isolation of trachea.
a. Schematic presentation of revascularized trachea after isolation. The fascial enwrapped tracheal segment is removed from the airway tract with preservation of the vascular pedicle of the fascia flap.
b. Incision of membranous trachea. A 2 cm segment of cervical trachea is isolated on the fascial vascular pedicle (arrow) and incised posteriorly. After isolation, the segment is opened posteriorly by longitudinal incision of the distal site of the fascia flap and by longitudinal incision of the membranous trachea. D=distal site of fascia flap; P=proximal site of fascia flap.
c. Incision of membranous trachea-axial section.
d. Tracheal patch-axial section.

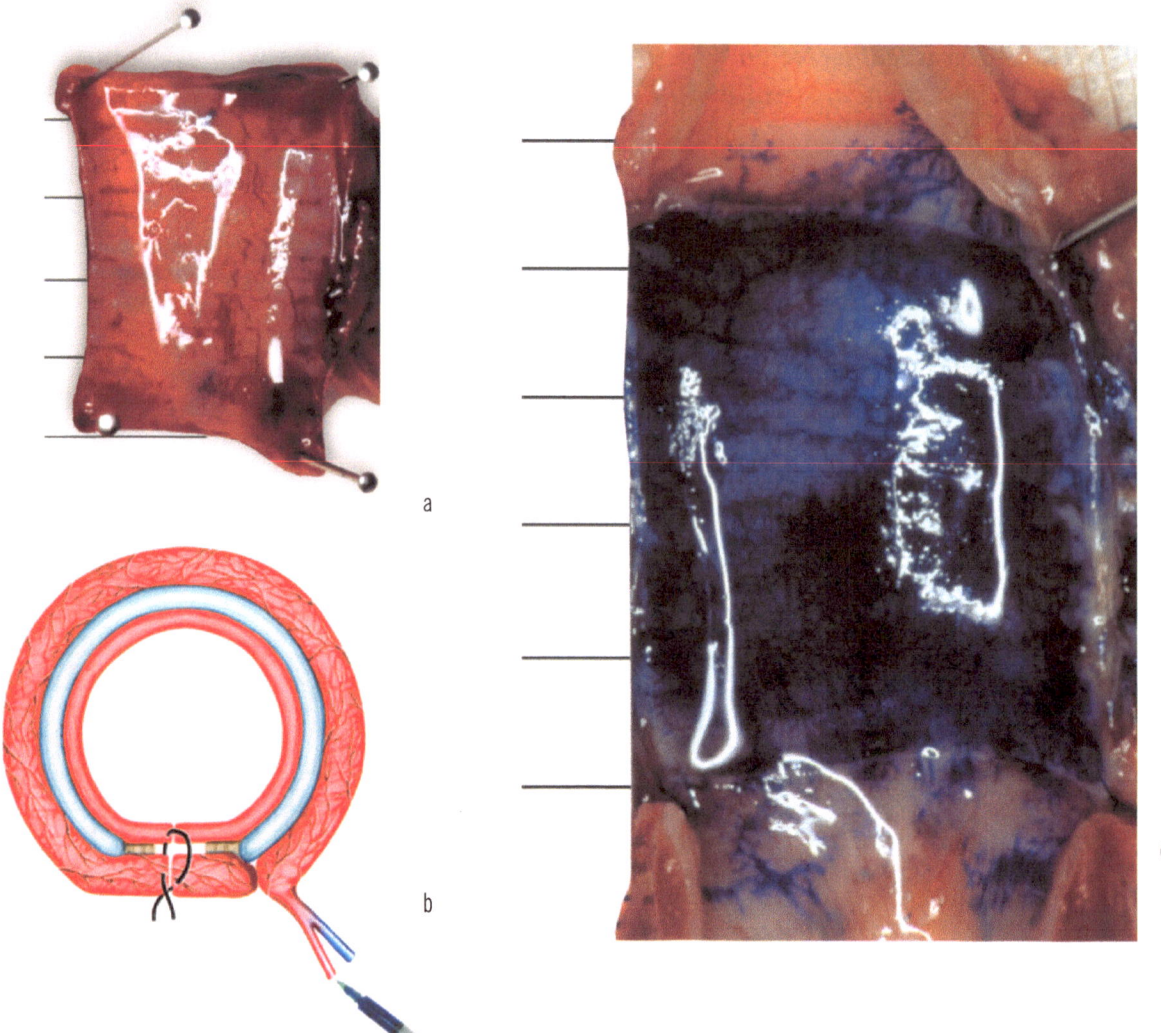

Figure 6. 11. Experimental model stage 2 – Re-introduction of isolated segment.

a. Revascularized trachea with exposition of mucosal lining. The tracheal patch is pinned onto cardboard with exteriorization of the respiratory mucosa. Note the normal appearance of the mucosal blood vessels.

b. Closure of isolated tracheal segment. The tracheal tube is closed by suturing of the membranous trachea and the incised fascia flap. The tube is reintroduced into its original position in the airway defect. After follow-up, the lateral thoracic artery is injected with blue silicone dye.

c. Macroscopy of reimplanted trachea after 1 month. The vascular pedicle of the fascia flap is injected with blue silicone 1 month after reimplantation of the exteriorized patch. The laryngotracheal complex is removed and incised posteriorly with visualization of the initial isolated patch (completely colored by blue silicone (Microfil®)). After follow-up, the surface area of the isolated segment can be identified because of the blue coloration of the mucosal lining.

The trachea can be isolated and reimplanted without influence on the surface area and without influence on the blood supply of the isolated segment.

This model lends itself for studying of the healing pattern of full thickness mucosal defects because standardized defects can be made on the exteriorized mucosa. This model allows for an exteriorization of the respiratory mucosa without influencing of the blood supply and without influencing the cartilaginous support of the trachea.

2B. Healing of full thickness patch defects

The healing of an anterior full-thickness mucosal defect was studied as visible in Fig. 6.12 and 6.13.

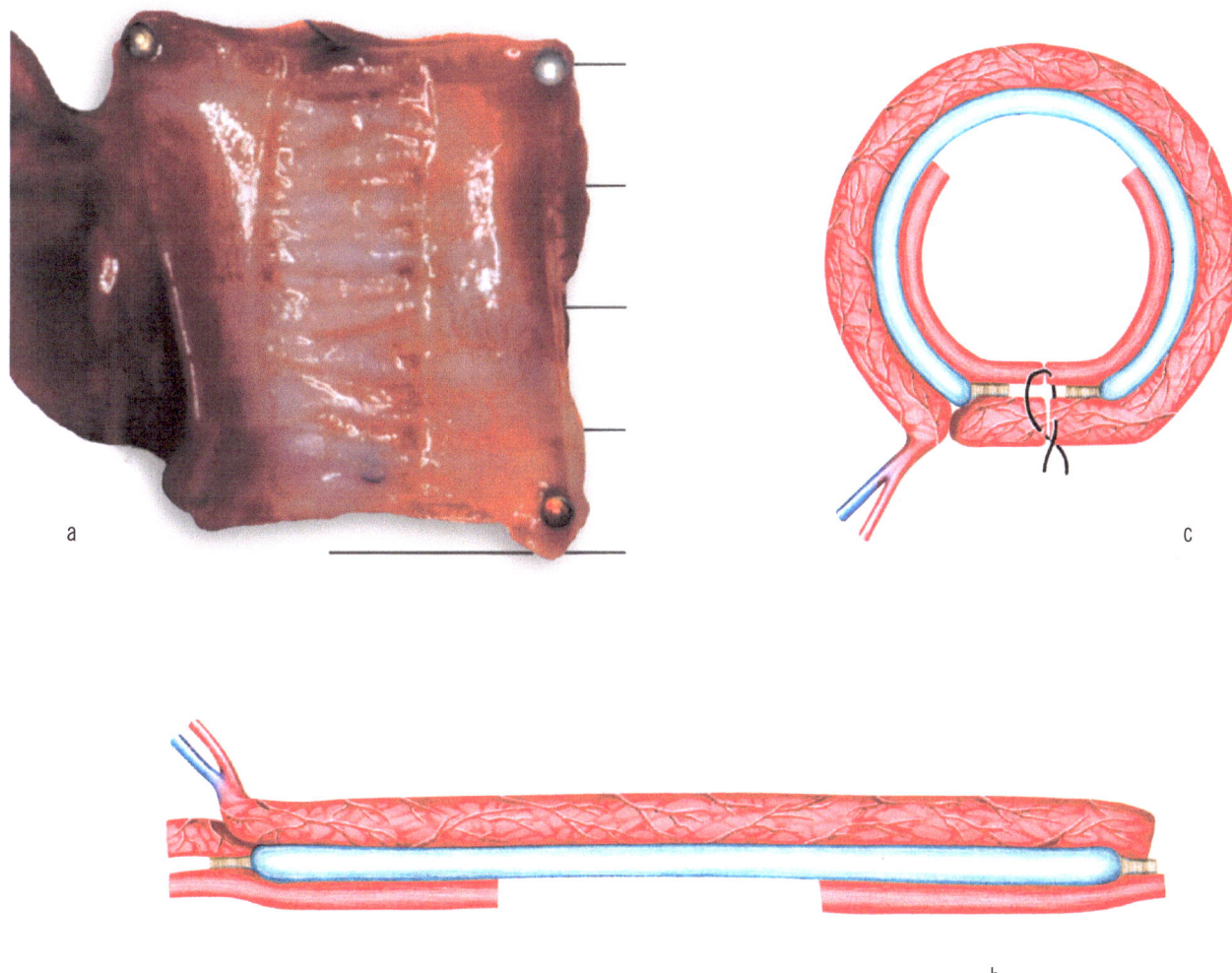

Figure 6.12. Anterior mucosal defect.
a. Macroscopy isolated patch with anterior defect. An anterior defect is made using a scalpel for mucosal incision and a microscissors for mucosal dissection. The anterior full-thickness defect, sharply demarcated from the intact mucosa, is visible.

b. Anterior defect-axial section.
c. Transformation of patch into tube. The patch is closed posteriorly and the tube is reintroduced into the airway tract.

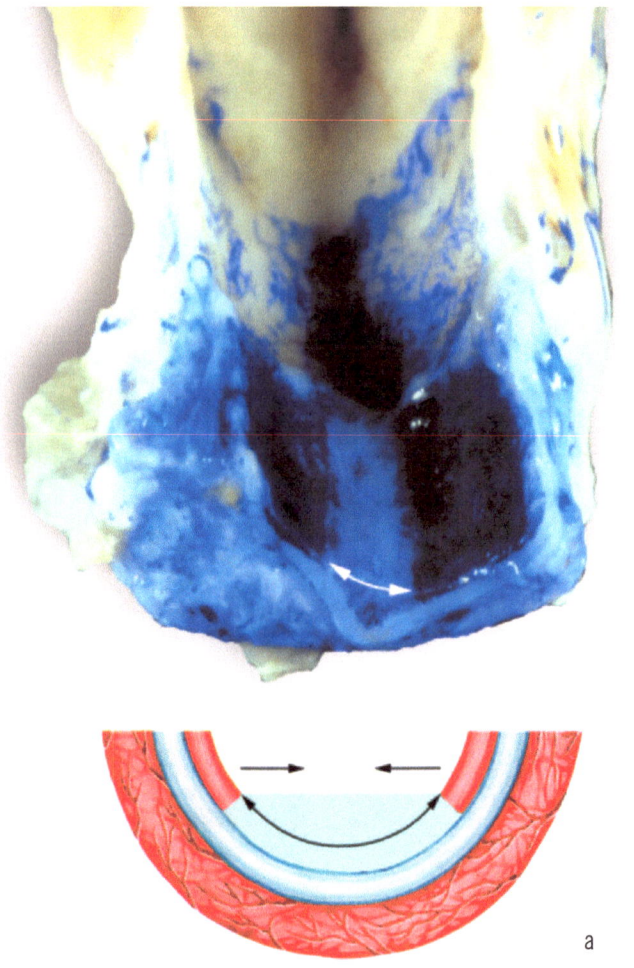

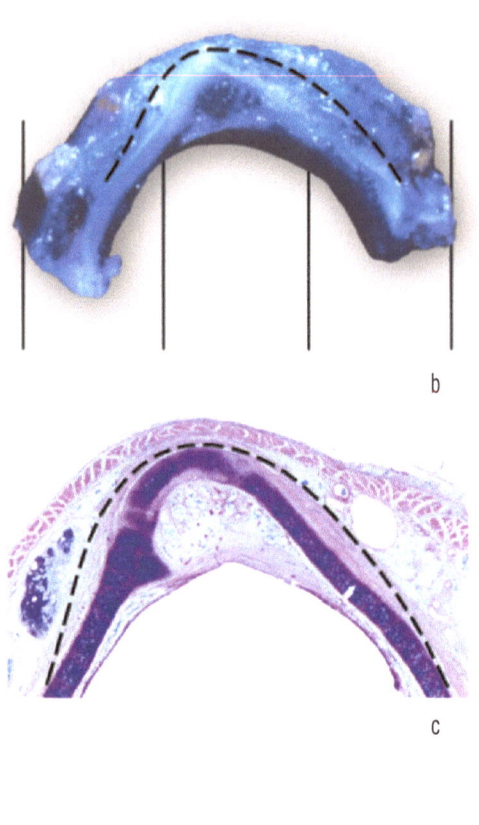

Figure 6.13. Anterior mucosal defect after 4 weeks healing.
a. Macroscopy of reimplanted trachea after 1 month. The vascular pedicle of the flap is injected with blue Microfil®. The upper half of the tracheal transplant (opened posteriorly) and the lower end of the larynx are visible. The intact mucosal lining (intensely colored with blue Microfil®) and the anterior scar are visible. The submucosal tissue is thickest in the center of the scar. The surface area of the defect (double white arrow) is reduced to 50% of the initial defect surface area (double black arrow). Granulation tissue formation and wound contraction forces (arrows) are responsible for the surface area reduction.
b. Axial section after healing. The initial shape of the cartilage ring is indicated by the dotted line.
c. Histology after healing. The surface area of the wound is reduced because of thickening of the lamina propria and because of wound contraction. The original shape of the cartilage ring is indicated by the dotted line (H.E. x 10).

The anterior mucosal defect showed a 50 % wound contraction. Macroscopical and histological examination showed that this major amount of surface area reduction could be attributed to a formation of granulation tissue and to wound contraction forces acting in the axial axis of the wound. The thickest layer of granulation tissue was seen in the middle of the scar.

2.C. Healing of full thickness circumferential defects

The same surgical steps as for the anterior patch mucosal defect may be made to evaluate healing of a circumferential mucosal defect. The mucosal lining of the isolated patch is completely removed during the second operation stage. After wounding, the tracheal patch is transformed into a completely denudated tube (Figure 6.14).

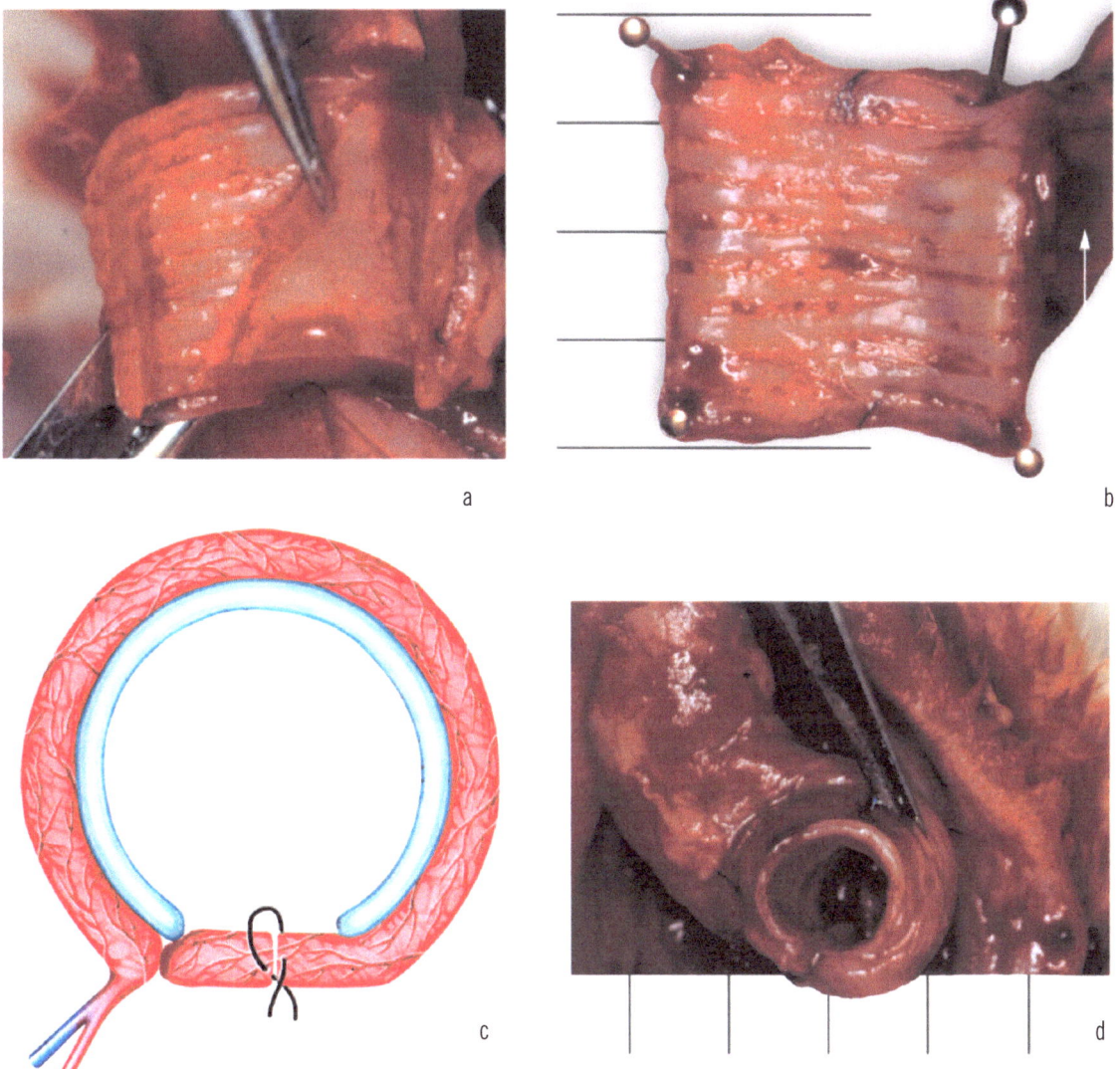

a

b

c

d

Figure 6.14. Full, circumferential tracheal defect.
a. Mucosal stripping. Isolated tracheal patch. The mucosal lining is completely removed after revascularization and after isolation of the tracheal segment.
b. Completely denuded patch. The patch consists of cartilage rings and intercartilaginous ligaments perfused by the fascial flap (arrow).

c. Schematic presentation denuded tube. The patch is transformed into a tube by posterior closure. This denuded tube will be re-implanted into the airway tract.
d. Macroscopy denuded tube after closure and before re-implantation in the airway.

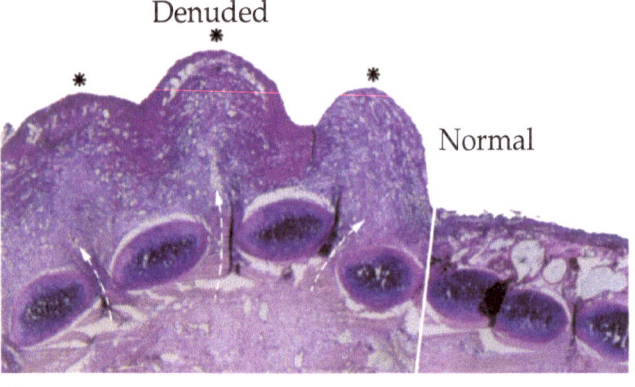

a

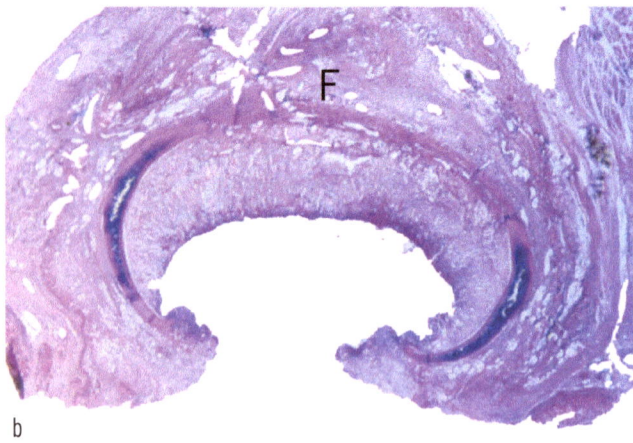

b

Figure 6.15.
Full, circumferential tracheal defect after 2 weeks healing.
a. Longitudinal histology. The place of the anastomosis between intact trachea and denuded trachea is visible (white line). The intact trachea shows a normal mucosal architecture with a lamina propria showing silicone injected blood vessels. The cartilage rings of the denuded trachea are intact and lined with a thick layer of granulation tissue. This granulation tissue is formed by angiogenic induction from the surrounding fascia flap. Vascularized tissue is growing through the intercartilaginous ligaments towards the airway lumen (arrows). The granulation tissue is not lined with epithelial cells and is thicker at the sites of the intercartilaginous ligaments (asterisks) (H&E, x 4).
b. Axial histology. Thick layer of granulation tissue has grown through the intercartilaginous ligaments (H&E, x 4). F=fascia flap.

Animals with a circumferential tracheal defect will show respiratory distress after an average period of 14 days due to excessive granulation tissue formation with obstruction of the airway lumen. Healing of circumferential mucosal defects is characterized by the formation of a thick layer of granulation tissue leading to respiratory distress (Fig. 6.15).

The loss of airway lumen during secondary healing of full-thickness mucosal defects is extensive. Granulation tissue formation is the main reason for the loss of airway lumen in tracheal wounds with preserved vascularization and cartilaginous support. A process of angiogenesis acting through the intercartilaginous ligaments forms the granulation tissue. The proliferation of vascularized connective tissue is blocked when the regenerated lamina propria becomes covered with respiratory epithelial cells.

Regeneration and migration of respiratory epithelium is relatively slow in full-thickness mucosal airway defect. In full-thickness mucosal wounds, the center of the scar will have the thickest lamina propria because this area is lastly covered with respiratory epithelium. Loss of airway lumen is the result of granulation tissue formation and of wound contraction forces acting in the direction of the upper surface of the granulating wound. Wound contraction is a basic biological process and occurs in an incompletely epithelialized defect. It has been defined as the mechanism by which the edges of a wound are drawn toward the center due to forces generated within that wound. Contraction is a vital aspect of open wound healing. The size of the tissue defect is reduced so that a lesser degree of connective tissue deposition and epithelialization is required. Myofibroblasts are the cells thought to be responsible for this phenomenon. The wound contraction forces acting during healing of the anterior mucosal wound resulted in a reduction of the curvature of the cartilage rings with further loss of airway lumen.

In the circumferential mucosal defect, reepithelialization is only possible by new growth of epithelium from the upper and lower anastomosis. Animals with a circumferential defect survived only a short period of 14 days because of excessive granulation tissue formation without signs of reepithelialization.

The problematic migration of respiratory cells from the wound margins seen in the anterior and in the circumferential mucosal defect is in contrast to optimistic reports in the literature concerning the possibility of respiratory epithelial cell migration (CHENG et al. 1997). Optimistic reports on migration of respiratory epithelium are usually based on the fast recovery of epithelium in small defects, on the fast recovery of epithelium in superficial mucosal wound healing with preservation of the basement membrane and on in vitro studies (ZAHN et al. 1992).

2.D. Healing of mucosal defects after mitomycin application

Formation of excessive amounts of granulation tissue is the major problem during healing of revascularized denuded segments of trachea. Granulation tissue formation results in obstruction of the airway lumen and leads to wound contraction, which may further diminish the airway lumen.

Mitomycin is known to prevent scarring and fibrosis after tracheal wounding (CORREA et al. 1999,

ELIACHAR et al. 1999). Mitomycin application may be used in an attempt to reduce the granulation tissue formation. The effect of Mitomycin application was studied on full-thickness patch mucosal defects (Fig. 6.16, 6.17) and on full-thickness circumferential mucosal defects (Fig. 6.18).

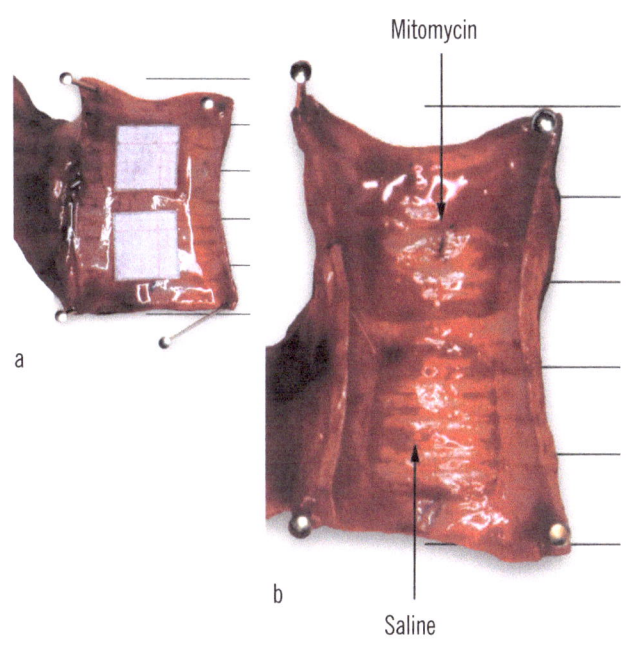

Figure 6.16.
Patch of denuded trachea treated with topical Mitomycin application.
a. Macrocopy of revascularized tracheal patch with outlining of mucosal defects.
b. Macroscopy of revascularized tracheal patch with defects. Two full-thickness mucosal defects (0.6 cm x 0.6 cm) are formed after revascularization and after isolation of the tracheal segment. The upper mucosal defect is treated with a single topical application of 0.5 ml (0.2 mg/ml) of Mitomycin whereas the lower mucosal defect is treated with saline. Drug delivery is via a soaked cotton pledget directly applied to the operative site for a duration of 5 minutes. The damaged tracheal patch is closed and placed inside the tracheal defect.

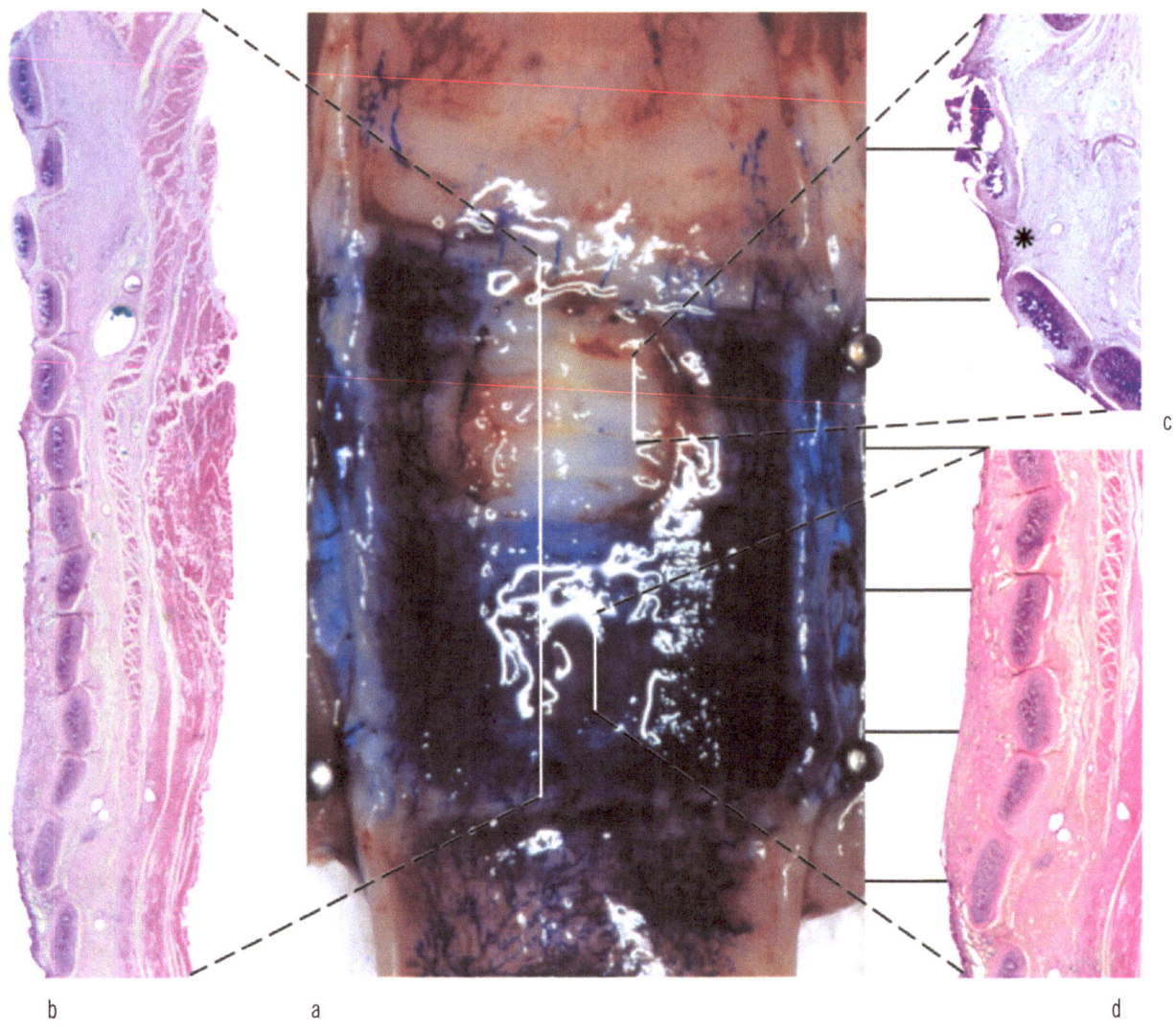

b   a   c   d

Figure 6.17.
Patch of denuded trachea treated with topical Mitomycin application after a 4 weeks healing period.
a. Macroscopy. The fascia flap was injected with blue Microfil®. The upper, Mitomycin-treated, defect is denuded over the majority of the initial defect area whereas the lower defect is completely healed.
b. Histology on longitudinal section overview. The defect treated with saline underwent secondary healing. The Mitomycin-treated defect has preserved its initial surface area and the cartilage rings are directly exposed to the airway lumen. Granulation tissue formation is completely blocked at the intercartilaginous ligaments (H&E, original magnification x 4).

c. Histology on longitudinal section-Detail of Mitomycin treated patch. The bare cartilage rings underwent partial necrosis and destruction (external side). The intercartilaginous space between two cartilage rings (asterisk) is lined with respiratory epithelium (H&E, original magnification x 10).
d. Histology on longitudinal section-Detail of patch treated with saline. The lamina propria contains smaller blood vessels and is slightly thicker than the lamina propria of the native trachea.

As shown in figure 6.17, untreated wounds are smaller than the wounds treated with Mitomycin. A single application of Mitomycin produces wounds that on average are 250% larger than controls, representing a 56% decrease in closure relative to that seen in control healing. Histological examination of the control patches shows a reepithelialized wound with a lamina propria that is slightly thicker than the lamina propria of the normal trachea. Histological examination of the Mitomycin-treated patches shows a blockage of angiogenesis at the sites of the intercartilaginous ligaments. The bare cartilage rings, that remain exposed to the airway lumen, will undergo necrosis with loss of support. Histological examination after 1 month reveals cartilage necrosis with respiratory epithelium between the necrotic cartilage rings. In contrast to the process of angiogenesis, migration of respiratory epithelial cells is not inhibited by the Mitomycin application.

Circumferentially denuded tracheal segments were treated with 1 ml of Mitomycin (0.2 mg/ml) as visible in fig. 6.18. After closure and replacement of the Mitomycin treated tube inside the airway tract, animals survived for a period of only 14 days.

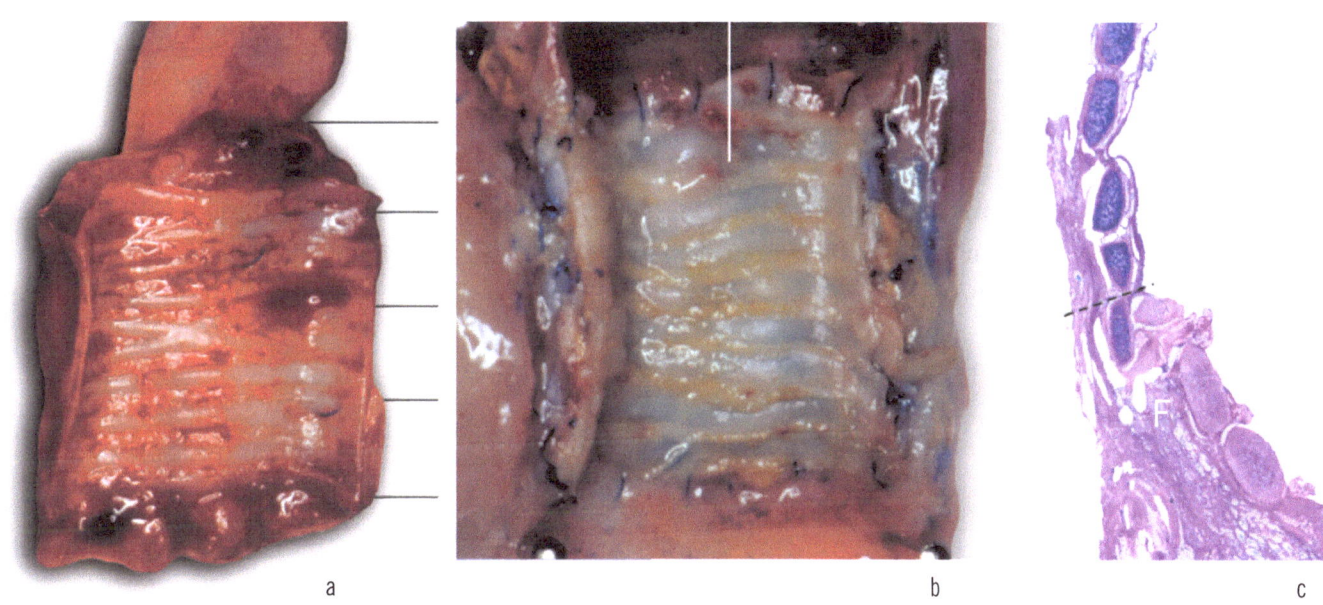

a   b   c

Figure 6.18. Circumferential defect with topical mitomycin application.
a. Macroscopy fully denuded segment. This segment is treated with 1 ml (0.2 mg/ml) of Mitomycin-local application during 5 minutes.
b. Macroscopy patch after 2 weeks follow-up. Macroscopy of denuded trachea 2 weeks after re-implantation. The fascia flap was injected with blue Microfil®. The fascial flap around the trachea is injected with blue silicone. The denuded segment shows bare cartilage rings (with loss of support) and intercartilaginous ligaments without signs of granulation tissue formation.

c. Histology on longitudinal section. The place of anastomosis between intact trachea and denuded trachea is indicated. The intact trachea shows a normal mucosal architecture with a lamina propria showing silicone-injected blood vessels. The cartilage rings of the denuded trachea are bare and are more eosinophilic (less vital) than the cartilage rings of the intact tracheal segment. The intensely vascularized fascia around the denuded segment is indicated with F (H&E, original magnification x 10).

After 14 days, animals with a denuded tube treated by Mitomycin showed respiratory distress because the bare cartilage underwent necrosis with loss of support. No granulation tissue will be formed at the luminal site of the Mitomycin treated cartilage segments. Topical application of Mitomycin blocks the angiogenic process and inhibits granulation tissue formation at the internal site of a mucosal defect. Mitomycin is known to act as an agent for scar inhibition and has gained wide acceptance in ophtalmology (SINGH et al. 1988, CHEN 1990) and otolaryngology (WARD et al. 1998) for procedures in which scarring is problematic. In this experimental model it was shown that the drug acts by blocking angiogenesis but without inhibition of the migration of respiratory epithelium. Mitomycin may have a negative influence on airway healing because the bare cartilage rings develop necrosis with loss of support. It seems that Mitomycin can safely and effectively be applied on scar tissue in the treatment of airway stenosis. In the clinical situation it is applicated in a concentration of 1 mg/ml during 3 minutes. However, warning is necessary when dealing with bare cartilage because of the risk for cartilage necrosis when granulation tissue formation is blocked.

3. Current limitations in laryngotacheal stenosis treatment

The limiting factor in laryngotracheal stenosis treatment concerns cases that are impossible to repair by segmental resection (tracheal resection, cricotracheal resection) or slide tracheoplasty. Such problems may be encountered when dealing with a re-stenosis after previous resection of tracheal segments and when dealing with acquired long segment (> 5 cm) tracheal stenosis. Cases with anastomotic failure (stenosis or dehiscence) are reported in most series of tracheal resection (WRIGHT et al. 2002). Some of them may be treated by a conservative approach (Mitomycin, stenting,...). If conservative treatment fails, tracheal

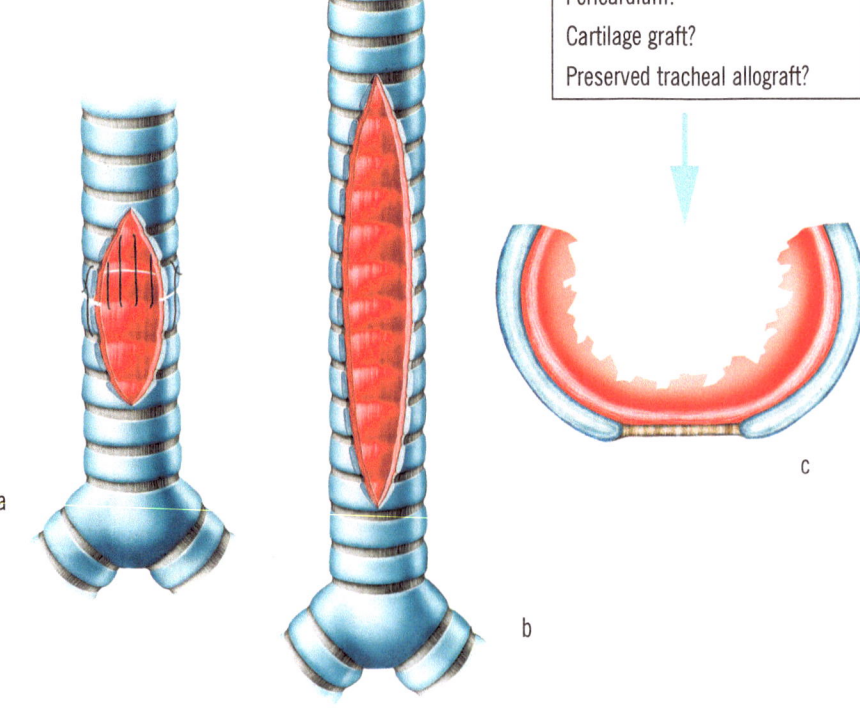

Figure 6.19.
Limiting factor in laryngotracheal stenosis treatment.
Situation after incision of recurrent (a) and long segment (b) stenosis.
c= axial section after longitudinal incision of restenosis and long segment stenosis.
The mucosal lining of the incised segment is scarred in cases of restenosis.

restenosis and long-segment stenosis may be treated by longitudinal incision of the stenotic segment and insertion of reconstructive tissue in the anterior airway defect (Fig. 6.19).

Tissues that are currently used for repair of anterior airway defects ('augmentation tracheosplasty') are pericardium (IDRISS et al. 1984, CHENG et al. 1997), cartilage (COTTON 1991, JAQUISS et al. 1995), and preserved tracheal allografts (HEBERHOLD et al. 1999).

Results obtained with these tissues are not constant and the healing mechanisms of the repair tissues are poorly understood. A devascularized mesenchymal patch of pericardium or cartilage without epithelial covering needs prolonged postoperative airway splinting, and is known for its proclivity to form troublesome granulations and the possibility of necrosis or collapse. Tracheal allograft reconstruction using cadaveric human tracheal allografts has been presented as a therapeutic option for patients with long segment tracheal stenosis and recurrent stenosis. Tracheal allograft reconstruction was introduced by Claus Heberhold (HEBERHOLD et al. 1999). The cartilaginous portion of the tracheal allograft is used as a patch reconstruction over a stented anterior airway defect. The healing mechanisms of preserved allografts are unclear.

4. Definition of optimal reconstruction of anterior airway defects

Research on composite tissue reconstruction was started in an attempt to find a reconstructive tissue matching the 'optimal tissue' as close as possible (Fig. 6.20). The optimal tissue combination is found in vascularized tracheal auto- and allografts but these transplants are not available when dealing with tracheal re-stenoses or long-segment stenoses.

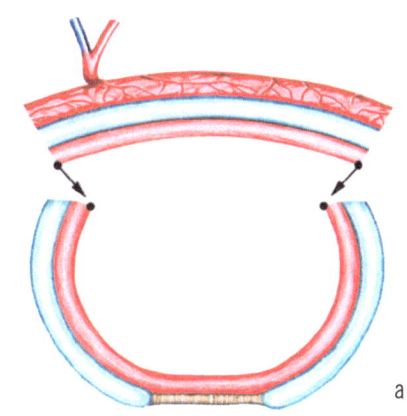

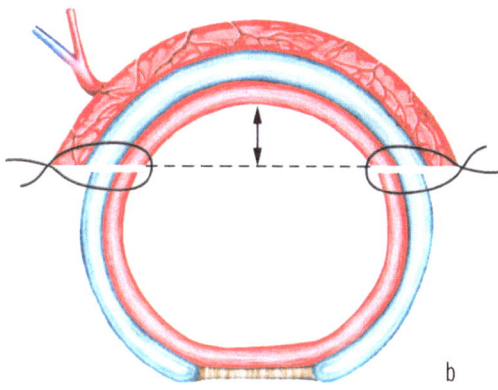

Figure 6.20.
Optimal reconstruction of anterior airway defect.
a. The optimal tissue consists of a respiratory mucosal lining and an elastic type of cartilage support. A vascular supply for the 2 tissue components is essential to keep the reconstruction viable.
b. The elastic nature of the cartilage component allows for insertion of the reconstructive tissue within the anterior airway defect with augmentation of the airway lumen (double arrow).

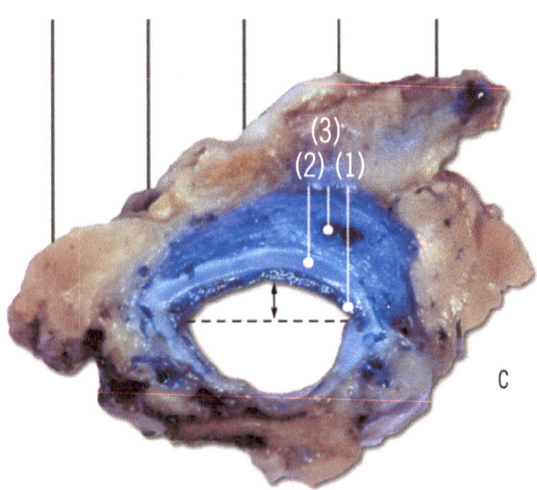

Figure 6.20. (continued).
Optimal reconstruction of anterior airway defect.
c. Experimentally, the optimal reconstruction is possible when using revascularized segments of tracheal allografts. The blue silicone injected reconstruction (consisting of respiratory mucosa (1), tracheal cartilage (2), and fascia (3)) repairs the anterior defect in an immunosuppressed animal.

The healing mechanisms of the different repair tissues for augmentation tracheoplasty were studied within our animal model. The objective was to look for autologous tissues that approached the results obtained with experimental, revascularized tracheal allotransplants in repairing anterior airway defects. Autologous tissues used for augmentation tracheoplasty in the experimental model are visible in Table 6.1.

Autologous tissues that provide for blood supply, mucosal lining, and cartilage support were evaluated individually and in several composite tissue associations.

The lateral thoracic fascia is a reconstructive tissue without lining and without support. It can be used as a soft tissue reconstruction for anterior airway defects (clinical examples of soft tissue reconstruction: periosteum (KRESPI et al. 1983), pericardium (IDRISS et al. 1984)). The lateral thoracic fascia can also be used as a vascular carrier for cartilage and mucosal grafts.

Ear cartilage can be used to study the healing of autologous cartilage grafts when placed in an anterior airway defect (clinical example of cartilage graft: rib cartilage (JAQUISS et al. 1995)). Tracheal cartilage without its mucosal lining was used as an experimental model to study the healing mechanism of preserved tracheal allografts (HEBERHOLD et al. 1999).

Buccal mucosa grafted to the vascularized fascia was used to study the epithelial lined soft tissue reconstruction without mucosal lining (clinical example of epithelial lined soft tissue reconstruction: myocutaneous flap (ELIACHAR et al. 1984, 1989).

The possibility of creating a composite tissue with the 3 individual tissue components (blood supply, cartilage, and mucosal lining) was evaluated within our experimental model.

Table 6.1. Autologous tissues used for experimental augmentation tracheoplasty

- Blood supply:
    vascularized soft tissue: lateral thoracic fascia.
- Cartilage component:
    -Ear cartilage.
    -Tracheal cartilage.
- Mucosal component: Buccal mucosa.

5. Airway reconstruction with vascularized soft tissue

Secondary healing after tracheal reconstruction will occur when using vascularized tissue without lining and without support. The effect of wound contraction during secondary healing in laryngo-tracheal reconstruction can be evaluated when using vascularized soft tissues (vascularized fascia flap) without epithelial lining. To evaluate secondary healing after airway reconstruction, vascularized fascia was used for the repair of anterior airway defects in rabbits (Fig. 6.21).

Healing of vascularized fascia within the airway is characterized by secondary healing as visible 1 month after reconstruction (Fig. 6.22).

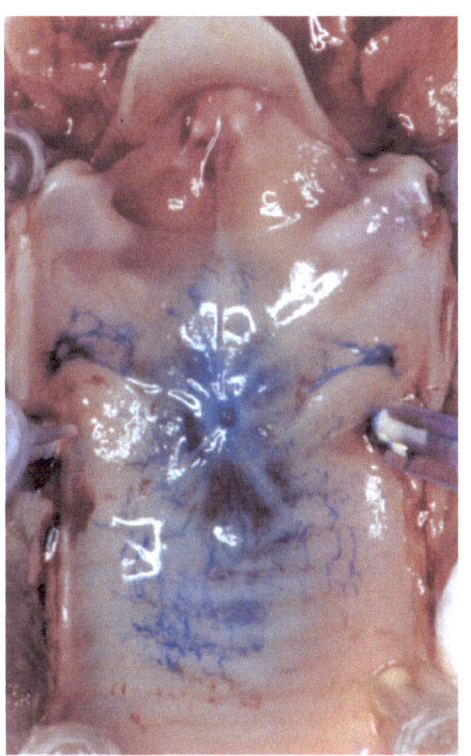

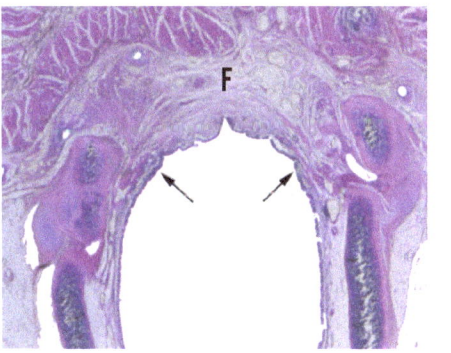

Figure 6.22.
Morphology after reconstruction with vascularized fascia.
a. Macroscopy fascia. Internal view after posterior longitudinal incision. The fascia is injected by blue silicone (Microfil®). Signs of wound contraction, that are most pronounced in the center of the patch, are visible.
b. Histology fascia. The contracted area of fascia is seen between arrows. Regenerated respiratory epithelium covers the contracted area. F= fascia flap (H&E original x 5).

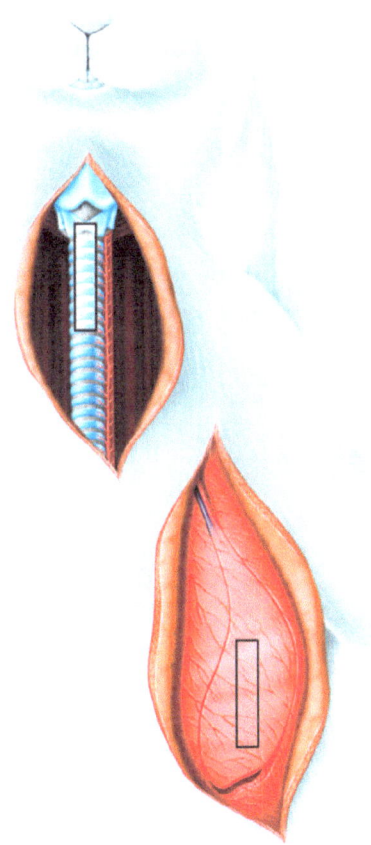

Figure 6.21.
Schematic presentation of anterior airway repair with vascularized fascia-overview.
An anterior defect is repaired with a patch of vascularized fascia of the same dimensions.

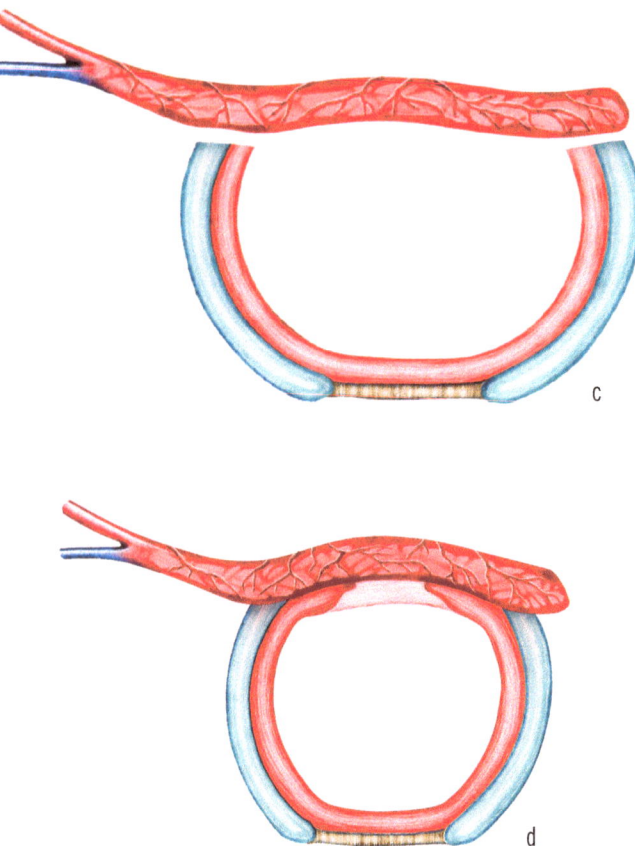

Figure 6.22. (continued)
Morphology after reconstruction with vascularized fascia.
c. Schematic presentation of fascial healing immediately after reconstruction.
d. Schematic presentation of fascial healing-situation after 1 month.
Healing of the fascia is characterized by re-epithelialization from the defect margins and by wound contraction of the reconstructed defect area (50% of initial defect area).

Defects repaired with non-epithelialized soft tissue will show a healing by secondary intention and will show a wound that will contract to about 50 % of the initial surface area of the defect. After healing, the non-epithelialized reconstruction will be lined with respiratory epithelium. Remucosalization starts at the margins of the graft with progressive migration of the epithelium to the center of the graft. The contracted surface area will become completely covered with respiratory epithelium. Soft tissue without epithelial lining will heal by secondary intention when used inside the airway. This tissue undergoes reepithelialization in combination with a wound contraction process and with a significant reduction of the reconstructed surface area. Vascularized periosteum (KRESPI et al. 1983, FRIEDMAN et al. 1987) is a clinical example of a soft tissue without epithelial lining. Because of the wound contraction process, soft tissue without epithelial lining is not a first choice option when augmentation of a stenotic airway is attempted.

Table 6.2. Tracheal repair with vascularized soft tissue without epithelial lining

- Absence of immediate support and lining.
- Re-epithelialization from margins.
- Granulation tissue formation.
- Wound contraction: 50% of defect area.
- Best result that can be obtained for anterior airway defect reconstruction:
  flat reconstruction with reduced (50%) surface area of defect.

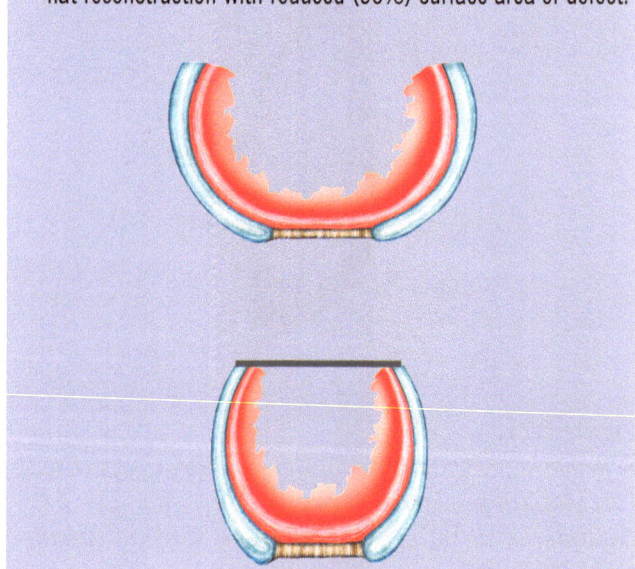

6. Airway reconstruction with cartilage grafts

6.A. Cartilage graft

The ear is a major source of cartilage in rabbits. In humans, cartilage grafts may be taken at the rib and at the outer ear. Cartilage grafts may be used to reconstruct an anterior airway defect (Fig. 6.23, 6.24).

Free cartilage grafts need re-mucosalisation to prevent graft necrosis. The process of re-epithelialisation originates from the margins of the defect.

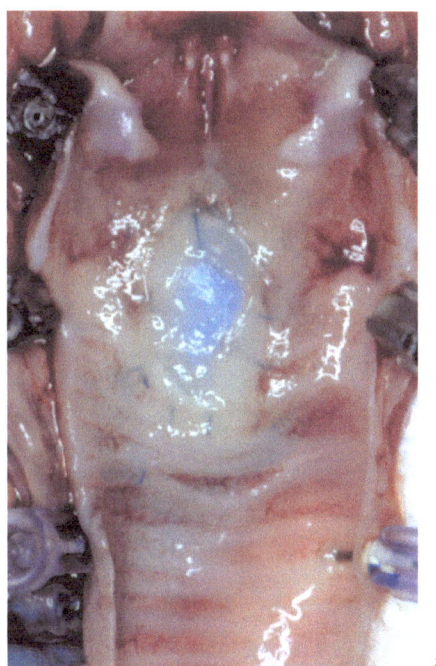

a

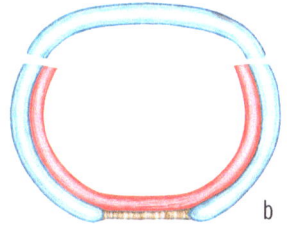 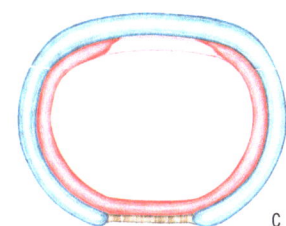

b   c

Figure 6.24.
Morphology after reconstruction with cartilage graft.
a. Free cartilage graft after a 4 week healing period.
Macroscopy of ear cartilage graft within an anterior airway defect. The sutures between graft and native airway are visible. The peripheral part of the graft is covered with respiratory epithelium while the central part of the graft is still bare.
b. Cartilage graft immediately after reconstruction.
c. Cartilage graft after healing.
Cartilage grafts are re-mucosalized from the margins. The peripheral part of the graft is remucosalized before the central part of the graft.

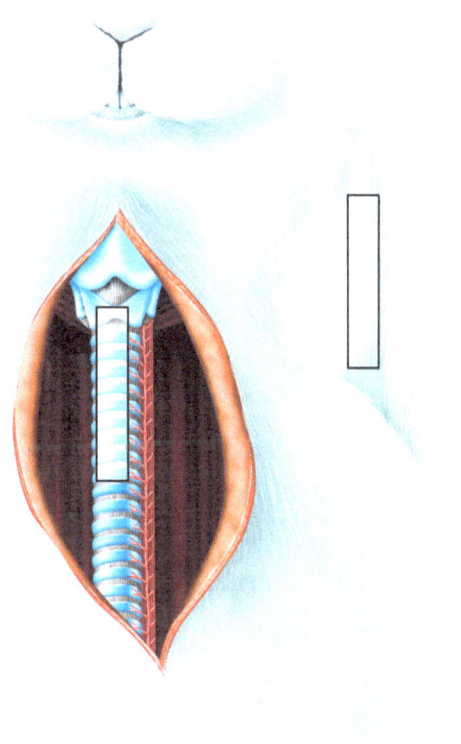

Figure 6.23.
Schematic presentation of anterior airway repair with cartilage graft-overview.
An anterior laryngotracheal defect is repaired with an ear cartilage graft.

Rib cartilage grafts are used in pediatric subglottic stenosis and in adult posterior glottic stenosis. In the pediatric population, an anterior cartilage graft can be used in combination with a posterior graft to resolve a subglottic stenosis (Fig. 6.25). This can be done for grade I-II (< 70%) subglottic stenosis.

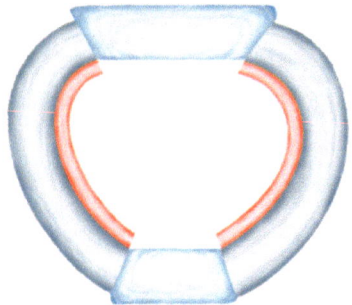

Figure 6.25. Free cartilage graft – Clinical indication. Subglottic stenosis in the pediatric population may be treated with cartilage grafts. An anterior and posterior costal cartilage graft with perichondrium on the luminal side is used. A stent is inserted intraluminaly over the tracheostomy tube to stabilize the posterior graft. In single-stage laryngotracheal reconstruction, a tracheostomy is avoided and an endotracheal tube is used as a stent for 7 days.

The status of the defect margins will be important in cartilage healing because the revascularization and re-epithelialization originates from these margins. Healing of cartilage grafts will be dependent on the size of the graft and the central part of the graft may undergo necrosis if a large patch of cartilage is used. Cartilage grafts are less reliable when dealing with a restenosis. The wound margins after longitudinal incision of a restenosis will show ischemia and ischemic wound margins are not the optimal environment for healing of cartilage grafts.

We developed the concept of 'vascularized cartilage' in an attempt to improve cartilage healing. The best results that may be obtained with cartilage grafts in repairing airway defects were

explored by using vascularized ear cartilage in rabbits. Free grafts of ear cartilage were attached to a vascular carrier and the composite tissue 'cartilage-blood supply' was transferred to an anterior airway defect 14 days after suturing the cartilage to the lateral thoracic fascia (Fig. 6.26).

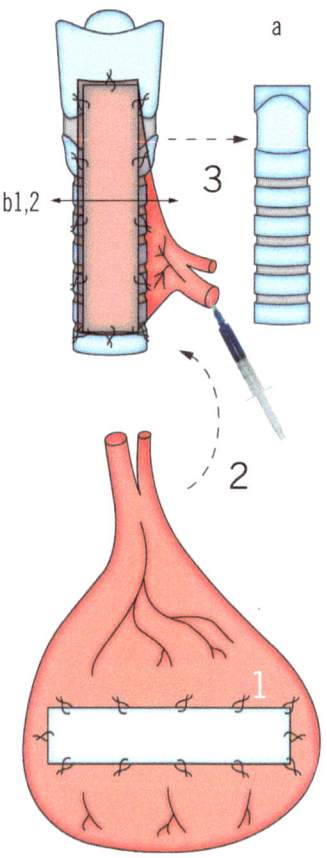

Figure 6.26.
Healing of a vascularized cartilage graft in an anterior airway defect.
a. Schematic presentation of anterior defect reconstruction with vascularized cartilage.
1. A free graft of ear cartilage is sutured to the lateral thoracic fascia flap.
2. The composite tissue is transferred to an anterior laryngotracheal defect 14 days after the grafting of the cartilage to the fascia flap.
3. Anterior wall of cricoid and trachea is resected to create anterior defect.
The reconstruction with vascularized cartilage is evaluated 4 weeks after repair of the anterior defect and after injection of the fascia flap with blue Microfil®.

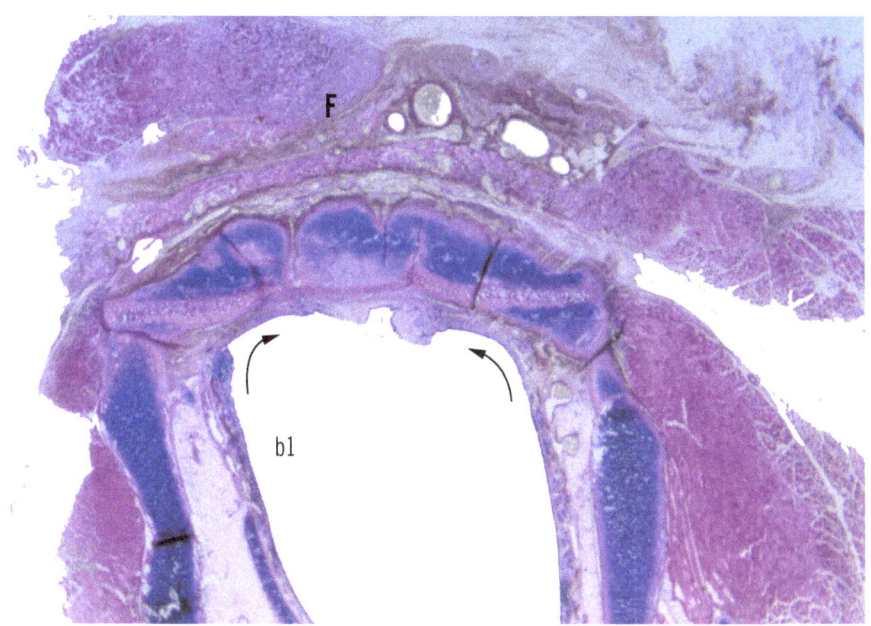

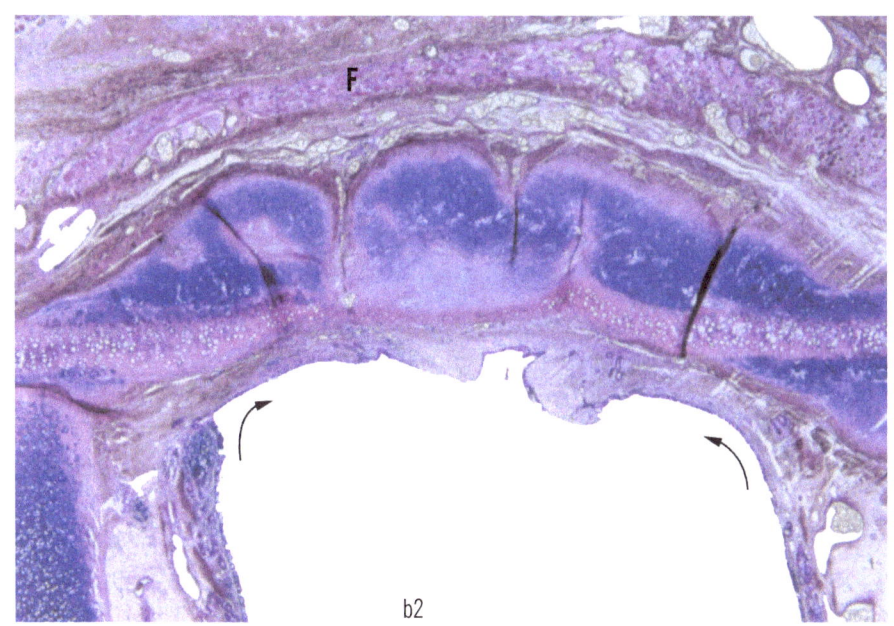

Figure 6.26. (continued)
Healing of a vascularized cartilage graft in an anterior airway defect.
b. Histology of reconstruction 4 weeks after reconstruction. (Hematoxylin-eosin, original magnification x 5 (b.1) x 10(b.2)). Secondary healing from the defect margins (arrows) has happened during the 4 week period. The vascularized fascia (F) is in direct contact with 1 site of the cartilage graft.

Healing of the composite tissue 'cartilage-blood supply' is not different from the healing of free cartilage grafts when used for repair of anterior airway defect in rabbits. Both reconstructions need coverage by a mucosal lining that migrates from the defect margins.

It can be hypothetized that the fascia flap within the composite tissue 'cartilage-blood supply' will protect the central part of the cartilage from undergoing necrosis when large grafts of cartilage are used . The hypothesis was tested in a model of circumferential tracheal repair. A tube of vascularized cartilage was produced in rabbits as visible in fig. 6.27.

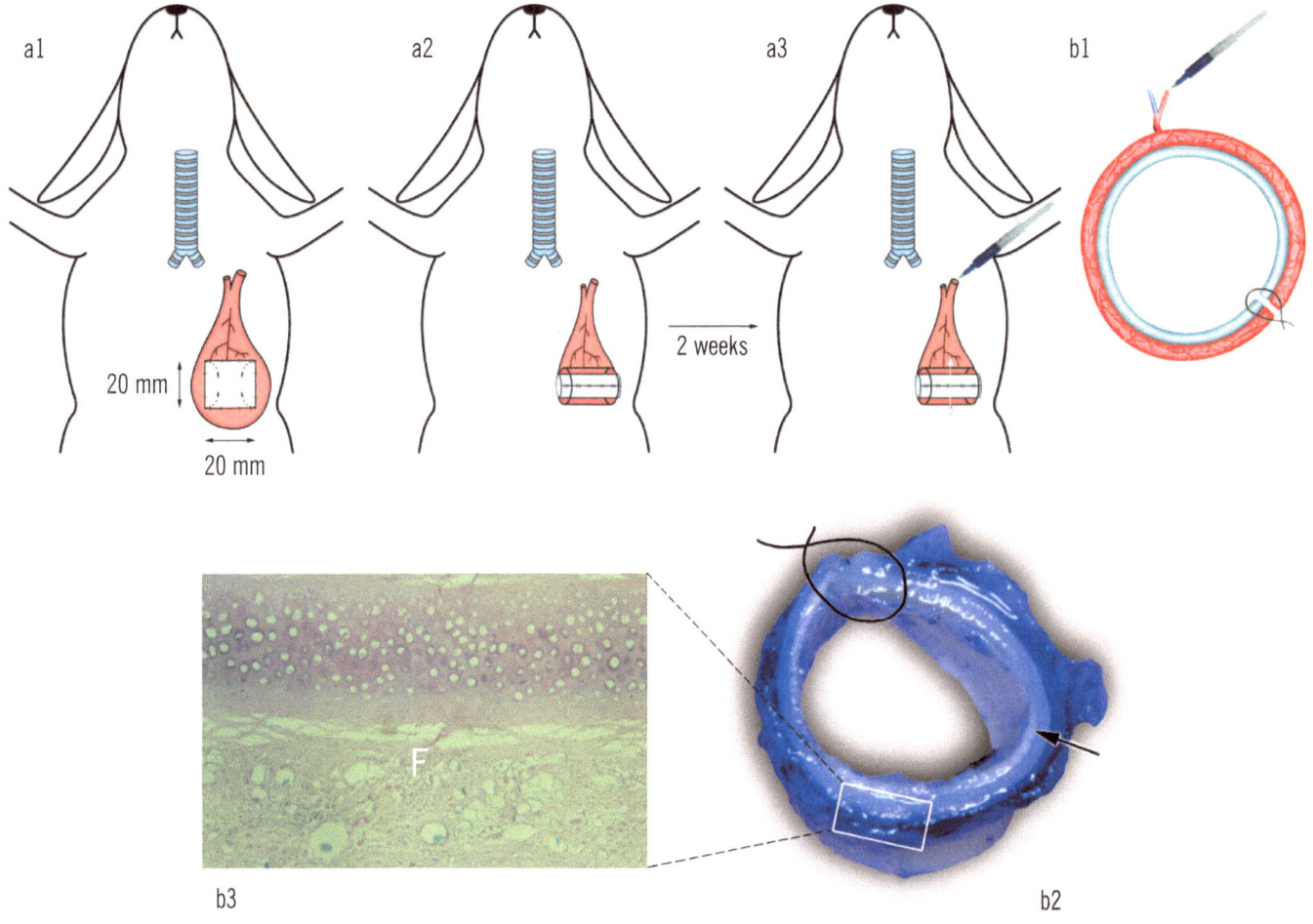

Figure 6.27.
Concept of a vascularized cartilage tube.

A segment of ear cartilage (20 x 20 mm) is transferred to the lateral thoracic fascia. The fascia is sutured to one side of the cartilage patch (a.1). The cartilage patch is made into a fascia-wrapped tube with a length of 20 mm (a.2). The tracheal tube is allowed to make vascular connections with the fascia during a 2 week period. The cartilage tube is sectioned for macroscopic evaluation after 2 weeks (a.3).
b.1. Axial section of cartilage tube. The vascular pedicle is injected with blue silicone dye.
b.2. Macroscopic view of vascularized cartilage tube after 2 weeks. The tube is well supported by healthy cartilage. The internal side of the tube is lined by perichondrium (arrow) and the external side of the tube is intensely connected with the fascia flap. The fascia is blue after injection of the vascular pedicle with blue silicone.
b.3. Histologic specimen of vascularized cartilage before reconstruction (H & E, original x 20). The cartilage shows a normal viability. The vascularized fascia (F) is in direct contact with one side of the cartilage graft. The blood vessels of the fascia flap are injected with blue silicone.

After 14 days, the cartilage tube was intensely connected to the surrounding fascia flap so that it could be used as a vascularized cartilage tube to replace a segment of cervical trachea (Fig. 6.28).

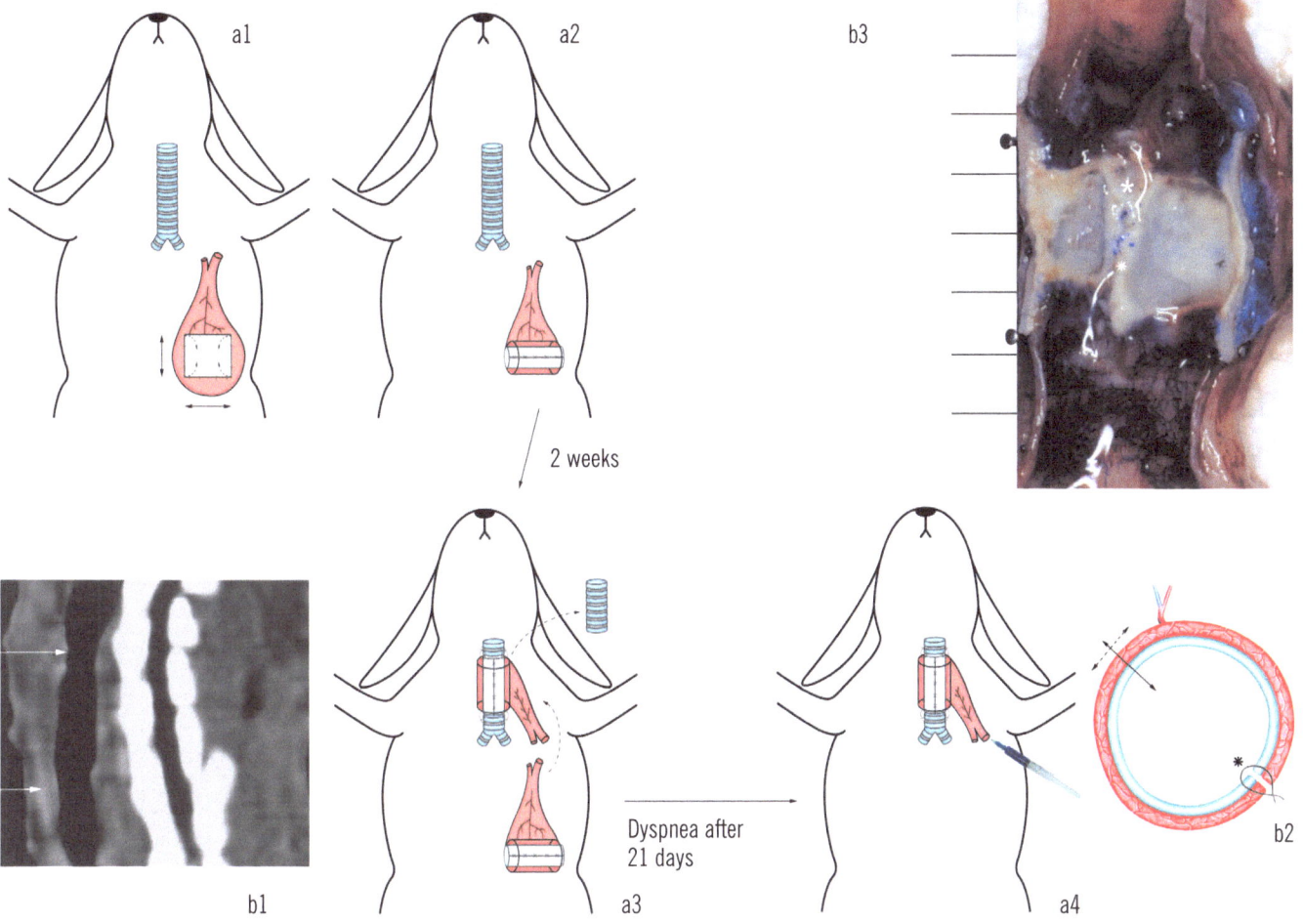

Figure 6.28.

Concept of tracheal replacement with vascularized tube of cartilage.

A segment of ear cartilage is transferred to the lateral thoracic fascia. The cartilage plate is sutured to the fascia with several sutures (a.1). The cartilage plate is made into a fascia-wrapped tube (a.2). The skin of the lateral thoracic area is closed.

The cartilage tube is transferred to the neck region with the surrounding fascial flap after 2 weeks. Two cm segment of cervical trachea is removed and the revascularized segment of cartilage (2 cm length) is sutured into the tracheal defect (a.3). The skin incisions are closed.

b.1. Computed tomographic scan sagittal reformation 1 week after transplantation shows the cartilage tube inside the airway (upper and lower anastomoses indicated by arrows).

Rabbits with a tracheal replacement will show dyspnea after a mean follow-up period of 21 days. The reconstruction is evaluated at the time of respiratory distress. The reconstruction is injected with blue Microfil® (a.4).

b.2. Axial section. The tracheal tube is removed, incised posteriorly (double arrow) and opened (dotted arrows) for macroscopic and histologic evaluation. The anterior suture line is indicated by an asterisk.

b.3. Macroscopy after longitudinal incision of cartilage tube. The mucosal areas that are supplied by the fascia flap are blue colored. The anterior suture line is indicated by an asterisk.

Animals with a segment of cervical trachea that was replaced by a composite graft consisting of a cartilage tube surrounded by vascularized fascia were followed until the first signs of respiratory distress (mean interval of 21 days). At that time, the animals were killed and the trachea removed after injection of the vascular pedicle of the fascia flap with blue silicone (Fig. 6.29).

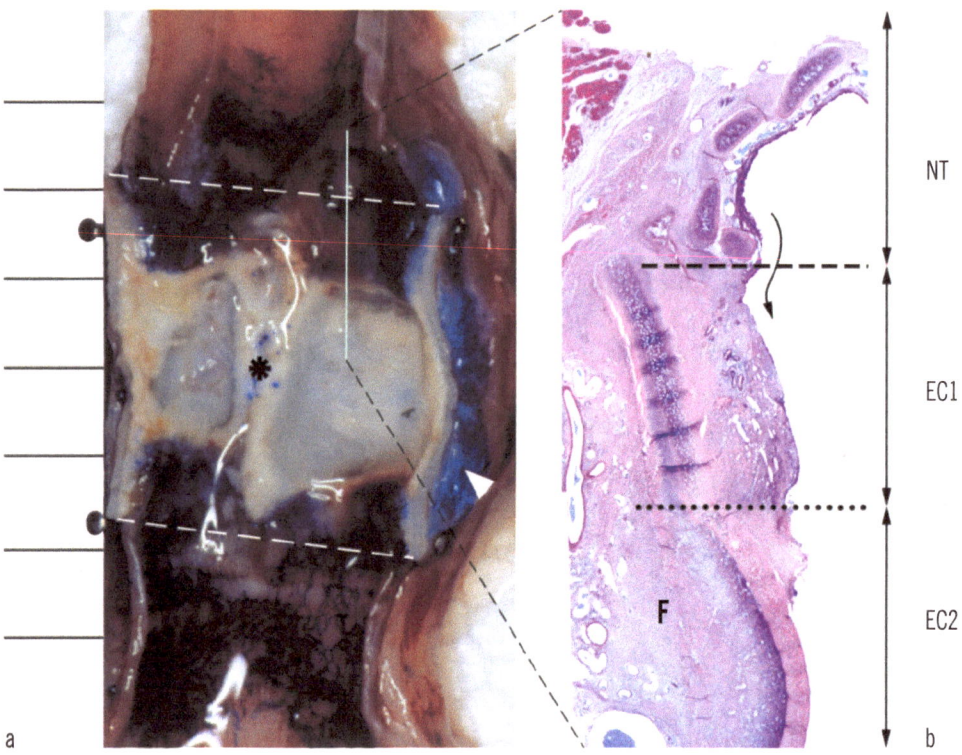

a   b

Figure 6.29.
Results of reconstruction with a tube of vascularized cartilage.
a. Macroscopic view after follow-up of segmental tracheal replacement with fascia-wrapped cartilage.
The artery of the fascia flap was injected with blue silicone before removal of the trachea. The trachea and the cartilage tube were opened posteriorly and pinned onto cardboard. White dotted lines indicate upper and lower anastomosis. The fascia flap around the cartilage tube is indicated with white arrowhead. An area of about 4 mm of the cartilage tube is lined with a blue colored mucosal lining at the upper and lower anastomosis. The middle 1.2 cm of the tube consists of bare cartilage. The regenerated lining of the cartilage tube has grown from the anastomotic sites of the native trachea. The blue coloration of the mucosal lining comes from collateral fascial blood supply at the anastomotic sites because direct growth of fascial blood vessels through the cartilage tube is not possible.

b. Histologic specimen after follow-up of segmental tracheal replacement with fascia-wrapped cartilage.
The lamina propria of the normal trachea (NT) consists of a well-vascularized (blue Microfil-injected blood vessels) connective tissue layer lined with ciliated epithelium. The lamina propria over the ear cartilage (EC1) at the anastomotic site consists of a thick layer of vascularized connective tissue lined with regenerated respiratory epithelium. The regenerated lamina propria consists of dense connective tissue with small blood vessels whereas the mucosal lining of the trachea consists of loose connective tissue with larger capillaries. The anastomotic site of the cartilage tube is re-mucosalized and consists of viable cartilage. The middle part of the cartilage tube (EC2) consists of bare cartilage with signs of necrosis (eosinophilic ground substance) and loss of support. F=Microfil-injected fascia flap (H&E original x 10).

Composite tissue consisting of cartilage and blood supply was used in an attempt to prevent necrosis when using large cartilaginous segments by establishing a connection with vascularized fascia at the outside of the graft. The vascularized fascia was intensely attached to the cartilage graft, but it could not prevent necrosis of bare cartilage with long-standing airway exposition. Cartilage tissue that was more than 4 mm separated from the defect margins underwent necrosis in spite of the connection with vascularized tissue at the outside of the cartilage graft. An explanation of this phenomenon can be found in the unique tissue characteristics of cartilage. For healing of a vascularized cartilage tube, regeneration of the lamina propria and regeneration of a respiratory lining has to come from the mucosal layer at the upper and lower anastomoses. Cartilage that is located in the middle of the tube is separated from the defect margins and shows long-standing airway exposure. The internal side of the bare cartilage in the middle of the tube is attacked by the hostile environment of the airway lumen and will undergo necrosis with loss of airway support. The fascia flap at the outside of the tube is not able to protect the internal side, because cartilage does not allow blood vessel growth through the cartilage graft. The revascularization and reepithelialization from the defect margins turned out to be very slow processes limited to a maximal distance of 4 mm after 3 weeks. The remucosalized areas at both anastomoses were characterized by viable cartilage and by a thick layer of vascularized connective tissue with regenerated epithelium on top. Airway exposure of bare cartilage during a period longer than 3 weeks resulted in necrosis. Only the remucosalized cartilage areas preserved their viability and support.

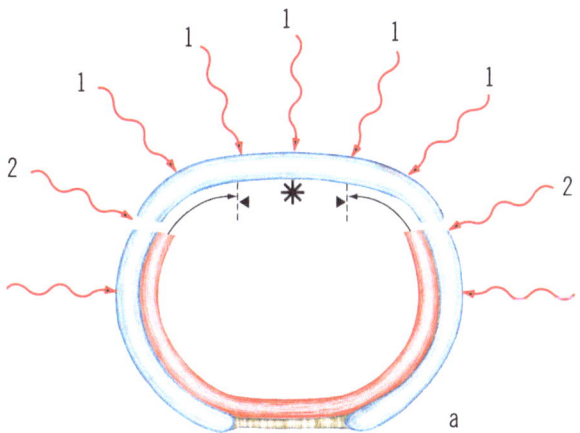
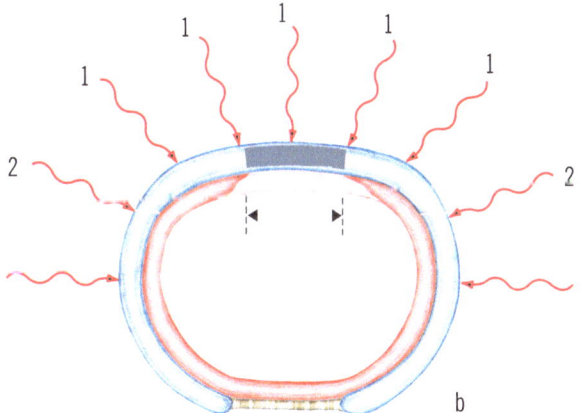

Figure 6.30.
Schematic presentation of cartilage healing.
Healing of cartilage graft inside airway defect a) before and b) after healing process. Graft remucosalization and revascularization occurs from the defect margins (black arrows). The middle part of the graft (between arrowheads) is most susceptible to undergo necrosis. Necrosis will result from airway exposition (asterisk) of the bare cartilage.
The cartilage graft will have the tendency to survive when the cartilage graft is small and the defect margins are well vascularized.

The cartilage graft will have the tendency to die when the cartilage graft is large and the defect margins are scarred.
Vascularized fascia (represented by red arrows) can improve cartilage vascularization at the outside of the graft (1) and may improve vascularization of scarred wound beds (2). Vascularized fascia cannot prevent necrosis of long-standing airway-exposed cartilage, because blood vessels of the fascia do not grow towards the internal side of the cartilage graft.

Transplant revascularization and re-epithelialization occurs over a maximal distance of 3-4 mm

Composite tissue consisting of 'cartilage graft + blood supply' is not superior to the avascular cartilage graft. Cartilage does not allow vessel ingrowth so that the surrounding fascia flap is unable to enhance the vascularity at the internal site of the cartilage. Both the 'vascularized cartilage' and 'the free avascular cartilage' graft are dependent on the margins of the native trachea for revascularization and remucosalization (Fig. 6.30). The findings of healing of cartilage are in agreement with a recent study on adenovirus-mediated ex vivo gene transfer of VEGF121 on angiogenesis and graft survival in a rabbit laryngotracheal reconstruction model with autologous auricular grafts. Angiogenesis was enhanced at the outside of the graft both at 1 and 10 weeks after treatment with VEGF 121 as compared to controls but no statistical improvement in graft survival was evident after treatment with VEGF121. Improved vascularization at the outside of the graft had no influence on survival of the cartilage graft (SAMADI et al. 2002).

6.B. Tracheal cartilage

Tracheal allograft reconstruction using cadaveric human tracheal allografts have been presented as a therapeutic option for patients with long segment tracheal stenosis and recurrent stenosis. Tracheal allograft reconstruction was introduced by Claus Heberhold (HEBERHOLD et al. 1999). The cartilaginous portion of the trachea is stored in acetone. Histologic studies have confirmed that all cells in the graft die and all major histocompatibility complex markers are lost. The cartilaginous portion of the trachea is then used as a patch reconstruction over a stented anterior airway defect. The healing mechanisms of preserved allografts are unclear.

The healing mechanism of cartilage composed of cartilage rings with intercartilaginous ligaments will be different from the healing of cartilage grafts. Cartilage grafts do not allow vessel ingrowth whereas cartilage rings connected with ligaments allow for vessel growth through the intercartilaginous ligaments. This ring-like cartilage design is available in tracheal allografts that may probably form an optimal tissue design for anterior airway repair.

To obtain some insight into tracheal allograft healing, an experimental model was developed with cartilage rings and intercartilaginous ligaments as reconstructive tissue for anterior airway defects. We first used revascularized patches consisting of autologous cartilage rings and intercartilaginous ligaments. This was done as visible in fig. 6.31.

Healing of a revascularized patch of autologous tracheal cartilage is characterized by a secondary intention healing. The anterior expansion of the airway lumen is lost during healing. The best result that can be obtained with tissue having the optimal cartilaginous design (vascularized segment of denuded trachea) is a flat reconstruction with preservation of the surface area of the defect. The luminal concavity provided by the cartilage ring is flattened by granulation tissue formation and the surface area of the defect may be reduced through wound contraction induced from the granulation tissue. This experimental model can be seen as an optimised healing model for the preserved tracheal allograft. They both consist of cartilage rings and intercartilaginous ligaments. Revascularized patches of autologous trachea consist of autologous, revascularized cartilage rings whereas preserved allografts consist of avascular, acetone preserved cartilage rings.

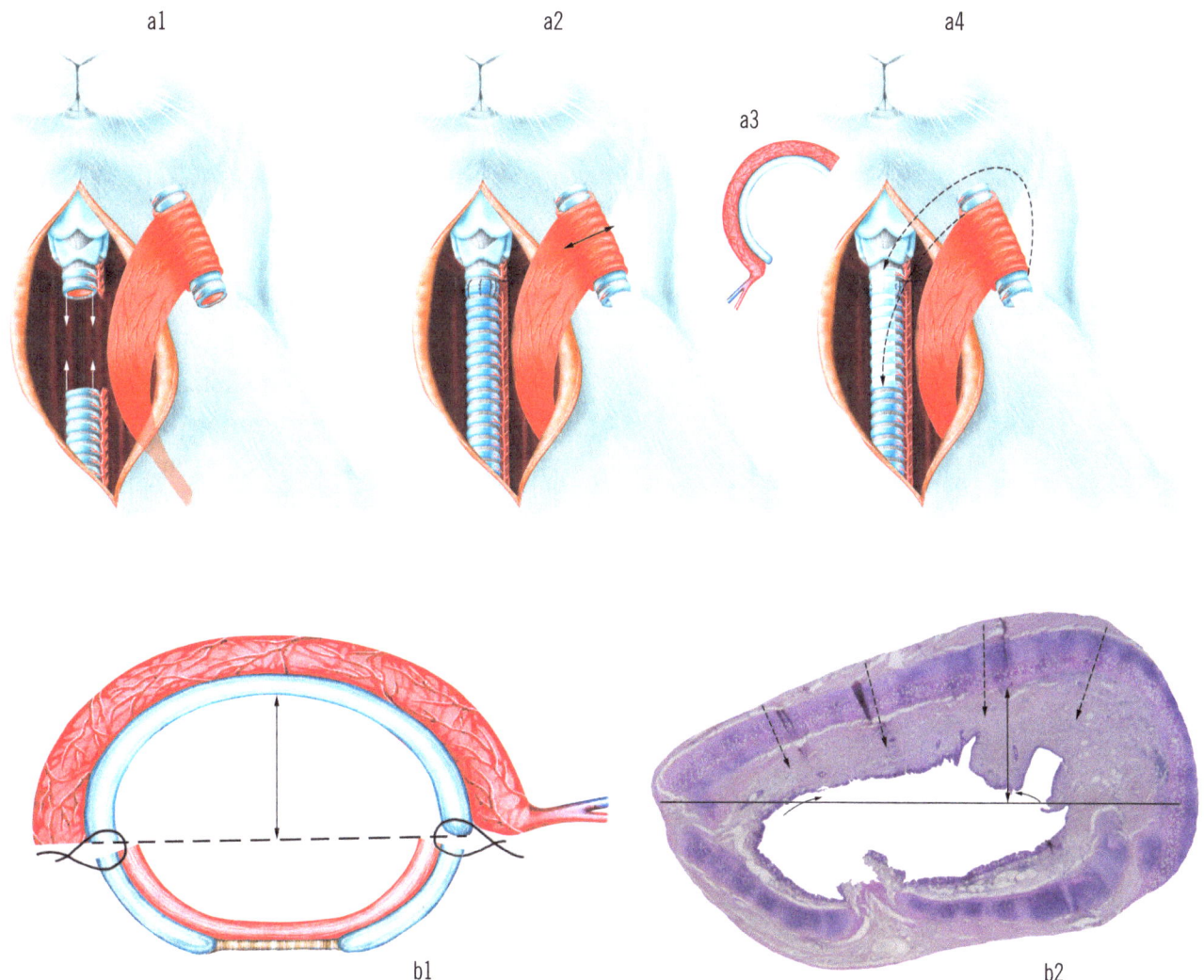

Figure 6.31.

Reconstruction of anterior airway defects with vascularized patches of cartilage consisting of rings and intercartilaginous ligaments.

a.1. A 1.5 cm segment of trachea is removed after 14 days of fascial wrapping.

The tracheal defect is closed by end-to-end anastomosis (arrows).

a.2. Situation after repair of the tracheal continuity. The revascularized tube is transformed into a patch by removal of the membranous trachea and by removal of a part of the cartilaginous ring. The mucosal lining of the patch is excised. An axial section through the tracheal patch (double arrow) shows the denuded segment of trachea (a.3).

a.4. An anterior laryngotracheal defect in created with a length of 1.5 cm. The denuded tracheal patch is used to repair the anterior defect.

b.1. Axial section after reconstruction. A denuded patch of vascularized trachea is used to repair an anterior airway defect with anterior expansion of the airway lumen (double arrow).

b.2. Axial histology 1 month after reconstruction (H.E. x 5). The cartilage shows a normal viability. The denuded patch is completely re-epithelialized. The submucosal layer of the patch is much thicker than the submucosal layer of the intact trachea. The luminal concavity provided by the cartilage ring (double arrow) is nearly completely lost after secondary healing.

Healing of vascularized cartilage occurs through the intercartilaginous ligaments (dotted arrows) and from the wound margins (arrows).

In our experimental setting, preserved tracheal allografts healed in a an unfavourable way when applied in experimental airway defects. Cryopreserved cartilage was used as reconstructive tissue to repair anterior airway defects in the rabbit (Fig. 6.32).

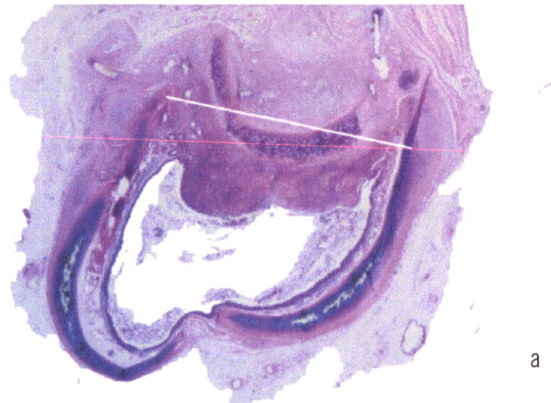

a

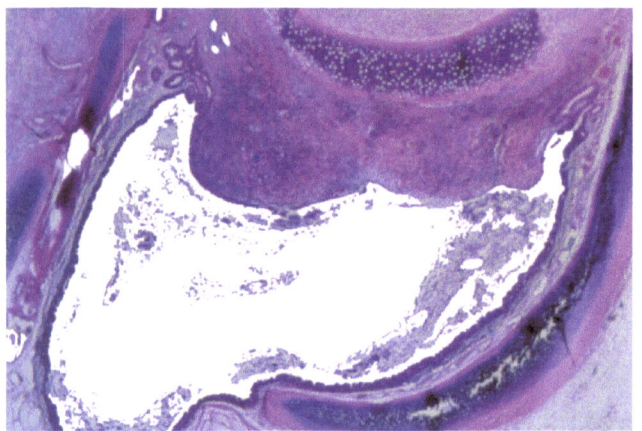

b

Cryopreserved tracheal allografts heal by secondary intention. Cryopreserved (or otherwise preserved) tracheal allografts should not be recommended for airway reconstruction because they heal in an unfavourable and unpredictable way. The use of tracheal allografts is usually promoted in combination with long-term stenting (JACOBS et al. 1999). Possible successes with the technique of transplantation with preserved allografts are difficult to understand and should be attributed to the long-term airway stenting. The working mechanism of long-term airway stenting is however also difficult to explain. The consideration that 'long-term airway stenting usually is advocated for unreliable laryngotracheal repair tissues' may be true for the preserved tracheal allograft.

Figure 6.32.
Cryopreserved tracheal allograft 1 month after repair of an anterior airway defect.
a. Anterior defect reconstructed with cryopreserved patch of tracheal allograft (H&E x 10).
b. Anterior defect reconstructed with cryopreserved patch of tracheal allograft (H&E x 4).
The healing mechanism of cryopreserved cartilage can be summarized as:
- Thick layer of granulation tissue on internal site of preserved allograft.
- Secondary healing over preserved allograft.
- Loss of support of the cryopreserved cartilage.
- Prolaps of reconstruction into airway lumen.

Table 6.3. Tracheal repair with autologous cartilage

- Absence of lining.
- Re-epithelialization from margins.
- Healing different for cartilage grafts and tracheal cartilage:
  - Cartilage graft prone to central necrosis.
  - Tracheal cartilage prone to granulation tissue formation.
- Best result that can be obtained for anterior airway defect reconstruction: flat reconstruction with full preservation of surface area of defect.

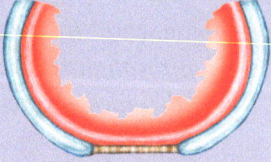
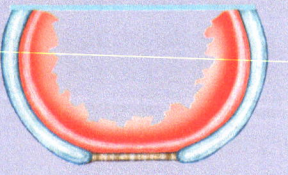

7. Airway reconstruction with a vascularized epithelial lining

7.A. Introduction

Another approach to reconstruction of anterior airway defects is to restore the epithelial lining. Free skin or mucosal grafts does not make sense in the repair of full-thickness airway defects. Skin carried by a muscle flap can be introduced into an airway defect and a clinical example is the 'Rotary door flap' (sternohyoid myocutaneous flap) described by Eliachar (ELIACHAR et al. 1984, 1989). In our experimental model we used buccal mucosa on a fascial vascular carrier for anterior airway repair. Would a vascularized mucosal lining be suitable for use inside anterior airway defects after incision of a restenosis or a long-segment stenosis?

7.B. Vascularized mucosa-experimental use

In rabbits, vascularized mucosa can be formed by using the lateral thoracic fascia flap as vascular bed and oral mucosa as full-thickness mucosa grafts (Fig. 6.33).

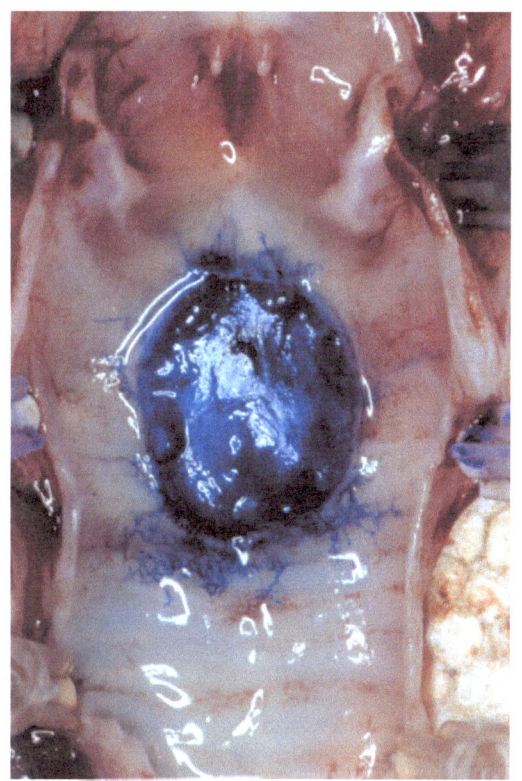

b

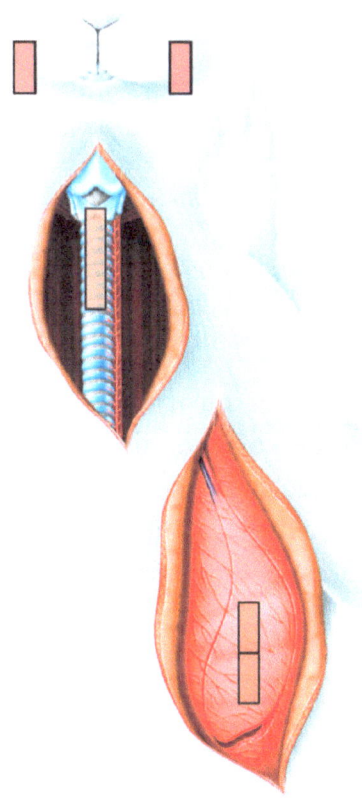

a

Figure 6.33.
Healing of vascularized mucosa-Experimental use.
a. Schematic presentation of mucosa-lined fascia. A fascia flap covered with buccal mucosa is used for laryngotracheal reconstruction in the following way:
-Full-thickness mucosal grafts are taken at the left and right buccal area.
-The mucosal grafts are sutured to the distal end of the fascial flap. The mucosa lined fascia is isolated on its vascular pedicle, rotated to the neck, and sutured into the anterior airway defect.
b. View on vascularized mucosa 1 month after reconstruction of anterior laryngotracheal defect. Fascia flap was injected with blue Microfil®. Oral mucosa is completely colored by Microfil®. The reconstruction shows primary healing with a sharp demarcation line between the oral and respiratory epithelial lining.

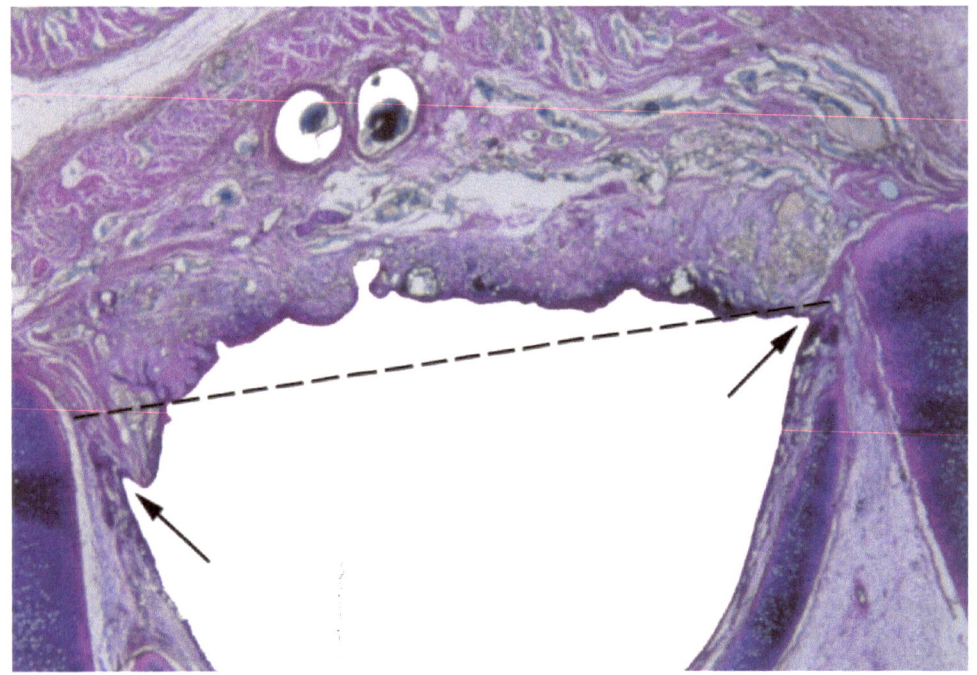

a

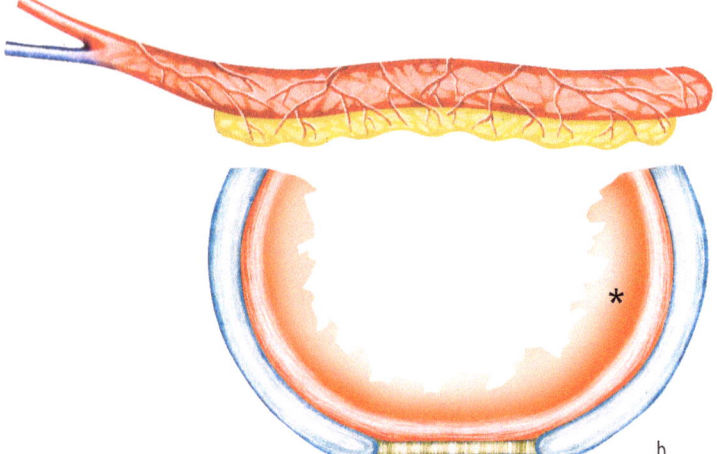

b

Figure 6.34.
Healing of vascularized mucosa-Histology after reconstruction.
a. Axial section. The intensely perfused fascia flap (blue Microfil® injected) is lined with squamous epithelium. A sharp transition area exists between oral and respiratory mucosa (arrows). A flat reconstruction between the margins of the defect will be provided when the size of the mucosal graft is similar to the size of the defect (H&E original x 5).
b. Schematic presentation of anterior airway defect after reconstruction. Mucosal lining of trachea may be scarred in the clinical situation (asterisk).

The mucosal lined reconstruction shows a primary healing with a complete take of the oral mucosa on the fascial vascular carrier and shows a preservation of the surface area of the reconstruction (Fig. 6.34).
The vascular supply and the epithelial lining of the graft makes the reconstructive patch independent from the defect margins for its healing. No revascularization and no re-epithelialization are necessary during healing and this may be advantageous in the clinical situation when a scarred wound bed is encountered. Wound healing with mucosal lined fascia is comparable to the wound healing seen when using skin lined flaps. A mucosal lining is however preferable for airway lining in order to prevent the crusting and desquamation seen when using skin grafts.

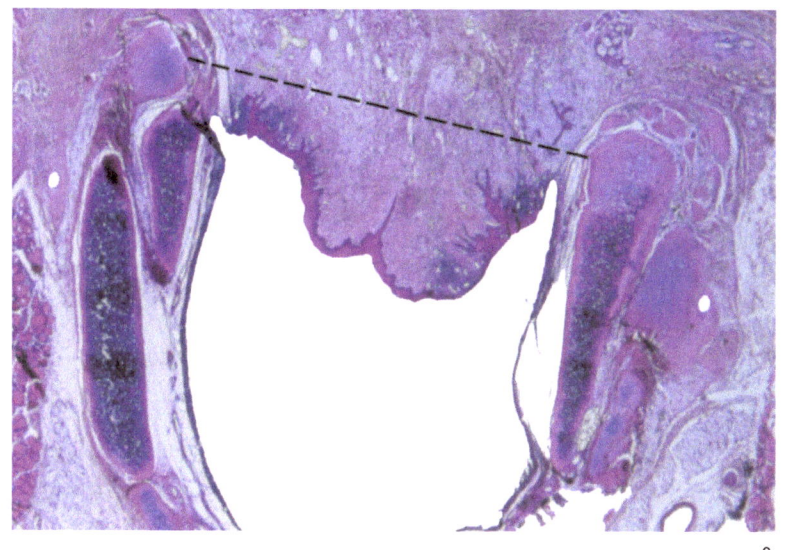

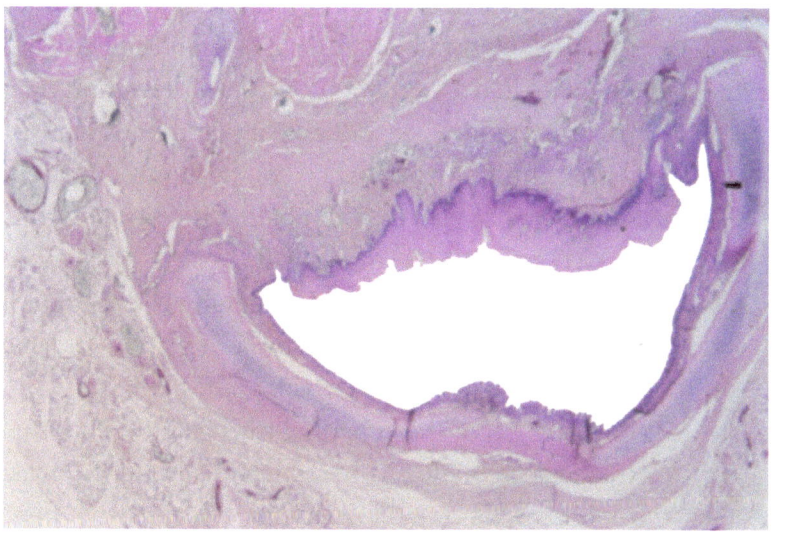

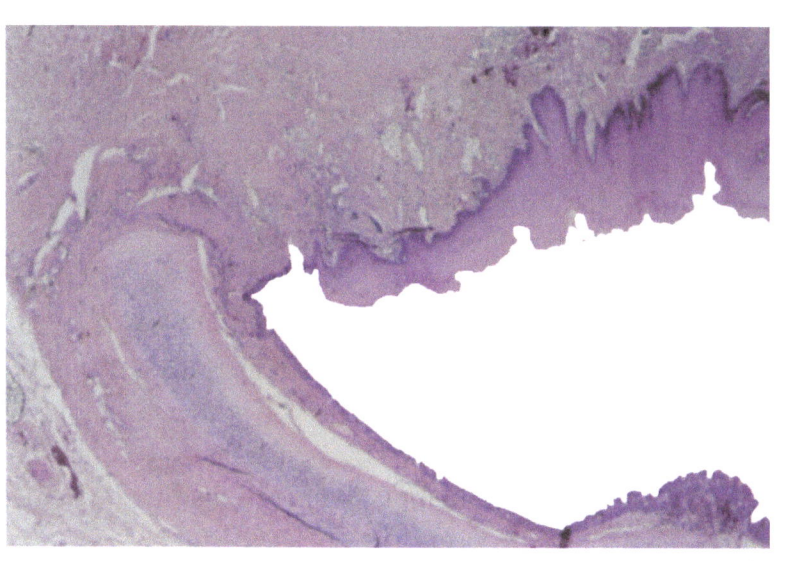

Figure 6.34.
Healing of vascularized mucosa-Histology after reconstruction (continued).
c. Section at cricoid level. Prolapse into the lumen will result if a bigger patch is sutured into the defect.

d. Section at tracheal level.

e. Section at tracheal level-Detail.
Transition between respiratory and oral mucosa is clearly visible.

A disadvantage of the mucosal lined fascia is the absence of supportive tissue. Essential when using a mucosal lined fascia flap into an airway defect is that the mucosal patch and the defect have a similar size. Prolapse into the airway will result if a mucosal patch, that is larger than the defect, is included.

Table 6.4. Mucosal component in airway reconstruction

- Primary healing
- One-stage reconstruction
- Can be used in clinical cases

Best result that can be obtained for anterior airway defect reconstruction:

flat reconstruction with full preservation of surface area of defect

The composite tissue ' mucosal graft + blood supply' was used in clinical cases of restenosis after previous tracheal resection. The mucosal lined fascia was preferred over the free cartilage graft because the introduction of a new blood supply into a scarred operative field was evaluated as advantageous.

7.C. Vascularized mucosa- clinical use

Use of the mucosal lined fascia is illustrated in 4 clinical cases of anastomotic stricture (restenosis) after segmental airway resection.

7.C.1 Case 1

An 18-year-old boy was admitted with severe laryngotracheal stenosis. The stenosis occurred after the patient was involved in a car accident 4 months earlier. At that time, the patient had been intubated for 3 weeks. After extubation, he underwent endoscopy and placement of a tracheotomy tube because of increasing dyspnea. He was found to have subglottic stenosis. The stenosis was initially treated by dilation and laser resection. He was referred presenting with a subglottic stenosis with complete obstruction of the lumen (Cotton grade 4) that started 1 cm below the vocal cords. On a computed tomography (CT) scan, the stenotic segment was estimated as having a length of 3 cm. The patient underwent a resection of the cricoid cartilage anteriorly, together with a resection of 4 cm of the proximal trachea including the tracheotomy site. The mediastinal trachea was mobilized and a suprahyoid release was performed. The mediastinal trachea was sutured to the cricoid cartilage posteriorly and to the thyroid cartilage anteriorly. Although the upper and lower airway segments were mobilized maximally, the anastomosis (Dexon 2-0) was still performed under some tension. The patient was extubated 1 day after the operation, and head flexion was maintained for 1 week. Five weeks after the operation, the patient underwent a replacement of the tracheotomy tube because of increasing dyspnea. On laryngoscopy a restenosis at the anastomosis was seen, with a 90% reduction of the airway lumen. Two attempts to remove the fibrotic tissue with a CO2 laser were not successful.

An augmentation tracheoplasty with a mucosal-lined fascia flap was decided on. The laryngotracheal complex was incised longitudinally starting at the caudal end of the anterior commissure and ending in the tracheostomy incision. The re-stenosis was located at the caudal cricoid level and had a length of 2 cm (Fig. 6.35).

The laryngotracheal complex was incised over 5 cm to allow for a sufficient expansion of the stenotic area. An elliptical anterior defect with a length of 5 cm and with a width of 1.5 cm was obtained. The tracheotomy tube was removed and the patient was intubated orally.

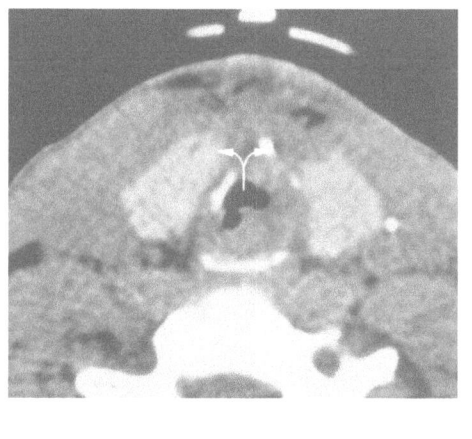

a

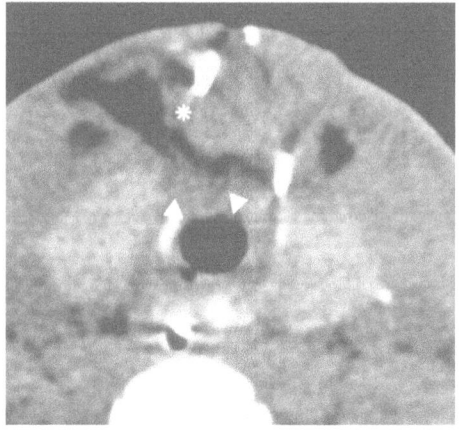

c

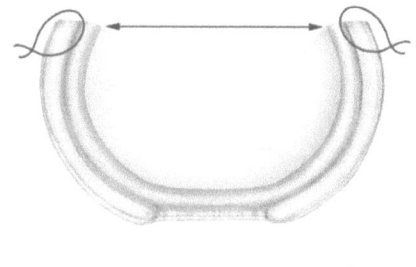

b

Figure 6.35. Vascularized mucosa-clinical use.
a. Preoperative CT scan. Axial CT scan through the anastomosis (area of caudal cricoid) after previous tracheal resection. The airway was incised anteriorly (white arrows) over a length of 5 cm and the stenotic area was expanded with creation of an anterior defect.
b. Schematic presentation of anterior airway defect after incision of the stenosis. The margins of the defect may be sutured to the surrounding tissues so that a maximal surface area of the defect (double arrow) is obtained. It is important that the anterior defect is not recoiling. Scarred mucosal lining.
c. Postoperative CT. The mucosal lined fascia is sutured in the anterior airway defect.
The full-thickness mucosa is visible between the arrowheads. The fascia flap is indicated by an asterisk. A flat reconstruction between the defect margins was obtained and this reconstruction was sufficient for normal respiration.

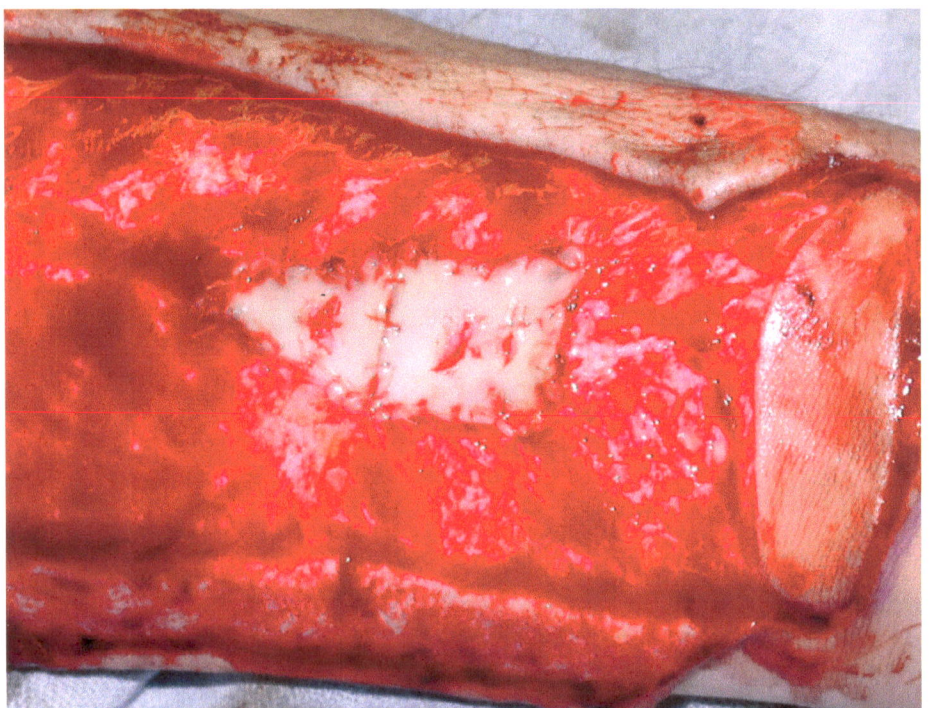

a

Figure 6.36.
Mucosa lined fascia flap.
a. Mucosal lined fascia. Two full thickness mucosal grafts were applied on the antebrachial fascia flap after elevation of the overlying skin (Dexon 6.0). Several sutures were placed in the middle of the mucosal graft to anchor it to the bed and to eliminate dead space. A mucosal covered area of 1.5 x 5 cm was obtained. The monitoring skin flap is visible at the distal flap site.

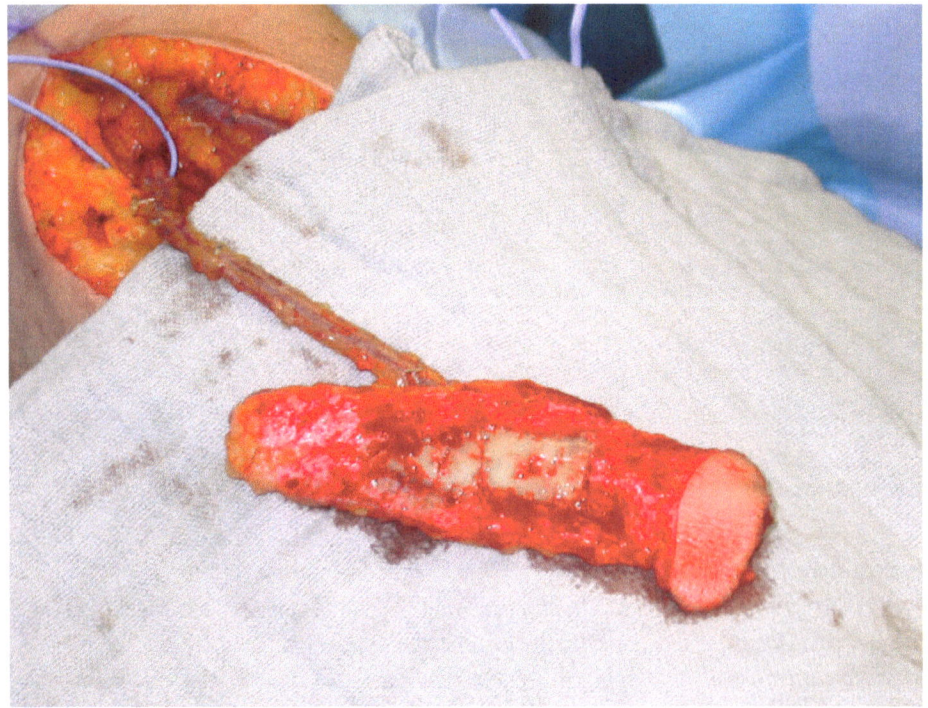

b

b. Mucosal lined fascia after flap dissection and isolation on the radial artery and vein.

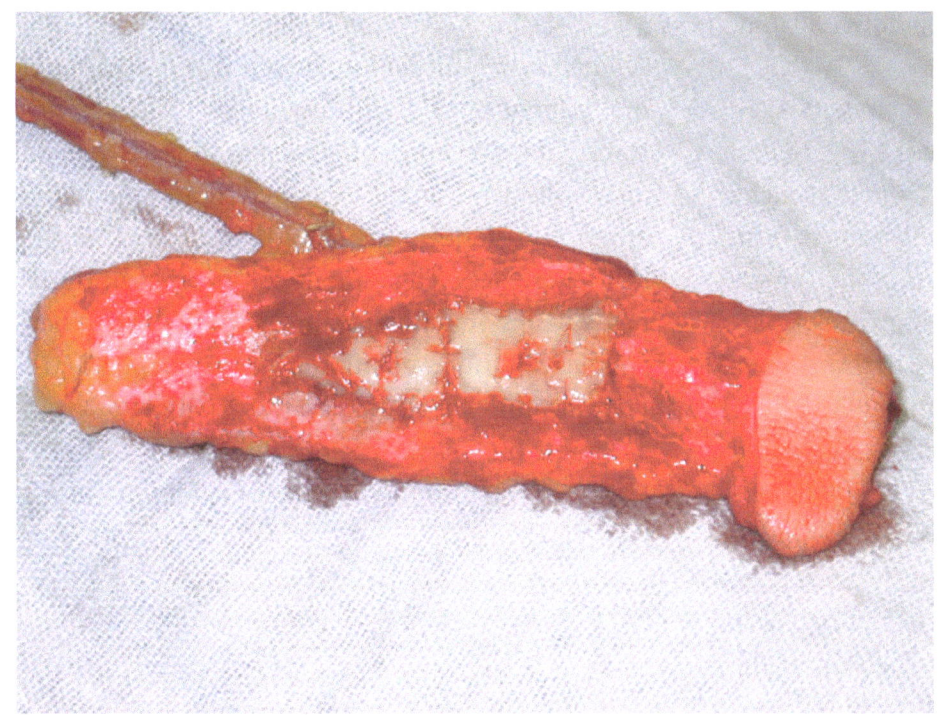

Figure 6.36. Mucosa lined fascia flap (continued).
c. Mucosal lined fascia after flap dissection and isolation on the radial artery and vein.

c

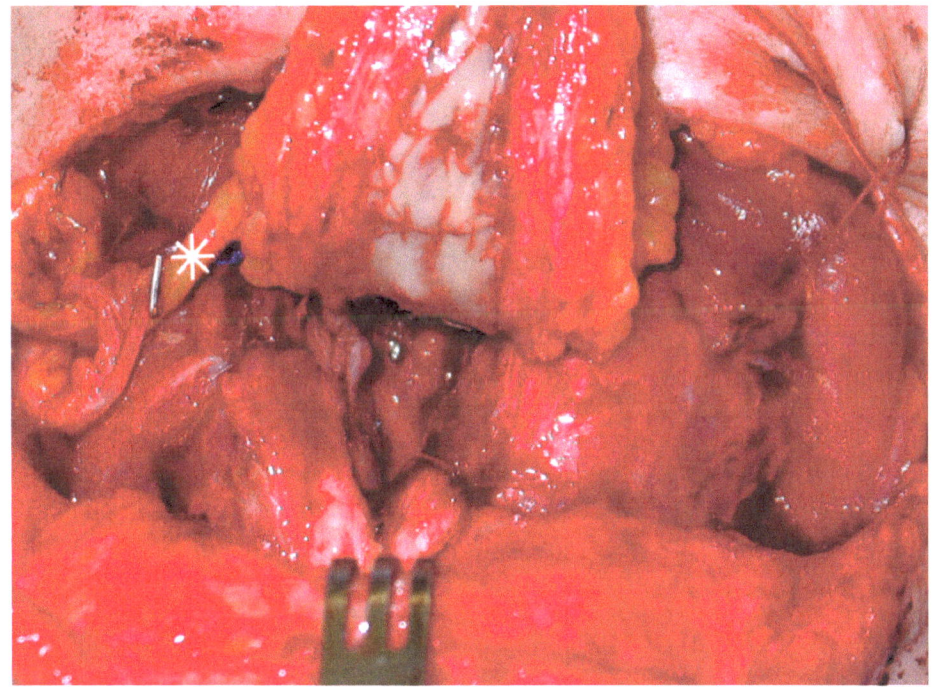

d. The mucosal lined fascia is sutured into the longitudinally incised tracheal defect from inferior to superior. The vascular pedicle is indicated with an asterisk.

d

The radial forearm fascia flap was used as the vascular carrier for the mucosal lining, because it provides fascial and fasciocutaneous tissue, vascularized by a long and reliable vascular pedicle consisting of the radial artery and vein.

A patch of fascia and subcutaneous tissue, measuring 8 x 5 cm, was exposed after a midline longitudinal incision of the radial forearm skin. A small strip of skin (measuring 2 x 6 cm) was included distally as a fasciocutaneous segment serving as a monitor for the postoperative viability of the flap (Fig. 6.36).

Two full-thickness mucosal grafts were harvested at the left and right buccal areas. The buccal mucosal defects were closed primarily. The mucosal grafts were trimmed and cleaned from underlying submucosal fat. Defatting the undersurface of the graft was done with a pair of scissors. The margins of the mucosal graft were secured to the fascia with interrupted sutures. A mucosa-covered area of 1.5 x 5 cm was obtained (6-0 Vicryl). The grafts were applied before dissection of the flap, because the stability of the undissected fascia allowed for easy suturing. After the mucosal grafts were applied, the fascial flap was dissected on its vascular pedicle. The skin at the donor defect was closed primarily. The mucosa-covered area of the fascia flap was sutured into the anterior airway defect with 3-0 Dexon. The distal end of the fascia flap was rotated over 180°, and the fasciocutaneous island was brought in the neck incision to serve as a monitor. The monitoring skin paddle was used as a visible control of the viability of the flap in the postoperative period. After insetting of the mucosa-lined patch, the fascia flap was revascularized by an end-to-end anastomosis between superior thyroid and radial artery and by an end-to-side anastomosis between internal jugular vein and radial vein. The patient was extubated without problems 5 days after the operation. A sufficient airway lumen with the mucosal-lined fascia in the anterior defect was seen on a postoperative CT scan (Fig. 6.35.c).

7.C.2. Case 2

A small subglottic airway lumen was encountered in 1 patient treated with the initial tracheal autotransplantation concept. The reason for the small airway lumen was the excessive shortening of the anterior-posterior patch length at the level of the caudal cricoid. The patient complained of dyspnea and the remaining radial forearm fascia flap was used as augmentation tissue. To obtain a primary healing, the fascia flap was grafted with full-thickness buccal mucosal grafts and this composite tissue was used to augment the airway lumen (Fig. 6.37).

Figure 6.37. CT scan at glottic, subglottic and cricoid level.
T3N0 tomor of left hemilarynx. Resection margins are indicated on the preoperative CT scan (1).
Revascularized trachea (3 levels) with indication of resection to form patch (2).
Postoperative CT scan (3 levels) with reconstruction (3).
a = glottic level.
b = subglottic level high and c = subglottic level low.
At the glottic level, the revascularized trachea is shortened to the desired length to obtain a patch position near the midline at the glottic level. It is desirable to include more of the cartilaginous trachea to obtain a good airway lumen subglottically. In this case, the revascularized trachea was shortened too much. A substenosis was obtained at the caudal cricoid level and at the anastomosis between reconstructed larynx and mediastinal trachea.
The stenotic area was expanded after longitudinal incision (arrows).
d. Mucosal lined radial forearm flap. Two full-thickness buccal mucosal grafts are sutured to the radial forearm fascia.
e. The mucosal graft is visible in the anterior airway defect.

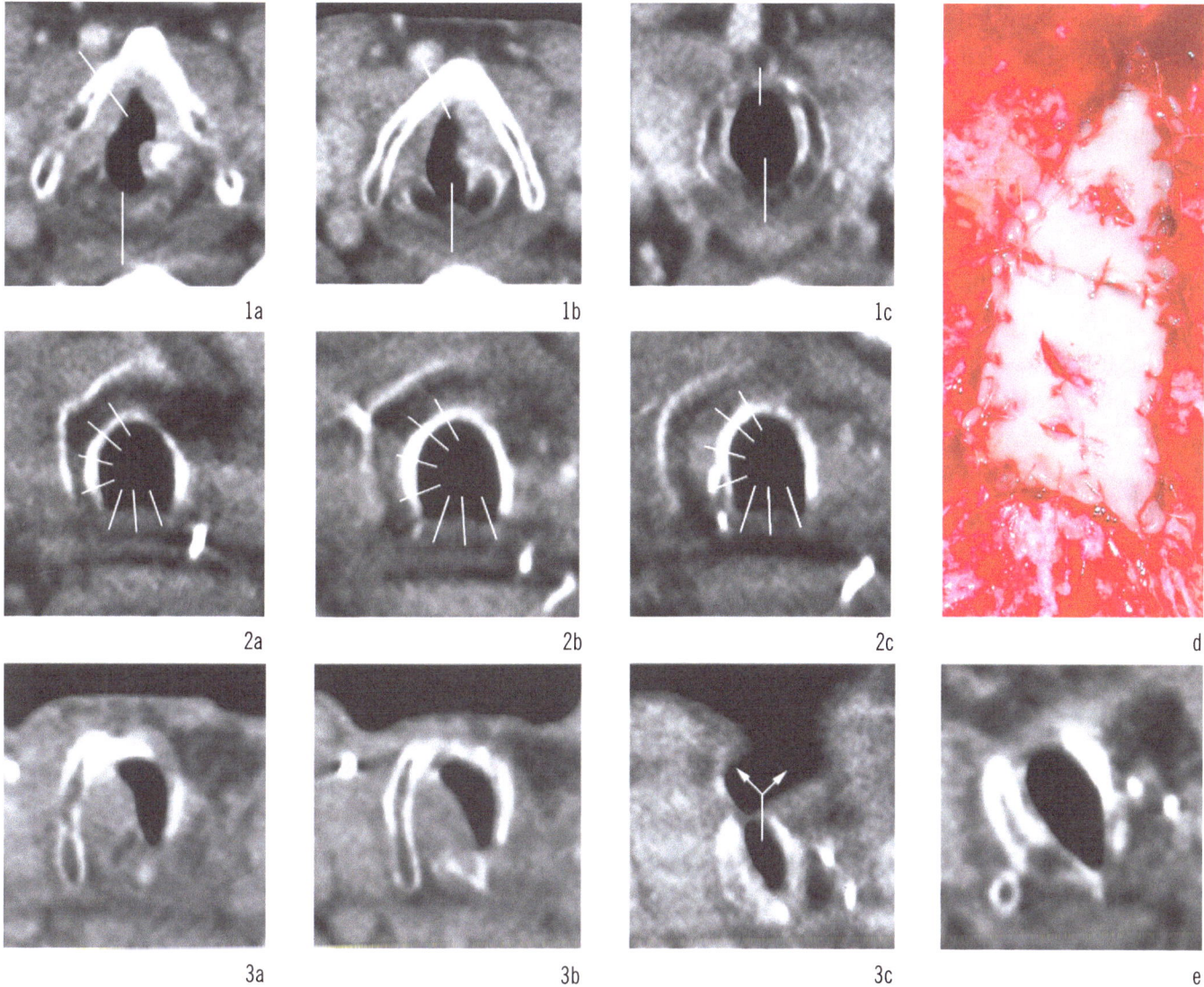

1a

1b

1c

d

2a

2b

2c

3a

3b

3c

e

The anterior suture line between tracheal patch and laryngeal remnant was incised longitudinally. The remaining radial forearm fascia flap was used as vascular carrier. A patch of fascia and subcutaneous tissue, measuring 8 by 5 cm, was exposed after a midline longitudinal incision of the radial forearm skin. Two full-thickness mucosal grafts were harvested at the left and right buccal areas. The buccal mucosal defects were closed primarily. The mucosal grafts were trimmed and cleaned from underlying submucosal fat. The margins of the mucosal graft were secured to the fascia using interrupted sutures. The grafts were applied before dissection of the flap because the stability of the undissected fascia allowed for easy suturing. After applying the mucosal grafts, the fascial flap was dissected on its vascular pedicle. The skin at the donor defect was closed primarily. The mucosal covered area of the fascia flap was sutured into the anterior airway defect with Dexon 3.0. After insetting of the mucosa lined patch, the fascia flap was revascularized by an end-to-end anastomosis between superior thyroid and radial artery and by an end-to-side anastomosis between internal jugular vein and radial vein. The patient was extubated without problems 5 days postoperatively. A sufficient airway lumen with the mucosal lined fascia in the anterior defect was seen on a postoperative CT scan (Fig. 6.38).

A mucosa-lined radial forearm fascial flap can be used successfully to close the airway defect after longitudinal incision and expansion of a stenotic area. The vascularized fascia allows for easy healing in a scarred operation field and the mucosal grafts allow for primary healing without wound contraction. A prerequisite for mucosal survival is that the margins and the central portion of the grafts are carefully sutured to the vascularized fascia.

A disadvantage of the mucosa-lined fascia is the absence of a cartilage component. Because support is lacking, a flat reconstruction between the margins of the anterior defect is the best result that can be obtained. Further expansion of the airway lumen by creating an anterior convexity is not possible, and this may be a drawback when a more extensive stenosis needs reconstruction. It was investigated whether the composite reconstruction 'mucosal lining-blood supply' could be improved by adding cartilage support to the mucosa-lined fascia flap (see 8. Airway reconstruction with vascularized mucosa and cartilage).

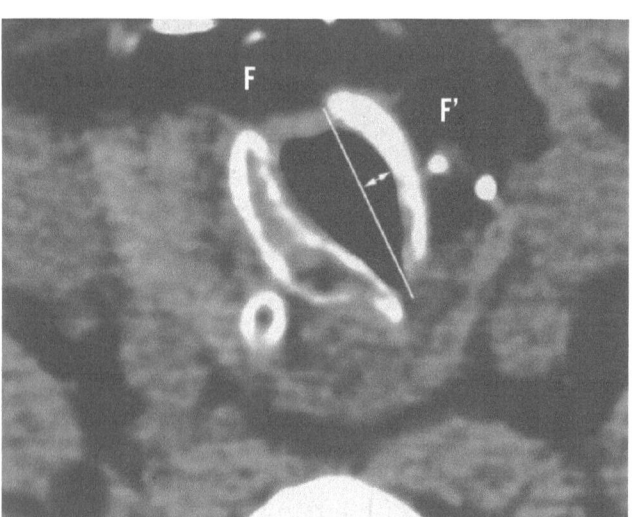
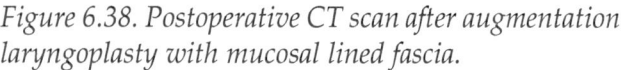
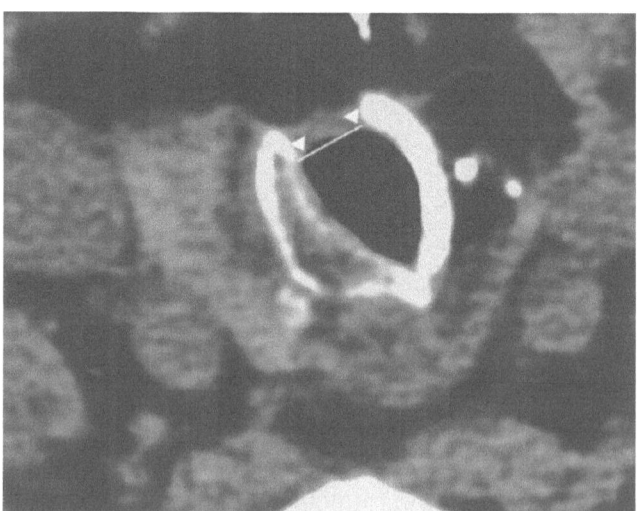

Figure 6.38. Postoperative CT scan after augmentation laryngoplasty with mucosal lined fascia.
The mucosal graft which is applied on the fascia flap and which augments the airway lumen is visible between arrowheads. F= fascia flap serving as a vascular carrier for the mucosal graft. F'=fascia flap serving as a vascular carrier for the tracheal patch. The flap used for tracheal autotransplantation was revascularized on the left side whereas the flap for lumen augmentation was revascularized on the right side.
This CT scan shows the difference between airway

reconstruction with mucosa lined fascia and airway reconstruction with revascularized segments of trachea.
The best result obtained with mucosa lined fascia (lining + blood supply) is a primary reconstruction of the anterior defect. The surface area of the defect is maintained; an additional anterior airway expansion is not possible. Revascularized trachea (lining + blood supply + cartilage support in the optimal tissue composition) succeeds in primary reconstruction with expansion of the airway lumen (double arrow).

7.C.3. Case 3 and 4

Two cases showed a stenosis in the area of the tracheostomy after previous surgery for posterior glottic stenosis treated by insertion of costal cartilage between the divided posterior cricoid. Segmental resection might be a possibility in these 2 cases. The 2 patients were treated with augmentation tracheoplasty rather than by segmental resection because of the previous surgery on the larynx.

Case 3 (female patient) showed a substenosis in the area of the former tracheostomy that developed progressively over a time period of 2 years (Fig. 6.39). In case 4, the tracheostomy could not be closed after correction of the posterior stenosis (Fig. 6.40). After removal of the Eliachar stent, which was in place for 6 weeks to support the posterior cartilage graft, it seemed that the airway at the site of the tracheostomy was to small to allow for simple closure. It was decided to expand the airway and to bring mucosa-lined fascia into the anterior defect.

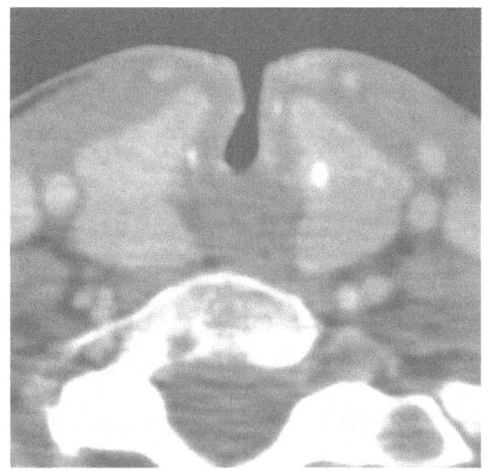

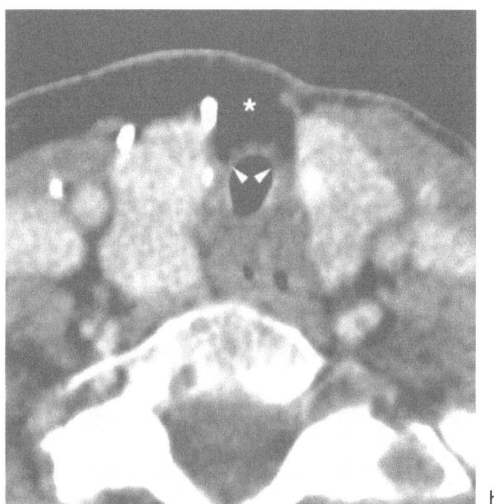

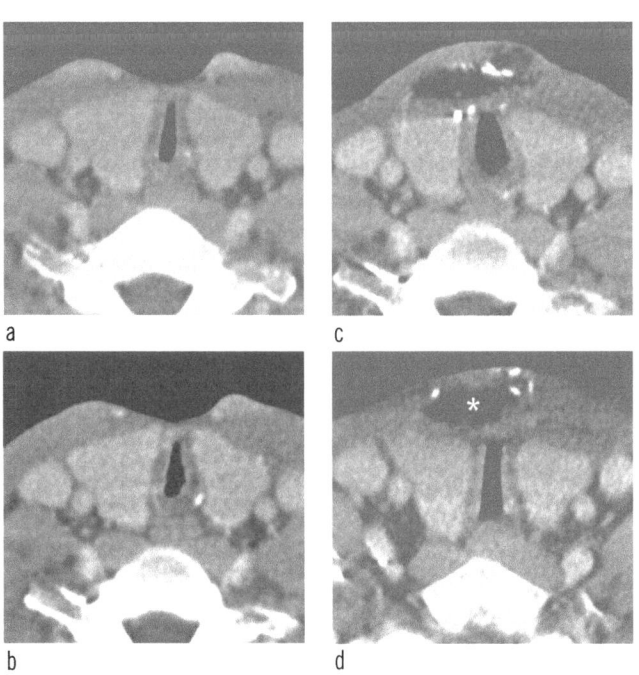

Figure 6.40. Case 4.
a. Preoperative. Tracheostomy can not be closed by skin inversion because of substenosis.
b. Postoperative. Situation after augmentation tracheosplasty. Buccal mucosa is visible between arrowheads. Fascia flap is indicated with asterisk.

Figure 6.39. Case 3.
a. and b. Preoperative. Substenosis in the area of the former tracheostomy.
c. and d. Postoperative. Airway expansion with mucosa-lined fascia. Fascia is indicated with an asterisk.

8. Airway reconstruction with vascularized mucosa and cartilage

8.A. Composite tissue consisting of cartilage and vascularized mucosa

An epithelial lined soft tissue flap can repair the surface area of an anterior defect. Cartilage support is however essential for obtaining an anterior expansion of the airway lumen. This support may be provided if an elastic piece of cartilage is sutured between the margins of an airway defect that is smaller than the cartilage segment. Elastic ear cartilage is available in large quantities in rabbits but only in small quantities in humans (Fig. 6.41). Fibrocartilage is available in much larger quantities in the human rib, but this type of cartilage has a low elasticity and is not suitable for 'additional expansion' of the airway lumen anteriorly.

Theoretically, 3 different designs are possible when elastic cartilage is added to a mucosal lined fascia flap. In a first design (Composite tissue concept 1), the cartilage graft is placed between inner and outer fascial layers. The full-thickness buccal mucosa graft is applied on the outer fascial layer after 180° rotation of the fascia flap. In this concept, both the cartilaginous and the mucosal components are well perfused by the fascial flap. The problem with this concept, however, is the low degree of support provided by the cartilage component. In order to obtain a convexity at the site of reconstruction, it is necessary to suture the margins of the elastic cartilage graft to the margins of a smaller airway defect. With the **composite tissue concept 1**, the margins of the mucosal graft are sutured to the margins of the defect, and as a consequence, the cartilage graft is located outside the defect without providing support to the reconstruction (Fig. 6.42).

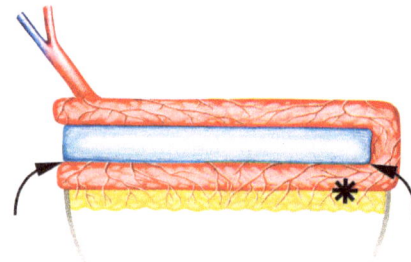

Figure 6.42. Composite tissue concept 1.
The composite tissue is formed by 180° rotation of the vascularized fascia. In this way, the cartilage is circumferentially covered and protected within a vascular bed. A full-thickness mucosal graft can be revascularized by capillary outgrowth from the inner layer of the vascularized fascia flap. One disadvantage of this concept is the low degree of support provided by the cartilage component. In order to obtain an anterior expansion of the airway lumen, the margins of the cartilage graft (arrows) need to be sutured to the margins of the defect. In this concept, the cartilage margin, which is wrapped with fascia, cannot be sutured to the margin of the defect without interfering with the blood supply to the inner fascial layer (asterisk).

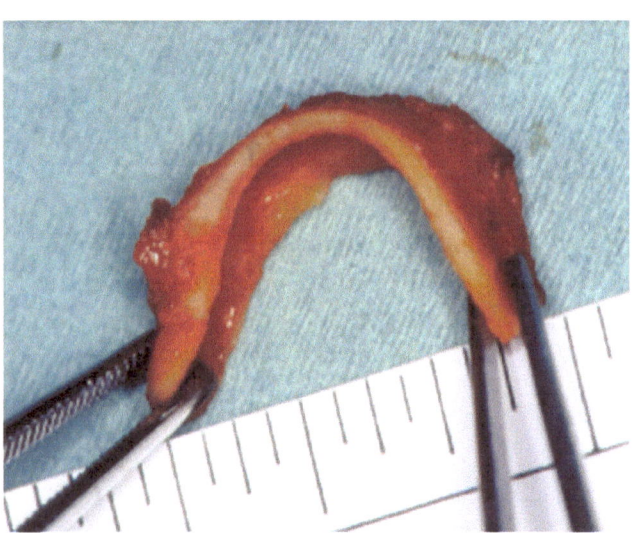

Figure 6.41. Cartilage support in airway reconstruction for additional lumen augmentation.
In humans, an auricular graft with dimensions approaching 2 x 5 cm may be harvested. Anterior convexity may be created if elastic cartilage with a length larger than the width of defect is sutured to the margins of that defect. Scale in Inches.

In the **composite tissue concept 2**, the mucosal graft is directly applied to the cartilage graft. This concept provides cartilage support but the mucosal graft cannot survive on the cartilage because the cartilage component will not allow for ingrowth of blood vessels. With this design, the only possibility to obtain survival of the mucosal graft is to use vascularized tracheal cartilage. Blood vessels can reach the mucosal graft through the intercartilaginous ligaments when using vascularized tracheal cartilage as supporting tissue (Fig. 6.43).

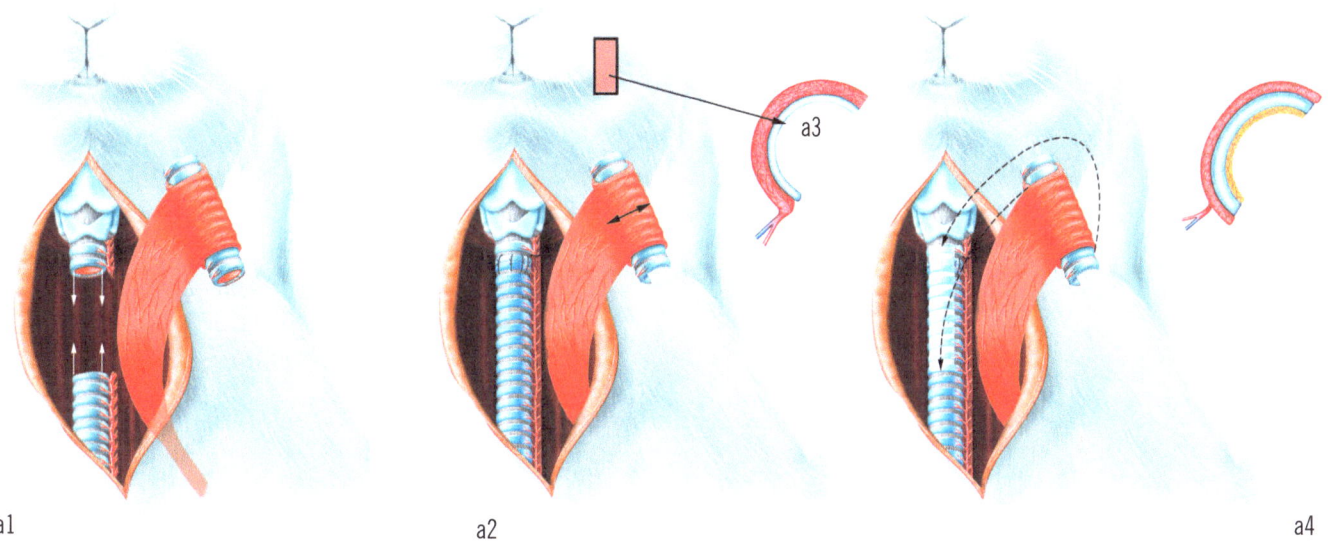

a1   a2   a4

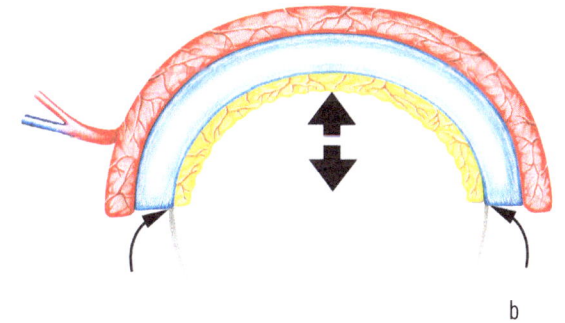

b

Figure 6.43.
Composite tissue concept 2.
a.1. A 1.5 cm segment of trachea is removed after 14 days of fascial wrapping.
The tracheal defect is closed by end-to-end anastomosis (arrows).
a.2. Situation after repair of the tracheal continuity. The revascularized tube is transformed into a patch by removal of the membranous trachea and by removal of a part of the cartilaginous ring. The mucosal lining of

the patch is excised. An axial section through the tracheal patch (double arrow) shows the denuded segment of trachea (a.3). After removal of the respiratory mucosal lining, the denuded patch is grafted with full-thickness buccal mucosa.
a.4. An anterior laryngotracheal defect is created with a length of 1.5 cm. The tracheal patch lined with buccal mucosa is used to repair the anterior defect.

b. Schematic presentation of composite tissue concept. Cartilage component is sutured to vascularized fascia and directly attached to mucosal graft. In this concept, the margins of the cartilage graft (single arrows) may be sutured to margins of defect with anterior expansion of the airway lumen (double arrow).

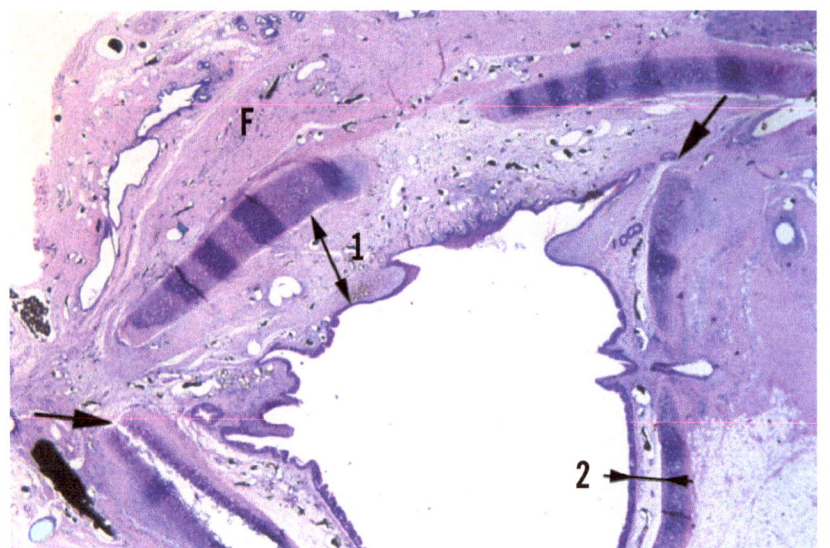

c1

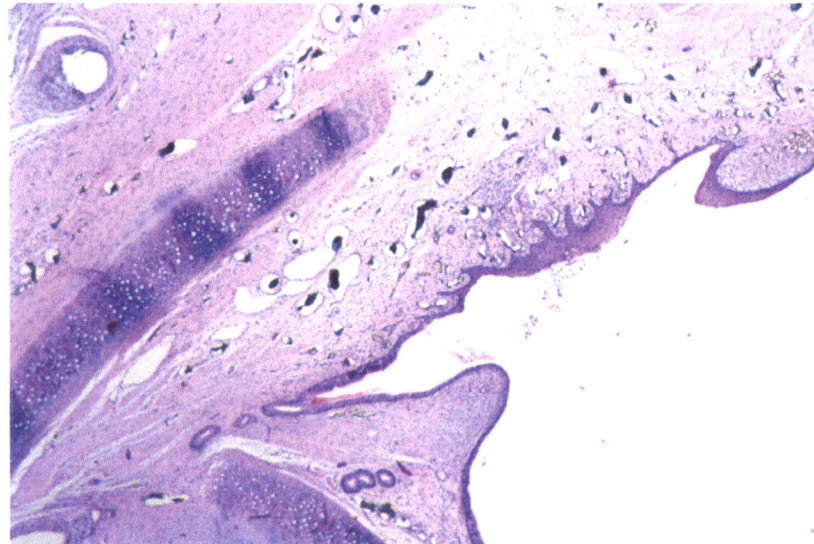

c2

Figure 6.43.
Composite tissue concept 2 (continued).
c. Composite tissue concept 2 with vascu-
larized cartilage-Histology axial section.
c.1. H&E, original magnification x 10. The
tracheal patch lined with buccal mucosa is
visible between arrows. The blood vessels
of the mucosal graft and the blood vessels
of the fascia flap (F) are injected with blue
Microfil®. Thickness of mucosal graft
(double arrow-1) is 3 times the thickness of
the respiratory epithelium (double arrow-
2).

c.2. H&E, original magnification x 20.
Blood vessels of fascia flap and mucosal
graft are filled with blue Microfil®.
Squamous epithelium is visible on top of
the mucosal graft.

The composite tissue concept 2 can provide for tissue with support, lining, and vascularization. This composite tissue concept is only a theoretical possibility because a cartilage framework consisting of cartilage rings and intercartilaginous ligaments is not available when dealing with a clinical case (re-stenosis, long segment stenosis) that needs tissue reconstruction of the airway tract.

When used for repair of anterior airway defects, the anterior expansion of the airway lumen is small because of the thickness of the oral mucosal graft. Circumferential airway reconstruction in rabbits will be impossible with this composite tissue because of the bulk provided by the full-thickness mucosal lining.

In the **composite tissue concept 3**, cartilage strips are applied on the fascia flap so that the mucosal grafts are located between the cartilaginous framework. With this concept, the airway lumen can be expanded at the sites where the cartilage strips are sutured to the margins of the defect (Fig. 6.44). This concept may give some additional airway lumen expansion by providing cartilage support at the most critical site of the stenosis. The composite tissue concept 3 may improve the concept of the 'mucosa-lined fascia'.

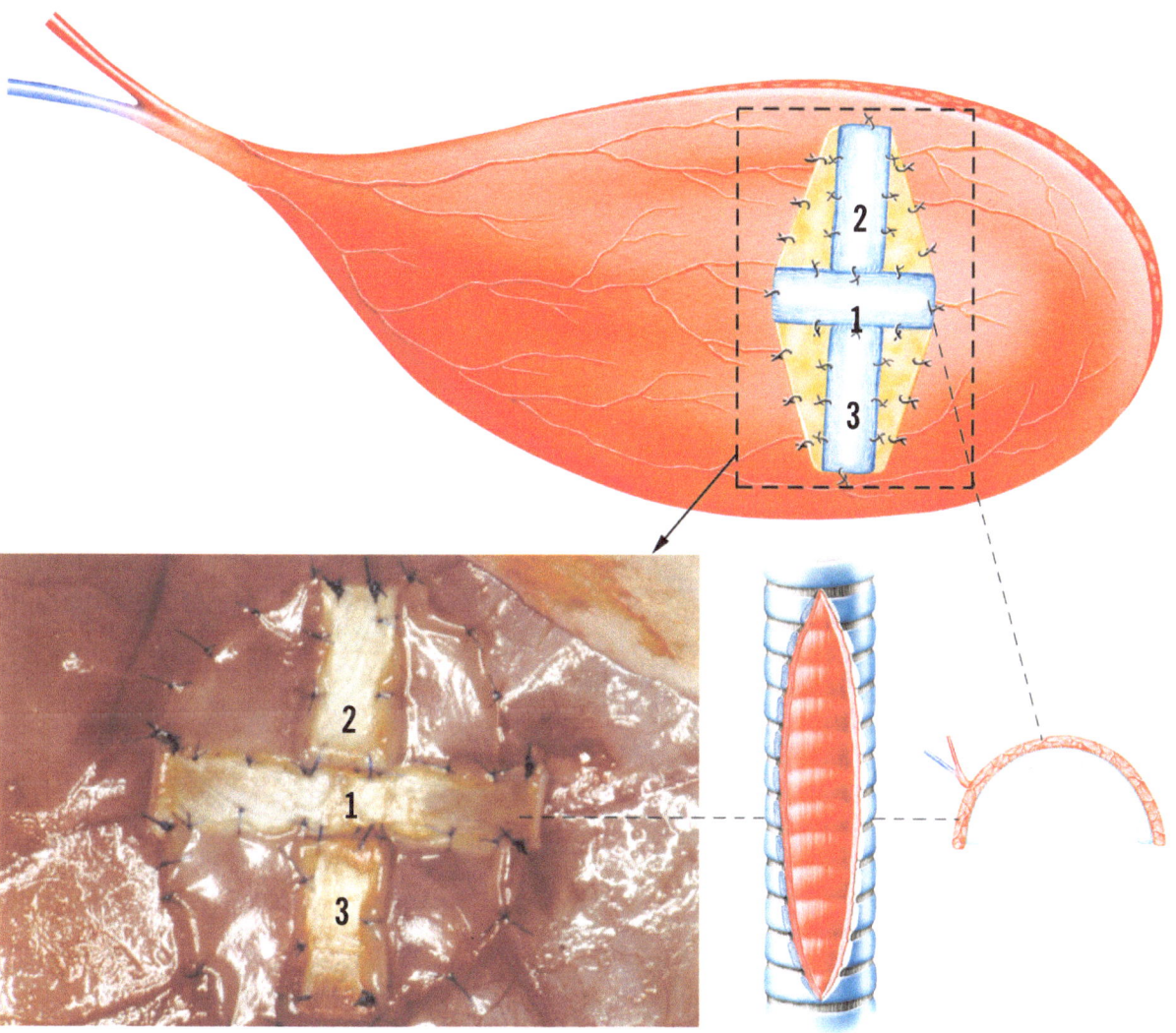

Figure 6.44. Composite tissue concept 3.
Cartilage grafts are sutured to the fascia flap between mucosal grafts. In this concept, 3 cartilage grafts are sutured to the fascial flap. The first cartilage graft (1) is sutured to the longitudinal axis of flap and will be used for airway lumen expansion. The other 2 cartilage grafts (2,3) are applied in the transverse axis of the fascia flap and give some longitudinal strength to the reconstruction. Cartilage grafts are sutured to each other. Four buccal mucosal grafts are sutured to the fascia flap and to the cartilage grafts to form a grafted area that will be used in anterior airway reconstruction. Anterior extension of the airway lumen will be obtained at the site of the cartilage graft (dotted line).

Healing of the composite tissue concept 3 will be without problems for the mucosal grafts. Full thickness mucosal grafts survive when carefully sutured to the fascia flap. Healing will be difficult for the cartilaginous framework of the composite tissue. For survival, the cartilage grafts need coverage by buccal mucosa. Secondary healing of the cartilage grafts will not occur inside the airway because the airway exposed cartilage will undergo necrosis before healing can take place. Flap prefabrication will be necessary to keep the cartilaginous component viable.

The principle of flap prefabrication may be used to improve the survival of the cartilage grafts. During flap prefabrication, the composite flap remains in the lateral thoracic area. With this technique, transfer of the composite flap is delayed until the cartilage grafts are sufficiently healed and covered with buccal mucosa (Fig. 6.45). After a 2 to 4 weeks healing period, the cartilage component is sufficiently healed so that the composite tissue can be transferred to an anterior airway defect.

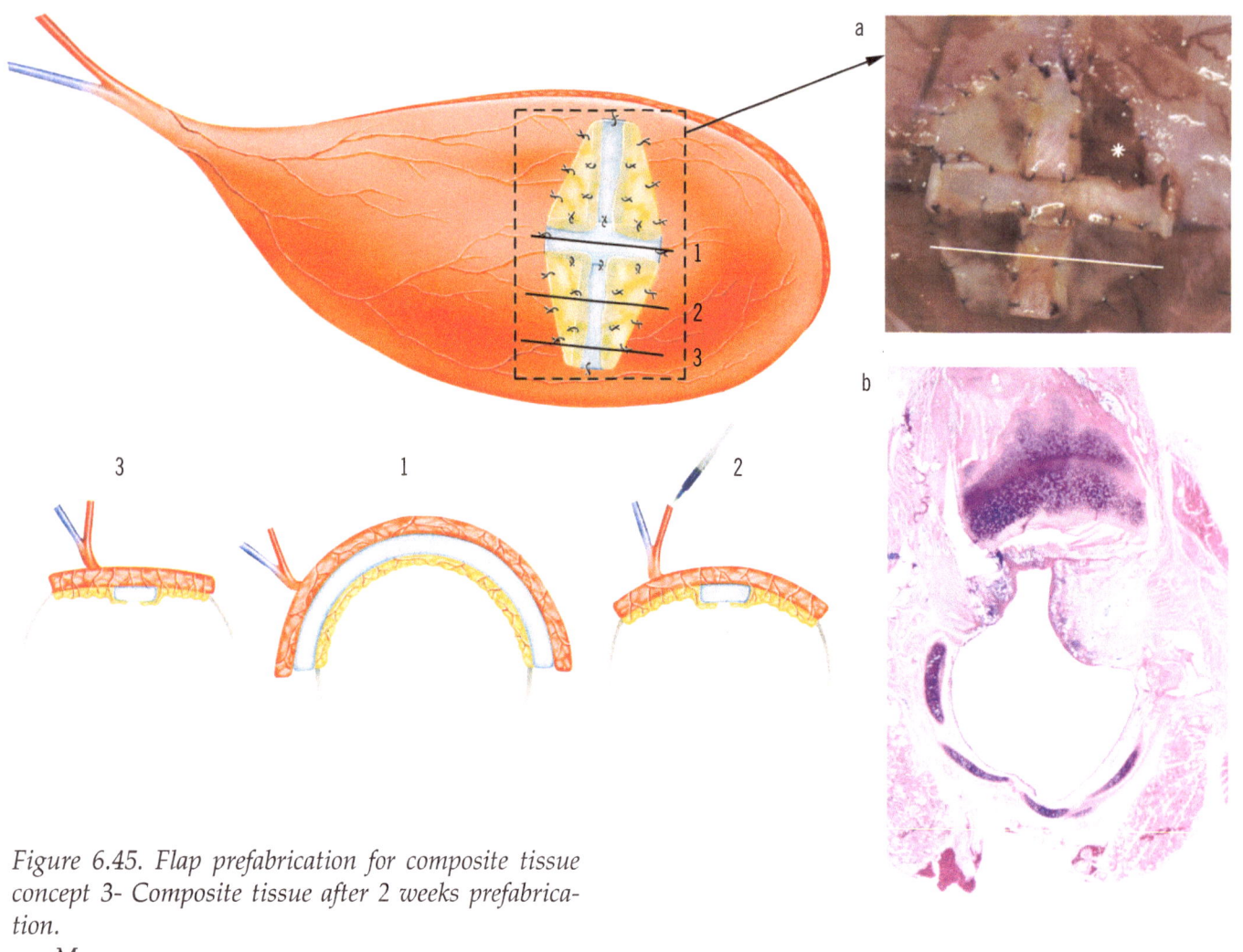

Figure 6.45. Flap prefabrication for composite tissue concept 3- Composite tissue after 2 weeks prefabrication.
a = Macroscopy
b = Histology

Figure 6.45. Flap prefabrication for composite tissue concept 3- Composite tissue after 2 weeks prefabrication (continued).
a. Situation 2 weeks after grafting of fascia with mucosa and cartilage. The full-thickness mucosal grafts show complete survival. Submucosal vessel ingrowth is visible (asterisk). Oral mucosa has begun to grow over edges of cartilage grafts. The composite tissue can be transferred to an anterior airway defect after 2 weeks of prefabrication. Anterior extension of the airway lumen will be obtained at the site of the cartilage graft (1) while a flat reconstruction will be obtained at both ends of the composite flap (3). Situation between convex and flat reconstruction will be seen at the site between middle and extremity of the flap (2).
b. shows the histology of a preformed composite tissue after repair of an anterior airway defect and after injection of the vascular pedicle with blue Microfil ® (H&E X 5). The anterior expansion of the airway lumen is visible. The reconstruction is lined with buccal mucosa. The blood vessels of the fascia flap are filled with Microfil®. The cartilage graft is completely covered with buccal mucosa.

8.B. Flap prefabrication for repair of a long segment laryngotracheal stenosis

The principle of prefabrication of the composite tissue has been used in a difficult clinical case of long segment stenosis. A 38-year-old man presenting with progressive stridor was urgently intubated. He was known to have laryngotracheal hypoplasia with episodes of dyspnea related to exercise. The present condition of extreme dyspnea was triggered by an upper airway infection. Because of the relatively small laryngeal inlet, a pediatric tube was used for intubation. Attempts to extubate the patient proved to be impossible, and a tracheotomy was placed after 1 week. After tracheotomy, the larynx and trachea were evaluated clinically and radiologically. On laryngoscopy, the glottic airway lumen was small with

a short anterior-posterior dimension. Vocal fold mobility was preserved, without signs of arytenoid ankylosis. A small airway lumen was found from the glottic level to the level of the tracheotomy. The length of the laryngotracheal stenosis measured 5.5 cm. The laryngeal cartilages had an abnormal form and shape, and they were intensely calcified. The mediastinal and thoracic parts of the trachea had a normal airway lumen (Fig. 6.46).

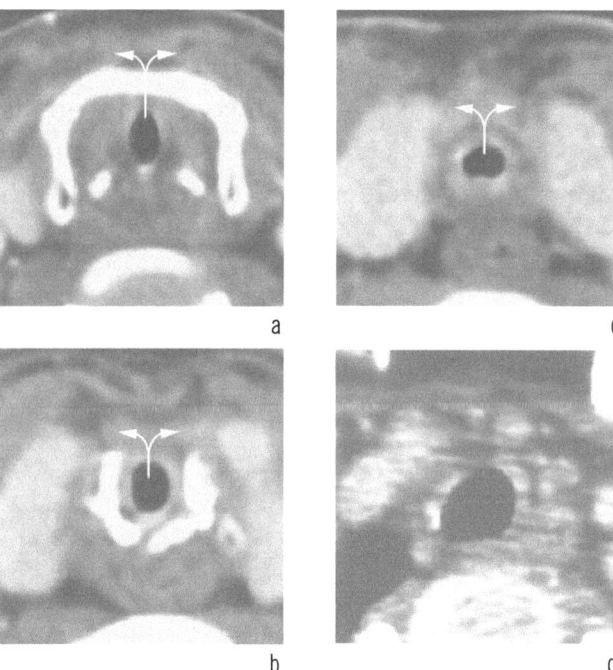

Figure 6.46. CT scan of laryngeal stenosis.
a. At glottic level. Thyroid cartilage is U-shaped, with short anterior-posterior length of glottic airway lumen.
b. At level of cricoid cartilage. Small airway lumen.
c. At level of cervical trachea. Small airway lumen.
d. At level of mediastinal trachea. At level of the upper mediastinum, airway lumen has a normal caliber.

For removal of the tracheotomy tube, a laryngotracheoplasty over a length of 5.5 cm was necessary. This intervention was also necessary for the patient to regain the ability to speak. The patient could not speak with the cannula because of a complete obstruction of the airway lumen above the tracheotomy site. Segmental airway resection or a slide tracheoplasty seemed impossible in this case because of involvement of the glottic level.

In a first operation stage, full-thickness mucosal grafts from the right and left buccal area, as well as auricular cartilage taken from both ears, were grafted to the left radial forearm fascia. Two auricular cartilages measuring 2 x 4 cm were obtained. Two cartilage grafts of 1 x 4 cm were sutured (4-0 Dexon) to the longitudinal axis of the fascia to allow for anterior expansion of the reconstructed airway lumen (Fig 6.47). Three cartilage grafts were sutured to the tranverse axis of the flap. The cartilage grafts were sutured to each other with 4-0 Prolene. Six full-thickness mucosal grafts were applied within the cartilaginous framework. A fascial area of 5.5 x 4 cm, grafted with mucosa and cartilage, was obtained after suturing the mucosal grafts to the fascia (4-0 Dexon). The grafted fascial area was sutured around a Gore-Tex tube to allow for secondary healing of the cartilage grafts in a convex shape. The forearm skin could not be closed over the preformed tissue, and a Gore-tex patch with paraffin gauze dressing was used to cover the tissue. The preformed tissue was inspected 20 days later under general anesthesia. The Gore-Tex was then removed, and the composite tissue was inspected. The sutures anchoring the grafts to the fascia were removed, except for the Prolene sutures between the different cartilage strips.

A progressive growth of blood vessels and buccal mucosa over the cartilage grafts could be seen (Fig. 6.48).

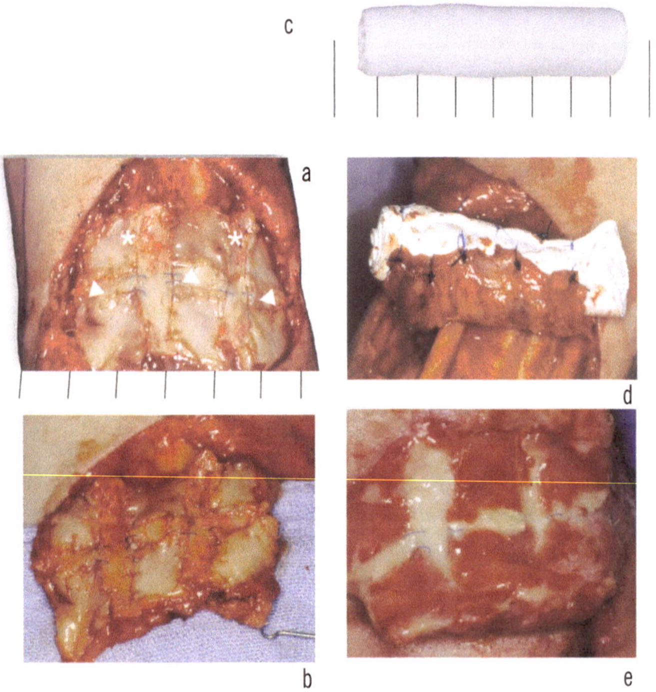

Figure 6.47.
Composite tissue for laryngotracheal reconstruction.
a. Composite tissue. Distal antebrachial fascia was grafted with cartilaginous framework. Two strips of auricular cartilage (asterisk) measuring 1 x 4 cm were applied in longitudinal direction of forearm to provide for anterior lumen expansion of reconstruction. Three shorter segments (arrowheads) were applied in transverse direction of forearm in order to give reconstruction some rigidity in longitudinal axis of reconstruction. Cartilage grafts were sutured to fascia (4-0 Dexon) and to each other (4-0 Prolene). Six mucosal grafts (1.2 x 1.2 cm) were sutured within cartilaginous framework with 6-0 Dexon. Patch had length of 5.5 cm (longitudinal axis of reconstruction; transverse axis of forearm) and width of 4 cm (transverse axis of reconstruction; longitudinal axis of forearm).
b. Distal site of preformed composite tissue was wrapped around Gore-tex tube (c) to hold cartilage grafts in convex shape during healing (d).
e. Situation of composite tissue after 20 days of prefabrication. Oral mucosa is growing over the cartilage grafts.

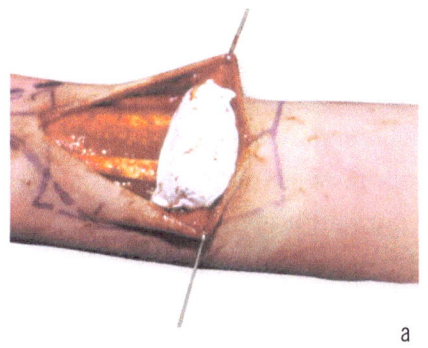 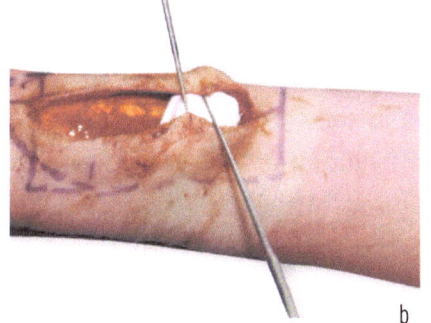 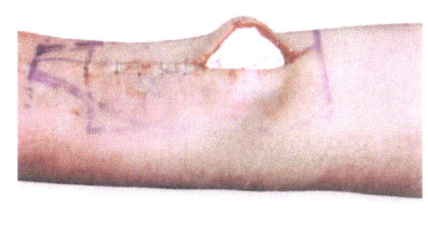

a   b   c

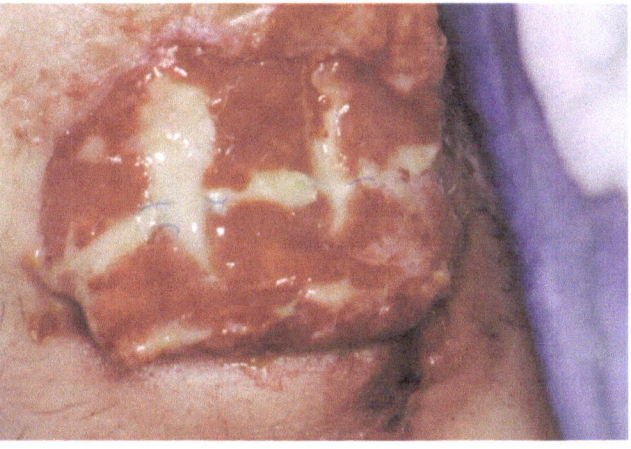

d

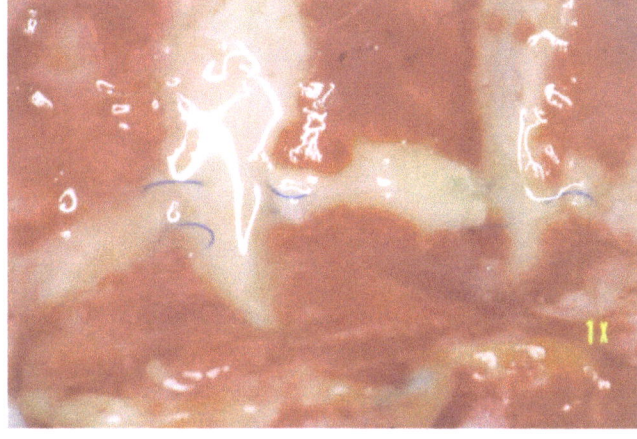

e

Figure 6.48. Flap prefabrication.
a., b., c. Preformed composite tissue-situation during waiting period.
Composite tissue flap is wrapped around tube. Skin defect cannot be closed, and whole reconstruction is protected with polytef (Gore-Tex) membrane.
d. Preformed composite tissue after 20 days. Cartilage

grafts are covered by oral mucosa at their margins. Note convex shape of composite tissue. Sutures anchoring grafts to fascia flap were removed, except for the Prolene sutures between cartilage grafts.
e. Preformed composite tissue after 20 days-Detail.

It was decided to transplant the preformed tissue 20 days after the initial operation. At that time, the cartilage strips were not completely re-epithelialized but they were sufficiently healed at the margins of the mucosal grafts to allow for transplantation. The forearm fascia was dissected on its vascular pedicle. The neck was opened, and the larynx and trachea were incised longitudinally from the level of the vocal folds to the level of the mediastinal trachea over a length of 5.5 cm. The anterior airway defect was expanded. The margins of the incised trachea were sutured to the strap muscles in order to maintain the expanded position of the incised anterior airway defect (Fig. 6.49. b, c). The tracheotomy tube was removed, and the patient was intubated orally. The composite flap was sutured in the anterior airway defect using 3-0 Dexon.

The flap was revascularized by suturing of the radial vessels to the superior thyroid artery (end-to-end) and to the internal jugular vein (end-to-side). A fasciocutaneous portion was included at the proximal site of the flap and sutured in the neck incision to serve as a monitor. The patient was extubated without problems 5 days after the operation. A CT evaluation performed 20 days after the operation showed a laryngotracheal airway lumen that was expanded by a factor of 3. The cartilage support was preserved and the reconstructed airway had a convex shape anteriorly (Fig. 6.49).

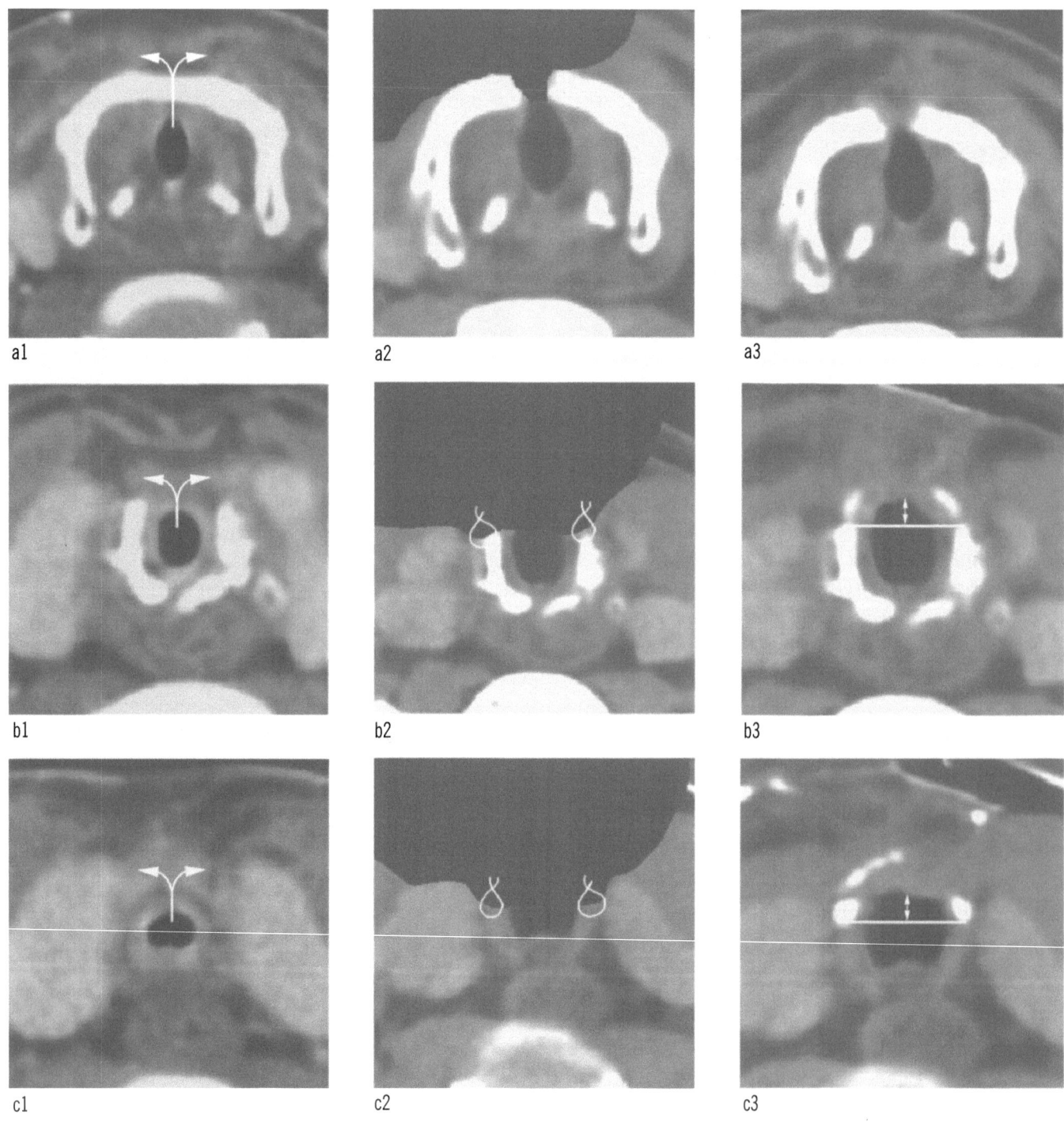

a1

a2

a3

b1

b2

b3

c1

c2

c3

Figure 6.49. Reconstruction of long airway stenosis with composite tissue.

a. At glottic level. Anterior commissure was incised and anterior defect was slightly expanded (arrows) (a.1). a.2. Simulation of intervention on CT scan. Upper end of composite tissue was inserted in anterior thyroid defect. This resulted in lengthening of the anterior-posterior diameter (a.3).

b. At level of cricoid cartilage. Airway was incised anteriorly and anterior defect was expanded (arrows) (b.1). b.2. Simulation of intervention on CT scan. Patch was placed in expanded anterior cricoid defect. Compared to a flat reconstruction between defect margins (white line), prefabricated composite reconstruction gives an additional anterior extension to reconstructed airway lumen. Surface area of airway lumen is augmented by a factor of 3 (b3).

c. At level of cervical trachea. Airway was incided anteriorly and anterior defect was expanded (arrows) (c.1). Some sutures (4-0 Prolene) were placed between margins of incised trachea and strap muscles to hold anterior defect in expanded position (c.2). Patch was placed in the expanded anterior tracheal defect. Note that strap muscles are displaced to margins of anterior tracheal defect. Compared to flat reconstruction between defect margins (white line), prefabricated composite reconstruction gives additional anterior extension to airway lumen. Surface area of airway lumen is expanded by factor of 3 (c.3).

d. Preformed composite tissue after 20 days at time of flap dissection. Incision of forearm skin and outlining of monitoring skin paddle is shown.

e. Postoperative view anterior neck. The monitor skin flap is visible in the neck incision.

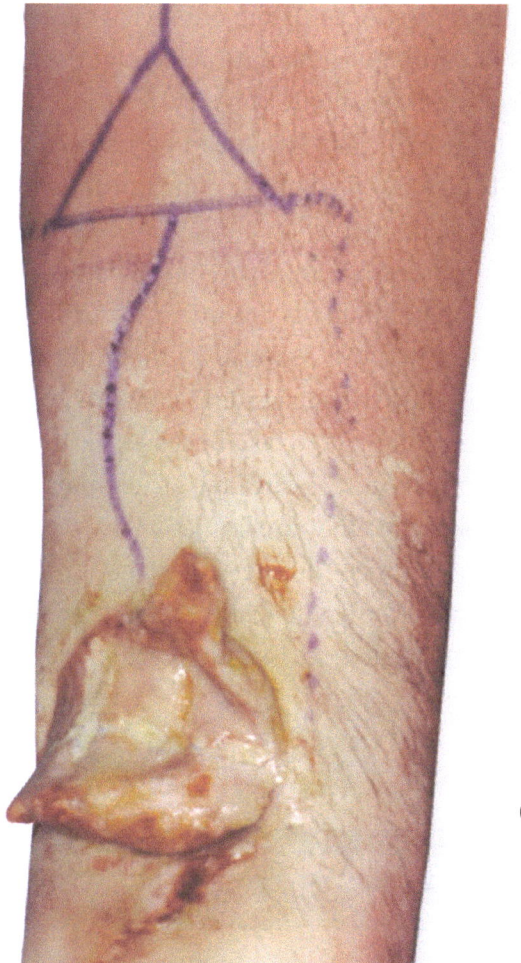

d

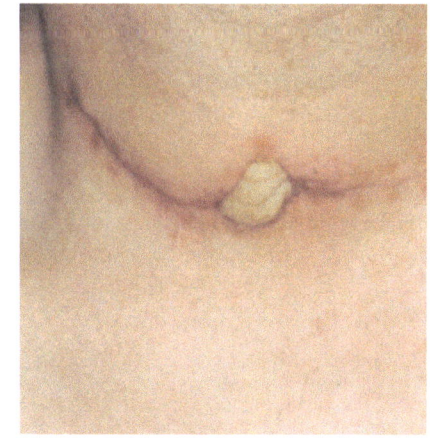

e

Composite tissue consisting of mucosal lining and strips of cartilage is the most adequate tissue that is currently available for airway wall reconstruction (Table 6.5). This tissue can be used to repair critical airway segments. Flap prefabrication needs to be done to allow for survival of the cartilage component. Overgrowth of the bare cartilage by the mucosal lining is essential for cartilage survival but is a slow process. In the clinical case, relining of the cartilage grafts (1 cm wide) was still incomplete after 20 days. Because of the slow remucosalization, the cartilage strips may undergo necrosis when they are immediately exposed to the airway lumen during a 1-stage procedure. After flap prefabrication, the cartilage grafts are sufficiently healed so that the cartilage support remains preserved.

Table 6.5. Composite tissue - fascia, buccal mucosa, elastic ear cartilage

- Primary healing
- Staged reconstruction
- Prefabrication during 1 month
- Small gain in anterior airway lumen expansion
- Is it worth the effort of flap prefabrication?

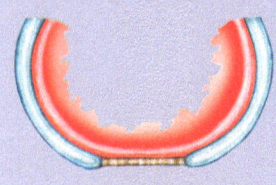 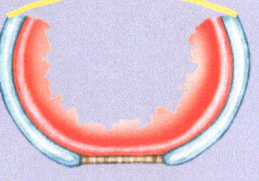

Table 6.6. Classification (from best (1) to worst (6) results) of reconstructive tissue for tracheal repair

1. Revascularized tracheal allografts (+ immunosuppression) and autografts (not available in cases of stenosis).
2. Cartilage graft-Oral mucosa-Blood supply (Prefabrication).
3. Buccal mucosa-Blood supply.
4. Cartilage graft.
5. Vascularized soft tissue.
6. Preserved tracheal allografts-synthetic material.

The combination 'buccal mucosa-fascia' can be used in a 1-stage operation and is our first choice option for the correction of restenoses and long segment stenoses (Table 6.6). Compared to the composite tissue 'buccal mucosa-fascia', the additional gain in airway lumen obtained with the combination 'buccal mucosa-cartilage-fascia' is small and one may wonder if the additional gain in airway lumen is worth the effort of flap prefabrication.

BIBLIOGRAPHY

Ahn ST, Mustoe TA. Effects of ischemia on ulcer wound healing: a new model in the rabbit ear. Ann Plast Surg 1990;24:17-23.

Bain WM, Harrington JW, Thomas LE, Schaefer SD. Head and neck manifestations of gastroesophageal reflux. Laryngoscope 1983;94:516-9.

Catty RMC. Healing and contraction in experimental full thickness wounds in the human. Br J Surg 1965;52:542-8.

Chen CW. Trabeculectomy with simultaneous topical application of Mitomycin-C in refractory glaucoma. J Ocul Pharmacol Ther 1990;6:175-82.

Cheng ATL, Backer CL, Holinger LD, Dunham ME, Mavroudis C, Gonzalez-Crussi F. Histopathologic changes after pericardial patch tracheoplasty. Arch Otolaryngol Head Neck Surg 1997;132:1069-72.

Correa AJ, Reinsch L, Sanders DL, Huang S, Deriso W, Duncavage JA, Garrett CG. Inhibition of subglottic stenosis with mitomycin C in the canine model. Ann Otol Rhinol Laryngol 1999;188:1053-60.

Cotton RT. The problem of pediatric laryngotracheal stenosis: a clinical and experimental study on the efficacy of autogeneous cartilage grafts placed between the vertically divided halves of the posterior lamina of the cricoid cartilage. Laryngoscope 1991;101(suppl 56).

Eliachar I, Marcovich A, Shai Y. Rotary door flap in laryngotracheal reconstruction. Arch Otolaryngol 1984;110:585-90.

Eliachar I, Roberts JJ, Welker KB, Tucker HM. Advantages of the rotary door flap in laryngotracheal reconstruction:is skeletal support necessary? Ann Otol Rhinol Laryngol 1989;98:37-40.

Eliachar R, Eliachar I, Esclamado R, Gramlich T, Strome M. Can topical Mitomycin prevent laryngotracheal stenosis? Laryngoscope 1999;109:1594-600.

Friedman M, Grybauskas V, Ioriumi DM, Skolnik E, Chilis T. Sternomastoid myoperiosteal flap for reconstruction of the subglottic larynx. Ann Otol Rhinol Laryngol 1987;96:163-9.

Grillo HC, Donahue DM, Mathiesen DJ, Wain JC, Wright CD. Postintubation tracheal stenosis: treatment and results. J Thorac Cardiovasc Surg 1995;109:486-92.

Grillo HC, Wright CD, Vlahakes GJ, MacGillivray TE. Management of congenital tracheal stenosis by means of slide tracheoplasty or resection and reconstruction, with long-term follow-up of growth after slide tracheoplasty. J Thorac Cardiovasc Surg 2002;123:45-152.

Heberhold C, Stein M, von Falkenhausen M. Long-term results of homograft reconstruction of the trachea in childhood. Laryngorhinootologie 1999;78:692-6.

Idriss FC, DeLeon SY, Ilbawi MN et al. Tracheopasty with pericardial patch for extensive tracheal stenosis in infants and children. J Thorac Cardiovasc Surg 1984;88:527-36.

Jacobs JP, Quintesseizza JA, Andrews T, Burke RP, Spektor Z, Deluis RE, Smith RJ, Elliott MJ, Heberhold C. Tracheal allograft reconstruction: the total North America and wordwide pediatric experiences. Ann Thorac Surg 1999;68:1043-51.

Jaquiss RDB, Lusk PR, Spray TL, et al. Repair of long segment tracheal stenosis in infancy. J Thorac Cardiovasc Surg 1995;110:1504-12.

Krespi YP, Biller HF, Baek SM. Tracheal reconstruction with a pleuroperiosteal flap. Otolaryngol Head Neck Surg 1983;91:610-14.

Monnier P, Savary M, Chapius G. Cricotracheal resection for pediatric subglottic stenosis: Update of the Lausanne experience. Acta Otorhinolaryngol Belg 1995;49:373-82.

Monnier P, Lang F, Savary M. Cricotracheal resection for adult and pediatric subglottic stenoses: similarities and differences. Operative Techniques in Otolaryngology-Head and Neck Surgery 1999;10:311-5.

Nordin U. The trachea and cuff-induced tracheal injury. Acta Otolaryngol, suppl 1977;345:1-77.

Pearson FG, Gullane P. Subglottic resection with primary tracheal anastomosis: Including synchronous laryngotracheal reconstruction. Semin Thorac Cardiovasc Surg 1996;8:381-91.

Rahbar R, Shapshay S, Healy G. Mitomycin: effect on laryngeal and tracheal stenosis, benefits, and complications. Ann Otol Rhinol Laryngol 2001:1-6.

Rethi A. An operation for cicatricial stenosis of the larynx. J. Laryngol Otol 1956;70:283-93.

Samadi DS, Jacobs IN, Walsh D et al. Adenovirus-mediated ex vivo gene transfer of human vascular endothelial growth factor in a rabbit laryngotracheal reconstruction model. Ann Otol Rhinol Laryngol 2002;111:295-301.

Singh G, Wilson MR, Foster CS. Mitomycin eye drops as treatment for pterygium. Ophtalmology 1988;95:813-21.

Stauffer JL, Olson DE, Petty TL. Complications and consequences of endotracheal intubation and tracheotomy. Am J Med 1981;70:65-76.

Ward RF, April MM. Mitomycin-C in the treatment of tracheal cicatrix after tracheal reconstruction. Int J Pediatr Otol 1998;44:221-6.

Wright CD, Graham BB, Grillo HC, Wain JC, Mathisen DJ. Pediatric tracheal surgery. Ann Thorac Surg 2002;74:308-14.

Zahn JM, Pierrot D, Chevillard M, Puchelle E. Dynamics of cell movement during the wound repair of human surface respiratory epithelium. Biorheology 1992;29:459-65.

CHAPTER 7

Other Vascularized Reconstructive Tissue for Laryngeal Repair

Epiglottic pull down in larynx reconstruction

Revascularization of the larynx as a treatment for chondroradionecrosis

Local skin flaps

Tracheostomy closure

Tracheal stenosis after laryngectomy

Multiple reconstructions using local, regional, or distal tissue have been described for use inside laryngeal defects. Three reconstructions using local tissues have proven reliable in specific situations. The epiglottic pull down technique can be used to reconstruct anterior laryngeal defects after frontal laryngectomy and the pectoralis major muscle can be used as a tool for laryngeal revascularization in cases of chondroradionecrosis. Flaps of neck skin may be used to close a tracheostomy or they may be used to expand a tracheal stenosis after laryngectomy.

1. Epiglottic pull down in larynx reconstruction

The term epiglottic laryngoplasty (SEDLACEK 1965, KAMBIC et al. 1976, TUCKER et al. 1979) refers to the reconstruction that is done by undermining the epiglottis and advancing it inferiorly and laterally to reconstruct the larynx following anterior hemilaryngectomy (Fig. 7.1, 7.2, 7.3).

The main utility of this procedure is for the management of selected carcinoma of the glottis invading the anterior commissure. Tumors originating in the anterior commissure are not an indication since they have a propensity for early invasion of the preepiglottic space.

Postoperative aspiration and breathy voice may be attributed to insufficient closure of the glottis anteriorly. Alternatively, tumors of the anterior glottis may also be treated by supracricoid laryngectomy (SCL) with cricohyoidoepiglottopexy (CHEP) (LACCOUREYE et al. 1997, 1998).

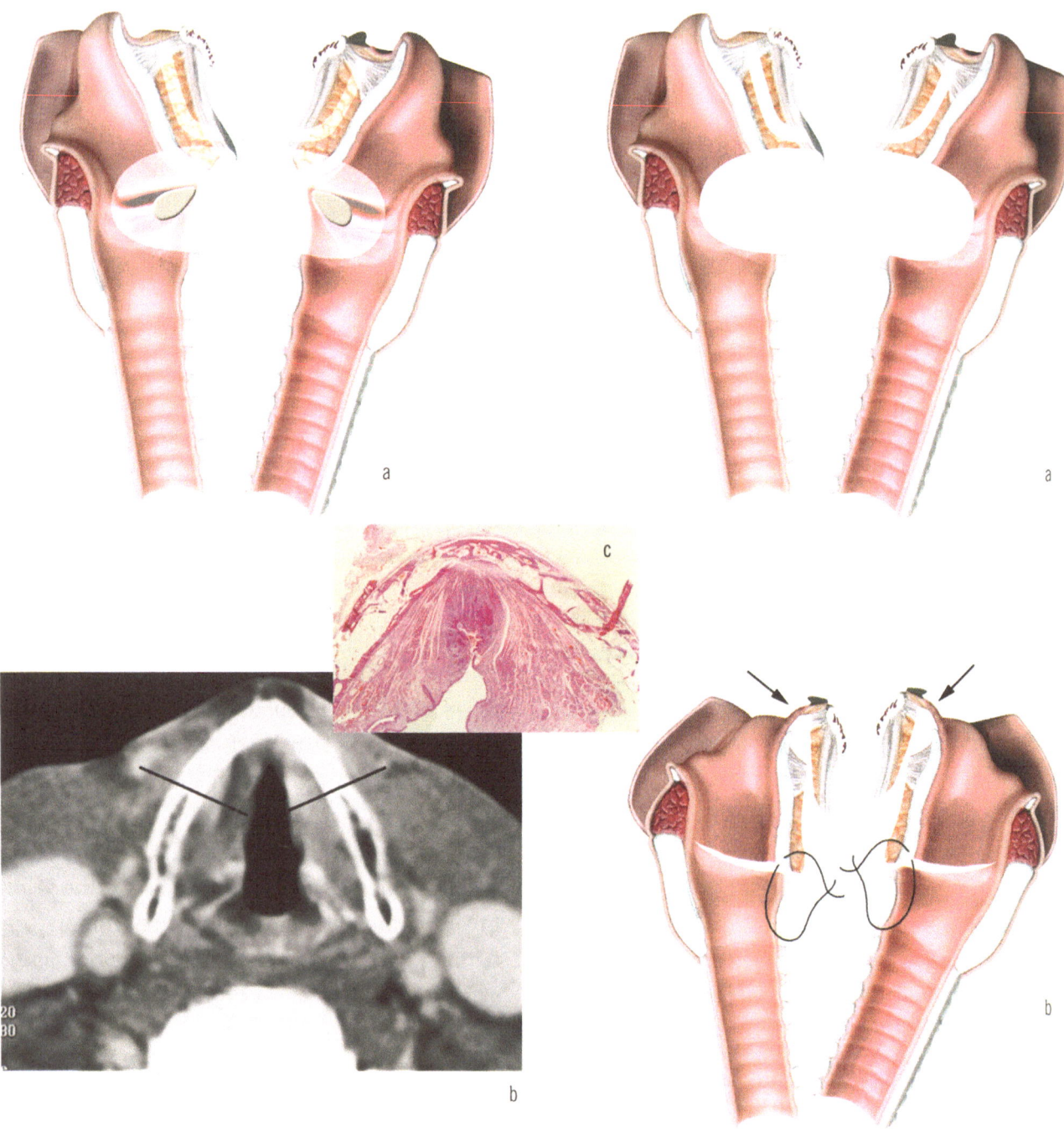

Figure 7.1. Frontal laryngectomy.
a. Laryngeal model-Indication for frontal laryngecto-
my. Tumor of the anterior glottis. Both false cords and
true cords are resected. One arytenoid can be included
in the resection.
b. Axial CT scan. Frontal hemilaryngectomy (black
lines) for tumor at anterior commissure.
c. Histology of resection specimen. Tumor visible in
anterior commissure.

Figure 7.2.
Laryngeal model-Epiglottoplasty.
An epiglottic flap is created by dissecting the fascia and
fat off the anterior surface of the epiglottis up towards
the vallecula (a). The epiglottis is sutured inferiorly to
the cut edge of the cricothyroid ligament and laterally
to the thyroid cartilage (b). The vallecular mucosa
(arrows) remains intact.

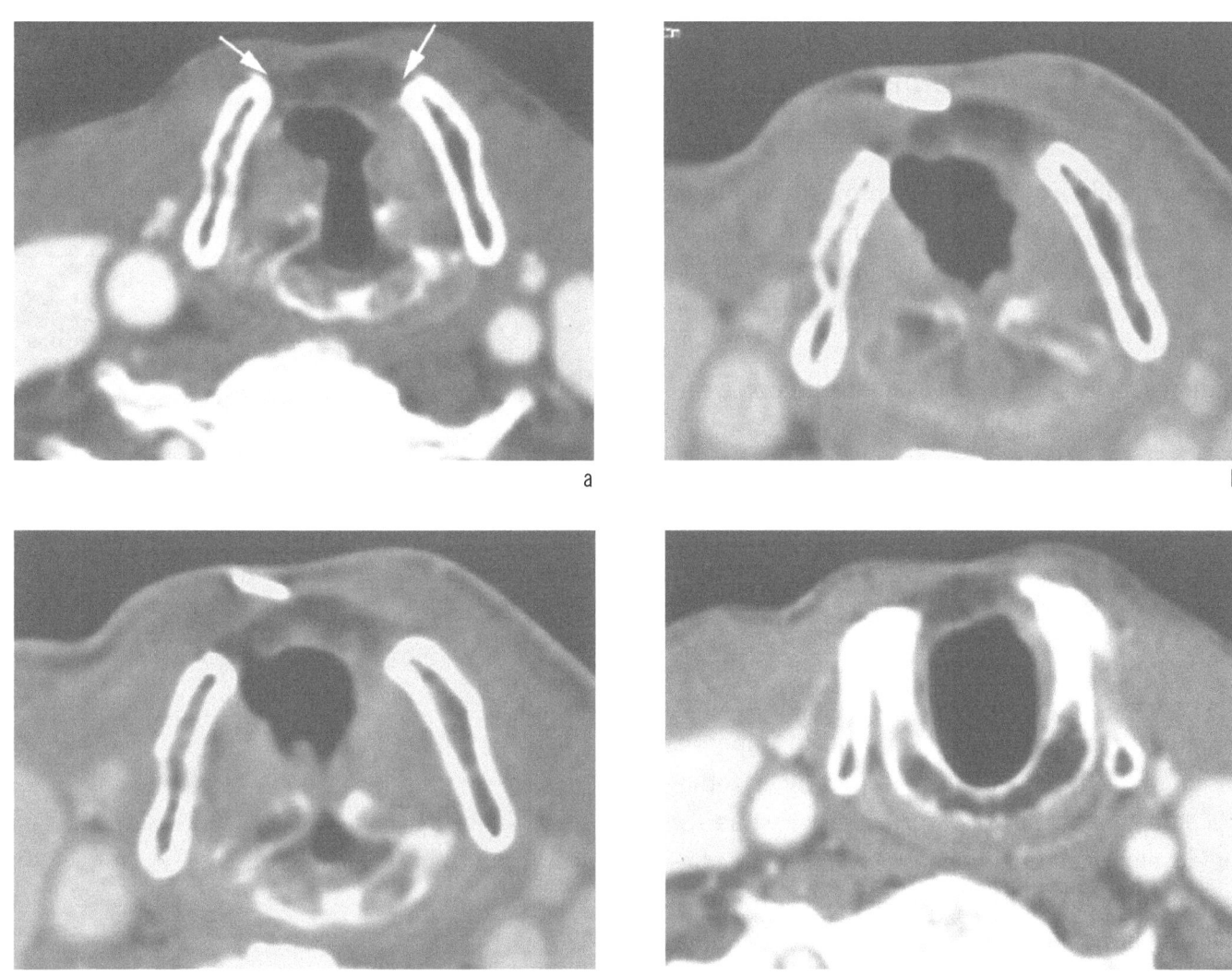

Figure 7.3. CT scan-postoperative.
a. Situation after reconstruction-glottic level. CT scan during quiet breathing. Epiglottis is visible between arrows.

b., c. Situation after reconstruction-glottic level. CT scan during phonation. Posterior closure by adduction of both arytenoids. Gap remains anteriorly.
d. Situation after reconstruction-subglottic level.

2. *Revascularization of the larynx as a treatment for chondroradionecrosis*

The pectoralis major flap has proven reliable in severe cases of chondroradionecrosis of the larynx. In these cases, the pectoralis major muscle serves as external cover and as a tool for larynx revascularization.

Radionecrosis of the larynx is an uncommon treatment complication, with an incidence of about 1% (PARSONS 1994) and cases of laryngeal necrosis occurring more than 10 years after radiation treatment have been described (O'BRIEN 1996). Recurrent tumor is not a concern after such a long delay, but one has to be aware that rarely second primary tumors may originate from an irradiated larynx (ERKAL et al. 2001). The late effects after radiation treatment are largely due to impaired vascular and lymphatic flow caused by endothelial damage and fibrosis. Certain risk factors for the development of laryngeal necrosis after radiation treatment have been described, including diabetes mellitus, arterial hypertension, and continued smoking.

Recent studies showed that even in advanced cases of laryngeal necrosis a functional larynx can be retained after intensive treatment with hyperbaric oxygen therapy (FELDMEIER et al. 1993; FERGUSON et al. 1987). In severe cases, surgical intervention with removal of necrotic tissue is indicated (BALM et al. 1993; McGUIRT 1997). If possible, the larynx is spared. The resultant wound is reconstructed with healthy, non-irradiated, well-vascularized tissue, improving the vascularization of the larynx. A pedicled pectoralis muscle is well suited for this purpose (Fig. 7.4).

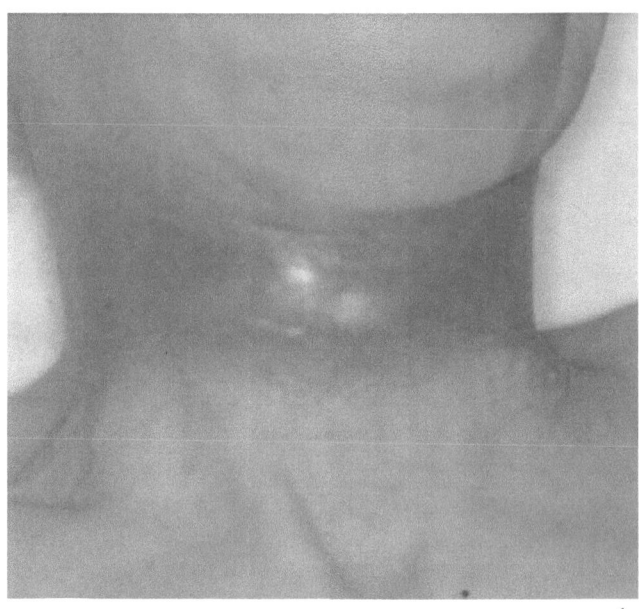

a1

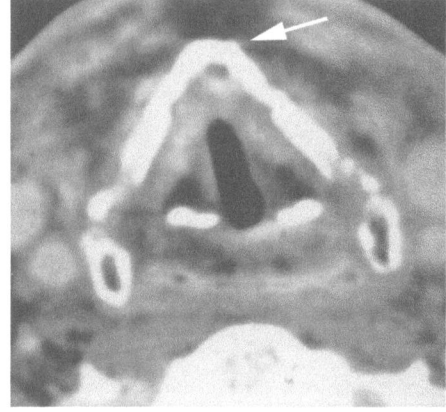

a2

Figure 7.4.
Treatment of chondroradionecrosis with pectoralis major muscle.
a. Preoperative situation.
Patient presenting with hoarseness, dyspnea and pain in the laryngeal region 14 years after radiotherapy for laryngeal cancer.
a.1. Anterior view. The patient present with inflammatory changes in the overlying skin and a cutaneous fistula is present.
a.2. Axial CT scan. Intra- and extralaryngeal soft tissue thickening is seen. Cutaneous fistula is indicated by arrow.

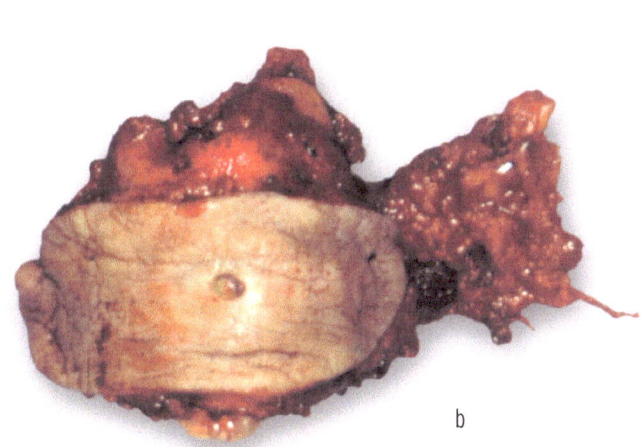

b

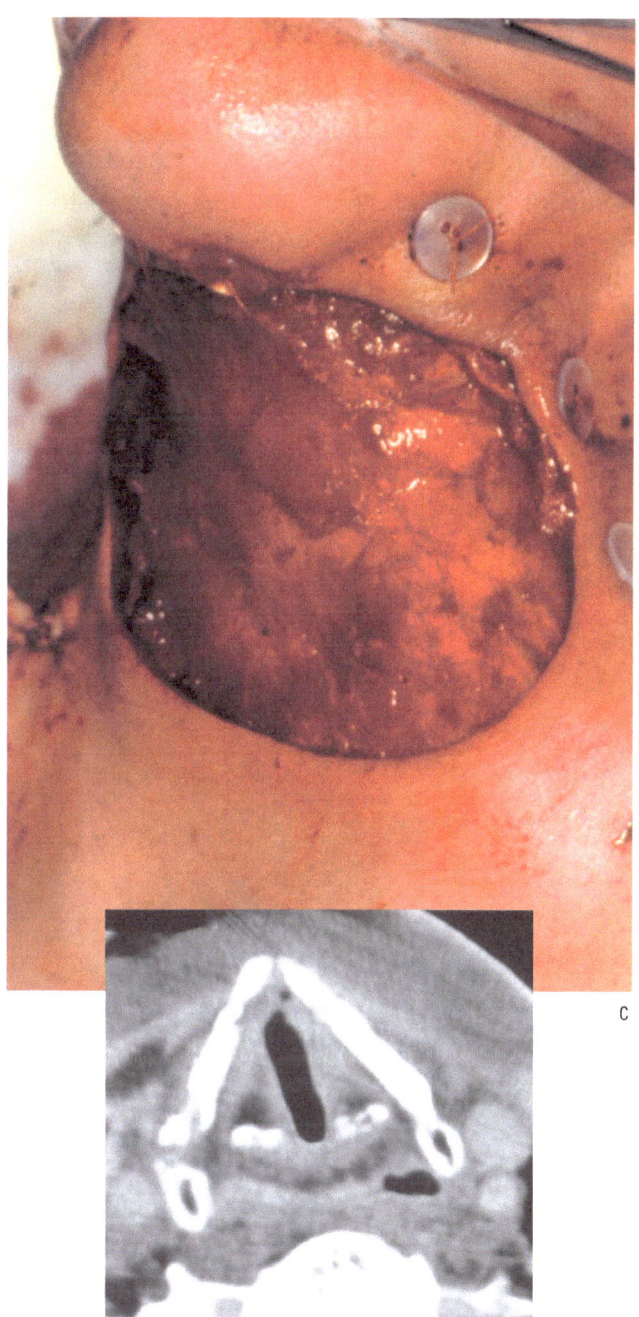

c

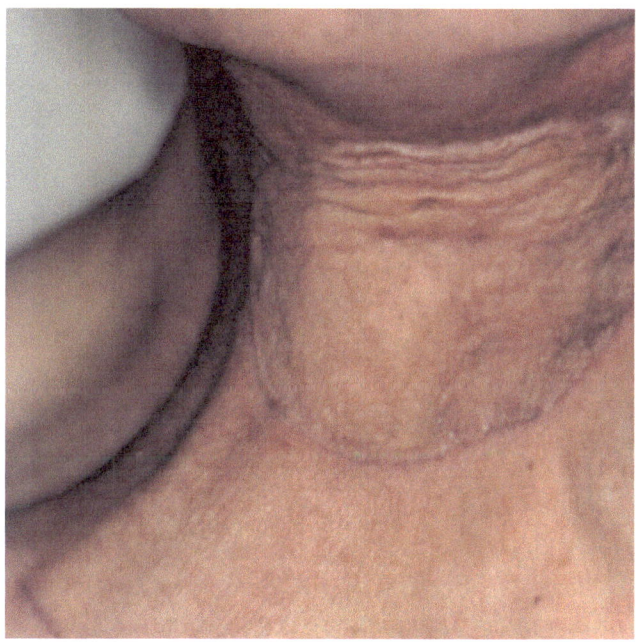

d

e

Figure 7.4. Treatment of chondroradionecrosis with pectoralis major muscle (continued).
b. Resection specimen. The soft tissues of the neck anterior from the big neck vessels are resected.
c. Neck defect repaired with pectoralis major muscle. The muscle will be grafted with a split-thickness skin graft.
d. Skin grafted pectoralis muscle after healing (better
color match than with myocutaneous flap).
e. Axial contrast enhanced CT image 3 months after transfer of pectoralis major flap. The laryngocutaneous fistula is closed by the overlying pectoralis major muscle. The internal site of the larynx shows a decongestion of its soft tissues.

3. Local skin flaps

3.A. Tracheostomy closure

The skin around the tracheostomy is the optimal tissue for closure of a long-standing tracheostomy. Clinical examples are visible in fig. 7.5, 7.6, 7.7 and 7.8.

Creating of an anterior convexity with reconstructive tissue without cartilage support is not possible. How the anterior augmentation of the airway lumen, visible in figure 7.5.b, can be obtained is explained in fig. 7.6 and 7.7.

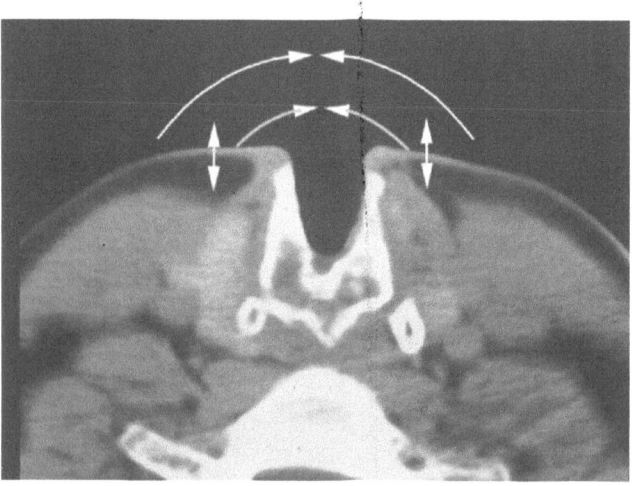

a

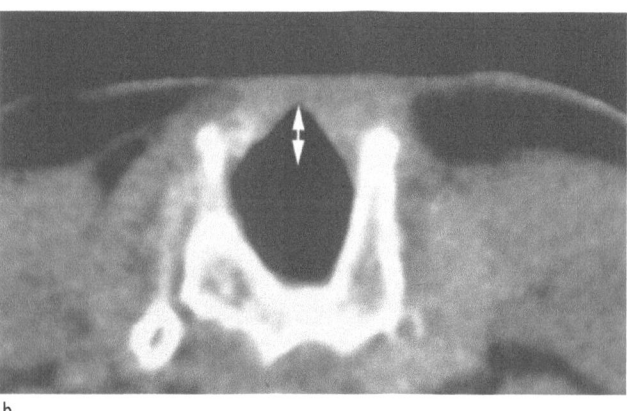

b

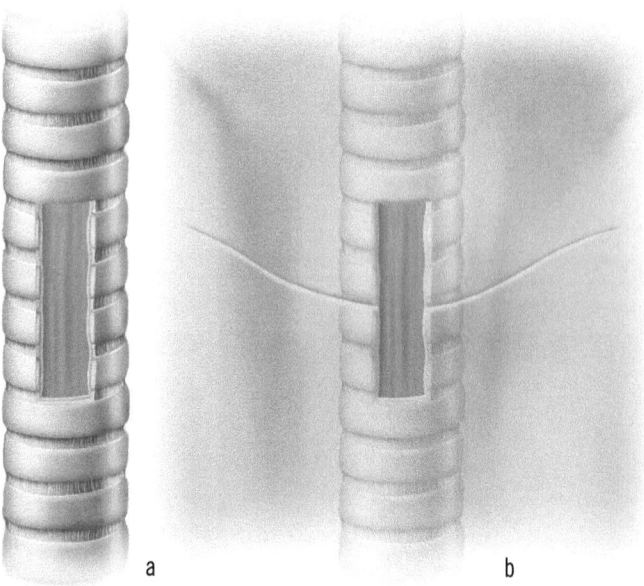

a   b

Figure 7.5.
Closure of a long-standing stomy.
a. Before closure. This patient had an anterior defect of the cricoid cartilage after a motor vehicle accident. There is a sufficient airway lumen and the anterior defect can be closed by inversion of the surrounding neck skin. The defect is closed in 2 layers (arrows).
b. After closure. The anterior defect is closed by skin. An anterior augmentation (double arrow) of the airway lumen is visible.

Figure 7.6.
Schematic presentation of tracheostomy closure with local skin flaps.
a. Anterior tracheal defect.
b. The neck skin is sutured to the defect to form a tracheostomy.
c. Closure of tracheostomy 6 weeks after formation of tracheostomy. Skin flaps are developed around the airway defect. The skin flaps are dissected. The edges of the flaps are removed (gray area).
d. The inverted skin flaps remain attached at the margins of the defect.
e. The upper and lower neck skin flap are undermined.
f. Situation after closure. A second layer closure is obtained by the upper and lower neck skin flap.

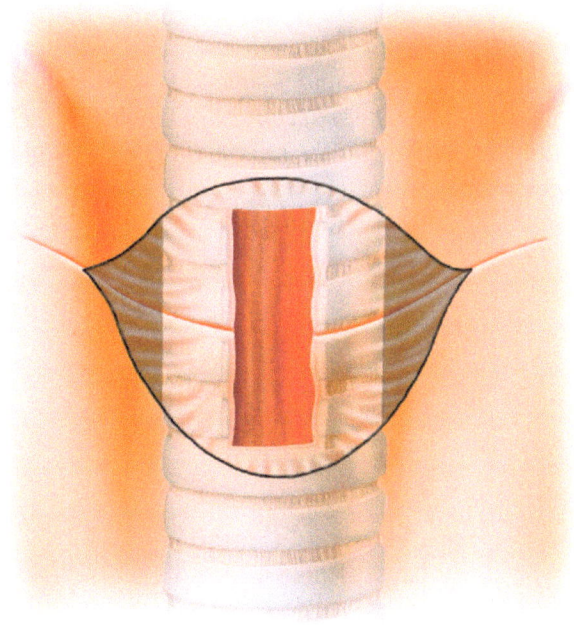

c

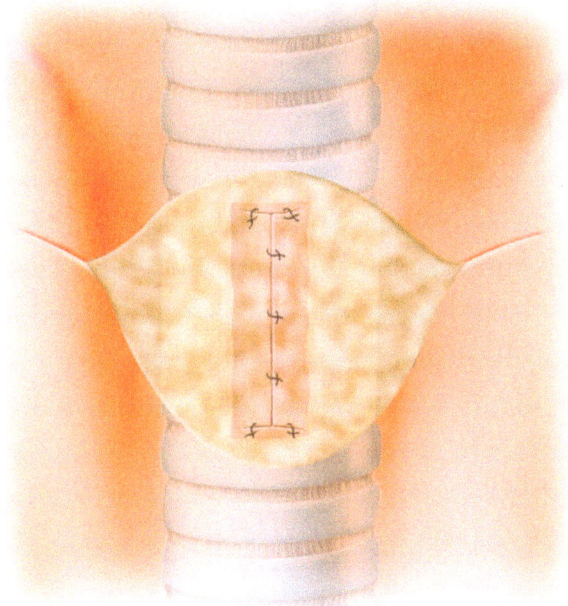

d

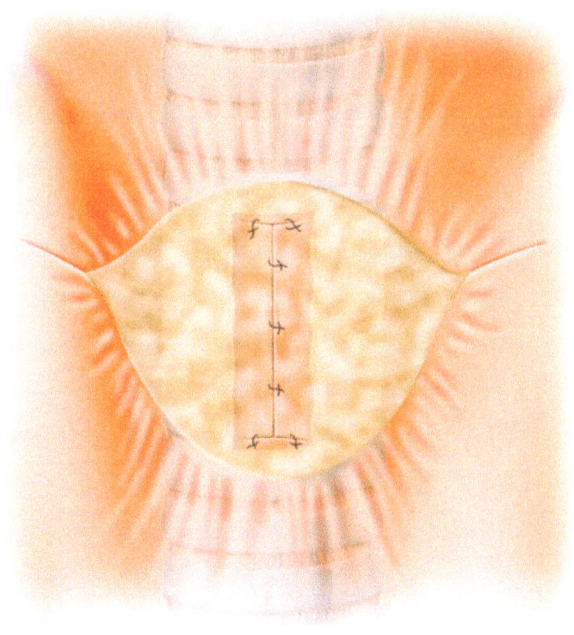

e

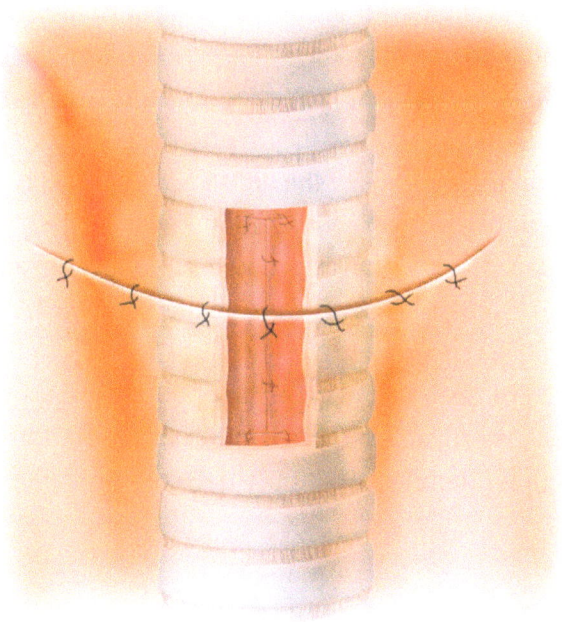

f

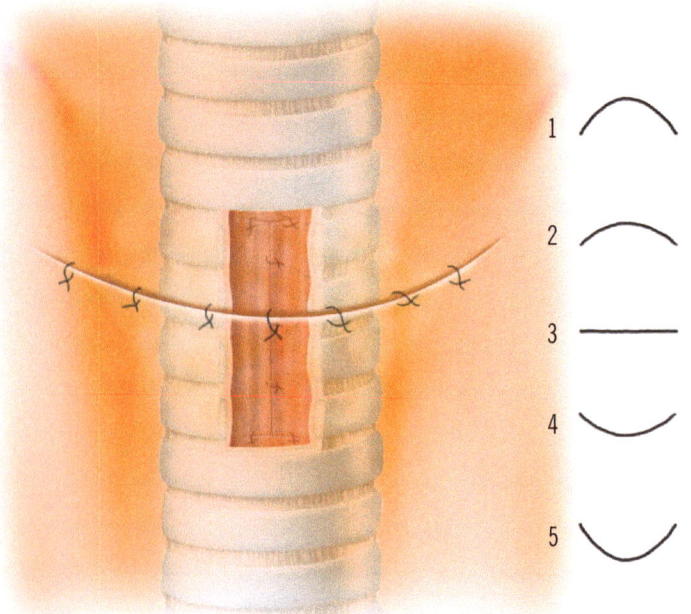

Figure 7.7. Closed tracheostome.

A cross section at 2 and 4 shows an anterior lumen augmentation. The skin convexity is obtained by the support provided by the proximal (1) and distal (5) intact tracheal cartilage ring. The cross section at 3 shows a flat reconstruction.

Anterior airway defects can be closed easily by surrounding neck skin as long as the airway lumen at the defect is sufficient for normal respiration. Important is a waiting period of at least 4 to 6 weeks between formation and closure of the tracheostomy because the inverted neck skin flaps rely on the margins of the defect for their survival. Ingenious reconstructions may be described for similar defects. They are however usually examples of reconstructive 'over acting' (HOMMA et al. 2003).

The neck skin can also facilitate the creation of a tracheostomy after tracheal autotransplantation to extended hemilaryngectomy defects (Fig. 7.8).

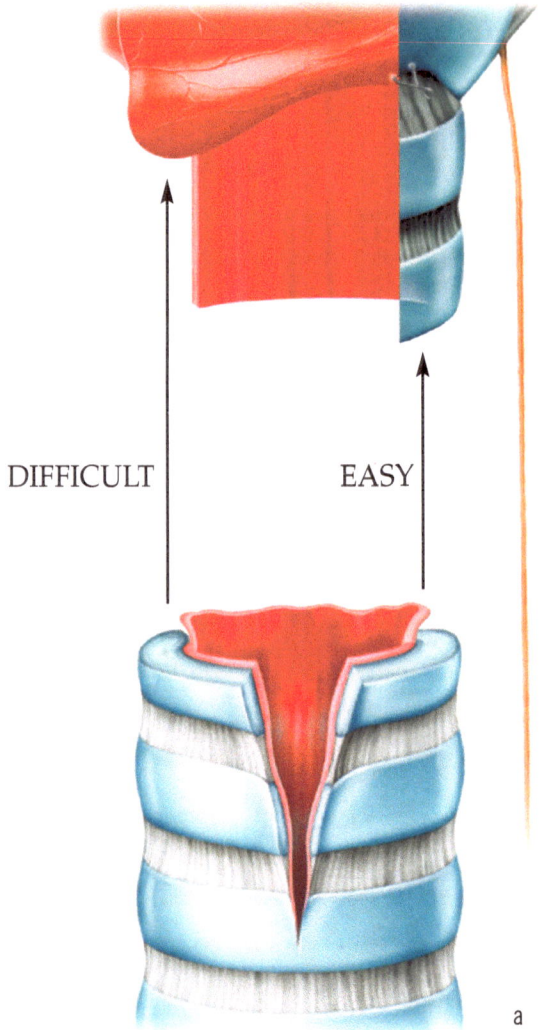

DIFFICULT   EASY

Figure 7.8.

The difficult tracheostomy after tracheal autotransplantation.

a. In some patients, mobilization of the mediastinal trachea after tracheal autotransplantation may be difficult; for example after radiotherapy.

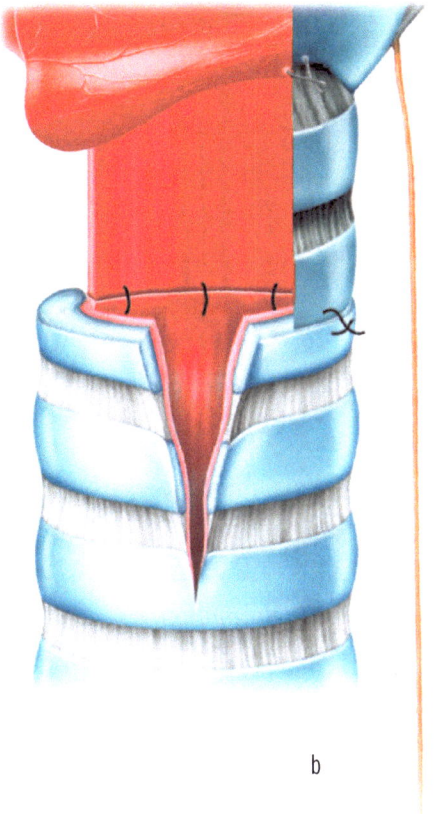

b

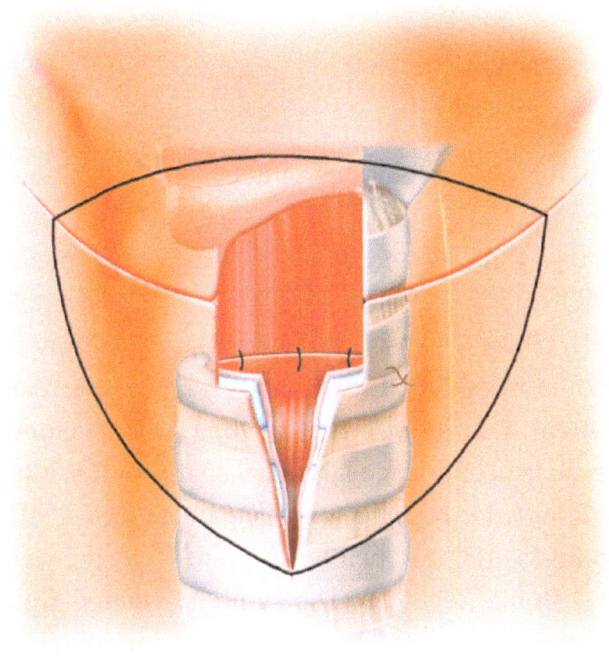

d

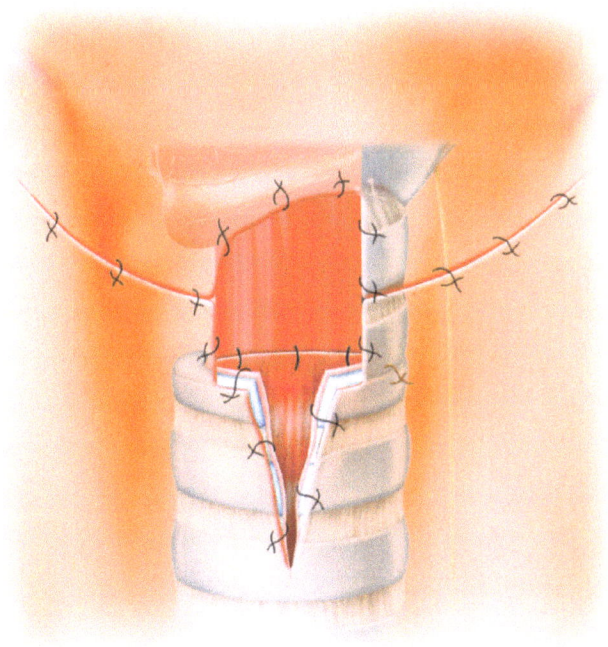

c

Figure 7.8.
The difficult tracheostomy after tracheal autotransplantation (continued).
b. The mediastinal trachea can be sutured to the tracheal cartilage remnant at the uninvolved side (gap of less than 2 cm).
c. The neck skin flaps are sutured to the trachea and to the reconstructed larynx.
d. After 4-6 weeks, the tracheostomy is closed by developing neck skin flaps that are inverted to close the airway opening.

3.B. Tracheal stenosis after laryngectomy

Local neck skin flaps can also be used to augment a stenotic tracheostomy after total laryngectomy. Augmentation consists in interrupting the line of circular scar contracture and inserting cutaneous flaps by using some form of Z-plasty (MONTGOMERY 1979, LORE 1988). An example of tracheal stenosis after total laryngectomy is shown in fig. 7.9. It concers a 74-year-old female patient who underwent a total laryngectomy because of end-stage laryngeal stenosis after intubation. After laryngectomy, she developed a 90% stenosis 1.5 cm below the level of the tracheostome (Fig. 7.9). The stenosis resulted from pressure excercised by the tracheal cannula. The stenosis was initially treated by laser and Mitomycin applications without success.

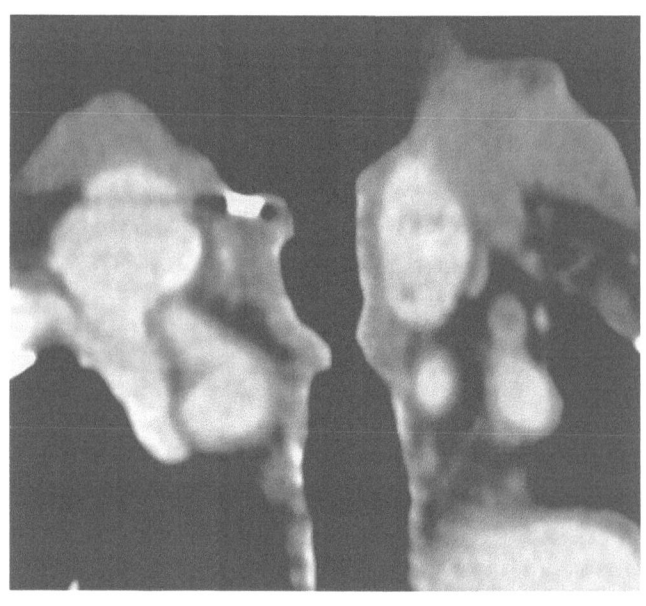

b. CT scan-Coronal reformation.
The stenosis is visible 1.5 cm below the tracheostomy.

The stenosis was treated by longitudinal incision of the upper 2 cm of trachea and insertion of the lower neck skin flap into the defect (Fig. 7.10, 7.11).

Figure 7.9.
Tracheal stenosis after laryngectomy-before correction.
a. CT scan-Sagittal refomation.

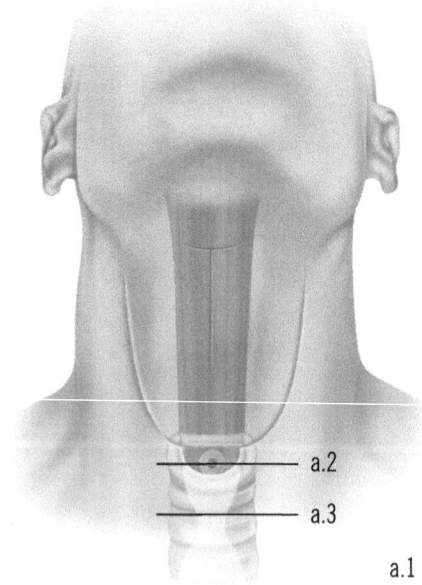

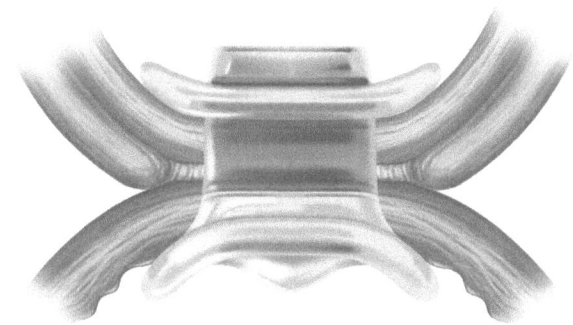

a.2

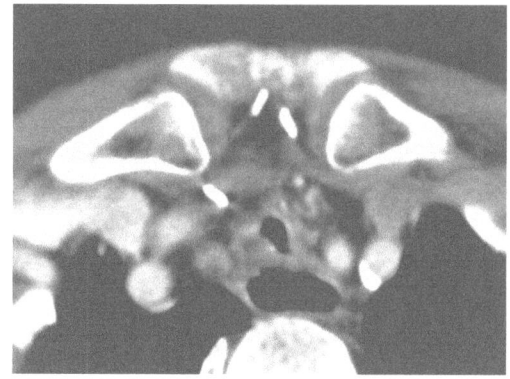

a.3

Figure 7.10. Tracheal stenosis after laryngectomy-correction.

a. a.1. Schematic presentation of stenosis.

a.2. Axial section at level of voice prosthesis.

a.3. CT axial section at level of stenosis.

b. Incision of neck skin and longitudinal incision of trachea.

c. Suturing of lower neck skin flap in anterior tracheal defect.

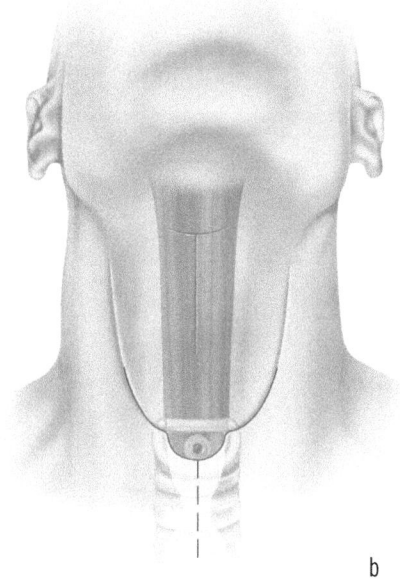

b

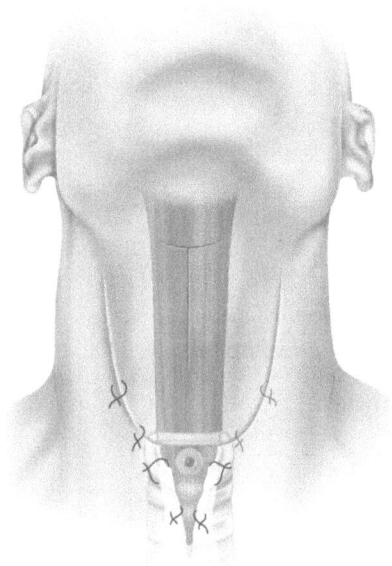

c

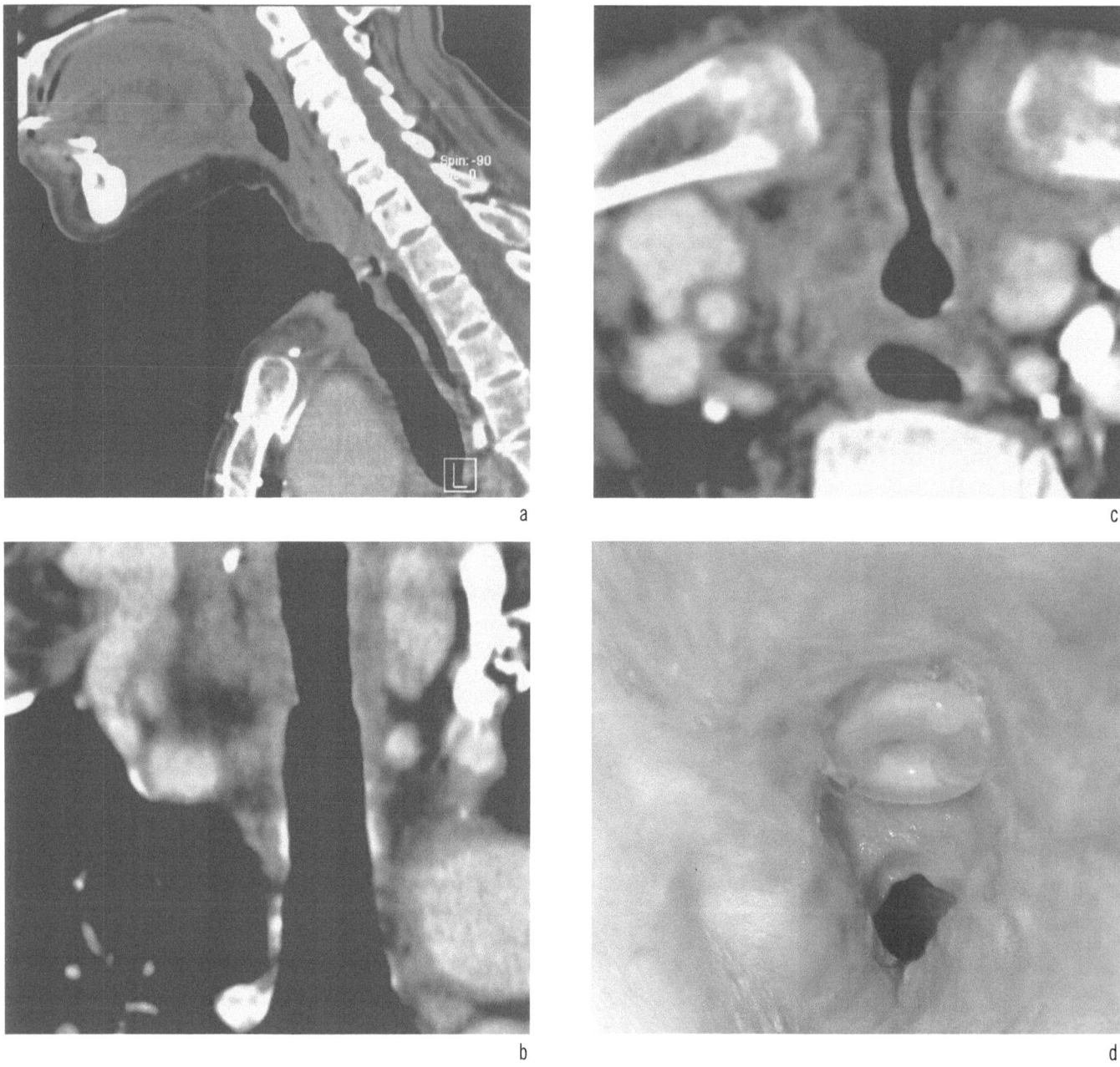

Figure 7.11. Tracheal stenosis after laryngectomy- after correction.
a. CT scan-Sagittal reformation.
b. CT scan-Coronal reformation.

c. Axial CT scan. Neck skin is sutured to tracheal incision.
d. Clinical picture.

BIBLIOGRAPHY

Balm AJ, Hilgers FJ, Baris G, et al. Pectoralis major muscle transposition: an adjunct to laryngeal preservation in severe chondroradionecrosis. J Laryngol Otol 1993;107:748-51.

Erkal HS, Mendenhall WM, Amdur RJ, et al. Synchronous and metachronous squamous cell carcinoma of the head and neck mucosal sites. J Clin Oncol 2001;19:1358-62.

Feldmeier JJ, Heimbach RD, Davolt DA, et al. Hyperbaric oxygen as an adjunctive treatment for severe laryngeal necrosis: a report of nine consecutive cases. Undersea Hyperb Med 1993;20:329-35.

Ferguson BJ, Hudson WR, Farmer JC Jr. Hyperbaric oxygen therapy for laryngeal radionecrosis. Ann Otol Rhinol Laryngol 1987;96:1-6.

Homma K, Himi T, Hoki K. A prefabricated osteocutaneous flap for tracheal reconstruction. Plast Rec Surg 2003;111:1688-93.

Kambic V, Radsel Z, Smid L. Laryngeal reconstruction with epiglottis after vertical hemilaryngectomy. J Laryngol Otol 1976;90:467-73.

Laccoureye O, Muscatello L, LaccoureyeL, et al. Supracricoid partial laryngectomy with cricohyoidoepiglottopexy for "early" glottic carcinoma classified as T1-T2N0 invading the anterior commissure. Am J Otolaryngol 1997;18:385-90.

Laccoureye O, Weinstein G, Naudo P, et al. Supracricoid partial laryngectomy after failed laryngeal radiation therapy. Laryngoscope 1998;106:495-8.

Loré JM. An atlas of head and neck surgery (3 rd ed.). W.B. Saunders Company, Philadelphia, 1988.

McGuirt WF. Laryngeal radionecrosis versus recurrent cancer. Otolaryngol Clin North Am 1997;30:243-50.

Montgomery WW. Surgery of the upper respiratory system (2 nd ed.). Lea and Febiger, Philadelphia, 1979.

O'Brien P. Tumour recurrence or treatment sequelae following radiotherapy for larynx cancer. J Surg Oncol 1996;63:130-5.

Parsons JT. The effect of radiation on normal tissues of the head and neck. In: Million RR, Cassisi NJ (eds) Management of head and neck cancer: a multidisciplinary approach. Lippincott, Philadelphia, pp 245-89.

Sedlacek K. (Reconstructive anterior and lateral laryngectomy using the epiglottis as a pedunculated graft). J Ceskoslovenka Otolaryngologie 1965;8:328-34.

Tucker HM, Wood BG, Levine H, et al. Glottic reconstruction after near total laryngectomy. Laryngoscope 1979;89:608-18.

CHAPTER 8

Progress in Head and Neck Reconstruction:

A historical overview based on blood supply of the reconstructive tissue

Autotransplantation of the trachea to extended hemilaryngectomy defects is based on vascular induction of a segment of trachea and is an example of flap prefabrication. Composite tissue reconstruction of tracheal defects is another application of flap prefabrication: composite tissue consisting of fascia, buccal mucosa and ear cartilage can be used for reconstruction of an anterior tracheal defect after a stage of prefabrication to allow for survival of the cartilage component.

The anatomy of the blood supply of the different repair tissues used in head and neck reconstruction will be reviewed in order to position the two laryngotracheal reconstructive prefabrication techniques within that field.

1. Introduction

The defect after major cancer ablative surgery in the head and neck region may be either due to loss of mucosa, skin, soft tissue, cartilage, bone or any combination of these tissues. The surgical defect created by resection of a tumor in the head and neck region may be repaired by primary closure if the loss of tissue is modest in nature. If primary closure is not feasible, then viable tissue should be brought over to repair the surgical defect.

Before the development of antibiotics, a conservative approach was generally taken to wound closure because of the risk of infection and the potential for tissue loss at the wound edges. Local wound care promoted healing through wound contraction (closure via secondary intention healing). The resultant scar was frequently associated with contracture and skin instability.

With the advent of antibiotics following the development of sulfonamides and penicillin in the mid-twentieth century, control of local wound infection permitted a more aggressive approach to wound closure. The use of split-thickness skin grafts allowed successful closure of large wounds. More complex wounds with circulatory impairment, chronic infection, and composite defects, however, were unsuitable for skin-graft coverage. The wounds could not be adequately managed until flaps were developed.

It soon became apparant that flaps could be transferred using normal tissue with intact circulation from an area of noninjury (donor site) to cover complex wounds.

The 2 most important considerations when using reconstructive tissue to close a defect within the head and neck area are to (1) restore form and function with (2) provide tissue that survives within the defect area.

This is a historical review of how head and neck reconstruction became influenced by the anatomy of the blood supply of the repair tissue and by the desire for preservation of form and function of the defect area.

2. The cutaneous circulation

Most of the reconstructive tissues used in the head and neck region consist of skin or have a cutaneous component. The cutaneous circulation (Fig. 8.1) has played an important role in the development of reconstructive techniques. The cutaneous system exists on three anatomic levels (fascia, subcutaneous fat, and skin) and is made up of five recognizable vascular plexuses (fascial, subcutaneous, cutaneous, dermal, and subepidermal) supplied by two types of cutaneous arteries (musculocutaneous and septocutaneous (through intermuscular septa)).

Figure. 8.1. The cutaneous microcirculation.
Anatomic levels: skin (A)-subcutaneous tissue (B) –fascia (C)-muscle (D).
Vascular plexuses: subepidermal (1), dermal (2), cutaneous (3), subcutaneous (4), fascial (5).
Musculocutaneous artery (MCA) and vein (MCV).
Septocutaneous artery (SCA) and vein (SCV).

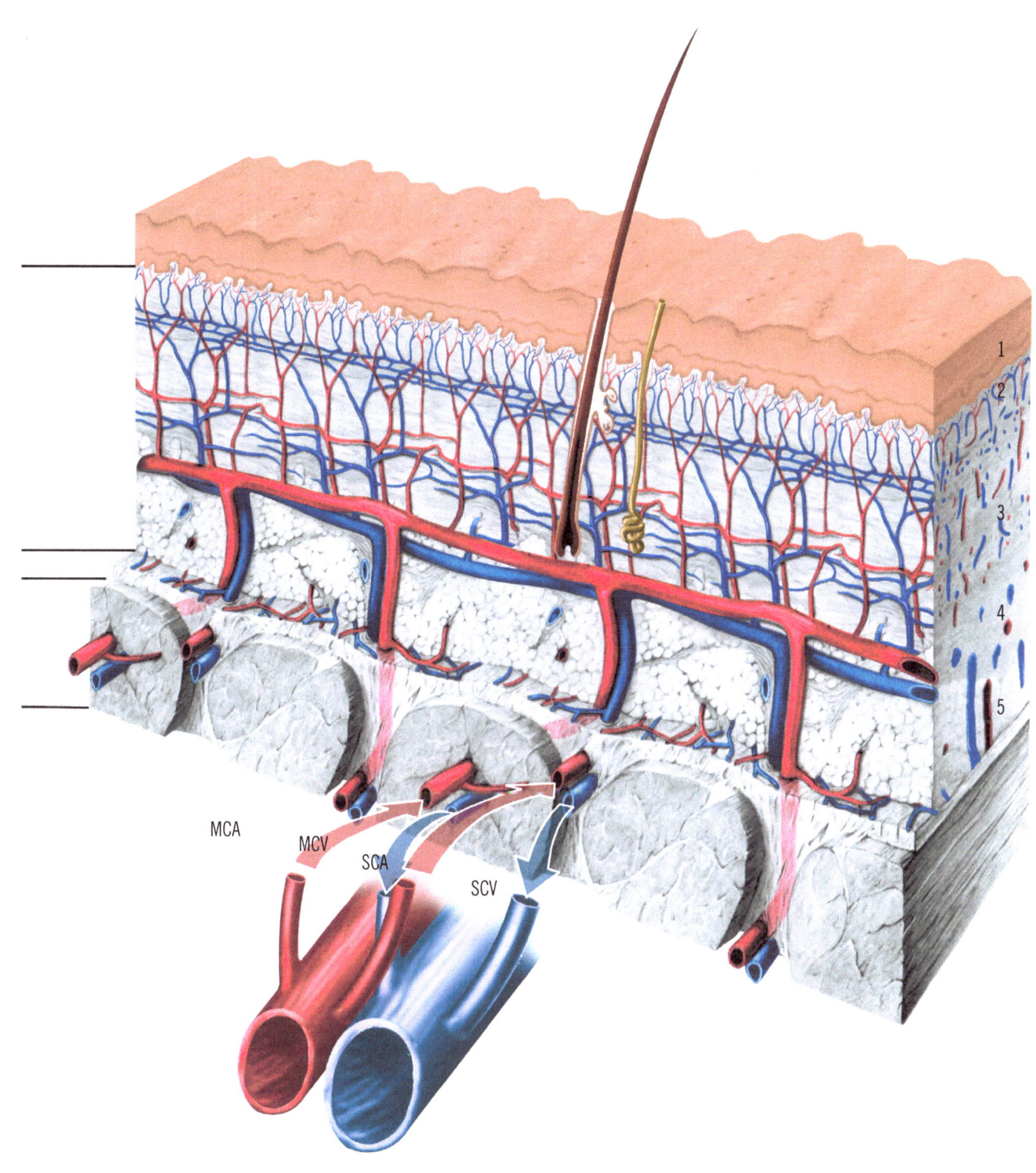

A

B

C

D

1
2
3
4
5

MCA

MCV

SCA

SCV

3. Skin grafts

The first reconstructive tissues consisted of skin grafts. Skin grafts are completely detached prior to being transferred to their recipient beds. In order to survive permanently they have to become reattached, and obtain a fresh blood supply from their new habitat. Depending on the thickness of the graft, 2 types of skin grafts can be distinguished (RUDOLPH 1979, PETRUZZELLI et al. 1994) (Fig. 8.2).

Split-thickness skin graft. Consists of epidermis and a variable portion of dermis. The graft is cut with a dermatome and leaves adnexal remnants, hair follicles, sebaceous glands and/or sweat gland apparatus as foci from which the donor site

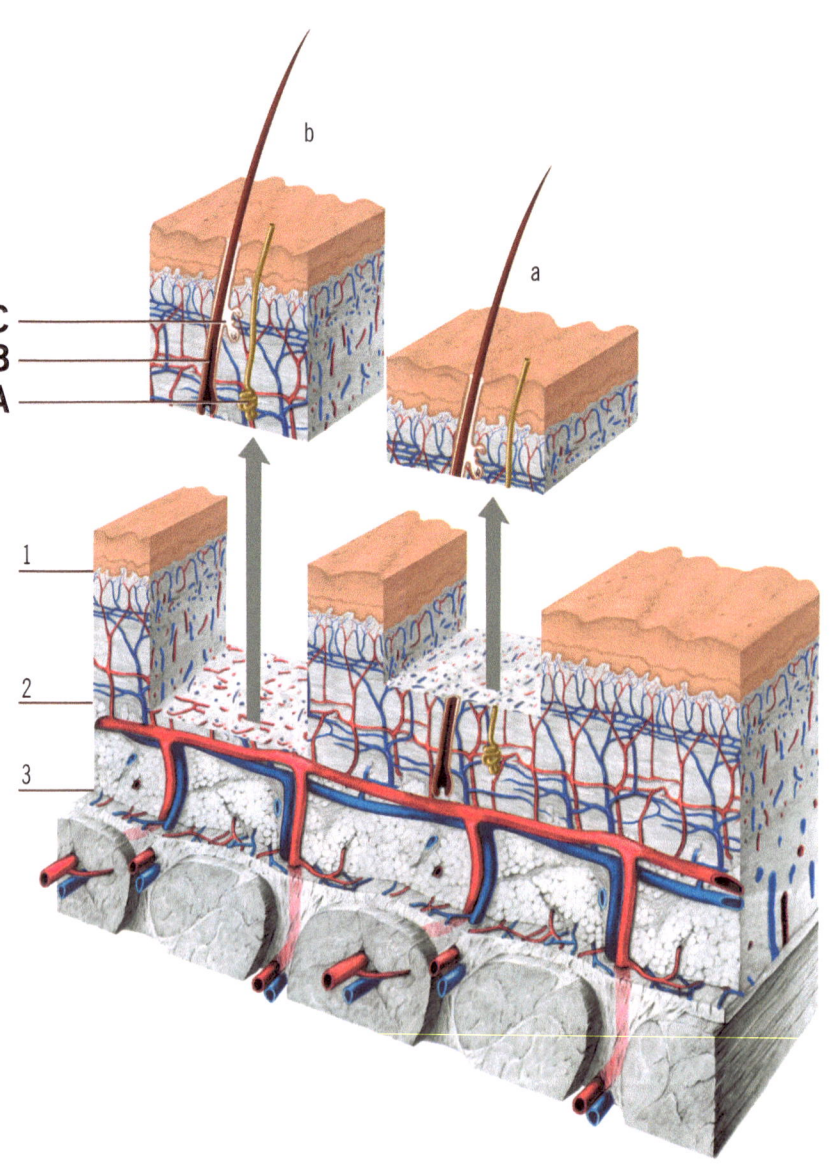

Figure 8.2. Skin graft.
a. Split thickness graft.
b. Full thickness graft
Epidermis(1), dermis (2)
Sweat gland (A), hair follicle (B),
sebaceous gland (C)
3. A skin flap contains the full-thickness
of the skin: epidermis, dermis, and subcu-
taneous tissue.

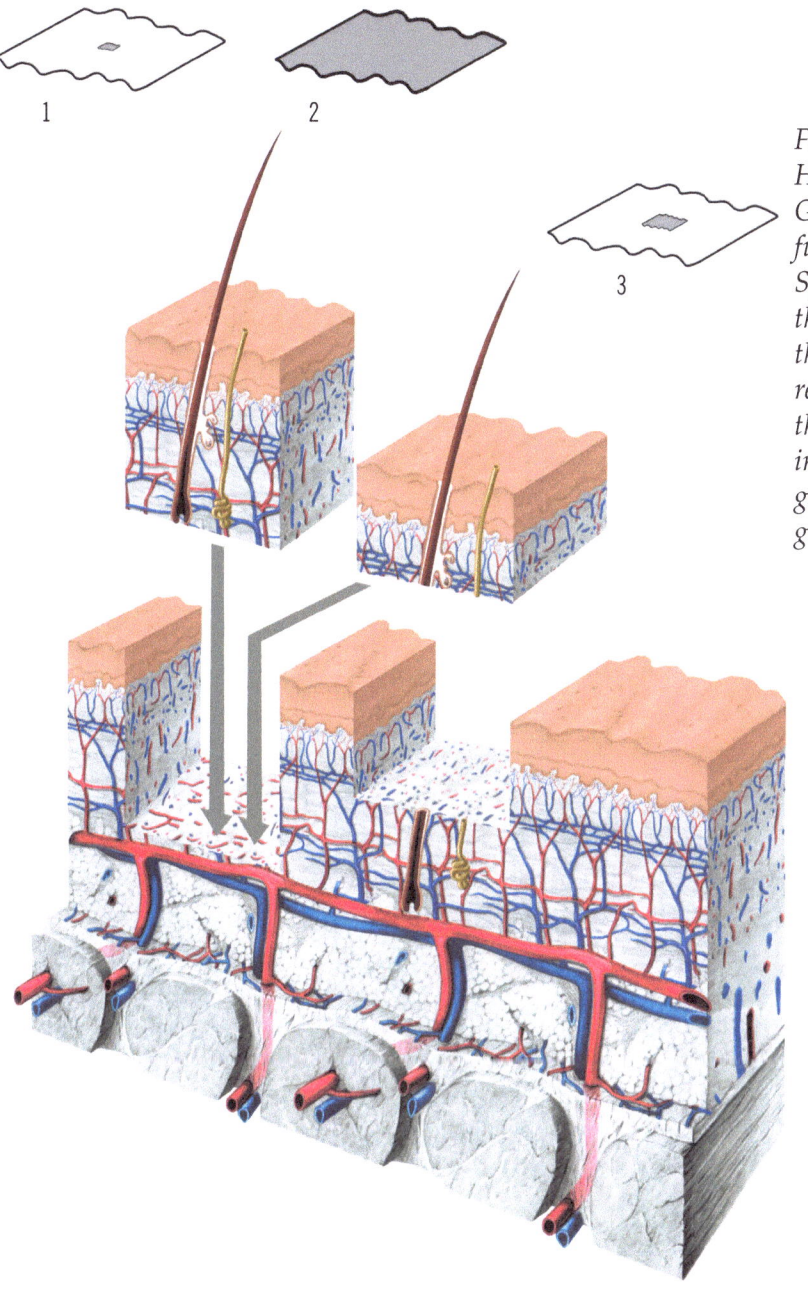

Figure 8.3.
Healing of full-thickness skin defect.
Granulating wounds contract most, while full-thickness grafted wounds do not contract. Split-thickness grafted wounds contract less than granulating wounds but more than full-thickness grafted wounds. Gray area shows remaining surface area after healing. A full-thickness skin defect can heal by secondary intention (1), by using a full-thickness skin graft (2) or by using a split-thickness skin graft (3).

can resurface. As a result the donor area heals spontaneously.

Full-thickness skin graft. Consists of epidermis and the full-thickness of dermis. The full-thickness skin graft is cut with a scalpel and leaves behind no epidermal elements in the donor area from which resurfacing can take place. The donor area has to be closed by direct suture or, if too large for

this, covered with a split-thickness skin graft.

Graft revascularization is achieved by the outgrowth of capillary buds from the recipient area to unite with those on the deep surface of the graft. The recipient bed should contain adequate blood supply and underlying soft tissue to allow for survival of the transplanted tissue.

Contractile fibroblasts, known as myofibroblasts, contract open wounds (GABBIANI et al. 1972, EHRLICH 1988). Skin grafting can affect this process, depending on the type of graft. On a similar wound, full-thickness grafts contract minimally, while split-thickness grafts contract significantly. The inhibitory effect of the full-thickness skin graft upon a contracting wound seems to be due to the inclusion of the full-thickness of the deep dermis, and appears to work via suppression of the myofibroblast population (RUDOLPH et al. 1979, RUDOLPH 1980) (Fig. 8.3).

After tumor resection in the head and neck region, defects are frequently not suitable for skin grafting. A skin graft cannot improve contour if a defect is devoid of subcutaneous tissue and cannot provide stable coverage of exposed bone devoid of periosteum (and cartilage devoid of perichondrium). In situations where the recipient bed is avascular, such as bone not covered by periosteum, or such as post radiotherapy, free skin grafts are not a reconstructive option (Fig. 7.4).

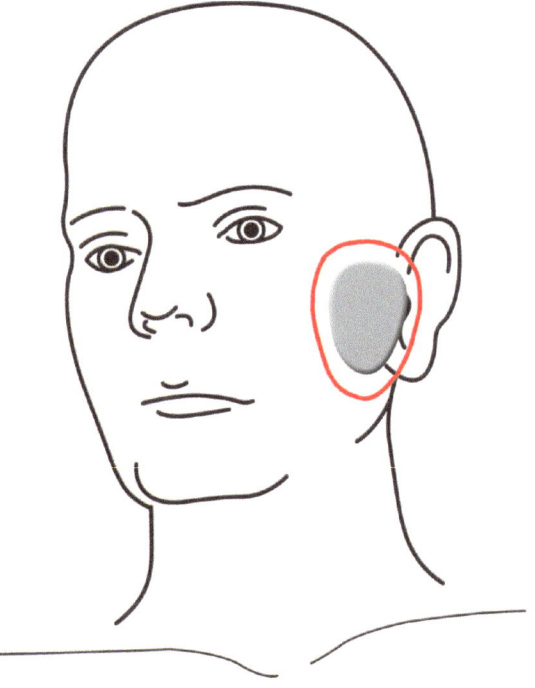

4. Random Pattern Flap

A flap, in contradistinction to a skin graft, contains within its substance a network of blood vessels, arterial, capillary and venous, and it is the effectiveness of the circulation through this network in perfusing the tissues of the flap at each stage of its transfer from donor to recipient which determines its survival. Because circulation of the transferred tissue is crucial for flap design and survival, the development of flap techniques has depended on defining the vascular anatomy of skin and underlying soft tissue. Initially the subdermal plexus was considered the source of blood supply to the skin. This network of arterial and venous channels was oriented parallel and adjacent to the skin surface. A random pattern flap based on this subdermal plexus was initially developed to allow elevation of a rectangular-shaped flap of skin and subcutaneous tissue with a length:width ration in the range of 2 to 1.5:1 (McGREGOR et al. 1970). Although limited in reach, this random pattern flap can be elevated and rotated to provide viable skin and subcutaneous tissue to close an adjacent wound (Fig. 8.5). Occasionally, the flap vascularity may be augmented using a so-called delay procedure, which consists of partially raising the skin flap for 2 to 3 weeks (McGREGOR et al. 1986, TAYLOR et al. 1992).

Figure 7. 4. Defect less suitable for skin grafting. Tumor of the parotid gland with skin invasion after previous irradiation. Tumor resection includes total parotidectomy with overlying skin and neck dissection. The outlined defect is less suitable for skin grafting and needs coverage by a flap.

Attempts to use a random pattern flap based on subdermal circulation distant from the wound site eventually resulted in the introduction of the tubed pedicle flap. The skin flap was attached to an arm carrier, which later required shifting the arm carrier of the random pattern flap from one body region (donor site) to another (recipient site) (McGREGOR et al. 1995). This ingenious use of the arm carrier allowed reconstruction of complex defects in the head and neck region (Fig. 8.6).

Despite the use of the arm carrier, the random pattern flap provided no new source of circulation when transferred to a distant site. Ultimately these flaps depended on the local wound environment for nourishment. Thus it is not surprising that many complex wounds reconstructed with random pattern flaps were subject to wound ulceration related to poor local wound circulation and inadequate bacterial resistance.

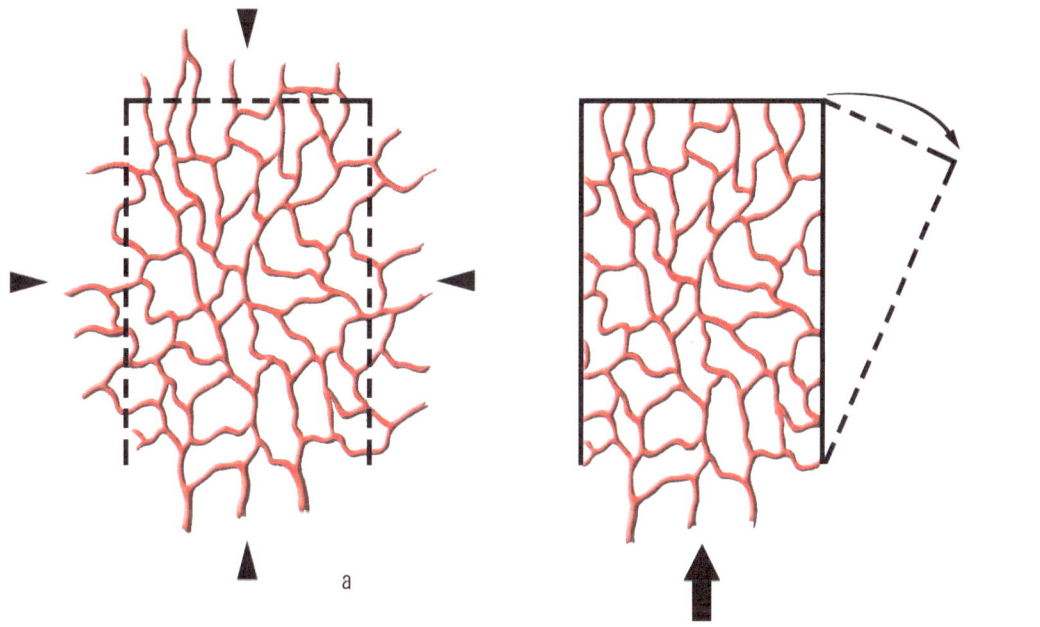

a

b

Figure 8.5. Random pattern flap.
a. Outline of flap design with 2:1 length:width ratio. A random pattern flap has insufficient pre-existing bias in the pattern of its arteries and veins to be of any value in the design of the flap. Because of the random nature of the vascular pattern of such a flap, it is subject to limitations in dimensions, particularly in the permissi-
ble length:breadth ratio. Arrowheads show direction of blood supply before elevation of the flap.
b. Situation after elevation of the flap. Short arrow shows direction of blood supply to the flap. Standard arc of rotation is indicated with long arrow.

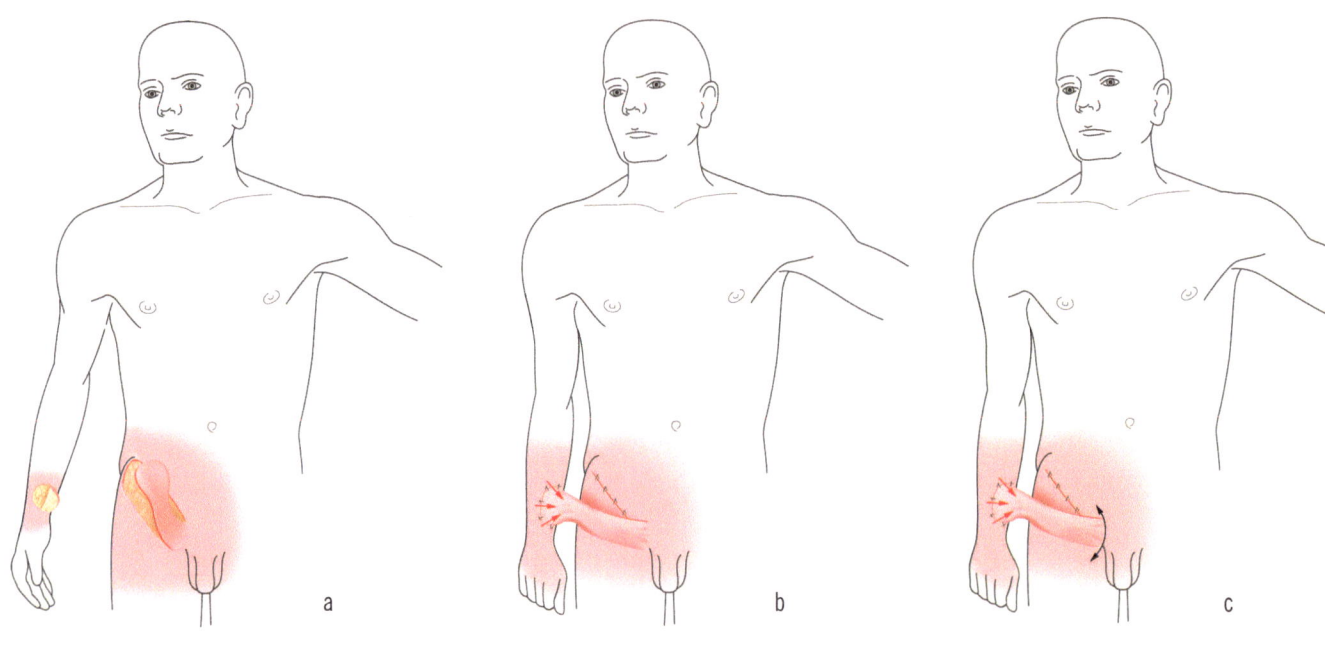

Figure 8.6.

Transfer of a tubed skin flap using a wrist carrier to defect in head and neck region.

When a single pedicled flap (a) is tubed, a circular raw surface is left when tubing is completed. A semicircular trap-door is outlined and raised on the side of the wrist. The effect is to create a circular raw surface corresponding in shape and dimensions to the raw surface left on the flap, as seen in a. The circular raw surface at the distal end of the flap is then sutured to the corresponding raw surface on the wrist (b). The next stage of transfer involves division of the flap at its base (c) 6 weeks after transfer to the wrist carrier. The distal end of the flap is sutured to the defect (d). Six weeks later the transfer is completed by detaching the flap from the wrist (e). Red arrows show direction of reperfusion of skin flap.

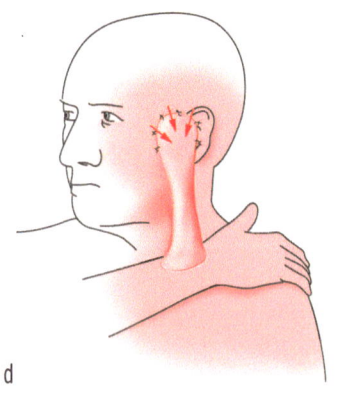

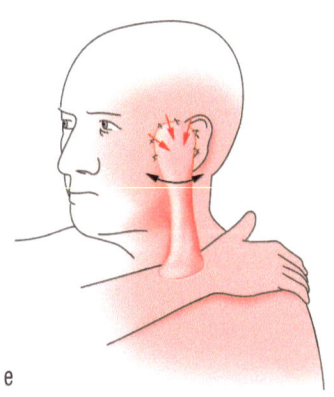

Table 8.1. The tubed skin flap based on a random pattern blood supply succeeds in restoration of soft tissue defects in the head and neck region
- Reconstruction after at least 3 operative stages.
- It takes several months before the defect is fully reconstructed.
- No new source of blood supply in the defect area.

5. *Axial Pattern Flap*

The need for longer flaps resulted in identification of specific vascular territories based on direct cutaneous vascular pedicles with an axial alignment of the flap based on the course of the superficial vascular pedicle (Fig. 8.7). Axial flaps based on this concept included lateral forehead (superficial temporal artery) and deltopectoral (internal mammary branches) flaps (Fig. 8.8.a). The avail- ability of these flaps had a tremendous impact on reconstruction, particularly in the head and neck. In 1963, McGregor first described the forehead flap. The forehead flap improved the ability to repair intraoral defcts (McGREGOR 1963). In 1965, Bakamjian first described the deltopectoral flap (BAKAMJIAN 1965). The deltopectoral flap allowed for a 2-stage reconstruction of the defect after radical parotidectomy (Fig.8.8.b) (BAKAMJIAN 1971).

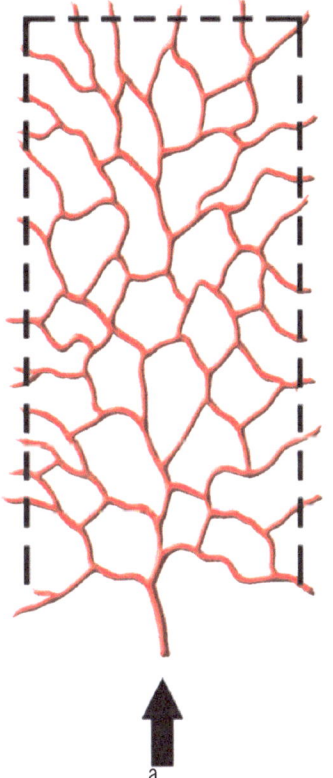
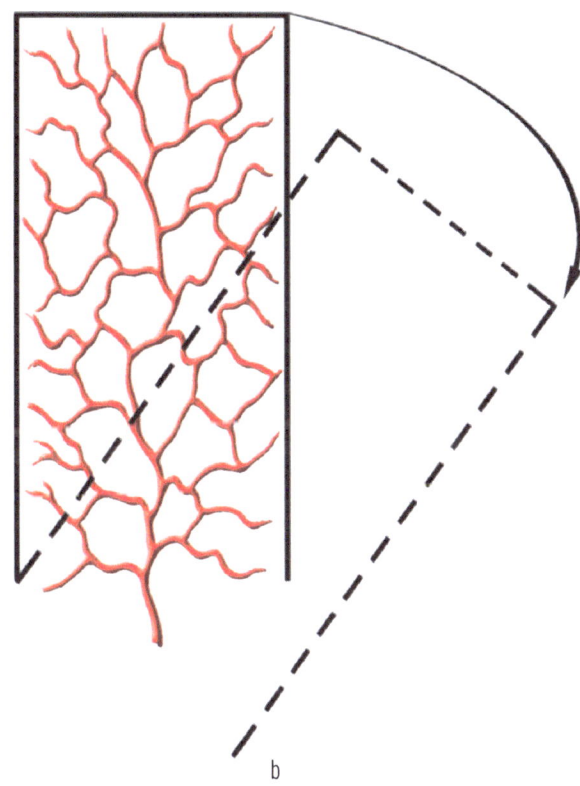

a

b

Figure 8.7. Axial pattern flap.
a. Outline of flap centered along axial course of vascular pedicle. Flap is designed along a pre-existing anatomically recognized arterio-venous system. Such a system running along the length of the flap allows it to be constructed as long as the territory of its axial arte- *ry with minimal regard to considerations of breadth. Arrow shows direction of blood supply before and after elevation of the flap.*
b. Arc of rotation after flap elevation.

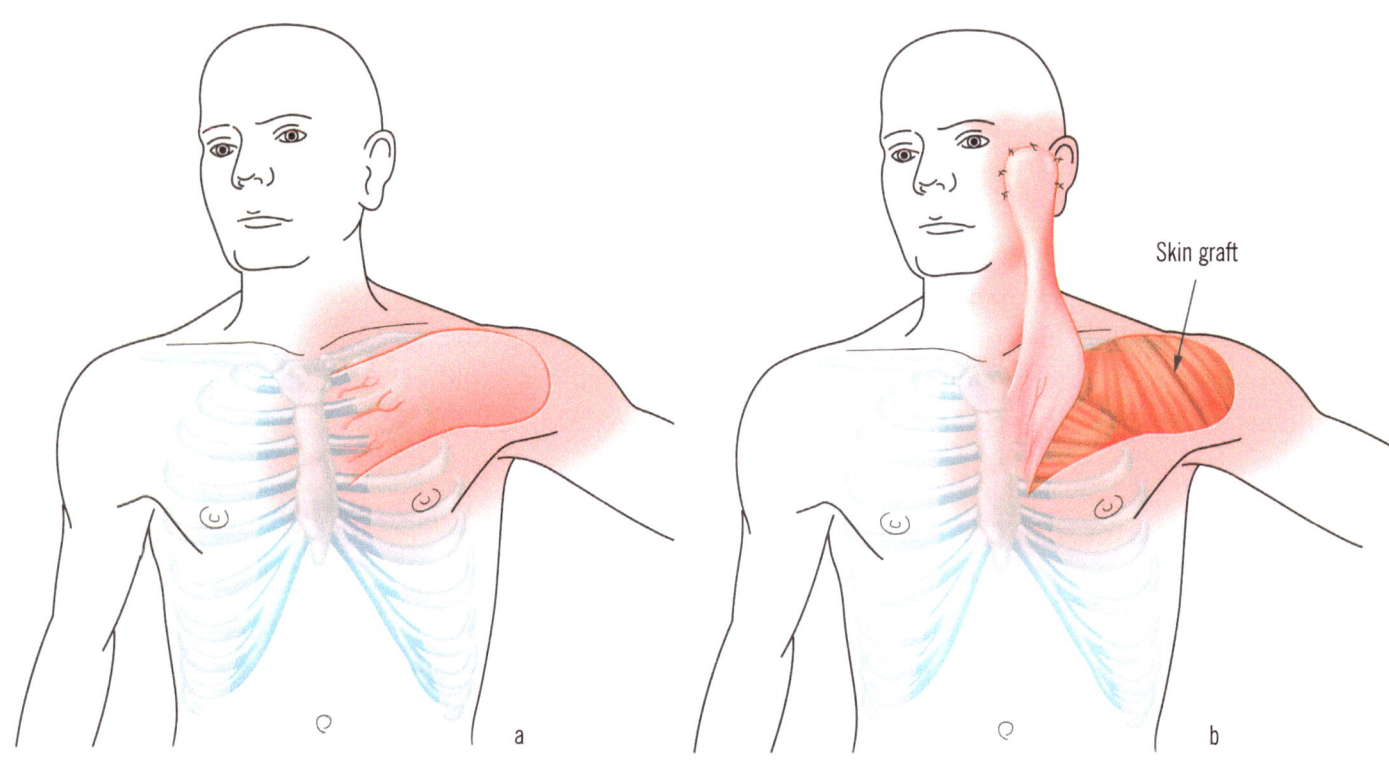

Figure 8.8. A deltopectoral flap.

a. Vascular anatomy and outline of the deltopectoral flap. The flap runs horizontally across the anterior chest wall towards the shoulder tip. The first three perforating branches of the internal mammary vessels provide its axial vascular basis.

b. Transposition of the flap to a head and neck defect *with skin grafting of the donor defect. A new source of blood supply is introduced into the defect area. 2-stage reconstruction of defect: the skin paddle is divided 4 to 6 weeks after inset of the flap. A split-thickness skin graft is applied on the defect area (arrow).*

Table 8.2. The axial pattern flap succeeds in restoration of soft tissue defects in the head and neck region

- Reconstruction in 1 stage; second operation necessary to divide the skin paddle.
- It takes 4 to 6 weeks for completion of the reconstruction.
- New source of blood supply in the defect area during healing period.

6. Pectoralis Major muscle and musculocutaneous flap

In 1979, Ariyan described the pedicled pectoralis major myocutaneous flap, which became the predominant method for reconstruction in head and neck cancer (ARIYAN 1979).

The pectoralis Major muscle was identified as a source of tissue that could be transposed as a flap based on its major vascular pedicle (thoracoacromial artery and vein). In addition, the important contribution of the muscle to skin circulation through musculocutaneous perforating vessels was recognized, thereby altering the approach to flap design. By releasing either the muscle origin, insertion, or both, muscle and musculocutaneous flaps with length:width ratios based on the muscle dimensions became a reality. Since the flap pedicle remains intact, the flap improves the circulation at the site of reconstruction.

Baek (BAEK et al. 1979) and Ariyan (ARIYAN 1979) first described the pectoralis major flap for use in head and neck reconstruction. The pectoralis major flap is used widely in reconstruction of head and neck defects because of its reliable blood supply and ease of harvest. The flap allows for a 1 stage reconstruction of the defect after radical parotidectomy (Fig. 8.9).

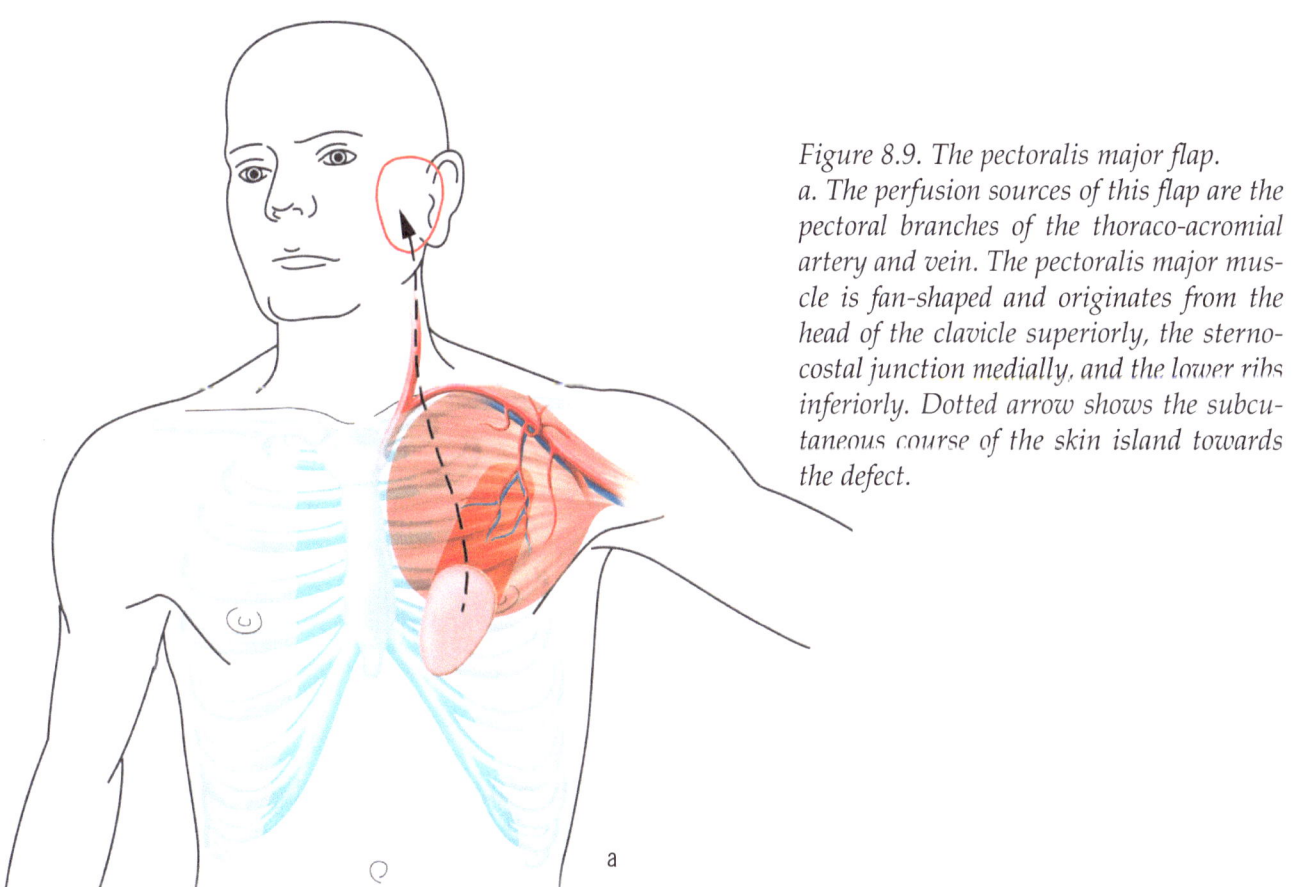

Figure 8.9. The pectoralis major flap.
a. The perfusion sources of this flap are the pectoral branches of the thoraco-acromial artery and vein. The pectoralis major muscle is fan-shaped and originates from the head of the clavicle superiorly, the sterno-costal junction medially, and the lower ribs inferiorly. Dotted arrow shows the subcutaneous course of the skin island towards the defect.

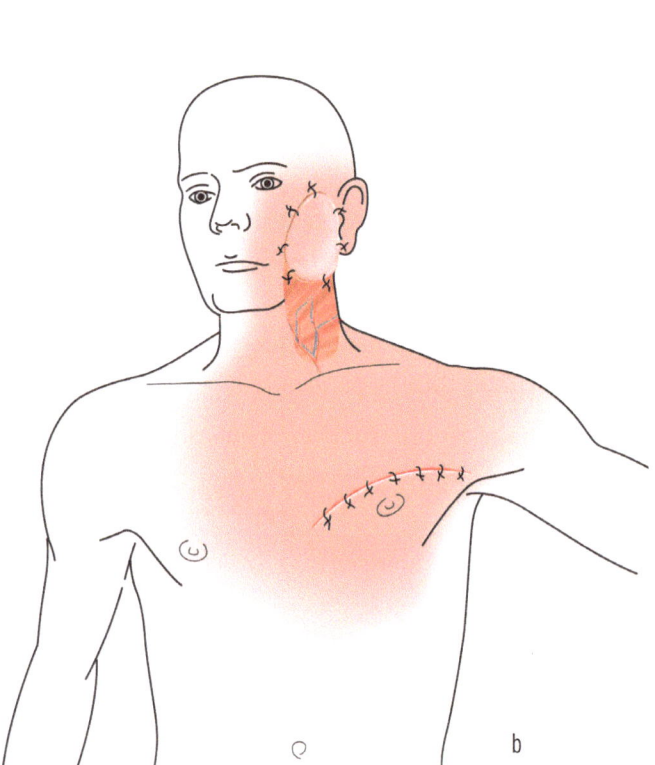

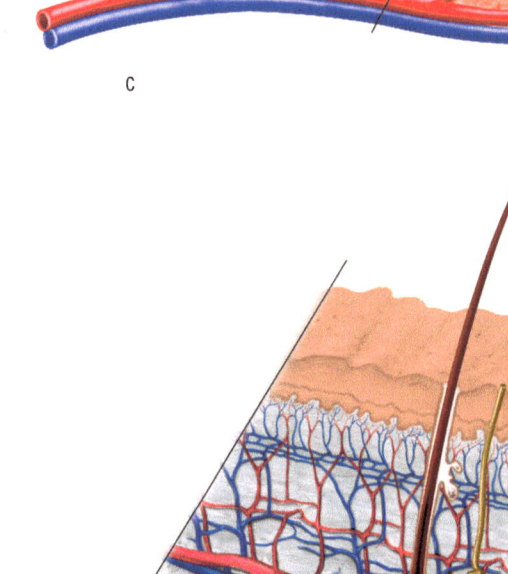

Figure 8.9. The pectoralis major flap (continued).
b. One-stage reconstruction of defect. The vascular pedicle and muscle is transposed subcutaneously towards the defect.
c. Vascular anatomy of myocutaneous flap. Muscle to skin circulation through musculocutaneous perforating vessels (asterisks).

Table 8.3. The pectoralis major myocutaneous flap succeeds in restoration of soft tissue defects in the head and neck region.

- Full reconstruction in 1 stage.
- New blood supply in the defect area.

Currently, the laryngopharyngectomy defect may be a good indication for use of the pectoralis myocutaneous flap (Fig. 8.10). Direct closure of the pharynx can be achieved primarily following laryngectomy. Primary closure of the pharynx requires at least 5 cm of the circumference of the pharynx to produce an adequate conduit. Anything less than 5 cm will require a skin 'patch'.

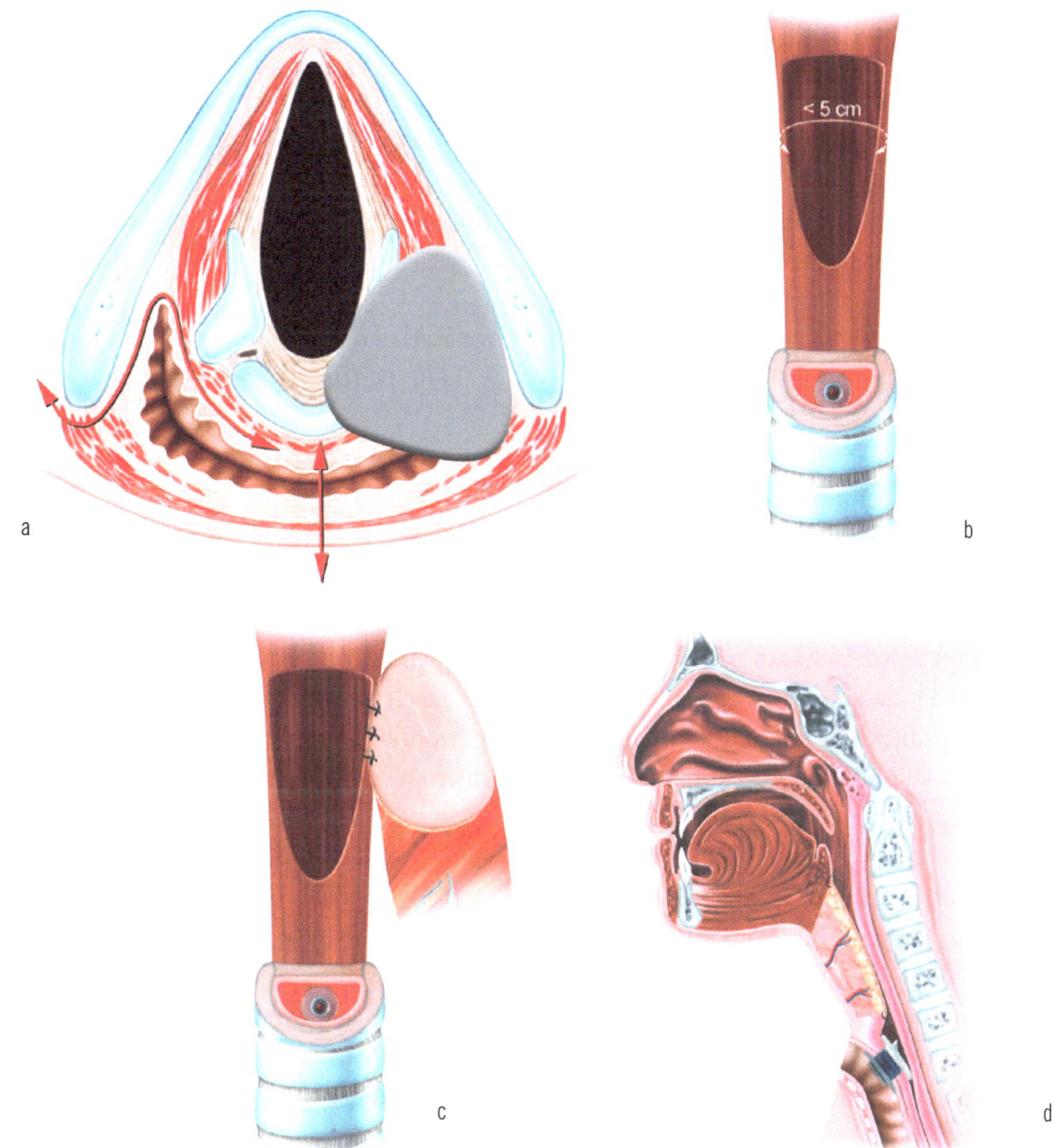

Figure 8.10. Use of the pectoralis major myocutaneous flap after laryngopharyngectomy.
a. Total laryngectomy with partial pharyngectomy. Extent of resection to remove tumor with extension to 1 side of hypopharynx is shown.
b. Hypopharyngeal defect following subtotal pharyngo-laryngectomy, leaving a posterior strip of mucosa of less than 5 cm.
c. Pectoralis flap being sutured into position.
d. Situation after total laryngectomy with repair of the anterior pharynx with a myocutaneous pectoralis major flap.

7. *Microvascular Composite Tissue Transplantation*

The emergence of microvascular techniques paralleled the development of the operating microscope, microinstruments, and sutures. Reliable anastomosis of vessels with external diameter of 0.5 to 2 mm became feasible with a patency rate of 95% or better. Different specialized tissues receiving blood supply from specific vessels are totally detached from the donor site and the artery and vein are reconnected at the recipient site by performing vascular anastomoses with the aid of magnification systems.

In 1973, Daniel and Taylor (DANIEL et al. 1973) reported the first successful free flap, the transplant of an autologous skin flap to the lower extremity using the operating microscope.

Since flaps are now specifically designed on known vascular pedicles, transplantation of composite tissue from the donor site to a distant site is possible based on anastomosis of the flap arterial and venous pedicles to suitable receptor vessels in proximity to the defect. The ability to transplant a flap to a distant site eliminates the necessity to select a flap with an arc of rotation that reaches the defect. The surgeon is thus able to transfer composite tissue based on flap suitability for defect coverage rather than proximity to the defect. In a one-step process, large amounts of different tissues can now be reliable transplanted to fill dead spaces and provide restoration of form, function, contour, and tension-free wound closure. In addition, free flaps are highly vascularized and thus can be used in an irradiated site or in patients who are prone to poor wound healing.

In expert hands, a successful flap transplant rate of 95 to 99% can be expected today, making free tissue transplant one of the most reliable forms of reconstructive tissue (KHOURI 1992, CORDEIRO et al. 1995).

Although many free flaps have been described for head and neck reconstruction, only 4 types of free flaps are required for reconstructing most of head and neck defects in the oncologic patient. These include fasciocutaneous flaps, musculocutaneous flaps, bone flaps, and jejunum.

7.A. *Fasciocutaneous free flap- The radial forearm flap*

The radial forearm flap popularized by Song et al. and known as the "Chinese flap" was reported in 1982 (SONG et al. 1982). In the forearm area, fascia supplies overlying subcutaneous tissue and skin in a more direct fashion. Direct branches from major vessels course through intermuscular septa to reach the deep fascia. These septocutaneous perforators supply the overlying skin and subcutaneous tissue. This relatively hairless flap has a long vascular pedicle and sensory nerves, and it has proven to be an invaluable source for intraoral and pharyngeal reconstruction (Fig. 8.11). In 1989, Urken and colleagues were the first to succesfully utilize a neurofasciocutaneous flap in head and neck reconstruction (MOSCOSO et al, 1994). The radial forearm free flap can be harvested to fit almost any shape of deformity in the tongue with less postoperative contracture and bulk, allowing for earlier return of speech and swallowing after surgery (SOUTAR et al. 1986, 1983) (Fig. 8.12).

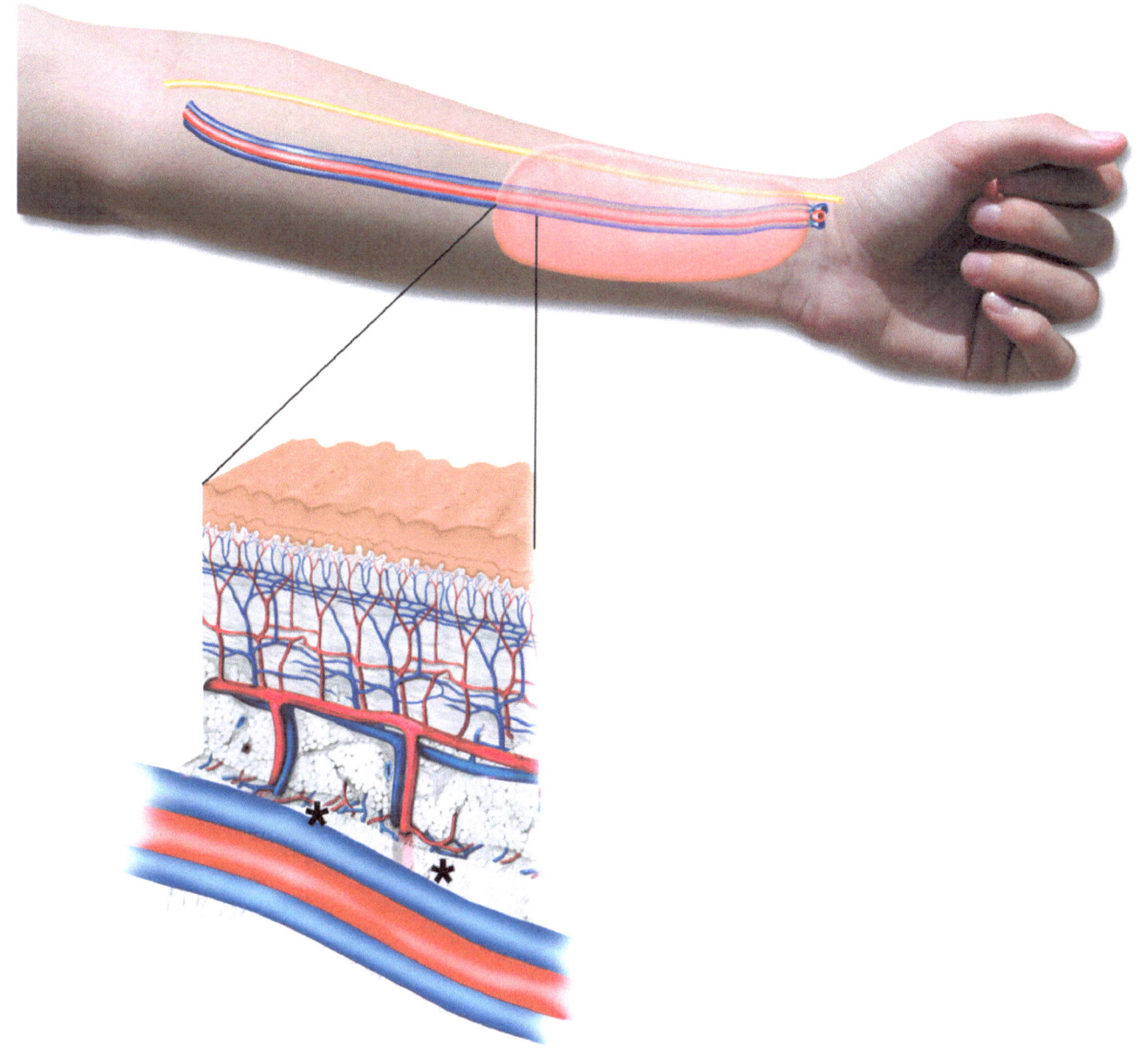

Figure 8.11. The radial forearm flap.
The radial forearm flap is supplied by multiple perfora-
ting segments (asterisk) from a major vessel (radial
artery) that courses through intermuscular septa.
The flap is based on the radial artery and 2 venae com-
mitantes. It consists of thin, pliable skin with minimal

soft tissue and a very long pedicle with large diameter.
In addition, a sensory nerve over the anterior forearm
skin (lateral antebrachial cutaneous nerve) can be
included within the flap, to provide sensory recovery at
the recipient site (URKEN 1990).

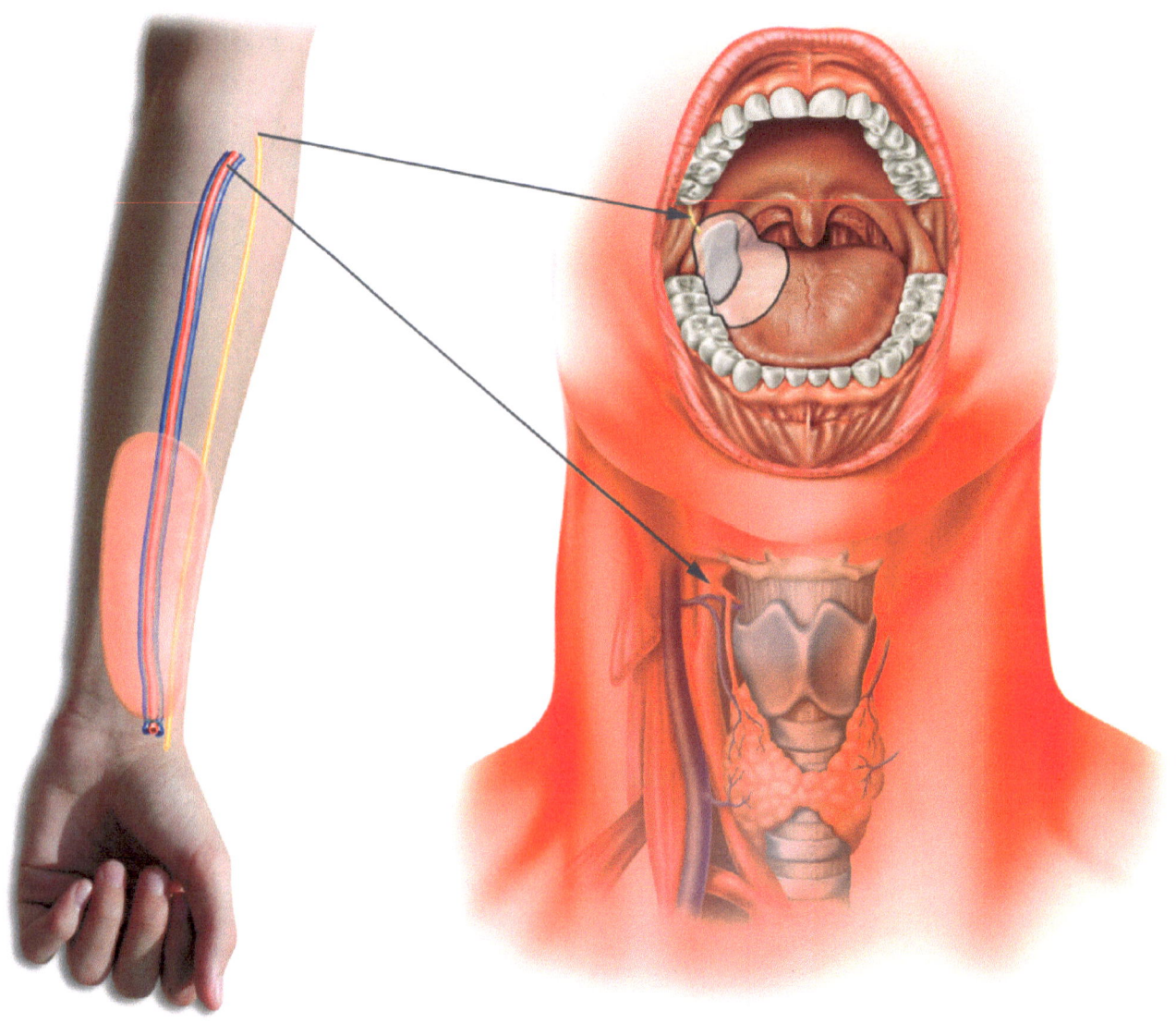

Figure 8.12. Use of the radial forearm flap for oropharyngeal reconstruction.
a. Extent of resection to remove a base of tongue tumor with extention to the tonsillar area. The stump of the lingual nerve (arrow) can serve as receptor for the lateral antebrachial cutaneous nerve. The lateral ante- *brachial cutaneous nerve will be anastomosed to the stump of the lingual nerve to provide sensory recovery in the forearm skin. The radial artery and 1 radial vein will be sutured to the superior thyroid vessels.*

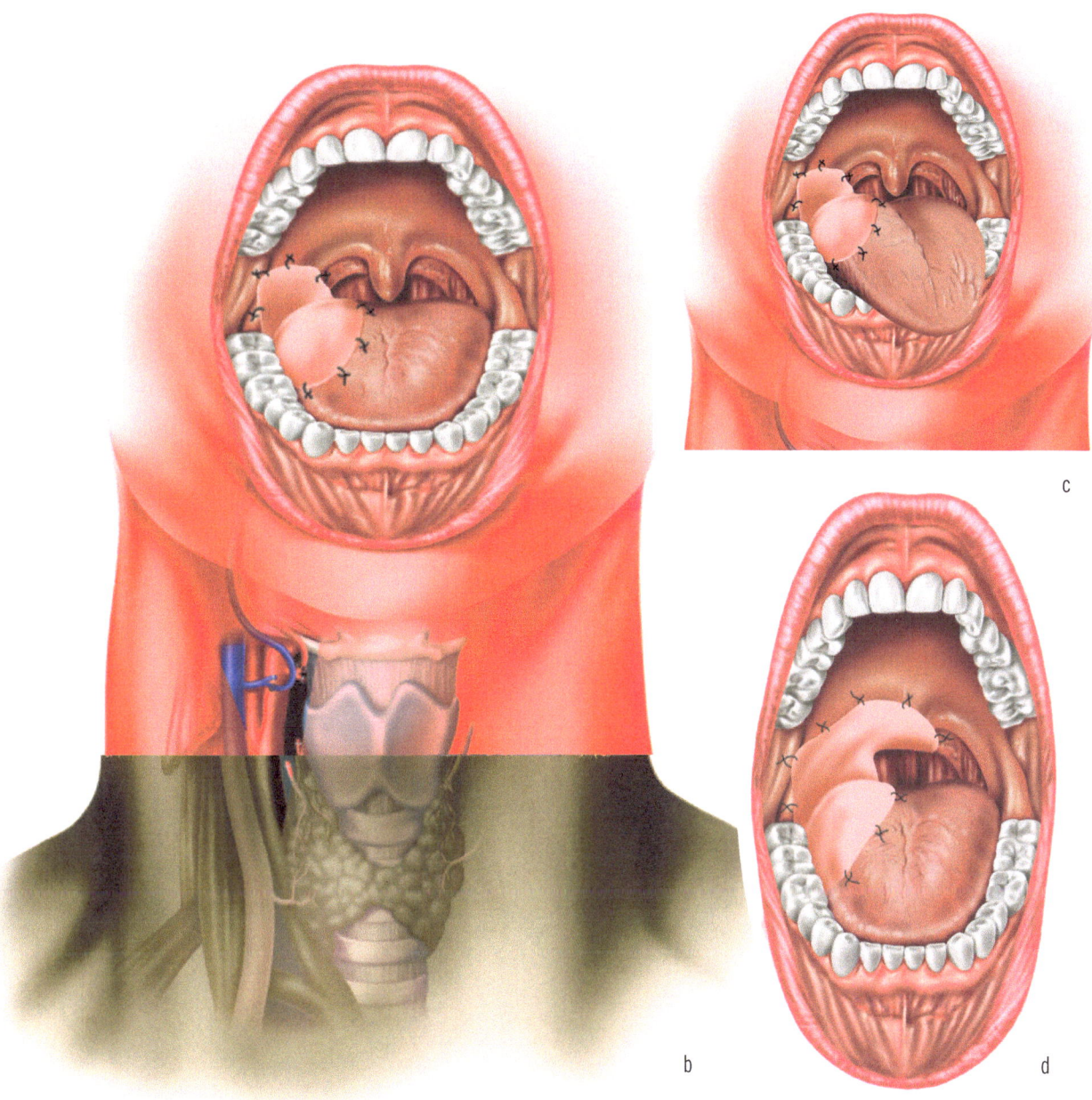

Figure 8.12. Use of the radial forearm flap for oropharyngeal reconstruction (continued).

b. Situation after reconstruction. The radial forearm flap succeeds in relining of the defect with good adaptation to the different anatomic planes. The radial artery is anastomosed to the superior thyroid artery (end-to-end) and 1 radial vein is anastomosed to the superior thyroid vein (end-to-end) (another possibility is an end-to-side anastomosis to the internal jugular vein).
c. The radial forearm skin allows for preservation of the

tongue mobility. Preservation of residual tongue volume and movement is crucial to the oral cancer patient's ability to chew, articulate, swallow and prevent drooling.
d. Reconstruction with the radial forearm flap can be extended to include half of the soft palate. The pliability of the flap allows for repair of the different anatomic planes (soft palate, tonsillar area, base of tongue).

7.B. Musculocutaneous free flap

The rectus abdominis (URKEN et al. 1991) and the latissimus dorsi muscle may be used. A free muscle or musculocutaneous flap can be developed for head and neck reconstruction (after wide excision of scalp, skull base defects, midfacial defects…). The vascular anatomy of a free musculocutaneous free flap is similar to that of the pectoralis major musculocutaneous flap. Free muscle and musculocutaneous flaps are indicated after total glossectomy, cranial base reconstruction, and repair of extensive scalp defects. A pedicled myocutaneous pectoralis major flap has definite drawbacks in tongue reconstruction. The tethering effect of the pedicle with its downward vector of pull on the reconstruction will not allow flap-to-palate closure during swallowing.

When the bulk of the tongue is removed a bulky flap is needed. A free myocutaneous flap such as the rectus abdominis flap can be used in total glossectomy defects (Fig. 8.13) (URKEN et al. 1991, NELIGAN et al. 1996, LYOS et al. 1999). To subserve tongue function (airway protection, swallowing, articulation) the donor tissue should be bulky, not only filling the oral cavity, but also creating a shelf above the laryngeal inlet to better direct the oral bolus down into the pharynx. Such bulk will allow a seal once the flap is in contact with the palate, possibly assisting in caudad propulsion of the food bolus. Such contact between flap and palate also greatly assists articulation.

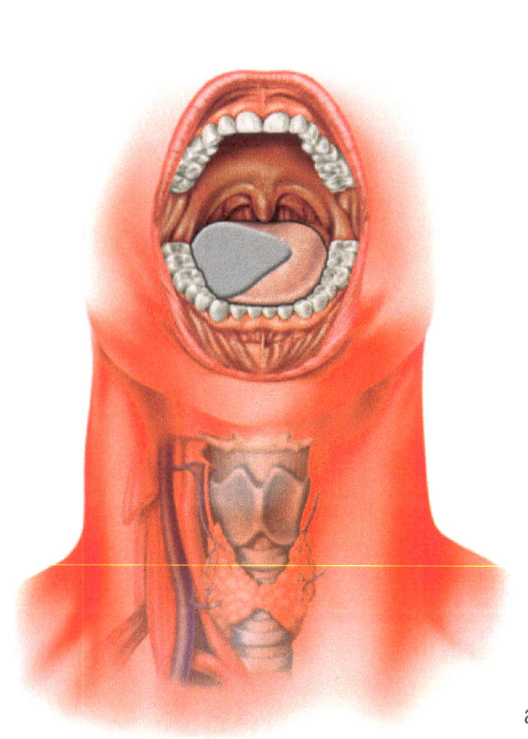

a

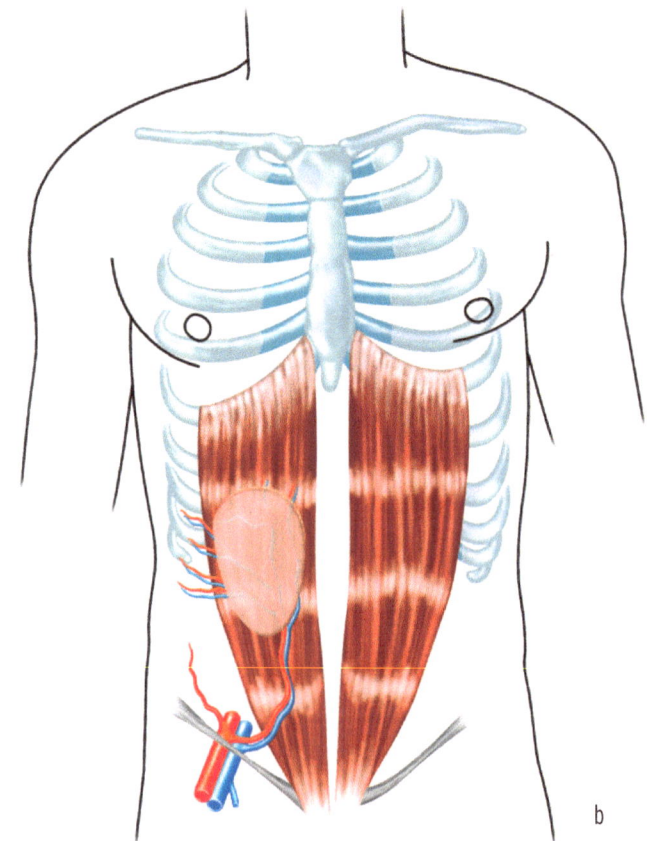

b

Figure 8.13. The rectus abdominis in reconstruction of total glossectomy defects.
a. Tongue tumor requiring a subtotal glossectomy.
b. The rectus abdominis flap is raised on the inferior epigastric vessels with a vertical skin paddle.
c. The myoctaneous flap restores tongue bulk. Revascularization of inferior epigastric vessels to neck vessels.
d. Sagittal section-total glossectomy.
e. Sagittal section-defect repaired with myocutaneous rectus abdominis flap.

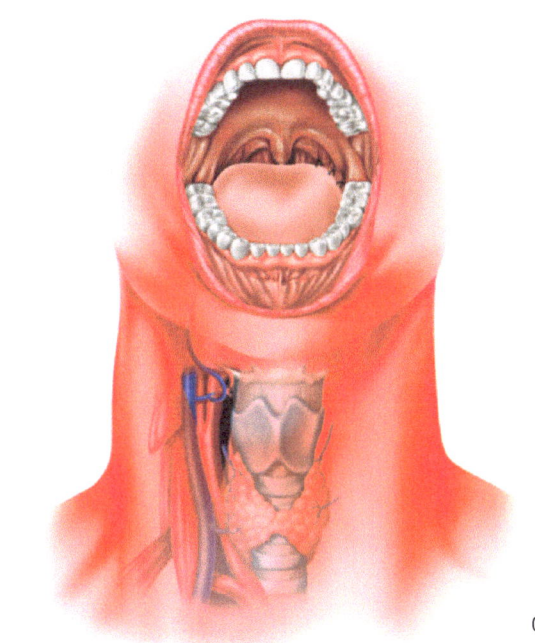

c

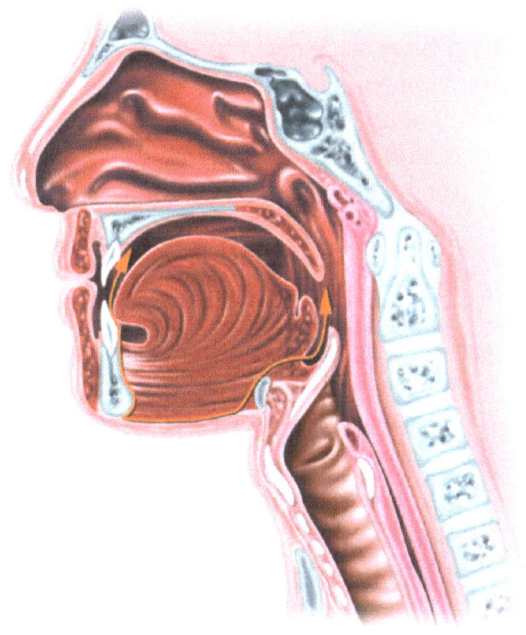

d

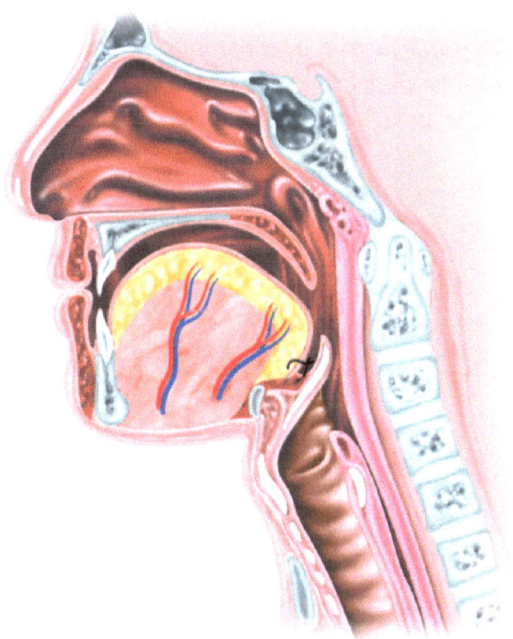

e

Cranial base reconstruction and repair of extensive scalp defects is not possible with a pectoralis major flap because of the limited arc of rotation of its pedicle. The free latissimus dorsi is a broad and flat muscle that is very useful to reconstruct extensive scalp defects (LIPA et al., 2004) (Fig. 8.14).

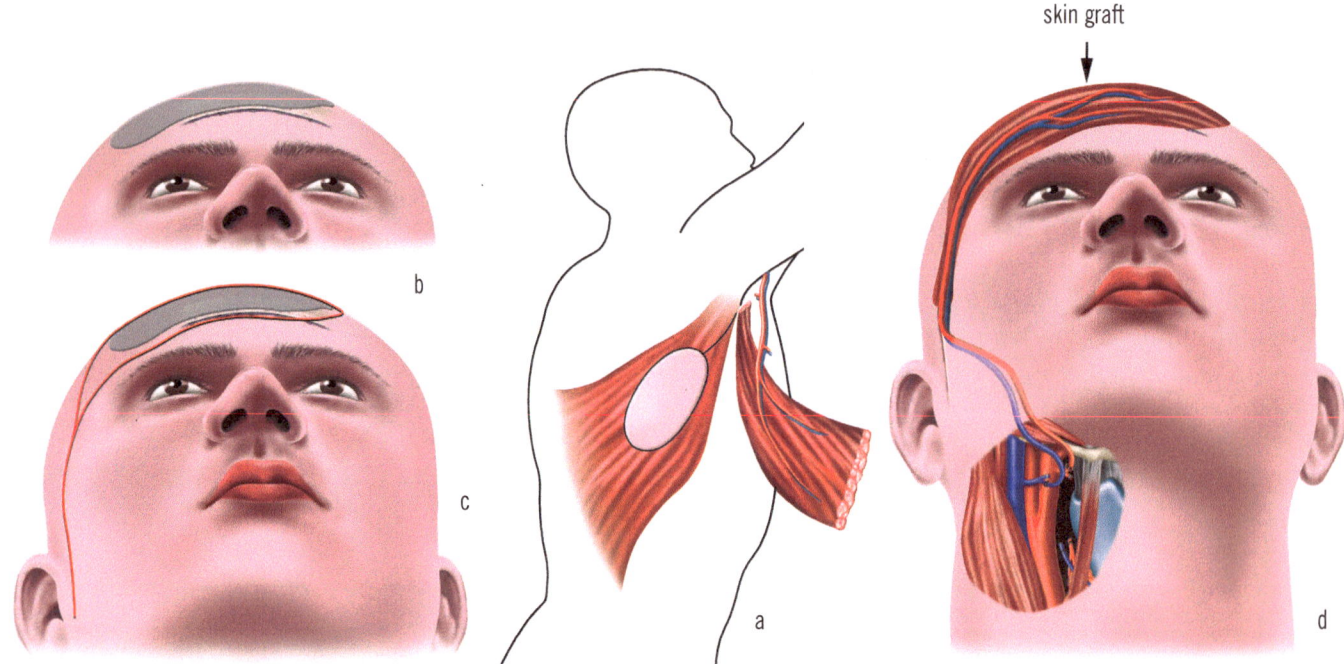

skin graft

Figure 8.14. Repair of extensive scalp defect with free latissimus dorsi flap.

a. The latissimus dorsi is a robust muscle flap that may be raised alone or with a skin paddle. The latissimus dorsi muscle is elevated on the thoracodorsal artery and vein.

b. Squamous cell carcinoma of the scalp and calvarium.

c. Scalp defect with full-thickness calvarian resection.

d. Reconstruction of scalp defect with latissimus dorsi muscle resurfaced with a split-thickness skin graft. Revascularization by suturing of thoracodorsal vessels to neck vessels. Alternatively, the superficial temporal vessels may be used as recipients.

7.C. Osseous free flap-Fibula

The fibula can be transferred as a free osseous or free osseocutaneous flap. The fibula is currently a favored donor site for mandibular reconstruction. Originally desribed in 1975 by Taylor, the bone stock is long, straight, strong, and easily accessed. TAYLOR et al. (1975) were first to report the successful transplant of the vascularized fibular bone flap for reconstruction of an open fracture of the lower extremity. For many years, the fibula flap was used only for long-bone reconstruction. Hidalgo pioneered the use of fibula free flaps for mandibular reconstruction in 1989, using multiple osteotomies to contour the flap in three dimensions (HIDALGO 1989) (Fig. 8.15, 8.16). Since then, the vascularized fibula flap has become a flap of choice for mandibular reconstruction (HIDALGO et al. 2002). The endosteal and periosteal branches of the peroneal artery supply the fibula bone. As much as 25 cm of fibula bone can be harvested in the adult, and the fibula's extensive periosteal vascular support allows the creation of multiple osteotomies for aesthetic and functional reconstruction of the mandible. Angle-to-angle defects of the mandible can be reconstructed using the fibula flap (Fig. 8.17).

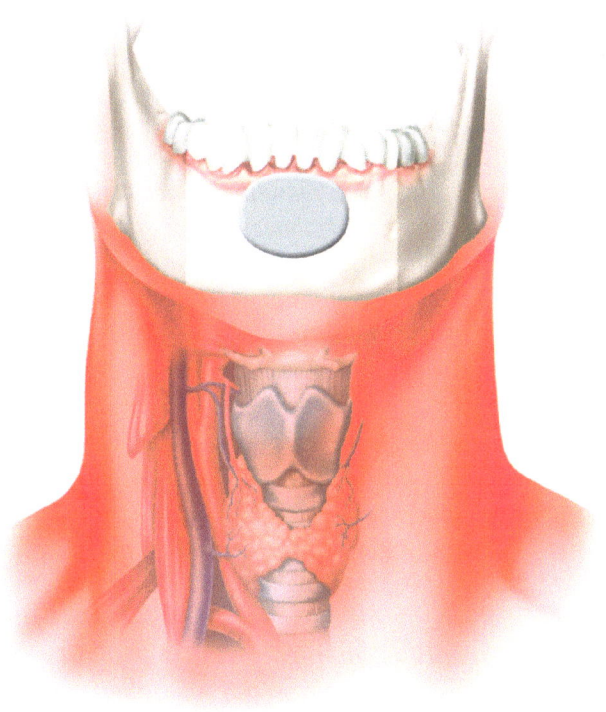

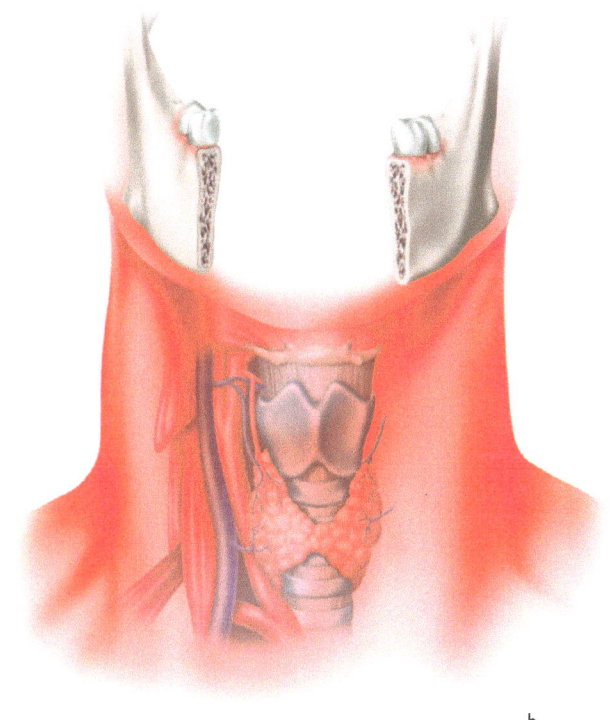

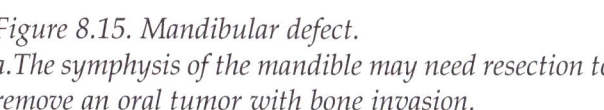

a

b

Figure 8.15. Mandibular defect.
a. The symphysis of the mandible may need resection to remove an oral tumor with bone invasion.

b. Anterior mandibular defect.

Figure 8.16. 'Andy Gump deformity'.
Total or partial loss of the mandible incurs serious functional, aesthetic, and psychological morbidity for patients. Prior to the development of advanced reconstruction options for mandibular defects, patients were left with terrible cosmetic deformities and poor function. The symphyseal resection produces the so-called "Andy Gump" deformity, named after the comic strip character with no chin. The unrepaired resection shows a patient with an unsupported and anesthetic lip and chin, severe retrogenia, incompetent lips, and malocclusion. Functional problems may include drooling, speech deficits, impaired deglutition, and possible repiratory compromise due to loss of the genial tubercle, which provides anchorage for the origin of the tongue and floor of mouth musculature.

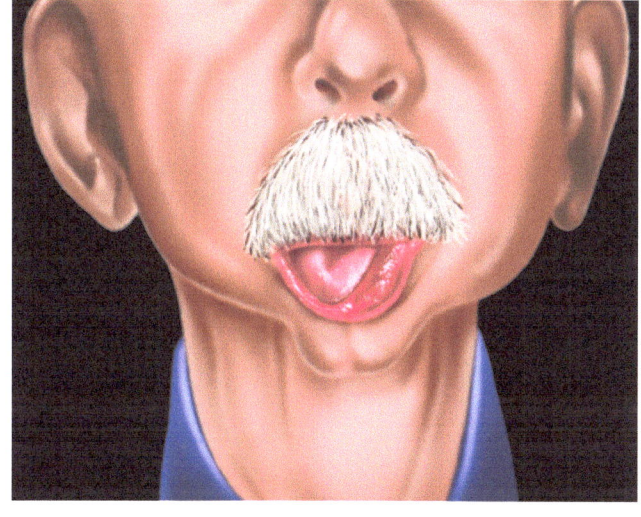

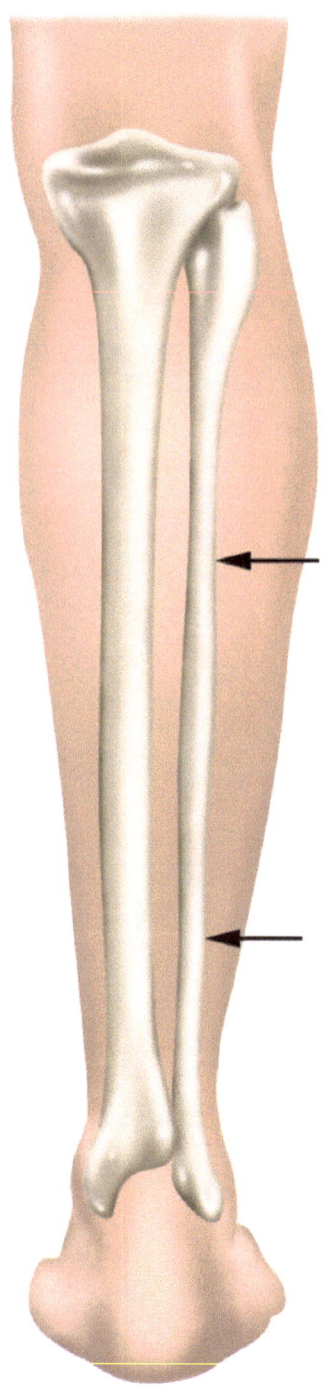
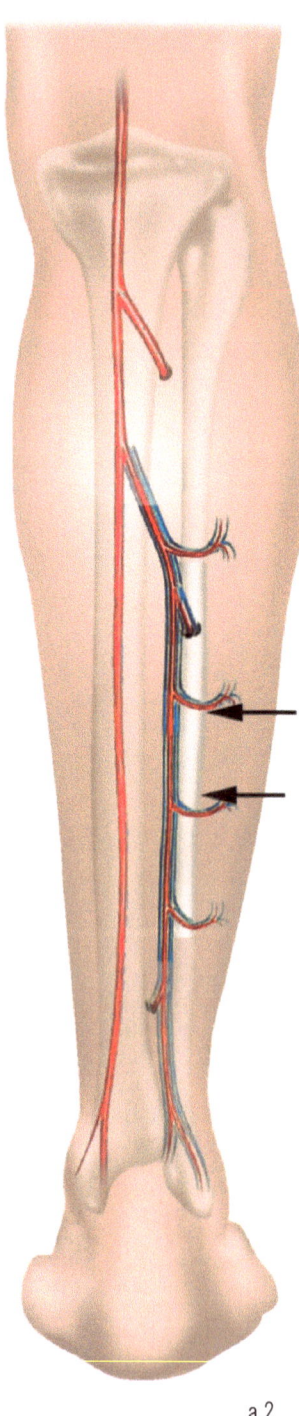

Figure 8.17.
Reconstruction with free fibula flap.
a. Donor site free fibula flap.
a.1. A segment of fibula (between 2 arrows) may be used for mandibular reconstruction. There is enough bone length available to reconstruct any length of mandibular defect.
a.2. A segment of fibula is taken with its blood supply (peroneal artery and veins) at the lower leg. The long bone is osteomized (arrows) to transform the bone in a convex shape comparable to the mandiblar arch. Osteotomies can be performed wherever necessary along the length of the graft. The periosteal blood supply is abundant and permits multiple osteotomies to be performed that are as little as 1 cm apart. Donor site morbidity is minimal provided that 8 cm of distal fibula are preserved for stability of the ankle.

a.1

a.2

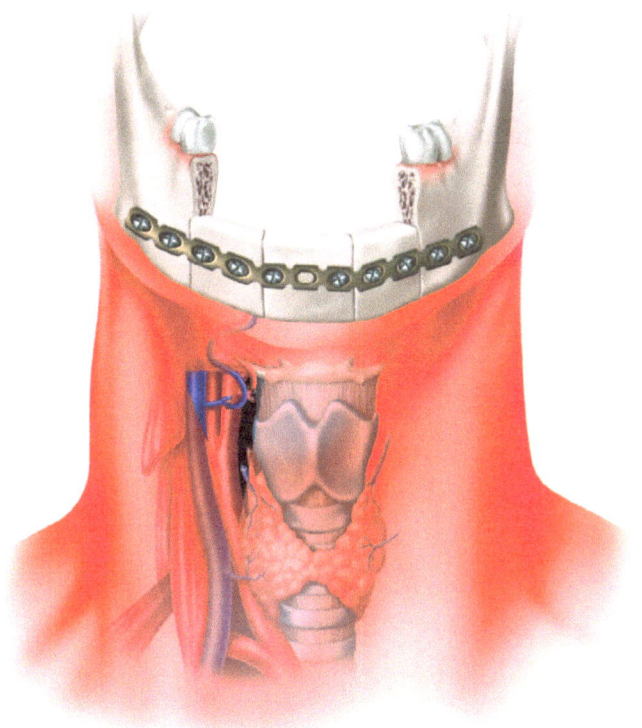

b.1

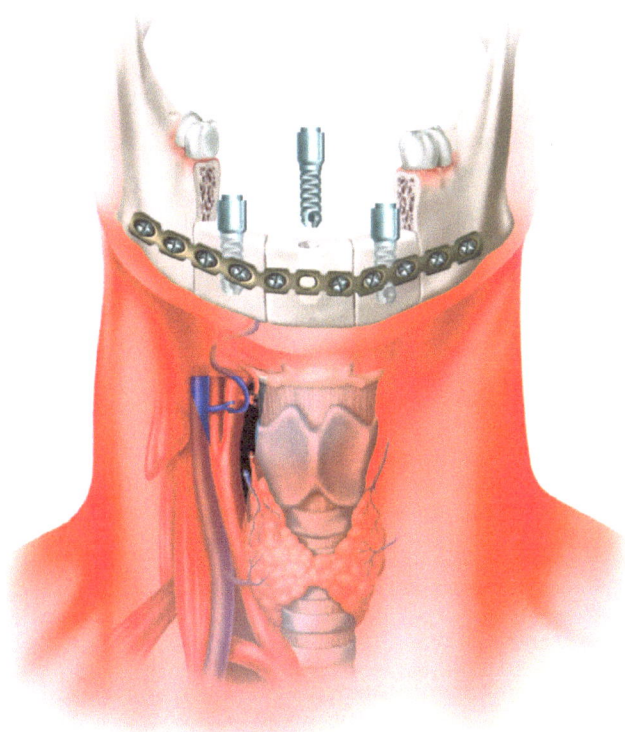

b.2

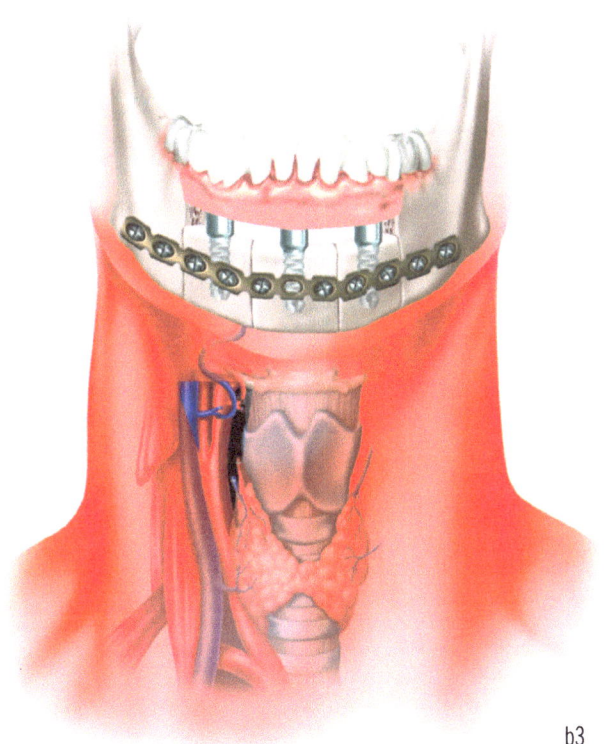

b3

Figure 8.17.
Reconstruction with free fibula flap (continued).
b.Defect repair with free fibula flap.
b.1. The anterior mandibular defect is repaired with the free fibula flap. The bicortical bone of the fibula accepts plates and screws for fixation. The peroneal artery is sutured to the superior thyroid artery; the peroneal vein is sutured to the superior thyroid vein.
b.2. Titanium implants are placed in the vascularized bone flap.
b.3. The osseointegrated implants support a dental prosthesis.

7.D. Visceral free flap-Free jejunal transplant (FJT)

Free jejunal transplant was the first autogenous tissue to be transplanted in humans. Seidenberg conducted a number of canine experiments involving FJTs to the head and neck to replace the pharyngoesophagus (SEIDENBERG et al. 1959). In 1959, they reported their experience with a patient who had undergone a pharyngoesophagectomy for recurrent cancer. Currently, the FJT has become one of the most useful flaps for reconstruction following pharyngoesophagectomy (SCHUSTERMAN et al. 1990) (Fig. 8.18).

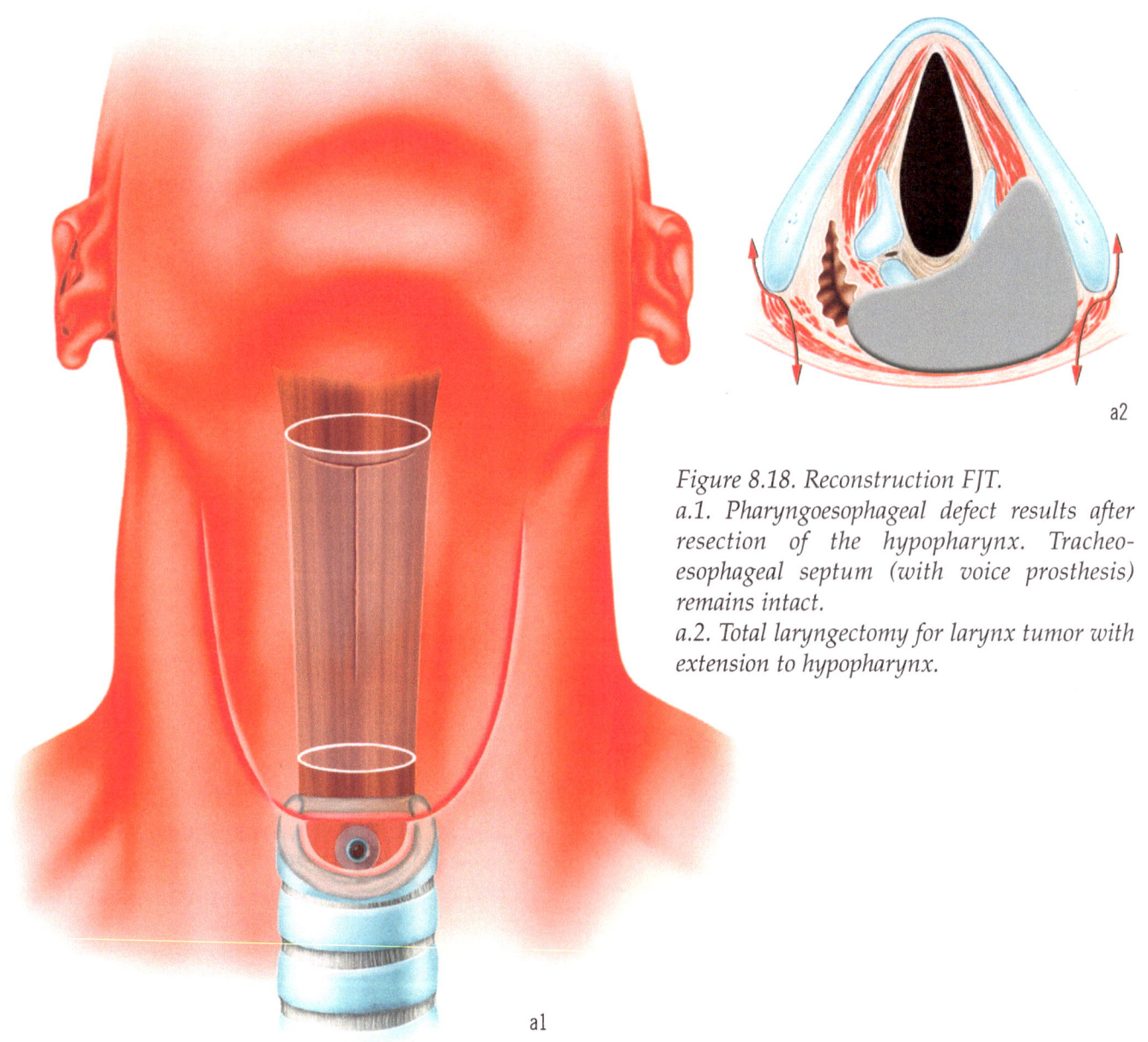

Figure 8.18. Reconstruction FJT.
a.1. Pharyngoesophageal defect results after resection of the hypopharynx. Tracheo-esophageal septum (with voice prosthesis) remains intact.
a.2. Total laryngectomy for larynx tumor with extension to hypopharynx.

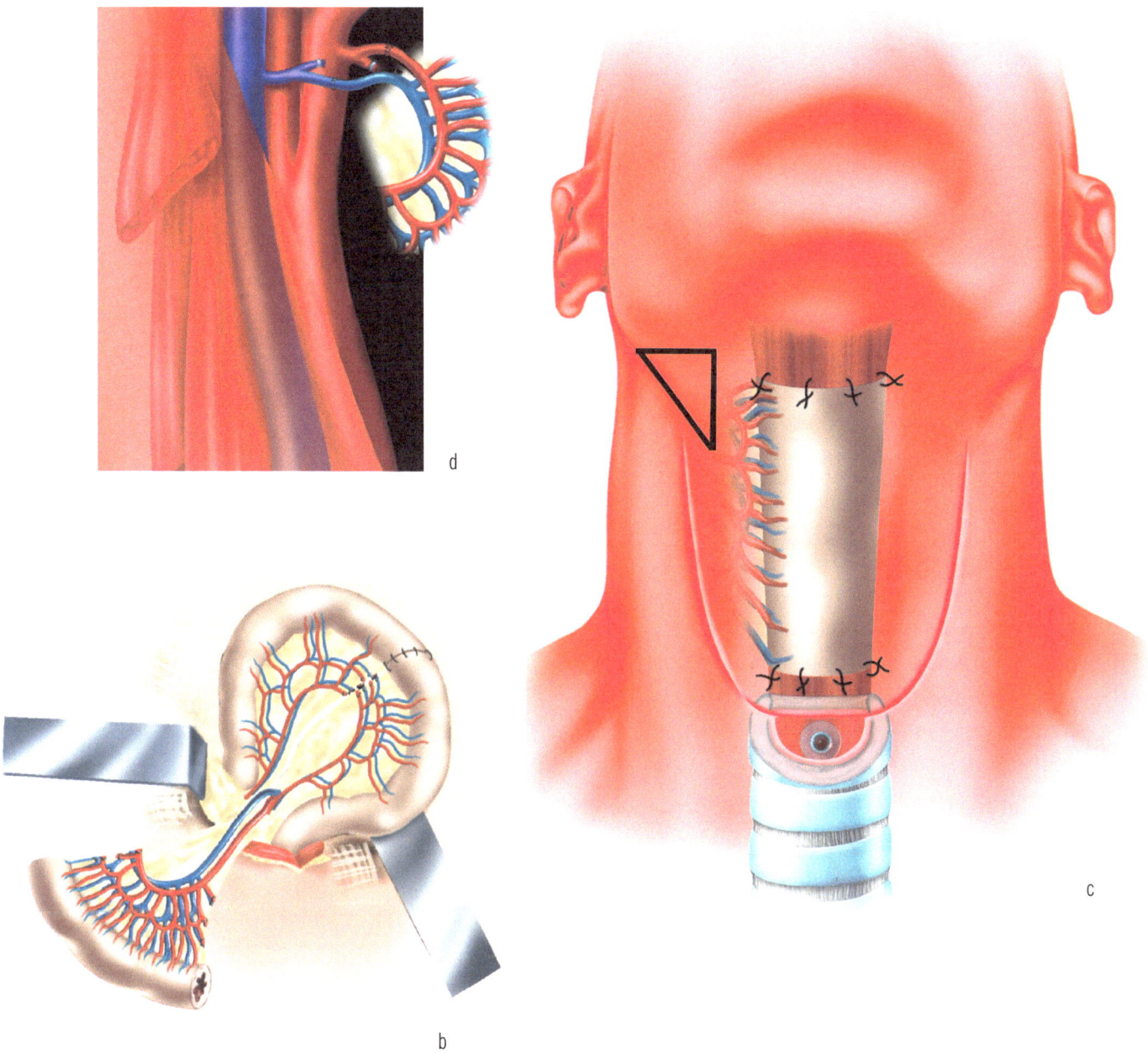

Figure 8.18. Reconstruction FJT(continued).
b. Donor site FJT. A segment of jejunum is isolated on
a vascular pedicle. Bowel continuity is reestablished.
c. Pharyngoesophageal defect is restored by FJT.
d. Vascular pedicle is anastomosed to superior thyroid
vessels.

Table 8.4 Progress made by free flaps in head and neck reconstruction

Fasciocutaneous flaps:
- Pliable, thin skin flap for oropharyngeal lining.
- Potential for sensate flap.

Myocutaneous flap
- Bulky reconstruction of tongue, scalp, and skull base defects (beyond the reach of a pectoralis flap).

Osseous flap:
- Vascularized bone.
- Support osseointegrated dental implants.

Visceral free flap:
- Vascularized tubes and patches of mucosa.

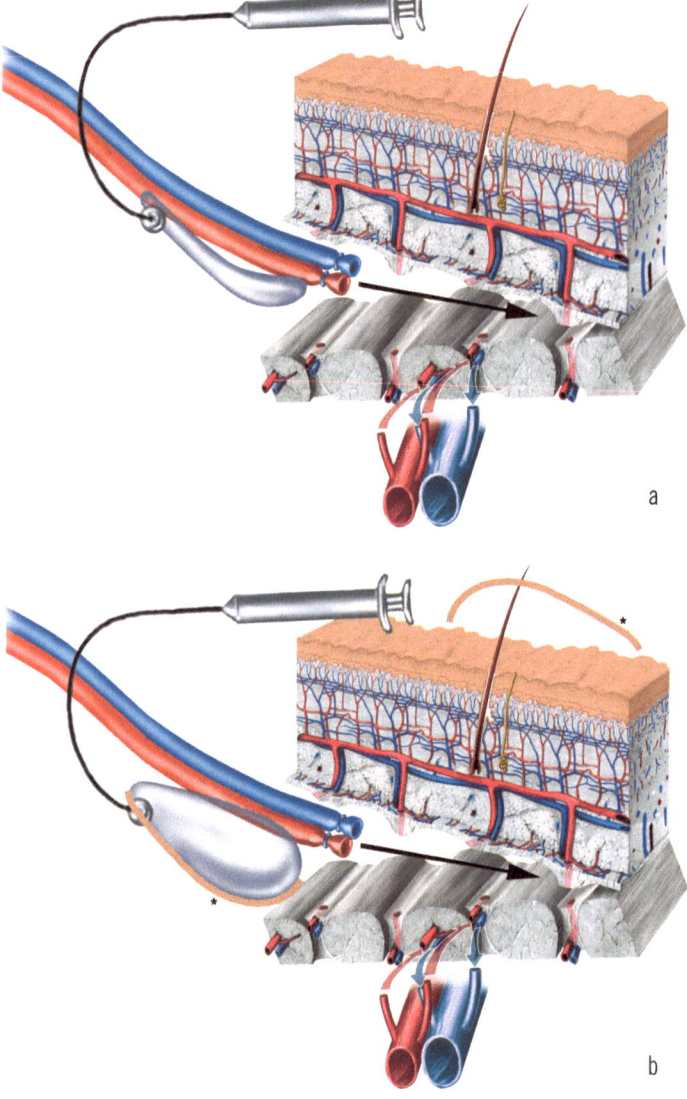

8. Flap prefabrication

Flap prefabrication and prelamination are evolving, new techniques that are useful in reconstructing complex defects of the head and neck. This approach was clinically first described by BAUDET at al. (1995).

Flap prefabrication involves the introduction of a new blood supply by means of a vascular pedicle transfer into a volume of tissue. After a period of revascularization, this volume of tissue may be transferred, based only on its implanted vascular pedicle. The transfer may be local transposition or by microsurgical transfer. Tissue expanders are frequently used as an aid. Prefabricated flaps allow the transfer of moderate-sized units of thin tissue to recipient sites throughout the body (Fig. 8.19). This technique for prefabrication is not always reliable for establishing a new dominant pedicle to a flap territory. With the numerous options available for safe flap selection, this technique for flap prefabrication is rarely required.

Flap prefabrication has been useful in patients recovering from extensive burn injury where thin donor sites are limited (PRIBAZ et al. 1999, 2001).

Figure 8.19. Example of flap prefabrication.
a. A suitable artery and vein are selected and buried in fascia or subcutaneous tissue in the planned flap territory. A tissue expander is introduced below the vascular pedicle. b. The tissue expander will augment the flap surface area (asterisks). In 6 weeks the flap is elevated based on the new vascular pedicle and either transposed or transplanted by microsurgery.

Flap prelamination refers to a technique in which additional tissue is added to an existing flap (without manipulation of its axial blood supply) to make a multilayered flap that may be used for complex, three-dimensional multilayered reconstructions. This technique may be used locally or at a distance, requiring microvascular transfer.

For instance if a nose is to be totally reconstructed it can be first created on a forearm with cartilage and bone grafts under the skin before it is transferred to the face (Fig. 8.20). This allows the surgeon to sculpt the tissue before transfer (PRIBAZ et al. 1999).

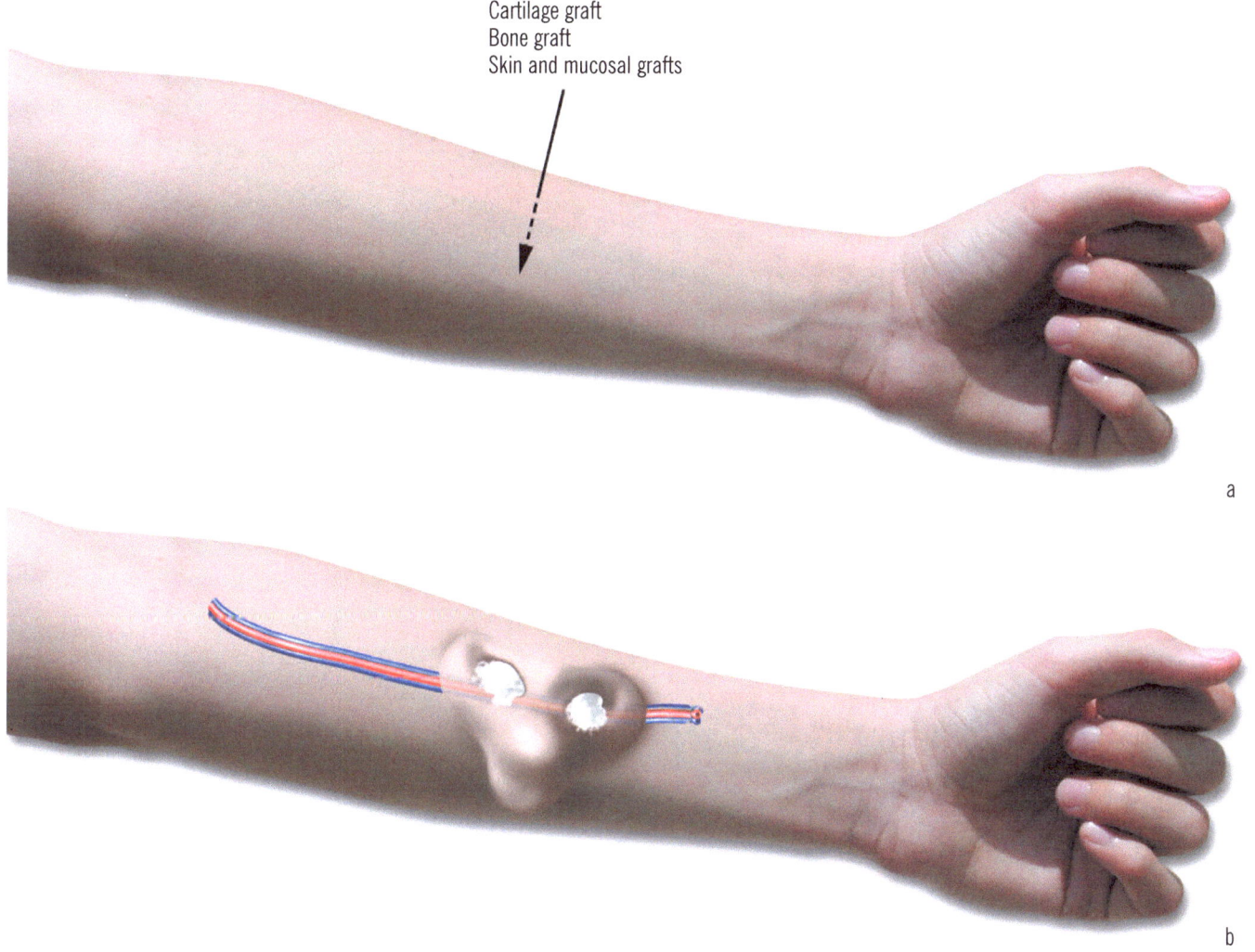

Cartilage graft
Bone graft
Skin and mucosal grafts

a

b

Figure 8.20. Example of flap prelamination.
a. Bone grafts, cartilage grafts and skin grafts are brought together on the radial forearm site.
b. A nose-like structure is created with the grafts and the forearm skin after several surgical interventions.

The prefabricated nose pedicled on the radial vessels can be used to restore the defect after total removal of the nose.

9. Flap prefabrication in laryngotracheal reconstruction

9.A. Flap prefabrication in laryngotracheal reconstruction

Tracheal autotransplantation to extended hemila-ryngectomy defects is an example of flap prefabrication with the use of the fasciocutaneous radial forearm flap (Fig. 8.21, 8.22, 8.23). Central to survival of the radial forearm flap is preservation of the numerous septocutaneous branches of the radial artery and inclusion of the deep fascia.

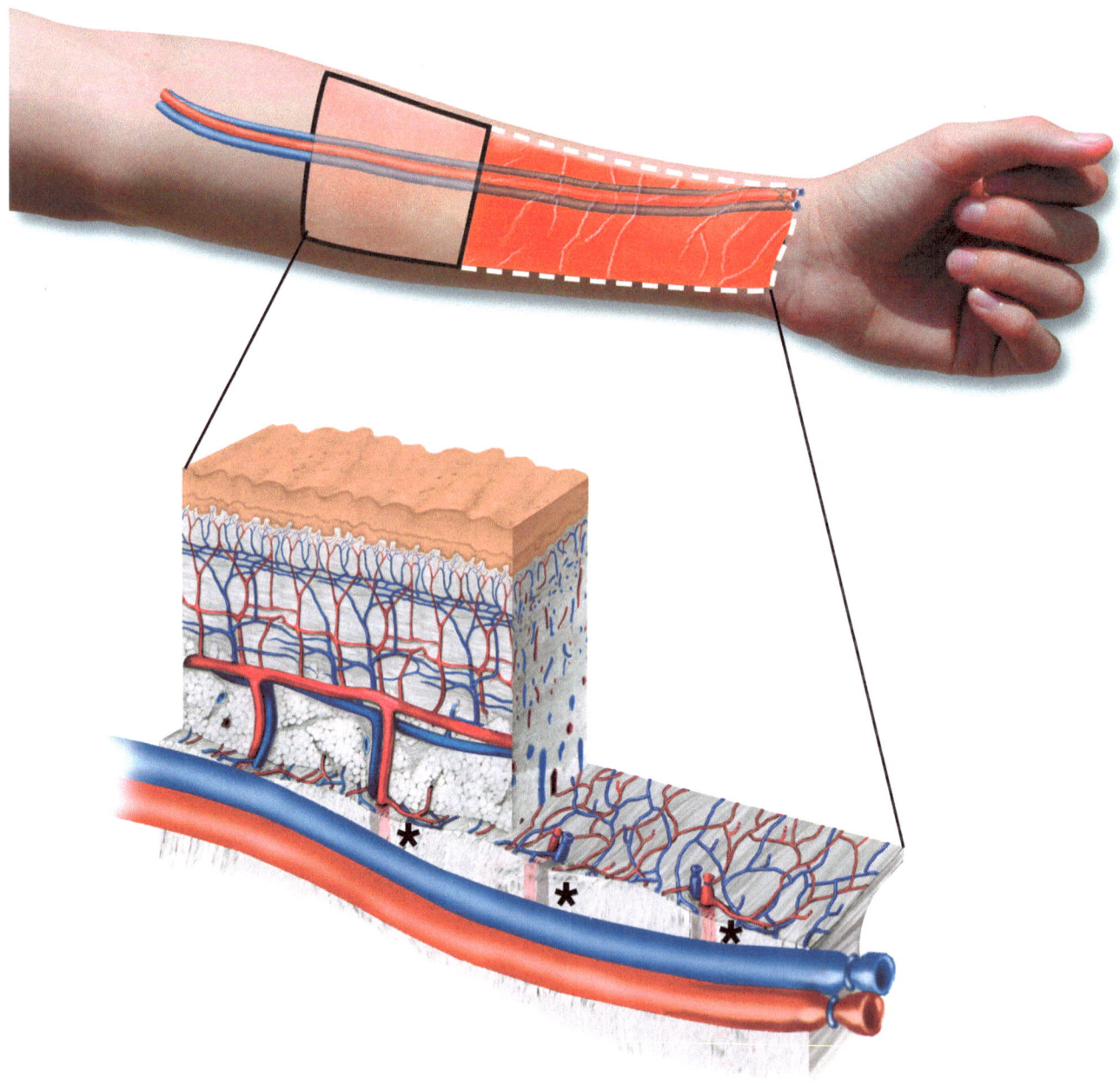

Figure 8.21. The radial forearm fasciocutaneous flap-Vascular anatomy.
The flap consists of a skin paddle and a fascial paddle.
The septocutaneous perforators (asterisks) supply the
overlying skin and subcutaneous tissue.

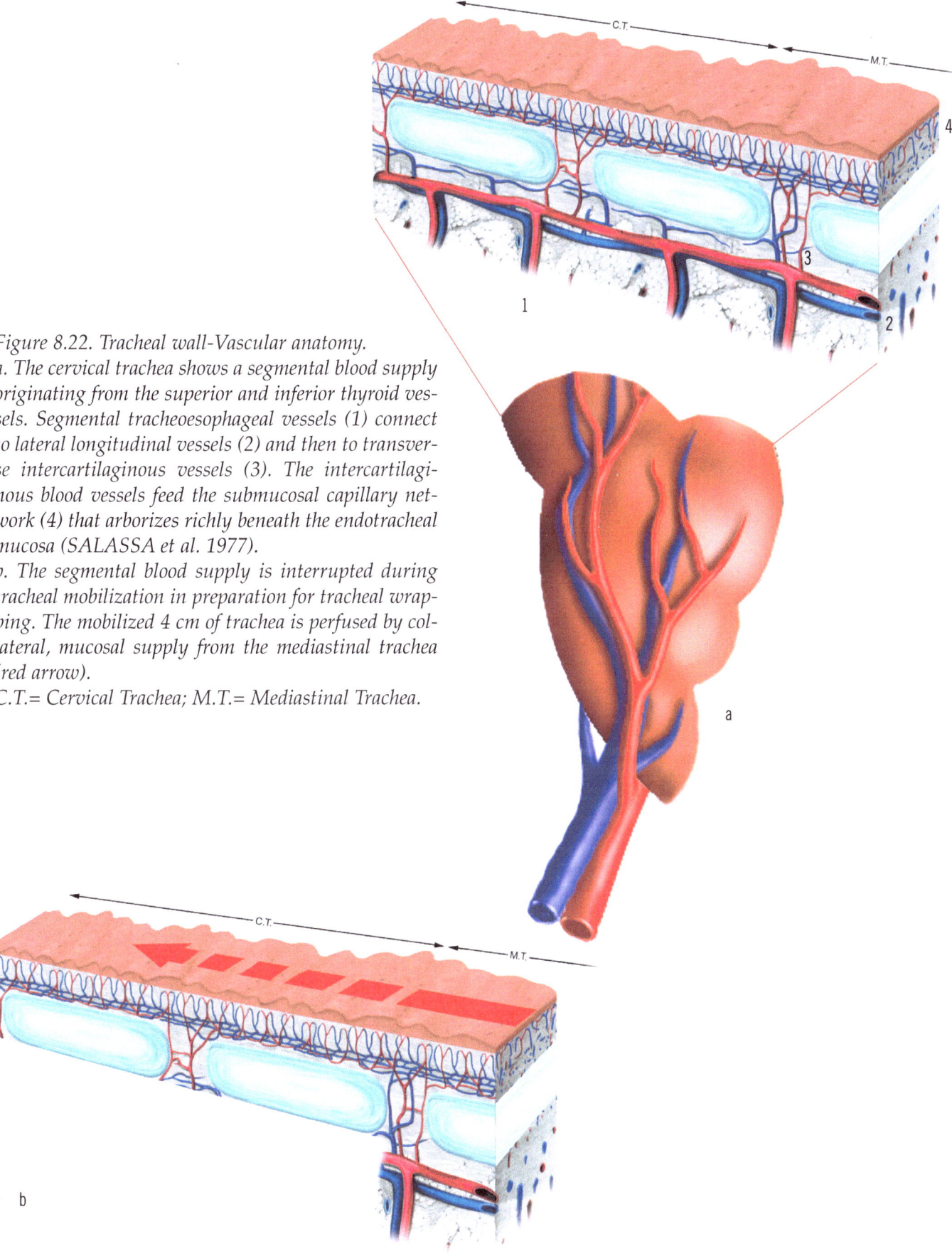

Figure 8.22. Tracheal wall-Vascular anatomy.
a. The cervical trachea shows a segmental blood supply originating from the superior and inferior thyroid vessels. Segmental tracheoesophageal vessels (1) connect to lateral longitudinal vessels (2) and then to transverse intercartilaginous vessels (3). The intercartilaginous blood vessels feed the submucosal capillary network (4) that arborizes richly beneath the endotracheal mucosa (SALASSA et al. 1977).
b. The segmental blood supply is interrupted during tracheal mobilization in preparation for tracheal wrapping. The mobilized 4 cm of trachea is perfused by collateral, mucosal supply from the mediastinal trachea (red arrow).
C.T.= Cervical Trachea; M.T.= Mediastinal Trachea.

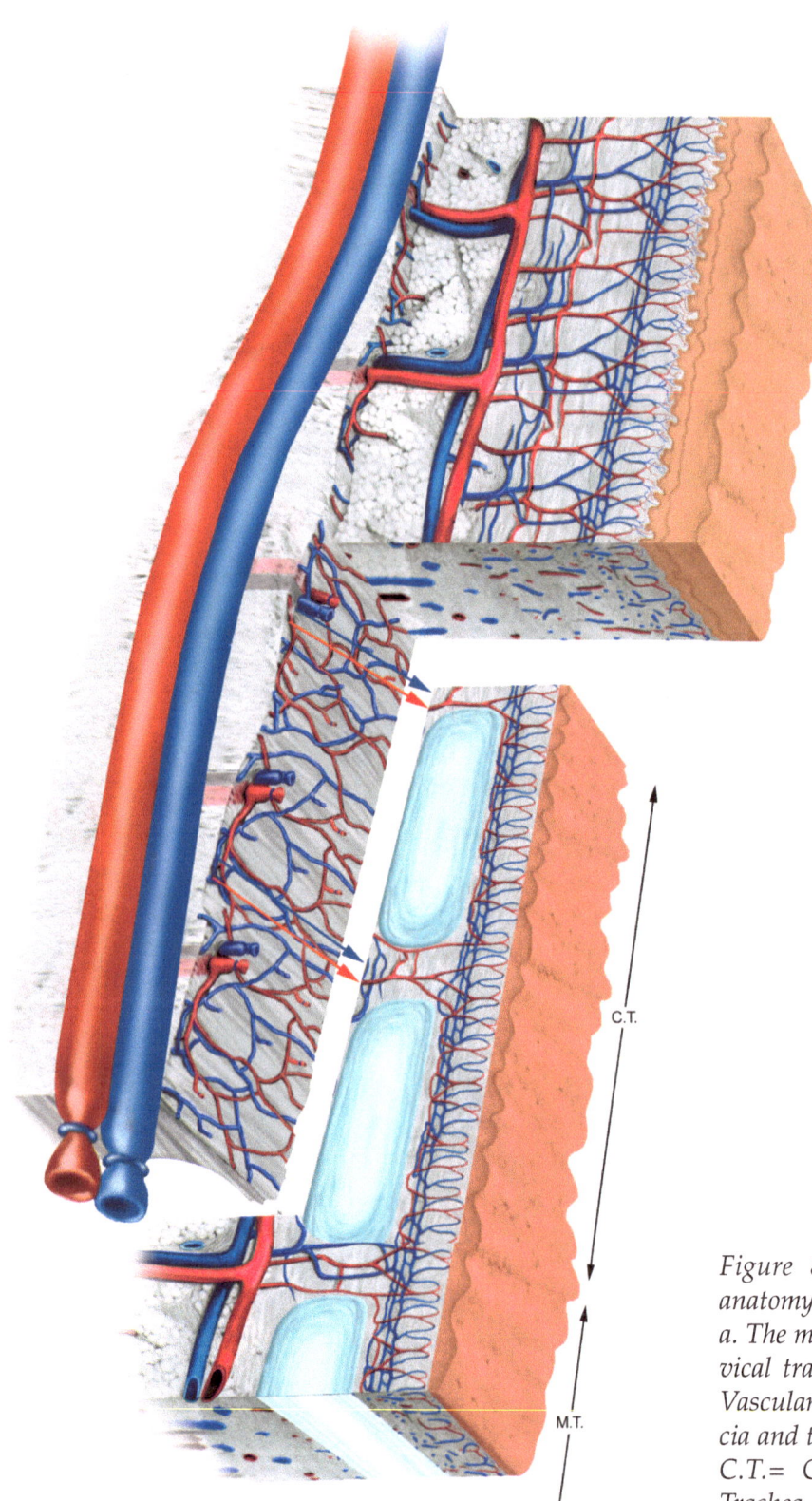

Figure 8.23. Tracheal prefabrication-Vascular anatomy.
a. The mobilized segment of trachea (4 cm of cervical trachea) is wrapped by the fascial paddle. Vascular connections will be formed between fascia and trachea (arrows).
C.T.= Cervical Trachea; M.T.= Mediastinal Trachea.

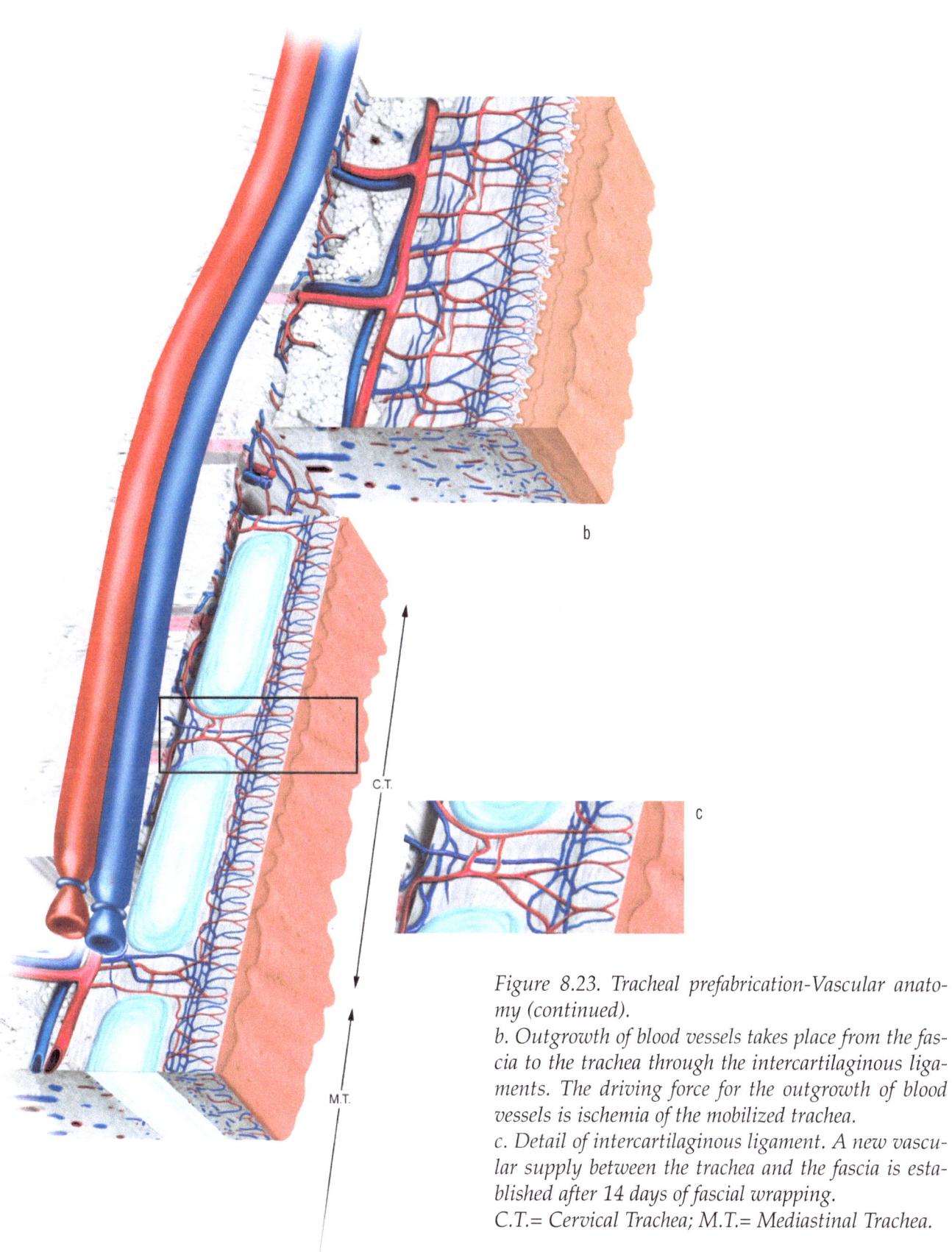

b

c

C.T.

M.T.

Figure 8.23. Tracheal prefabrication-Vascular anatomy (continued).

b. Outgrowth of blood vessels takes place from the fascia to the trachea through the intercartilaginous ligaments. The driving force for the outgrowth of blood vessels is ischemia of the mobilized trachea.

c. Detail of intercartilaginous ligament. A new vascular supply between the trachea and the fascia is established after 14 days of fascial wrapping.

C.T.= Cervical Trachea; M.T.= Mediastinal Trachea.

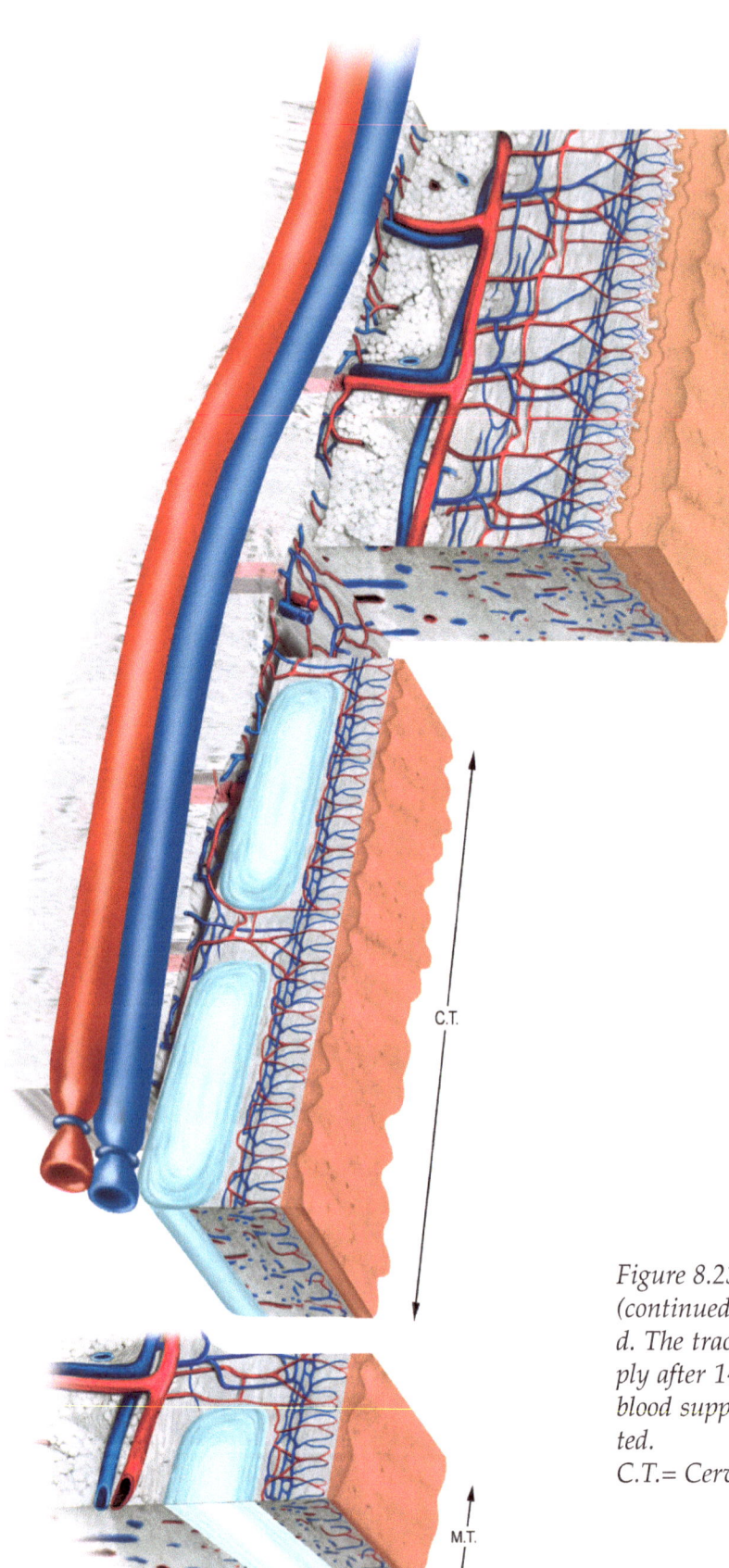

Figure 8.23. Tracheal prefabrication-Vascular anatomy (continued).

d. The trachea can be mobilized on its new blood supply after 14 days. At that time, the collateral, mucosal blood supply from the mediastinal trachea is interrupted.

C.T.= Cervical Trachea; M.T.= Mediastinal Trachea.

C.T.

M.T.

The morphology of the trachea is ideally suited for indirect revascularization with radial forearm fascia. Tissue ischemia is needed to induce a new blood supply. Tissue with a normal blood perfusion will not obtain a new blood supply after fascial wrapping (Fig. 8.24). The characteristic anatomy of the tracheal's blood supply (SALASSA et al. 1977) allows for tissue ischemia without the risk for necrosis. Tissue ischemia is a well known stimulus for revascularization. Ischemia stimulates central blood vessel ingrowth and acts as an angiogenic stimulus (KNIGHTON et al. 1981).

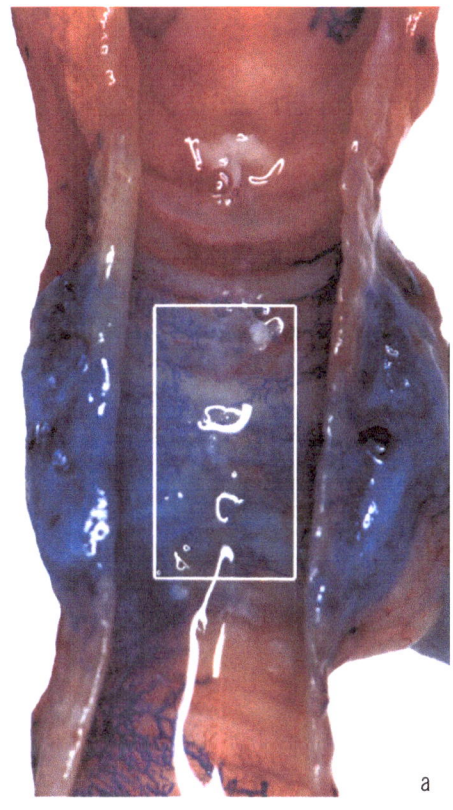

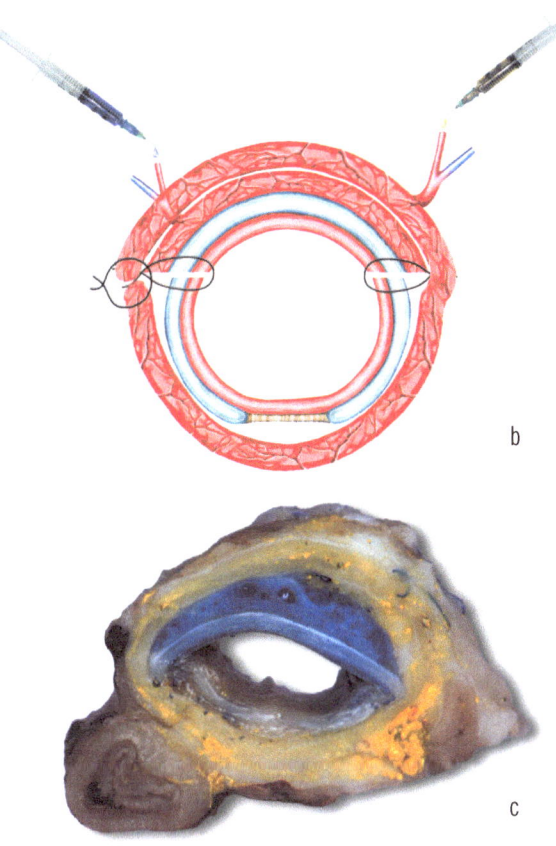

Figure 8.24. Ischemia as driving force for tracheal prefabrication-Experimental evidence.

a. Internal view of the rabbit's trachea after 2 weeks of fascial wrapping and after injection of the fascia with blue Microfil®. The vascular induction process is visualized by the blue silicone injected blood vessels at the intercartilaginous ligaments. The revascularized trachea (outlined patch) can be used to repair an anterior airway defect.

b. After flap prefabrication (with the left lateral thoracic fascia) during 14 days, a tracheal patch autotransplant was used to repair an anterior tracheal defect. At the time of autotransplantation, the reconstructed trachea was circumferentially wrapped with the right lateral thoracic fascia flap. After a 4 week follow-up period, the lateral thoracic vessels were injected with

Microfil® (left side with blue Microfil®, right side with yellow Microfil®) and the trachea was harvested for evaluation of outgrowth of blood vessels from fascia to trachea.

c. Most of the vascular connections are visible between autotransplant and fascia. Outgrowth of blood vessels from the autotransplant to the margins of the defect (blue colored vessels) are also visible.

Nearly no yellow colored vascular connections are visible. The trachea had no vascular needs after reconstruction and no vascular connections were formed between the reconstructed trachea and the circumferential fascial wrapping.

9.B. Flap prelamination in laryngotracheal reconstruction

Tracheal reconstruction with the use of composite tissue (buccal mucosa, vascular supply, cartilage) is an example of flap prelamination. Flap prelamination is necessary to allow for survival of the cartilage component (Fig. 8.25).

Figure 8.25.
Flap prelamination for tracheal reconstruction.
a. Buccal mucosa and cartilage grafts are brought together with the radial forearm fascia.
b. After 4 weeks, the cartilage grafts will be sufficiently covered with mucosa so that the reconstruction can be transplanted to an anterior tracheal defect.

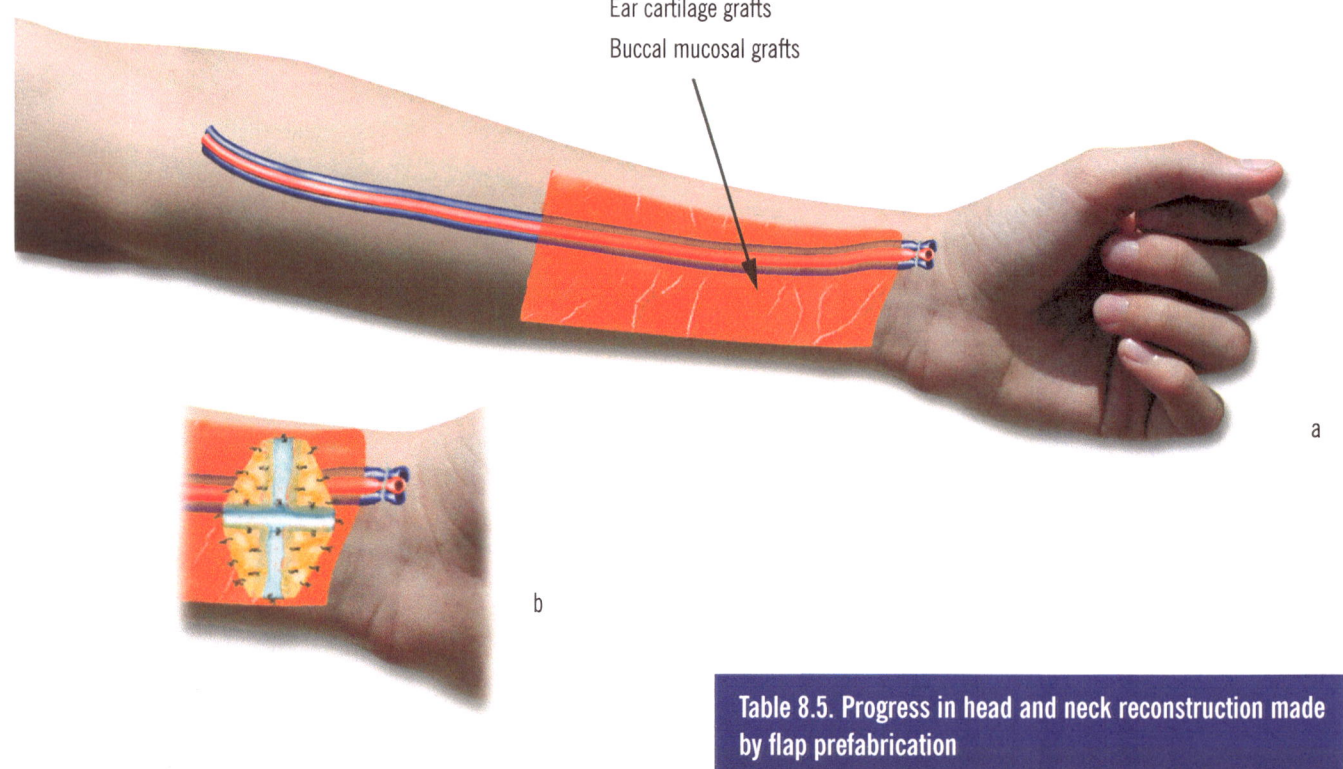

Ear cartilage grafts
Buccal mucosal grafts

a

b

Table 8.5. Progress in head and neck reconstruction made by flap prefabrication
Flap prefabrication:
- Production of thin skin flap after extensive burn injury.
- Vascular induction of trachea.
Flap prelamination
- Prefabrication of complex composite tissue (nose, ear).
- To facilitate ingrowth of skin grafts (ROHNER et al. 2003) and mucosal grafts (DELAERE et al. 2001).

10. Composite tissue allotransplantation

With the increasing knowledge that composite tissue transplantation can be maintained with similar regimens as for solid organ transplants, the evolution of reconstructive microsurgery has moved into the era of composite tissue allotransplantation. The first composite tissue allotransplant in the head and neck was a larynx which was performed in Cleveland, USA (STROME et al, 2001). Composite tissue allografting, or CTA, differs from organ transplantation in that the larynx unlike the kidney, heart or liver, is a combination of many different tissues (mucosa, cartilage, muscle, blood vessels, nerves, lymphatics). There is speculation that all of these different tissues require different mechanisms and levels of immunosuppression, so that CTAs become a more complicated problem than organ transplantation (THOMAS et al. 2000). The current focus for composite tissue allotransplantation is to minimize the toxicity of immunosuppression and the induction of tolerance. If these goals can be achieved, we will enter an era in which composite tissue allo transplantation will revolutionize the field of reconstructive microsurgery.

BIBLIOGRAPHY

Ariyan S. The pectoralis major myocutaneous flap. A versatile flap for reconstruction in the head and neck. Plast Reconstr Surg 1979;63:73.

Baek S, Biller HF, Krespi Y, Lawson W. The pectoralis major myocutaneous island flap for reconstruction of the head and neck. Head Neck 1979;1:293.

Bakamjian VY. A two-stage method for pharyngoesophageal reconstruction with a primary pectoral skin flap. Plast Reconstr Surg 1965;36:173.

Bakamjian VY, Long M, Rigg B. Experience with the medially based deltopectoral flap in reconstructive surgery of the head and neck. Br J Plast Surg 1971;24:174.

Baudet J, Pelissier P, Casoli V. 1984-1994: ten years of skin flaps. Prefabricated flaps. Ann Chir Plast Esthet 1995;40:597-605.

Daniel RK, Taylor GI. Distant transfer of an island flap by microvascular anastomosis. Plast Reconstr Surg 1973;52:111-4.

Cordeiro P, Hidalgo D. Conceptual considerations in mandibular reconstruction. Clin Plast Surg 1995;22:61-9.

Ehrlich HP. Wound closure: Evidence of cooperation between fibroblasts and collagen matrix. Eye 1988;2:149-57.

Gabbiani G, Hirschel BJ, Ryan B, et al. Granulation tissue as a contractile organ. J Exp Med 1972;135:719-34.

Hidalgo DA. Fibula free flap: a new method of mandible reconstruction. Plast Reconstr Surg 1989;84:71-9.

Hidalgo DA, Pusic AL. Free-flap mandibular reconstruction: a 10-year follow-up study. Plast Reconstr Surg 2002;110:438-49.

Khouri R. Free flap surgery: the second decade. Clin Plast Surg 1992;19:757-61.

Knighton DR, Silver IA, Hunt TK. Regulation of wound healing angiogenesis: effect of oxygen gradients and inspired oxygen concentration. Surgery 1981;90:262-5.

Lipa JE, Butler CE. Enhancing the outcome of free latissimus dorsi muscle flap reconstruction of scalp defects. Head & Neck 2004;26:46-53.

Lyos AT, Evans GR, Perez D, Schusterman MA. Tongue reconstruction: outcomes with the rectus abdominis flap. Plast Reconstr Surg 1999;103:442-7.

McGregor I. The temporal flap in intraoral cancer; its use in repairing the post-excisional defects. Br J Plast Surg 1963;16:318.

McGregor IA, Jackson IT. The extended role of the deltopectoral flap. Br J Plast Surg 1970;23:173.

McGregor IA, Morgan RG. Axial and random pattern flaps. Br J Plast Surg 1973;26:202.

McGregor IA, McGregor AD. Fundamental techniques of plastic surgery. Churchill Livingstone 1995.

Moscoso JF, Urken M. Radial forearm flaps. Otolaryng Clin North Am 1994;27:1119- 40.

Neligan PC, Mulholland S, Irish J, et al. Flap selection in cranial base reconstruction. Plast Reconstr Surg 1996;98:1159-66.

Petruzzelli GJ, Johnson JT. Skin grafts. Otolaryg Clin North Am 1994;27:25-37.

Pribaz JJ, Fine N, Orgill DP. Flap prefabrication in the head and neck: a 10-year experience. Plast Reconstr Surg 1999;103:808-20.

Pribaz JJ, Weiss DD. Free flap reconstruction of the nose. Operative Tech Plast Reconstr Surg 1999;6:240.

Pribaz JJ, Fine NA. Prefabricated and prelaminated flaps for head and neck reconstruction. Clin Plast Surg 2001;28:261-72.

Pribaz JJ, Fine NA. Prefabricated and prelaminated flaps for head and neck reconstruction. Clin Plast Surg 1999;6:240.

Rohner D, Jaquiéry C, Kunz C, Bucher P, Maas H. Maxillofacial reconstruction with prefabricated osseous free flaps: A 3 year experience with 24 patients. Plast Rec Surg 2003;112:748-57.

Rudolph R. Inhibition of myofibroblasts by skin grafts. Plast Reconstr Surg 1979;63:473-80.

Rudolph R, Fisher JC, Ninneman JL. Skin grafting. Boston, Little, Brown, 1979.

Rudolph R. Contraction and the control of contraction. World J Surg 1980;4:279-87.

Salassa JR, Pearson BW, Payne WS. Gross and microscopical blood supply of the trachea. Ann Thor Surg 1977;24:100-7.

Seidenberg G, Rosenak S, Hurwitt E, et al. Immediate reconstruction of the cervical esophagus by a revascularised isolated segment of jejunal segment. Surgery 1959;149:162.

Schusterman MA, Shestak K, de Vries EJ, et al. Reconstruction of the cervical esophagus: free jejunal transfer versus gastric pull-up. Plast Reconstr Surg 1990;85:16-21.

Song R, Gao Y, Song Y, Yu Y, Song Y. The forearm flap. Clin Plast Surg 1982;9:21-6.

Soutar DS, Scheker LR, Tanner NSB, McGregor IA. The radial forearm flap: a versatile method for intraoral reconstruction. Br J Plast Surg 1983;36:1.

Soutar DS, McGregor IA. The radial forearm flap in intraoral reconstruction: the experience of 60 consecutive cases. Plast Reconstr Surg 1986;78:1.

Strome M, Stein J, Esclamado R et al. Laryngeal transplantation and 40-month follow-up. New Engl J Med 2001;344:1676-9.

Taylor GI, Miller G, Ham F. The free vascularized bone graft: a clinical extension of microvascular techniques. Plast Reconstr Surg 1975;55:533-9.

Taylor I, Corlett R, Caddy C, Zelt Z. An anatomic review of the delay phenomenon II. Clinical applications. Plast Reconstr Surg 1992;89:408.

Thomas F, Ray P, Thomas JM. Immunological tolerance as an adjunct to allogeneic tissue grafting. Microsurgery 2000;20:435-40.

Urken ML, Turk J, Weinberg H, Vickery C, Biller HF. The rectus abdominis free flap in head and neck reconstruction. Arch Otolaryngol Head Neck Surg 1991;117:857-66.

Urken ML, Weinberg H, Vickery C, Biller HF. The neurofasciocutaneous radial forearm flap in head and neck reconstruction: a preliminary report. Laryngoscope 1990;100:161.

Subject Index